NEUROLOGY
Neonatology Questions and Controversies

NEUROLOGY
Neonatology Questions and Controversies

Series Editor

Richard A. Polin, MD
Professor of Pediatrics
College of Physicians and Surgeons
Columbia University
Vice Chairman for Clinical and Academic Affairs
Department of Pediatrics
Director, Division of Neonatology
Morgan Stanley Children's Hospital of NewYork-Presbyterian
Columbia University Medical Center
New York, New York

Other Volumes in the Neonatology Questions and Controversies Series

NEUROLOGY

Neonatology Questions and Controversies

Jeffrey M. Perlman, MB, ChB
Professor of Pediatrics
Division of Newborn Medicine
Department of Pediatrics
Weill Cornell Medical College
Division Chief, Newborn Medicine
NewYork-Presbyterian Hospital
New York, New York

Consulting Editor
Richard A. Polin, MD
Professor of Pediatrics
College of Physicians and Surgeons
Columbia University
Vice Chairman for Clinical and Academic Affairs
Department of Pediatrics
Director, Division of Neonatology
Morgan Stanley Children's Hospital of NewYork-Presbyterian
Columbia University Medical Center
New York, New York

SECOND EDITION

SAUNDERS

1600 John F. Kennedy Blvd.
Ste 1800
Philadelphia, PA 19103-2899

NEUROLOGY: Neonatology Questions and Controversies   ISBN: 978-1-4377-3611-3

Notice

Knowledge and best practice in this field are constantly changing. As new research and experience broaden our understanding, changes in research methods, professional practices, or medical treatment may become necessary.

Practitioners and researchers must always rely on their own experience and knowledge in evaluating and using any information, methods, compounds, or experiments described herein. In using such information or methods they should be mindful of their own safety and the safety of others, including parties for whom they have a professional responsibility.

With respect to any drug or pharmaceutical products identified, readers are advised to check the most current information provided (i) on procedures featured or (ii) by the manufacturer of each product to be administered, to verify the recommended dose or formula, the method and duration of administration, and contraindications. It is the responsibility of practitioners, relying on their own experience and knowledge of their patients, to make diagnoses, to determine dosages and the best treatment for each individual patient, and to take all appropriate safety precautions.

To the fullest extent of the law, neither the Publisher nor the authors, contributors, or editors assume any liability for any injury and/or damage to persons or property as a matter of products liability, negligence or otherwise, or from any use or operation of any methods, products, instructions, or ideas contained in the material herein.

Library of Congress Cataloging-in-Publication Data
Neurology: neonatology questions and controversies / [edited by] Jeffrey Perlman.—2nd ed.
    p. ; cm.—(Neonatology questions and controversies)
  Includes bibliographical references and index.
  ISBN 978-1-4377-3611-3 (hardback)
  I. Perlman, Jeffrey M.   II. Series: Neonatology questions and controversies.
  [DNLM: 1. Infant, Newborn, Diseases.   2. Nervous System Diseases.   3. Infant, Newborn.
WS 340]
  LC classification not assigned
  618.92'8—dc23

                                                                    2011052864

Senior Content Strategist: Stefanie Jewell-Thomas
Content Development Specialist: Lisa Barnes
Publishing Services Manager: Anne Altepeter
Team Manager: Hemamalini Rajendrababu
Project Manager: Divya Krish
Designer: Ellen Zanolle

Printed in the United States

Last digit is the print number: 9 8 7 6 5 4 3 2 1

Contributors

Joseph B. Cantey, MD
Department of Pediatrics
University of Texas Southwestern
   Medical Center
Dallas, Texas
   *Neonatal Meningitis: Current Treatment
   Options*

Rowena G. Cayabyab, MD
Assistant Professor of Clinical Pediatrics
Department of Pediatrics
Division of Neonatal Medicine
Keck School of Medicine
University of Southern California,
   Los Angeles
Attending Neonatologist
Department of Pediatrics
Good Samaritan Hospital
Neonatologist
Division of Neonatal Medicine
Children's Hospital Los Angeles
Los Angeles, California
   *Cerebral Circulation and Hypotension
   in the Premature Infant: Diagnosis and
   Treatment*

Keung-kit Chan, MBBS, MRCPCH
Resident Specialist
Department of Pediatrics
Kwong Wah Hospital
Kowloon, Hong Kong
   *Neonatal Hypotonia and
   Neuromuscular Disorders*

Basil T. Darras, MD
Associate Neurologist-in-Chief
Professor of Pediatrics
Department of Neurology
Director, Residency Training and
   Neuromuscular Programs
Harvard Medical School
Children's Hospital Boston
Boston, Massachusetts
   *Neonatal Hypotonia and
   Neuromuscular Disorders*

Jahannaz Dastgir, DO
Department of Neurology
Harvard Medical School
Children's Hospital Boston
Boston, Massachusetts
   *Neonatal Hypotonia and
   Neuromuscular Disorders*

Linda S. de Vries, MD, PhD
Professor
Department of Neonatology
Wilhelmina Children's Hospital
Utrecht, The Netherlands
   *Amplitude-Integrated EEG and Its
   Potential Role in Augmenting
   Management Within the NICU*

Lisa Eiland, MD
Assistant Professor of Pediatrics
Weill Cornell Medical College
Adjunct Faculty
Laboratory of Neuroendocrinology
Rockefeller University
New York, New York
   *Pain and Stress: Potential Impact on the
   Developing Brain*

Petra S. Hüppi, MD
Professor
Department of Pediatrics
University of Geneva Chief, Division of
   Development and Growth
Department of Pediatrics
University Children's Hospital
Geneva, Switzerland Visiting Scientist
Department of Child Neurology
   Harvard Medical School
Children's Hospital of Boston
Boston, Massachusetts
   *Magnetic Resonance Imaging's Role in
   the Care of the Infant at Risk for Brain
   Injury*

Ericalyn Kasdorf, MD
Fellow in Neonatology
NewYork-Presbyterian Hospital
New York, New York
   *General Supportive Management of
   the Term Infant with Neonatal
   Encephalopathy Following Intrapartum
   Hypoxia-Ischemia*

David Kaufman, MD
Associate Professor of Pediatrics
University of Virginia Medical School
University of Virginia Children's
   Hospital
Charlottesville, Virginia
   *Neonatal Meningitis: Current Treatment
   Options*

David W. Kimberlin, MD
Professor
Department of Pediatrics
University of Alabama at Birmingham
Birmingham, Alabama
   *Neonatal Herpes Simplex Virus and
   Congenital Cytomegalovirus Infections*

Abbot R. Laptook, MD
Professor
Department of Pediatrics
The Warren Alpert Medical School of
   Brown University
Medical Director
Neonatal Intensive Care Unit
Women and Infants Hospital of Rhode
   Island
Providence, Rhode Island
   *The Use of Hypothermia to Provide
   Neuroprotection for Neonatal Hypoxic-
   Ischemic Brain Injury*

Gregory A. Lodygensky, MD
Professor of Pediatrics
Division of Neonatal and Pediatric
   Intensive Care
University Children's Hospital
Geneva, Switzerland
   *Magnetic Resonance Imaging's Role in
   the Care of the Infant at Risk for Brain
   Injury*

Claire W. McLean, MD
Assistant Professor of Pediatrics
Keck School of Medicine
University of Southern California
Division of Neonatal Medicine
Attending Neonatologist
Children's Hospital Los Angeles
Los Angeles, California
   *Cerebral Circulation and Hypotension
   in the Premature Infant: Diagnosis and
   Treatment*

Caroline C. Menache, MD
Pediatric Neurologist
University Children's Hospital
Geneva, Switzerland
   *Magnetic Resonance Imaging's Role in the
   Care of the Infant at Risk for Brain Injury*

Laura R. Ment, MD
Professor
Departments of Pediatrics and
   Neurology Associate Dean
Yale University School of Medicine
New Haven, Connecticut
   Perinatal Stroke

Eliza H. Myers, MD
Department of Pediatrics
Yale University School of Medicine
New Haven, Connecticut
   Perinatal Stroke

Shahab Noori, MD
Associate Professor of Pediatrics
Keck School of Medicine
University of Southern California
Attending Neonatologist
Division of Neonatology and Cancer for
   Fetal and Neonatal Medicine
Department of Pediatrics
Children's Hospital Los Angeles
Los Angeles, California
   *Cerebral Circulation and Hypotension
   in the Premature Infant: Diagnosis and
   Treatment*

Jeffrey M. Perlman, MB, ChB
Professor of Pediatrics
Division of Newborn Medicine
Department of Pediatrics
Weill Cornell Medical College
Division Chief, Newborn Medicine
NewYork-Presbyterian Hospital
New York, New York
   Introduction
   *Intraventricular Hemorrhage and White
   Matter Injury in the Preterm Infant*
   *General Supportive Management of
   the Term Infant with Neonatal
   Encephalopathy Following
   Intrapartum Hypoxia-Ischemia*

Pablo J. Sánchez, MD
Professor
Department of Pediatrics
University of Texas Southwestern
  Medical Center
Attending Physician
Parkland Health and Hospital System
Attending Physician
Children's Medical Center
Dallas, Texas
  *Neonatal Meningitis: Current Treatment
  Options*

Mark S. Scher, MD
Professor of Pediatrics and Neurology
Case Western Reserve University
  School of Medicine
Chief, Division of Pediatric Neurology
Director, Fetal/Neonatal Neurology
  Program
Department of Pediatrics
Rainbow Babies and Children's Hospital
University Hospitals of Cleveland
Cleveland, Ohio
  *Diagnosis and Treatment of Neonatal
  Seizures*

Istvan Seri, MD, PhD
Professor of Pediatrics
Head, Division of Neonatal Medicine
Keck School of Medicine
University of Southern California
Director, Center for Fetal and Neonatal
  Medicine
Children's Hospital Los Angeles
Los Angeles, California
  *Cerebral Circulation and Hypotension
  in the Premature Infant: Diagnosis and
  Treatment*

Steven M. Shapiro, MD, MSHA
Professor of Neurology
Virginia Commonwealth University
Richmond, Virginia
  *Hyperbilirubinemia and the Risk for
  Brain Injury*

Toshiki Takenouchi, MD
Instructor
Department of Pediatrics
Keio University School of Medicine
Tokyo, Japan
  *Intraventricular Hemorrhage and White
  Matter Injury in the Preterm Infant*

Mona C. Toet, MD, PhD
Department of Neonatology
  Wilhelmina Children's Hospital
  Utrecht, The Netherlands
  *Amplitude-Integrated EEG and Its
  Potential Role in Augmenting
  Management Within the NICU*

Betty R. Vohr, MD
Professor of Pediatrics
Director, Neonatal Follow-up
The Warren Alpert Medical School of
  Brown University
Women and Infants Hospital of Rhode
  Island Providence, Rhode Island
  *Long-Term Follow-Up of Very Low-
  Birth-Weight Infants*

Andrew Whitelaw, MD, FRCPCH
Professor of Neonatal Medicine
Department of Clinical Science
University of Bristol
Consultant Neonatologist
Neonatal Intensive Care Unit
Southmead Hospital
Bristol, United Kingdom
  *Posthemorrhagic Hydrocephalus
  Management Strategies*

Jerome Y. Yager, MD
Professor and Director of Research
Department of Pediatrics
University of Alberta Professor and
  Head
Pediatric Neurosciences
Department of Pediatrics
Stollery Children's Hospital
Edmonton, Alberta, Canada
  *Glucose and Perinatal Brain Injury:
  Questions and Controversies*

Santina Zanelli, MD
Assistant Professor of Pediatrics
University of Virginia Medical School
University of Virginia Children's
  Hospital
Charlottesville, Virginia
  *Neonatal Meningitis: Current Treatment
  Options*

Series Foreword

Richard A. Polin, MD

"Medicine is a science of uncertainty and an art of probability."

—William Osler

Controversy is part of everyday practice in the NICU. Good practitioners strive to incorporate the best evidence into clinical care. However, for much of what we do, the evidence is either inconclusive or does not exist. In those circumstances, we have come to rely on the teachings of experienced practitioners who have taught us the importance of clinical expertise. This series, "Neonatology Questions and Controversies," provides clinical guidance by summarizing the best evidence and tempering those recommendations with the art of experience.

To quote David Sackett, one of the founders of evidence-based medicine:

> *Good doctors use both individual clinical expertise and the best available external evidence and neither alone is enough. Without clinical expertise, practice risks become tyrannized by evidence, for even excellent external evidence may be inapplicable to or inappropriate for an individual patient. Without current best evidence, practice risks become rapidly out of date to the detriment of patients.*

This series focuses on the challenges faced by care providers who work in the NICU. When should we incorporate a new technology or therapy into everyday practice, and will it have positive impact on morbidity or mortality? For example, is the new generation of ventilators better than older technologies such as CPAP, or do they merely offer more choices with uncertain value? Similarly, the use of probiotics to prevent necrotizing enterocolitis is supported by sound scientific principles (and some clinical studies). However, at what point should we incorporate them into everyday practice given that the available preparations are not well characterized or proven safe? A more difficult and common question is when to use a new technology with uncertain value in a critically ill infant. As many clinicians have suggested, sometimes the best approach is to do nothing and "stand there."

The "Questions and Controversies" series was developed to highlight the clinical problems of most concern to practitioners. The editors of each volume (Drs. Bancalari, Oh, Guignard, Baumgart, Kleinman, Seri, Ohls, Maheshwari, Neu, and Perlman) have done an extraordinary job in selecting topics of clinical importance to everyday practice. When appropriate, less controversial topics have been eliminated and replaced by others thought to be of greater clinical importance. In total, there are 56 new chapters in the series. During the preparation of the "Hemodynamics and Cardiology" volume, Dr. Charles Kleinman died. Despite an illness that would have caused many to retire, Charlie worked until near the time of his death. He came to work each day, teaching students and young practitioners and offering his wisdom and expertise to families of infants with congenital heart disease. We are dedicating the second edition of the series to his memory. As with the first edition, I am indebted to the exceptional group of editors who chose the content and edited each of the volumes. I also wish to thank Lisa Barnes (content development specialist at Elsevier) and Judy Fletcher (global content development director at Elsevier), who provided incredible assistance in bringing this project to fruition.

Preface

The discipline of newborn neurology continues to be of great academic and clinical interest, with continual advances being made in basic and clinical research. As our understanding of the mechanisms contributing to brain injury continues to grow, it has been paralleled by the introduction of targeted strategies in several instances. The second edition of this volume has been expanded with three additional chapters, including the potential contribution of stress and viral infections to neonatal brain injury and the diagnostic role of amplitude EEG in the neonatal intensive care unit. The contributing authors are all outstanding clinicians, as well as researchers, who have developed expertise that relates directly or indirectly to neonatal neurologic problems.

Although this volume is not all-inclusive, the goal is that the information contained in it will facilitate patient care and serve as a stimulus for future research.

Jeffrey M. Perlman, MB, ChB

/

Contents

CHAPTER 1

Introduction

Jeffrey M. Perlman, MB, ChB

The perinatal period represents a clinical setting of potential risk for injury to developing brain secondary to many causes, with the chance for long-lasting, profound neurocognitive deficits. Ongoing research continues to advance our understanding of the basic mechanisms contributing to perinatal brain injury, which in turn in several instances has facilitated the introduction of targeted strategies. The second edition of this book again addresses some of the prominent factors and events contributing to brain injury as well as describes some of the novel treatment options that have been introduced. Three new chapters have been added related to neonatal herpes simplex and congenital cytomegaloviral infections (Chapter 12), pain and stress and the potential impact on the developing brain (Chapter 13), and the potential role of the amplitude-integrated EEG in augmenting management in the critically ill neonate (Chapter 15).

The remaining chapters are updates, so I will only highlight advances in each area where applicable. Importantly, the incidence of severe intraventricular hemorrhage remains a prominent problem in extremely premature infants. Thus 21% of infants born at 23 weeks of gestation and 13% to 14% of those born at 24 to 25 weeks of gestation still have the most severe forms of hemorrhage (Chapter 3). Therapeutic hypothermia continues to show a neuroprotective effect when administered within 6 hours, and the number need to treat, based on the three large randomized studies, is 9 (Chapter 5). An important experimental observation suggests that inhalational xenon, when used in conjunction with hypothermia, has added neuroprotective effects. It will be important to determine whether this observation can be translated clinically (Chapter 6). The potential role of targeted novel anticonvulsants in the treatment of neonatal seizures is on the horizon, awaiting clinical trials (Chapter 8). What defines hypoglycemia and who should be treated has troubled clinicians for decades. In Chapter 9 an argument is made that lower concentrations of glucose than previously tolerated are not associated with adverse long-term sequelae; however, these have all been retrospective observations. In Chapter 12 the approach to the management of the two most common and potentially treatable viruses—herpes simplex and cytomegalovirus—and the impact on brain is highlighted. The potentially important adverse impact of pain and stress on developing brain is discussed in Chapter 13. There is increasing use of amplitude-integrated electroencephalography in neonatal intensive care units—for example, to facilitate entry of candidate infants for therapeutic hypothermia as well as for the diagnosis of seizures, Chapter 15 provides the reader with a comprehensive overview of this methodology and its potential uses. The remaining chapter updates are all outstanding in their depth and comprehensive reviews and make for compelling reading.

The primary goal of this second edition is that after reviewing each chapter, the reader will have a clearer management strategy that is based on an understanding of the underlying pathophysiology. A desired secondary goal is that the highlighted gaps in knowledge will serve as a strong stimulus for future research.

CHAPTER 2

Cerebral Circulation and Hypotension in the Premature Infant: Diagnosis and Treatment

Claire W. McLean, MD, Shahab Noori, MD, Rowena G. Cayabyab, MD, and Istvan Seri, MD, PhD

- ● Definition of Hypotension
- ● Pathogenesis and Diagnosis of Pathologic Cerebral Blood Flow
- ● Treatment Strategies
- ● Summary and Recommendations

As the field of neonatology has progressed over the last few decades, better monitoring and more effective interventions have been developed for supporting the respiratory, fluid and electrolyte, and nutritional abnormalities frequently encountered in very low-birth-weight (VLBW) infants. However, the ability to effectively and continuously monitor the hemodynamic changes at the level of systemic and organ blood flow and tissue perfusion remains very limited despite the advances achieved with the use of targeted neonatal echocardiography and other bedside organ and tissue perfusion monitoring modalities, such as electrical impedance velocimetry, near-infrared spectroscopy (NIRS), visible light spectroscopy, and laser Doppler technology as well as the use of amplitude-integrated EEG (aEEG) to follow changes in brain activity. With the improvements in hemodynamic monitoring and a better understanding of the principles of developmental cardiovascular physiology has come the realization of how little is actually known about circulatory compromise and its effect on organs, especially brain, blood flow, blood flow–metabolism coupling, and long-term outcomes. Although we can continuously and reliably monitor systemic blood pressure and there are myriad interventions for "normalizing" it, blood pressure is the only dependent component among the hemodynamic parameters regulating tissue perfusion and is determined by changes in the two independent variables, cardiac output and systemic vascular resistance (SVR). Accordingly, in addition to monitoring and maintaining perfusion pressure (blood pressure), the goal is to preserve normal systemic and organ blood flow and tissue oxygenation especially to the vital organs—that is, the brain, heart, and adrenals. In this regard, when it comes to the brain, medicine is at an even greater disadvantage. For instance, measuring cerebral blood flow (CBF) is more complex than measuring systemic blood flow (left ventricular output), although continuous assessment of cardiac output in neonates at the bedside has remained a significant challenge. In addition, even assessment of systemic blood flow becomes very complicated when shunting through the fetal channels (ductus arteriosus and foramen ovale) occurs during the first few postnatal days in the VLBW neonate. Also, clinical evidence of ischemia cannot be detected in the brain as easily as in other organs—for example, the heart, liver, and kidneys. Seizures are a clear sign of a pathologic process, but they can be difficult to recognize in the VLBW population, although the use of aEEG might be helpful. In addition, by the time seizures are present, irreversible injury may have already occurred. Most importantly, the clinician faces the formidable task of effectively supporting and protecting the enormously complex developmental processes that are occurring in the brain of a VLBW infant during the postnatal transitional period and beyond. Yet detection of changes in CBF and cerebral function in a timely manner is difficult, and the understanding of how to manage the hemodynamic disturbances that affect CBF, flow-metabolism coupling, brain function, and structure and, ultimately, neurodevelopmental outcome, is limited.

The intent of this chapter is to review the available information on the definition of systemic hypotension and the pathogenesis, diagnosis, and treatment of early cerebral perfusion abnormalities in the VLBW infant that have been shown to precede intracranial hemorrhage and periventricular white matter injury (PWMI). Because CBF, flow-metabolism coupling, and cerebral oxygenation in this population are such a complex topic, we focus our discussion on the first postnatal days, during which the cardiorespiratory transition from fetal to extrauterine life occurs. We discuss some of the modalities that are being explored for identifying changes in CBF and cerebral oxygenation at the bedside. Once a pathologic process is identified, provision of a coherent, safe, and effective means of treating that process is crucial. We present a rational treatment for the pathologic processes underlying clinically evident brain injury in the VLBW infant based on the most up-to-date monitoring and clinical evidence available. Unfortunately, only a little evidence exists with regard to the appropriateness and effectiveness of the current approaches to treatment of neonatal hypotension and cardiovascular compromise. In an area as controversial and complex as this one, it is important to always highlight what is not known. Our goal is to provide the practitioner with recommendations for diagnosis and treatment that should be considered guidelines only. Finally, although the understanding of both normal and pathologic processes in the preterm brain is improving, evidence for a definitive clinical approach remains scant.

Definition of Hypotension

Hypotension, defined by population-based normative data, occurs in up to 50% of VLBW infants admitted to the neonatal intensive care unit. Hypotension in the immediate postnatal period is thought by many to be one of the major factors contributing to central nervous system injury, eventual cerebral palsy, and poor long-term neurologic outcome in VLBW neonates. Indeed, the *association* between hypotension and brain injury and poor neurodevelopmental outcome is well documented[1-8] and forms the basis of therapeutic efforts to normalize blood pressure. However, *causation* has never been demonstrated between hypotension and poor neurodevelopment. In other words, one cannot infer that long-term neurodevelopmental outcomes will improve if hypotension is rigorously avoided.

In addition, retrospective studies have raised concerns by finding an association between treated hypotension and poor neurodevelopmental outcomes.[9,10] However, it remains unclear whether hypotension, its treatment, or both were responsible for the documented association. Indeed, a follow-up study[11] to the original randomized prospective trial[12] comparing the effectiveness of dopamine and epinephrine in increasing blood pressure and CBF in hypotensive VLBW neonates during the first postnatal day found that neonates who responded to dopamine or epinephrine had long-term neurodevelopment outcomes comparable to those of age-matched normotensive controls, and that patients who did not respond to vasopressor-inotrope treatment had worse long-term outcome. These findings suggest that treatment of neonatal hypotension, when carefully titrated, may actually be effective and not harmful. However, because the primary outcome measure of the original study[12] was not long-term neurodevelopmental outcome, the follow-up study[11] may have not been appropriately powered to put this concern definitely to rest. Finally, results of a recent study support the notion that the careful treatment of neonatal hypotension might not be harmful as it found that low blood pressure in extremely preterm infants during the first 72 hours of postnatal life, regardless of treatment, was independently associated with poor neurodevelopmental outcome.[13]

In clinical practice, hypotension is usually defined as the blood pressure value below the 5th or 10th percentile for the gestational age– and postnatal age–dependent normative blood pressure values (Fig. 2-1).[14-16] However, there is no consensus

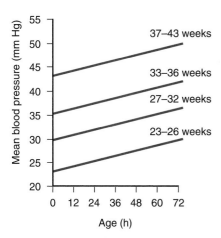

Figure 2-1 Gestational age– and postnatal age–dependent normogram for mean blood pressure values in preterm and term neonates during the first 3 postnatal days. The normogram is derived from continuous arterial blood pressure measurements obtained from 103 neonates with gestational ages between 23 and 43 weeks. Because each line represents the lower limit of 80% confidence interval of mean blood pressure for each gestational age group, 90% of infants for each gestational age group will have a mean blood pressure equal to or greater than the value indicated by the corresponding line (the lower limit of the confidence interval). (From Nuntnarumit P, Yang W, Bada-Ellzey HS. Blood pressure measurements in the newborn. *Clin Perinatol.* 1999 26:981-996.)

among neonatologists about the acceptable lower limit of systemic mean or systolic arterial blood pressure, and most units have different guidelines for the initiation of treatment of hypotension.

From a pathophysiologic standpoint, three levels of functional alterations of increasing severity can be used to guide the definition of hypotension on the basis of later findings in the literature (Fig. 2-2). However, it is important to keep in mind that no prospectively collected information is available on mortality and morbidity associated with these different blood pressure thresholds.

First, the mean blood pressure associated with the loss of CBF autoregulation is the generally accepted definition of hypotension (autoregulatory blood pressure threshold).[17] Indeed, there is considerable information in the literature indicating that CBF autoregulation is functional in normotensive but not in hypotensive VLBW neonates in the immediate postnatal period (Fig. 2-3).[5,18,19] Autoregulation is the ability of arteries to constrict or dilate in response to an increase or decrease, respectively, in the transmural pressure to maintain blood flow relatively constant within a range of arterial blood pressure changes (see Fig. 2-2). However, in the neonate, this response has a limited capacity. In addition, the autoregulatory blood pressure range is narrow in the neonatal patient population and the 50th percentile of the mean blood pressure is relatively close to the lower autoregulatory blood pressure threshold. In other words, small decreases in blood pressure may result in loss of CBF autoregulation, especially in the preterm infant.[18] Findings now suggest that the autoregulatory blood pressure threshold is around 28 to 30 mm Hg even in the extremely LBW (ELBW) neonate during the first postnatal day (Fig. 2-4).[18,19] At this blood pressure, however, cellular function and structural integrity are unlikely to be

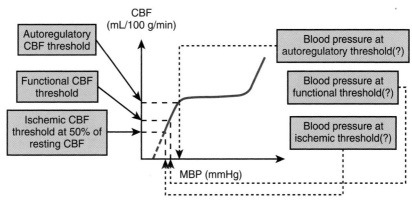

Figure 2-2 Definition of hypotension by three pathophysiologic phenomena of increasing severity: autoregulatory, functional, and ischemic thresholds of hypotension. *CBF,* Cerebral blood flow; *MBP,* mean blood pressure.

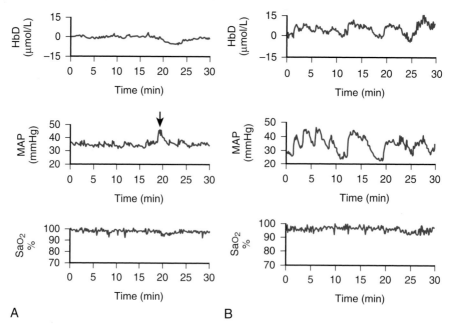

Figure 2-3 Intact and compromised cerebral blood flow (CBF) autoregulation in very low-birth-weight (VLBW) neonates in the immediate postnatal period. Changes in cerebral intravascular oxygenation (HbD = HbO_2 − Hb) correlate with changes in CBF. **A,** Changes in HbD (i.e., CBF), mean arterial pressure (MAP), and oxygen saturation (SaO_2) in a 1-day-old, 28-week gestational age (GA) preterm infant whose subsequent head ultrasound findings remained normal. No change occurs in CBF in relation to the sudden increase in MAP associated with endotracheal tube suctioning *(arrow)*. **B,** Changes in HbD (CBF), MAP, and SaO_2 in a 1-day-old 27-week GA preterm infant whose subsequent head ultrasound revealed the presence of periventricular white matter injury. Changes in blood pressure are clearly associated with changes in CBF. (From Tsuji M, Saul PJ, duPlessis A, et al. Cerebral intravascular oxygenation correlates with mean arterial pressure in critically ill premature infants. *Pediatrics.* 2000;106:625.)

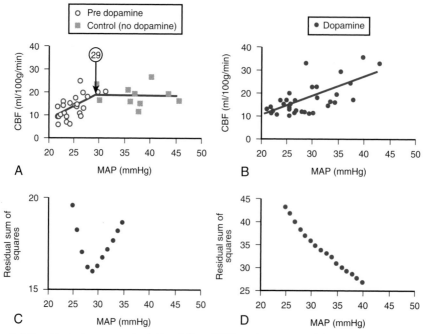

Figure 2-4 Relationship between cerebral blood flow (CBF) and mean arterial pressure (MAP) in hypotensive and normotensive extremely low-birth-weight (ELBW) neonates during the first postnatal day and the effect of dopamine on this relationship. **A** and **B,** MAP (mm Hg) and CBF (mL/100 g/min) measured by near-infrared spectroscopy (NIRS) in normotensive ELBW neonates not requiring dopamine (Control, *closed squares*; n = 5) and hypotensive ELBW neonates before dopamine administration (Predopamine, *open circles*; n = 12). The lower threshold of the CBF autoregulatory blood pressure limit (29 mm Hg; **A**) is identified as the minimum of residual sum of squares of the bilinear regression analysis **(B).** **C** and **D,** MAP (mm Hg) and CBF (mL/100 g/min) in the formerly hypotensive ELBW neonates after dopamine treatment *(filled circles)*. No break point is evident in the CBF-MAP curve in ELBW neonates receiving dopamine **(C),** because no minimum is identified by the bilinear regression analysis **(D).** (From Munro MJ, Walker AM, Barfield CP. Hypotensive extremely low birth weight infants have reduced cerebral blood flow. *Pediatrics.* 2004;114:1591.)

affected, because increased cerebral fractional oxygen extraction (CFOE), micro-vascular vasodilation, and a shift in the hemoglobin-oxygen dissociation curve to the left can maintain tissue oxygen delivery at levels appropriate to sustain cellular function and integrity.[20,21]

If blood pressure continues to fall, it reaches a value at which cerebral function becomes compromised (functional blood pressure threshold). Data from later reports suggest that the functional blood pressure threshold may be around 22 to 24 mm Hg in the VLBW neonate during the first postnatal days (Fig. 2-5).[21,22] However, caution is needed when interpreting these findings, which were obtained in a small number of preterm infants, because their clinical relevance is unclear. Furthermore, the relationship between cerebral electrical activity, neurodevelopmental outcome, and the threshold of CBF associated with impaired brain activity is not known.

Finally, if blood pressure decreases even further, it reaches a value at which structural integrity becomes compromised (ischemic blood pressure threshold). On the basis of findings in immature animals, it is assumed that the ischemic CBF threshold is around 50% of the resting CBF.[18] Although it is unclear what blood pressure value represents the ischemic CBF threshold in the VLBW neonate during the first postnatal day, it may be below 20 mm Hg (see Fig. 2-2).[23,24] It is important to emphasize that the situation is further complicated by the fact that these numbers represent moving targets for the individual patient. Indeed, other factors, such as $PaCO_2$ levels, the presence of acidosis, preexisting insults (asphyxia), and underlying pathophysiology (sepsis, anemia), have an impact on the critical blood pressure value at which perfusion pressure and cerebral oxygen delivery cannot satisfy cellular oxygen demand to sustain autoregulation, then cellular function, and finally struc-tural integrity.

At present, continuous monitoring of blood pressure and assessment of indirect signs of tissue perfusion (urine output, capillary refill time, and lactic acidosis) remain the basis for identifying the presence of cardiovascular compromise. However,

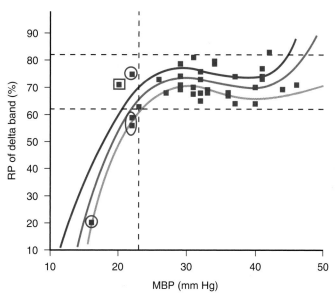

Figure 2-5 Relationship between mean blood pressure (MBP) and cerebral electrical activity in very low-birth-weight neonates during the first 4 postnatal days. Shown is the relationship between MBP and the relative power (RP) of the delta band of the electroencephalogram, showing line of best fit with 95% confidence interval (N = 35; R^2 = 0.627; P < 0.001). *Horizontal dotted lines* represent the normal range of the relative power of the delta band (10th-90th percentile), whereas the *vertical dotted line* identifies the point of intercept. The *open square* identifies the infant with abnormal cerebral fractional oxygen extraction (CFOE), and the abnormal elec-troencephalogram records are *circled*. (From Victor S, Marson AG, Appleton RE, et al. Relationship between blood pressure, cerebral electrical activity, cerebral fractional oxygen extraction and peripheral blood flow in very low birth weight newborn infants. *Pediatr Res.* 2006;59:314-319.)

adequate blood pressure may not always guarantee adequate organ perfusion in VLBW neonates during the first postnatal day.[25] Indeed, blood pressure, the product of systemic blood flow and systemic vascular resistance, only weakly correlates with superior vena cava (SVC) flow in VLBW neonates during the immediate postnatal adaptation.[26] SVC flow has been used as a surrogate for systemic blood flow in the VLBW neonate during the immediate postnatal period, when shunting through the fetal channels prohibits the use of left ventricular output to assess systemic blood flow.[27] The finding that adequate blood pressure may not always guarantee adequate systemic blood flow in these patients may be explained at least in part by the notion that the cerebral vascular bed, especially of the 1-day-old ELBW neonate, may not be of high priority and thus it will constrict rather than dilate in response to a decrease in the perfusion pressure (discussed in detail later).[28-30]

Pathogenesis and Diagnosis of Pathologic Cerebral Blood Flow

Fluctuations in CBF are implicated in the pathogenesis of periventricular-intraventricular hemorrhage (P/IVH) and PWMI in the VLBW infant.[1,29,31,32] Both systemic and local (intracerebral) factors play a role in the pathogenesis of these central nervous system injuries and therefore are important in diagnosis. In addition, the level of maturity, postnatal age, and intercurrent clinical factors (e.g., infection/inflammation, vasopressor-resistant hypotension) need to be considered. In this section, we briefly discuss monitoring parameters that are currently in widespread clinical use (systemic arterial pressure and arterial blood gas sampling) and then delve into the emerging field of bedside monitoring of systemic and organ blood flow, especially CBF and brain activity. We review most of the existing technologies, including echocardiography and Doppler ultrasound, impedance electrical cardiometry (IEC), NIRS, and aEEG, and discuss the applicability and limitations of these modalities. We do not discuss the use of magnetic resonance imaging (MRI) for assessing CBF in the neonatal patient population, because this topic is addressed in Chapter 16.

A logical place to begin the discussion on monitoring CBF in the VLBW infant is to ask, "What is the normal CBF in the VLBW infant?" Several investigators have addressed this issue. It is clear from these studies that CBF is lower in preterm infants than in adults, corresponding to the lower metabolic rate of the preterm brain. Using xenon-133 clearance, Greisen[33] found that, in 42 preterm infants with a mean gestational age of 31 weeks, CBF was 15.5 ± 7.2 mL/100 g/min during the first postnatal week, a value three to four times lower than that in adults.[33] Interestingly, patients enrolled in this study who were receiving mechanical ventilation had lower CBF than their nonventilated counterparts and those receiving CPAP (11.8 ± 3.2 vs. 19.8 ± 5.3 and 21.3 ± 12 mL/100g/min, respectively). Cerebral blood flow in this study was not consistently affected by postnatal age, gestational age, birth weight, mode of delivery, $PaCO_2$, hemoglobin concentration, mean blood pressure, or phenobarbital therapy. In contrast, subsequent publications by the same group of authors investigating CBF reactivity in preterm infants during the first three postnatal days showed that, as expected, $PaCO_2$ and hemoglobin concentration significantly affect CBF in this patient population.[34-36]

Using positron emission tomography (PET) to measure CBF, Altman and colleagues[37] found lower values for CBF in preterm and term neonates compared to those obtained by the use of xenon-133 clearance.[37] More importantly, they reported that in a series of one term and five preterm infants with CBF between 4.9 and 10 mL/100g/min, the term neonate and three of the preterm infants had normal neurodevelopmental outcome at 24 months.[37] Therefore, the neurodevelopmentally safe lower limit of CBF in the neonate may be between 5 and 10 mL/100/min. Finally, because CBF is affected by many factors other than blood pressure, it is not possible to define the blood pressure value consistently associated with a decrease of CBF below this safe limit that results in ischemic brain injury.

Kluckow and Evans,[27] using SVC blood flow as a surrogate for systemic blood flow and CBF in well preterm neonates younger than 30 weeks of gestation who were receiving minimal ventilatory support, established normal values of SVC flow during the first 48 postnatal hours. Of note is that the extent to which SVC flow is representative of systemic or cerebral blood flow in preterm neonates during the first postnatal days is not known. In a subsequent study that included sick preterm infants younger than 30 weeks of gestation, the same group found that 38% of infants had a period of low SVC in the first 24 (mostly 12) postnatal hours.[25] The incidence of low SVC flow was significantly related to the level of immaturity and was more than 70% in very preterm neonates—that is, of gestational age less than 27 weeks. The sudden increase in the peripheral vascular resistance caused by the loss of the low-resistance placental circulation, the complex process of cardiorespiratory transition to the postnatal circulatory pattern, and myocardial and autonomic central nervous system immaturity have been proposed to contribute to these findings. Indeed, these factors may explain why many of these very preterm neonates struggle to maintain normal systemic blood flow during the first 12 to 24 postnatal hours. Importantly, a proportion of the very preterm babies with extremely low SVC flow were found to have systemic blood pressures in the normal range (i.e., equal to or greater than their gestational age in weeks), a finding supported by subsequent studies of this group of researchers.[26,38,39] Because normal blood pressure and decreased organ blood flow to nonvital organs are the hallmarks of the compensated phase of shock and because a portion of SVC flow represents blood returning from the brain, a vital organ, it is conceivable that the vascular beds of the cerebral cortex and white matter are low-priority vessels and function similar to those of nonvital organs in the very preterm neonate during the immediate postnatal period. This hypothesis, which is supported by earlier studies in different animal models[40,41] and observations in the human neonate,[28,29] may explain why SVC blood flow may be decreased in some very preterm neonates who have normal systemic blood pressure. Most babies with documented low SVC flow in the first 24 to 48 hours that do not go on to have P/IVH or PWMI are more mature (28 vs. 25-26 weeks of gestation). Thus, for preterm babies of less than 30 weeks of gestation, low systemic blood flow (and CBF) may be necessary but not sufficient to cause intracranial pathology. Importantly, all patients studied had an increase in SVC flow by 24 to 36 hours, and all P/IVHs occurred after the SVC flow had increased. Findings of a later prospective observational study by our group using echocardiography and NIRS confirm and expand these observations.[42] In this study, very preterm neonates who were presented with lower systemic blood flow and higher cerebral vascular resistance during the first 12 postnatal hours were at a higher risk for the development of P/IVH. Importantly, the bleeding occurred only after cardiac output and brain blood flow had increased. Taken together, these findings implicate an ischemia-reperfusion cycle in the pathogenesis of P/IVH in very preterm neonates during the immediate transitional period.

The methods used to assess systemic and cerebral blood flow in VLBW neonates in the immediate transitional period have significant limitations. When SVC flow is used to assess systemic and cerebral blood flow, measurements are operator-dependent owing to the uncertainties associated with the accurate measurement of vessel diameter and flow velocity. The fluctuations in vessel size during the cardiac cycle and the pattern of low flow velocity in the SVC are the major factors contributing to these technical difficulties. In addition, the shape of the SVC, the lack of data on the magnitude of the contribution of CBF to SVC flow, and the lack of a documented association between $PaCO_2$ and SVC flow in this patient population call for some caution in the interpretation of these findings.

Kehrer and associates[43] measured blood flow in both internal carotid and vertebral arteries and used the sum of the flow in the four arteries supplying the brain to assess the changes in CBF volume in preterm infants of 28 to 35 weeks of gestation over the first 2 postnatal weeks. Although the technique has significant limitations, the findings suggest that a steep rise in CBF occurs from the first to the second postnatal days and that this pattern is independent of gestational age. Thereafter,

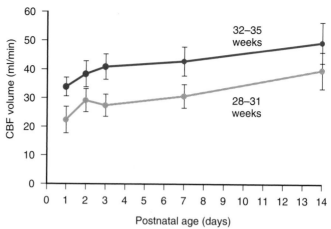

Figure 2-6 Changes in cerebral blood flow (CBF) volume in preterm neonates during the first 14 days after delivery. Shown is the development of CBF volume with increasing postnatal age in two different gestational age groups (28-31 and 32-35 weeks). The mean and 95% confidence interval are also shown (analysis of variance [ANOVA]; n = 29, P < 0.0001). (From Kehrer M, Blumenstock G, Ehehalt S, et al. Development of cerebral blood flow volume in preterm neonates during the first two weeks of life. *Pediatr Res.* 2005;58:927-930.)

CBF continues to rise gradually (Fig. 2-6). Because there is not a significant increase in brain weight during the first 48 postnatal hours, the investigators inferred that the observed increase in CBF during that period was secondary to increased cerebral perfusion per unit weight of tissue. On the other hand, the more gradual increase over the ensuing 2 weeks is likely due to a combination of both increased brain weight and increased perfusion.[43] The investigators studied only healthy preterm infants with normal brains, whereas the series of investigations by Evans, Kluckow, and their colleagues[25,26,38,39] included a group of preterm infants who were sicker and had a higher incidence of significant intracranial pathology. Nevertheless, the results of the two groups are complementary as they provide evidence for a decreased CBF in the first postnatal day, followed by a significant increase by the second post-natal day. It is tempting to speculate that the low CBF in the study by Kehrer and associates[43] during the first postnatal day represents a decrease from that in the fetus, but this might not be the case because findings of a later study suggest that a decrease in SVC flow and left cardiac output in very preterm neonates occurs by 12 hours of postnatal age and not immediately after birth.[44] Taken together, results of these studies suggest that low CBF in the first postnatal day and the ensuing reperfusion is a physiologic phenomenon occurring in most (if not all) very preterm neonates and that this phenomenon is a necessary but not sufficient cause of intracranial pathology (P/IVH or PWMI) in this patient population.

The ultimate goal is to improve neurodevelopmental outcome in preterm infants, and because low SVC flow in the early postnatal period has been implicated not only in the development of P/IVH and PWMI but also in impaired neurologic outcome at 3 years,[6] those infants most at risk in the immediate postnatal period must be identified. It is clear from the large number of epidemiologic and hemody-namic studies that the level of immaturity is one of the most important predisposing factors for the occurrence of more abrupt changes in CBF and the increased vulner-ability during postnatal adaptation and for poor neurologic outcome. Therefore, assessment of CBF during the first 24 to 48 postnatal hours in the most immature and vulnerable patients is important. However, owing to the technical difficulties associated with reliable and continuous assessment of CBF, clinical practice currently relies on indirect measures for diagnosis of changes in cerebral perfusion. For instance, the notion that a pressure-passive cerebral circulation exists in most sick preterm neonates has led to the use of systemic blood pressure as the only surrogate measure for cerebral perfusion. However, in the compensated phase of shock, main-tenance of normal systemic blood pressure is not the equivalent of adequate nonvital organ blood flow, and the forebrain might not be a vital organ in the very preterm neonate immediately after delivery (see earlier). Therefore, the sole reliance on blood pressure in the assessment of CBF in this patient population during the first postnatal day may not be adequate.

In addition to blood pressure, monitoring of the indirect clinical indicators of tissue perfusion such as urine output, capillary refill time (CRT), and acid-base status are important. Although these indirect clinical indicators by themselves are fairly nonspecific for evaluating systemic flow, using CRT and blood pressure together results in greater sensitivity. Indeed, when blood pressure and CRT are less than 30 mm Hg and 3 seconds, respectively, the sensitivity for identifying low systemic blood flow is 86%.[45] In addition, avoidance of both hypocapnia and hypercapnia is of utmost importance because of the effect on CBF.

If the monitoring commonly used now in clinical practice at the bedside is not sufficient to tell the whole story on CBF, what can be added? Fortunately, most of the interest in organ blood flow monitoring has focused on the cerebral circulation. This interest has led to the development of a multitude of techniques for monitoring both CBF and systemic perfusion. The most frequently used techniques for CBF monitoring are Doppler ultrasound and NIRS, and aEEG has been used for monitoring cerebral function. The gold standard for monitoring systemic perfusion in the clinical practice is echocardiography, and novel approaches have recently also been developed, including IEC. We briefly discuss each of these modalities in the following sections with a primary focus on those that can be performed noninvasively at the bedside.

Doppler Ultrasound

Velocity of blood flow can be measured through the use of the Doppler principle, which states that the change in frequency of reflected sound is proportional to the velocity of the passing object (in this case, blood). The calculated velocity needs to be corrected for the angle between the vessel and the emitted sound beam (angle of insonation), and the straightforward idea is complicated by the fact that arterial blood is pulsatile and its speed varies within the vessel (i.e., it is faster in the center of the vessel). It is important to recognize that speed of blood (distance traveled per unit time) in a vessel means little by itself; we are really interested in the absolute blood flow (volume per unit time). Thus, volumetric measurements are crucial. Investigators have used several different volumetric indices, including SVC, internal carotid artery, and vertebral artery flow, as previously discussed.[27,43] The limitations of SVC flow measurements were discussed earlier. In general, major technical problems with volumetric measurements include but are not restricted to the small size of the vessels, the motion of vessel wall, and whether or not an angle of insonation of less than 20 degrees can be achieved. In addition to volumetric measurements of vessel blood flow, right ventricular and left ventricular outflow measurements have been studied. Both are fraught with pitfalls in the very preterm neonate in the immediate postnatal period, because the patent foramen ovale (PFO) and patent ductus arteriosus (PDA) create shunts that confound measurements of the right ventricular and left ventricular flows, respectively. It is believed that right ventricular output may be a more reliable indicator of systemic blood flow during the immediate postnatal period with the fetal channels open, because shunting by the patent foramen ovale is less significant than PDA shunting during the first 24 hours after delivery.[46] Indeed, right ventricular output and systemic blood pressure have been correlated with EEG parameters (brain function) in VLBW infants in the immediate postnatal period.[47]

Ultrasound techniques are noninvasive and widely accessible in the intensive care setting, and they can be done at the bedside. However, all ultrasound measurements depend on operator skill and have their significant limitations. As for the issues related to operator skills, centers utilizing these methods to diagnose pathologic CBF in neonates must have a rigorous quality control system in place with neonatologists well trained in functional echocardiography and available at the bedside at any time.[48]

With regard to the limitations to the use of vascular Doppler ultrasonography in assessing organ blood flow, the most important limitation is the small size of the artery of interest (e.g., middle or anterior cerebral artery), which precludes accurate measurement of its diameter. Because the estimation of blood flow (Q) depends on assessment of mean velocity of the blood (V) and the vessel diameter (D) (Q = V $[\pi D^2/4] \times 60$), any small error in measuring the diameter will translate into a significant error in estimating the actual blood flow. Therefore, instead of directly measuring blood flow, investigators often use changes in various Doppler-derived indices, such as mean blood flow velocity or the pulsatility or resistance index, as surrogates for changes in blood flow. This approach is based on the premise that the vessel diameter remains constant despite the changes in blood flow. However, this concept in not universally accepted.[46] Nevertheless, both animal and human studies have shown an acceptable correlation between these indices and other measures of blood flow.[49-52]

As for the technical aspect of vascular Doppler ultrasonography, one must pay special attention to consistently scan the same segment of the vessel with the same angle of insonation. Because the vessel diameter may vary at different sites, the measured velocity may also be different. With regard to the angle of insonation, one should try not to exceed 20 degrees, because with a higher angle, the velocity is significantly underestimated. Although, most new ultrasound systems have the capability to correct for the angle of insonation, using the same angle of insonation for repeated measurements will ensure better reproducibility of the data. Finally, although normative data for the Doppler ultrasonography–derived indices for various vessels are available, the previously described limitations require caution in interpretation of a single measurement. Rather, repeated measurements and the use of trends over time are thought to be more informative of the hemodynamic status and the changes in organ blood flow.

Impedance Electrical Cardiometry

Impedance electrical cardiometry is a noninvasive and continuous bedside method of measuring beat-to-beat left ventricular output on the basis of detection of changes in thoracic electrical bioimpedance (Aesculon; Cardiotronic, La Jolla, CA) caused by the changes in the orientation of the red blood cells in the ascending aorta during systole and diastole normalized for the body mass of the patient.[53] The method has been validated against thermodilution and other direct methods of cardiac output measurement and has shown excellent correlation in adults and children.[53,54] Although its clinical utility in neonates is still untested, preliminary data from our group show a very good correlation with traditional echocardiographic quantitation of left ventricular output in term[55] and preterm (unpublished data) neonates. However, further validation of this technique using cardiac output measurement methods more accurate than echocardiography, such as magnetic resonance imaging, is needed before the use of IEC can be recommended in the neonatal patient population. In conclusion, IEC represents an interesting potential means to obtain continuous, noninvasive data in absolute numbers on stroke volume and cardiac output at the bedside in neonates.

Near-Infrared Spectroscopy

NIRS has received much attention since its first use in newborns in 1985,[56] and numerous papers have been published describing its use. Basically, it involves emission of light of a specific wavelength (near-infrared range, 600-900 nm), from one optode which then travels through tissue and is detected on the other side by another optode. Because of the presence of compounds whose absorption of NIR light depends on oxygen status (chromophores such as hemoglobin and cytochrome aa_3), the absorption during passage through brain can be measured, and oxygenation indices calculated. The newborn skull and tissues overlying the brain are thin, so most of the signal received is representative of brain tissue. In the VLBW neonate, the biparietal diameter is such that essentially the whole brain can be seen by the traveling light, and results can be interpreted as global. Different wavelengths of light can be used to assess different parameters, such as oxyhemoglobin, deoxyhemoglobin, and cytochrome aa$_3$ oxidase. Through induction of a small but rapid change in arterial oxygen saturation in the subject, CBF can be calculated with the use of Fick's principle. This method assumes that during the measurement period, cerebral blood volume (CBV) and cerebral oxygen extraction remain constant.

Because the measurement depends on inducing a small but sudden change in arterial oxygen concentration, the technique may not be feasible in babies with severe lung disease (in whom no change in oxygen saturation occurs with an increased FIO$_2$) and in infants with normal lungs in whom oxygen saturation is 100% when they breathe room air. To get around this problem, an injected tracer dye such as indocyanine green has been used instead of oxygen, with similar results.[57] Some instruments use the tissue oxygenation index (TOI), which is the weighted average of arterial, capillary, and venous oxygenation and theoretically allows the measurement of cerebral hemoglobin oxygen saturation without manipulation of FIO$_2$ or use of dye. However, this index also has significant potential for inaccuracy, with an intrameasurement agreement in a single subject as large as −17% to +17%.[58] Indeed, reproducibility of NIRS measurements in general has been an ongoing issue for investigators, especially in the detection of focal changes in cerebral hemodynamics. This is a significant problem, because focal hemodynamic changes are at least as likely as global changes to contribute to neuropathology.

Despite these limitations, NIRS has been validated through comparison with xenon-133 clearance in human newborns.[59] Xenon-133 clearance is the experimental model gold standard, utilizing arteriovenous differences in clearance rates of an inert radioisotope and giving a global measurement of CBF. An algorithm allowing for continuous monitoring of regional tissue oxygen saturation in absolute numbers has been developed for adult, pediatric, and neonatal use.[60] Although NIRS represents a practical solution and information on its use in neonates has been encouraging,[61] accumulation of more data and prospective studies looking at both short- and long-term outcomes are needed to provide an evidence-based utilization of NIRS in neonatal medicine.

Amplitude-Integrated EEG (Cerebral Function Monitoring)

There is evidence to support the use of aEEG in asphyxiated infants in the first several hours after birth, because it is one of the most accurate bedside methods to establish a neurologic prognosis.[62] For this reason, it has been used to select candidates for enrollment in head-cooling neuroprotection trials. This technology uses a single-channel EEG recording with biparietal electrodes. Frequencies lower than 2 Hz and higher than 15 Hz are filtered selectively, and the amplitude of the signal is integrated. The signal is then recorded semilogarithmically with slow speed, effectively compressing hours of EEG recording into shorter segments that reflect global background activity and major deviations from baseline (e.g., seizures). Studies have shown that aEEG correlates well with conventional EEG[63] and has the distinct advantage of being easily applied and interpreted by nonneurologists. In a later study, normal aEEG findings in the first 72 postnatal hours in asphyxiated term neonates have been shown to be prognostic of normal neurologic outcome at 2 years of age.[64] Coupled with early neurologic examination, simultaneous aEEG improved specificity and positive predictive value of abnormal results for abnormal neurologic outcome at 18 months of age.[65]

Significantly less information has been gathered about the use of aEEG in the preterm population. However, some typical patterns of background activity for preterm infants have been established, and a number of studies exist that point to its applicability in this group. For instance, in preterm infants with a large P/IVH, aEEG findings during the first postnatal week are predictive of survival and intermediate-term neurologic outcome.[66]

Before aEEG can be incorporated into routine clinical use, data on tracings in normal premature infants in the immediate postnatal period as well as longitudinal development of mature brain activity must be collected and evaluated. Two studies by one group of investigators have attempted to do just that.[67,68] A group of clinically

2

and ultrasonographically normal infants with gestational ages between 23 and 29 weeks were studied with aEEG in the first two postnatal weeks. With increasing gestational and postnatal age, the occurrence of continuous activity increased and discontinuous low-voltage activity was less likely to be seen. The number of bursts per hour also decreased with increasing gestational age. Although the investigators offered these findings as a foundation for neurodevelopmental prognosis in VLBW infants, they also represent an important starting point for cerebral function monitoring in the immediate postnatal period.

West and colleagues[47] examined the relationships among echocardiographic blood flow findings, mean arterial blood pressure, and aEEG findings in the first 48 hours after birth in preterm infants (<30 weeks of gestation). They found that low right ventricle output, used as a surrogate for systemic blood flow, in neonates with shunting across the fetal channels at 12 hours of postnatal life correlated with low aEEG amplitude whereas low mean blood pressure (<31 mm Hg) correlated with low EEG continuity. However, there was no relationship between aEEG amplitude and SVC flow. Although preliminary in nature, this study at least succeeds in drawing an association between a parameter in wide clinical use (blood pressure monitoring) and two more experimental modes of CBF monitoring (Doppler ultrasonography and aEEG). Taken together with evidence that early aEEG in preterm infants can be helpful in predicting long-term neurodevelopmental outcome, it is reasonable to suggest that aEEG merits further study in the VLBW population as a means of identifying infants at risk for low CBF and/or for pathologic fluctuations in CBF.

Summary

Methods capable of diagnosing altered CBF and the associated changes in brain function in the VLBW population in the first hours to days after delivery are still largely in the experimental arena. It is unlikely that one monitoring parameter will be sufficient to encapsulate the whole picture of real-time continuous assessment of cerebral blood flow and oxygen delivery. To do that in the future, we need to employ an approach to similar that previously and currently used in clinical practice. That is, hands-on clinical assessment must be used in combination with a variety of technologies, ranging from the conventional (heart rate, blood pressure, O_2 saturation) to the advanced (Doppler ultrasonography, IEC, NIRS, aEEG). Both systemic and cerebral blood flow, as well as oxygen delivery and extraction, will have to be evaluated simultaneously and continuously to enable more informed minute-to-minute decisions about how, when, and what to treat to be made. This goal has not been achieved, but even now experimental technologies are giving an insight into more commonly used monitoring parameters, and as the understanding of these new methods expand, it is likely that some will be incorporated into routine clinical use in the not too distant future.

Figure 2-7 shows an example of the information a comprehensive hemodynamic bedside monitoring and data acquisition system developed by our research program can convey in real time at the bedside.

Treatment Strategies

In the previous section we focused on newer experimental modalities for monitoring CBF in the VLBW neonate, with a primary emphasis on those that could be performed at the bedside noninvasively. As mentioned earlier, functional Doppler echocardiography, IEC, NIRS, and aEEG are not yet currently appropriate for widespread routine clinical use for CBF monitoring, as their application and interpretation require specialized technology and further study to determine the significance and reproducibility of results. By extension, application of these methods in clinical practice must eventually be shown to improve long-term neurologic outcome. However, results of studies using these experimental strategies can be useful for tailoring routine care because they give a glimpse of how mean arterial pressure and systemic blood flow affect CBF. This section focuses on how routinely monitored

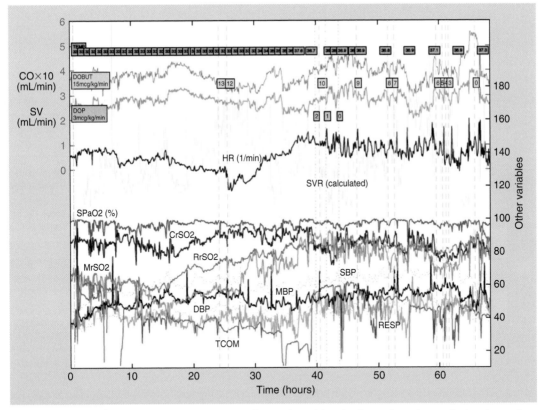

Figure 2-7 Hemodynamic parameters continuously monitored by the hemodynamic monitoring tower in a term, 3-day-old neonate with hypoxic-ischemic encephalopathy undergoing rewarming from therapeutic whole-body hypothermia. Parameters continuously monitored included arterial oxygen saturation (SpaO$_2$; %); heart rate (HR; beats/min); respiratory rate (RESP; L/min); systolic blood pressure (SBP, mm Hg), diastolic blood pressure (DBP; mm Hg), mean blood pressure (MBP; mm Hg); beat-to-beat cardiac output (CO; mL/min) and stroke volume (SV; mL/min) using impedance electrical cardiometry, cerebral (CrSO$_2$), renal (RrSO$_2$) and muscle (MrSO$_2$) mixed venous tissue oxygen saturation using near-infrared spectroscopy NIRS, and transcutaneous CO$_2$ (TCOM, mm Hg). These parameters are depicted on the *y*-axis, and age after delivery in hours is shown on the *x*-axis. Rewarming was started at 30 hours of monitoring. Core temperature (TEMP) is shown in *small boxes* and dopamine (DOP) and dobutamine (DOBUT) doses are depicted over the cardiac output and stroke volume data. Automatically calculated systemic vascular resistance (SVR; mm Hg × min/mL) is also depicted. See text for details.

indices, such as arterial blood pressure, acid-base status, and oxygenation, as well as commonly used medications, presence of a PDA, and intercurrent infection may affect CBF, as suggested by studies using the aforementioned CBF monitoring techniques. We discuss management options, including evidence for when and how to treat systemic hypotension and clinical signs of systemic organ hypoperfusion. Ultimately we propose a rational treatment strategy for maintaining brain perfusion and oxygenation in the VLBW infant in the first few postnatal days.

Systemic Hypotension

There are several clinical approaches to diagnosis and treatment of neonatal hypotension. First, as mentioned earlier, in a small group of ELBW infants, Munro and colleagues (see Fig. 2-4)[20] identified a mean arterial pressure of 28 to 30 mm Hg as a breakpoint, below which autoregulation appeared to be absent. Use of dopamine to raise the mean blood pressure resulted in a normalization of the CBF in these hypotensive infants. Thus, treatment of hypotension with dopamine quickly restores normal blood pressure and CBF. However, CBF autoregulation was not immediately restored. Indeed, findings of an earlier study suggest that it may take up to 1 hour for CBF autoregulation to be restored following treatment of systemic hypotension.[69]

However, if a mean blood pressure of 28 to30 mm Hg or higher is considered normal in all infants, many will be treated whose overall hemodynamic status does not indicate a need for treatment or may receive a treatment modality (volume, vasopressors/inotropes, or inotropes) that does not specifically address the underlying pathophysiology of their cardiovascular compromise.

The most widespread approach to the definition and treatment of hypotension in the VLBW neonate during the immediate transitional period is use of a mean blood pressure that equals the gestational age in numerals. There are two major concerns with this approach. First, if the autoregulatory blood pressure breakpoint is truly at 28 to 30 mm Hg for this patient population, blood pressure at the level of the gestational age in the more immature and thus vulnerable preterm neonates will be out of the autoregulatory range. Second, as discussed earlier, some of these immature neonates, even with normal blood pressure, have low systemic and presumably cerebral blood flows,[21] because their cerebral vasculature may constrict rather than dilate in the compensated phase of shock.[28-30,40,41] Because low SVC flow (used as a surrogate of CBF) in the first postnatal day is a known risk factor for P/IVH and poor neurodevelopmental outcome,[6] it is important to identify these infants at risk, and this identification cannot be accomplished with blood pressure monitoring alone. As discussed earlier, the combined use of blood pressure and indirect clinical signs of tissue hypoperfusion (blood pressure 30 mm Hg or less and CRT 3 seconds or less[45]) may help to identify patients with low systemic and thus low cerebral blood flow. If functional echocardiography is available, VLBW neonates who are normotensive (their blood pressure is equal to or higher than their gestational age in numerals) but have low systemic blood flow may be identified. As this presentation mostly occurs during the first 6 to 12 hours postnatally, targeted use of functional echocardiography to measure SVC blood flow may be the best direct approach currently available to detect low systemic perfusion. However, even if one can diagnose low systemic blood flow during the first hours after delivery, at present we do not have a truly effective treatment modality to improve systemic blood flow in this patient population. In addition, as mentioned earlier, hypotension defined by the gestational age–based criterion in VLBW neonates appears to be a risk factor for poor neurodevelopmental outcome and it is not known whether treatment with vasopressors or inotropes does[11] or does not[9] ameliorate the risk. Thus, one could speculate that some of the hypotensive infants may have been treated too late to make a difference or that the most widely applied treatment approach is ineffective in some neonates to ameliorate the hypotension- and/or low CBF–associated brain injury.

Finally, because of the uncertainties surrounding the definition of hypotension and the relationship between blood pressure and CBF in the VLBW neonate in the immediate postnatal period, as well as the potential side effects of vasopressor use and the lack of evidence that treatment of hypotension improves neurodevelopmental outcome, some authorities advocate that hypotension in the VLBW neonate during the first postnatal day(s) be treated only if there is clear evidence of organ hypoperfusion (i.e., lactic acidosis). We would argue, however, that by the time lactic acidosis can be detected, cerebral ischemia is likely to have occurred, provided that the brain has also contributed to the production of lactate. Therefore, this approach carries the theoretical risk of allowing significant cerebral hypoperfusion to occur. However, most neonatologists agree that once the fetal channels are closed and the blood pressure–CBF relationship is restored after the first few days following delivery, blood pressure becomes a more reliable indicator of vital organ perfusion even in the most immature neonate, and hypotension should be treated promptly with careful titration of the most appropriate vasopressor/inotrope or inotrope to avoid sudden changes in systemic blood pressure and blood flow.

Treatment of Hypotension Associated with PDA

A PDA with significant left-to-right shunting often manifests as hypotension,[46,70] which is a common presentation in VLBW infants in the immediate postnatal transition period. It has been demonstrated that shunting through a nonconstricting PDA in the first 6 hours after delivery is primarily left to right and is highly associated with a low SVC flow state.[27,71] Treatment of the PDA before 6 hours of postnatal life with indomethacin induces ductal constriction by 2 hours of drug administration, but this effect is not associated with simultaneous improvements in systemic blood flow.[72] Indomethacin decreases CBF via a direct cerebrovascular vasoconstrictive effect that is independent of the drug's inhibitory action on prostaglandin synthesis.[73] It is possible that the documented decrease in severe P/IVH with early indomethacin use is due to this localized cerebral vasoconstrictive effect during a time when reperfusion may occur[72] and has less to do with improving the preceding low systemic blood flow state by closure of the ductus. However, this notion is not supported by the findings of a meta-analysis comparing the effectiveness, side effects, and hemodynamic effects of indomethacin and ibuprofen.[74] According to the findings of the meta-analysis, although ibuprofen does not induce cerebral vasoconstriction to a degree comparable to that seen with indomethacin, there is no difference in the incidence of P/IVH in VLBW neonates treated with indomethacin and those treated with ibuprofen.

Cardiovascular management of the hemodynamically unstable, hypotensive VLBW neonate with a large PDA should focus on measures that induce stepwise and reversible increases in pulmonary vascular resistance until pharmacologic or, if this fails, surgical closure of the PDA takes place. Such measures may include the avoidance of hyperventilation and respiratory (or metabolic) alkalosis and maintenance of a oxygen saturation value at the lower end of the acceptable range. It should also be remembered that high doses of vasopressors might preferentially increase systemic vascular resistance and thus left-to-right shunting through the ductus; although blood pressure may be maintained in an acceptable range, systemic perfusion could become even more compromised. Therefore, administration of high doses of dopamine or epinephrine should be avoided unless systemic blood flow can be repeatedly assessed with the use of functional echocardiography.

Treatment of Hypotension Associated with Other Causes

For hypotension due to causes such as septic shock, adrenal insufficiency, and hypovolemia, every effort should be made to treat the underlying cause and support the cardiovascular status. Although there are very little experimental data regarding the response of CBF to vasopressor medications in the hypotensive VLBW infant, some evidence is accumulating.

Dopamine is the first-line medication for many neonatologists because of its beneficial cardiovascular and renal effects.[75] It effectively increases blood pressure in the preterm infant, but its effect on organ blood flow is less well described. As mentioned earlier, evidence now indicates that despite its effect on increasing blood pressure and renal perfusion, dopamine does not have a selective vasoactive action on the cerebral circulation in normotensive VLBW neonates.[76,77] However, in hypotensive VLBW infants, the dopamine-induced increase in blood pressure is associated with an increase in CBF.[11,20,69] This finding suggests once again that cerebrovascular autoregulation is impaired in hypotensive preterm infants and that effective treatment of hypotension is associated with an increase in CBF and a delay in the restoration of CBF autoregulation (see earlier).

Are other vasopressors more effective in restoring normal CBF in this population than dopamine? A randomized controlled trial compared the cerebrovascular, hemodynamic, and metabolic effects of dopamine and epinephrine using a stepwise titration of the two medications to achieve optimum blood pressure in VLBW neonates in the first 24 postnatal hours.[11] Both medications increased cerebral perfusion in the medium-dose range, with epinephrine being slightly more effective in infants of less than 28 weeks of gestation and dopamine being more effective in those of greater than 28 weeks of gestation. Because both medications were effective at increasing blood pressure and CBF and this is the only peer-reviewed publication available on the cerebrovascular effects of epinephrine in VLBW neonates, there is no reason to choose one vasopressor over the other for this particular application.

As for inotropes and lusitropes, there has been growing interest in the potential use of milrinone, a selective phosphodiesterase III inhibitor, in neonates and infants who have undergone cardiac surgery and in VLBW neonates with low systemic blood flow during the first postnatal day. Milrinone effectively decreases the incidence of low cardiac output in infants following cardiac surgery.[78,79] Because the low-flow state in preterm infants immediately after birth is in many ways similar to the low cardiac output syndrome in postoperative cardiac patients, this drug has potential both as treatment and prophylaxis of low systemic blood flow (and presumably low CBF) in the VLBW patient population. A pilot study examined the safety, efficacy, and optimal dosing of milrinone in infants of less than 29 weeks of gestation during the first hours of postnatal life.[80] At the applied dose, milrinone appears to be relatively safe in the 1-day-old VLBW neonate. A randomized controlled trial revealed, however, that milrinone is ineffective to prevent the occurrence of low systemic blood flow in the 1-day-old VLBW neonate,[81] so the routine use of milrinone in this population cannot be recommended. Dobutamine, another sympathomimetic amine with direct positive inotropic and mild vasodilatory effects, effectively increases cardiac output and blood pressure in the VLBW neonate, especially when the cardiovascular compromise is caused by myocardial dysfunction.[82] Virtually no data are available on the cerebrovascular effects of dobutamine in the VLBW neonate.

Beyond the presentation of different forms of neonatal shock treated by vasopressors/inotropes, inotropes, and lusitropes, there has been increasing recognition that vasopressor-resistant hypotension frequently develops in the VLBW population. This presentation is thought to be due to cardiovascular adrenergic receptor downregulation and the higher incidence of relative adrenal insufficiency in the VLBW neonate.[83-86] A prospective observational study examining the hemodynamic effects of low-dose hydrocortisone administration in preterm neonates with vasopressor resistance and borderline hypotension found no independent effect of this treatment modality on CBF.[86]

Impact of Provision of Intensive Care on Systemic and Cerebral Hemodynamics

In addition to the impact of the hemodynamic changes on CBF during the postnatal transition, the effects of all interventions must be considered at all times. They include ventilatory maneuvers, the use of medications other than vasopressors/inotropes or inotropes, and invasive procedures. Premature infants with a median gestational age of 31 weeks have been reported to have a decrease in CBF velocity (and thus presumably in CBF) in response to transient hyperoxia.[87] This occurs without a decrease in $PaCO_2$, implicating hyperoxia directly in the decrease in CBF. Hypocarbia is a well-described cause of cerebral vasoconstriction, and a negative association between $PaCO_2$ and CBF and CFOE has been demonstrated in VLBW infants during the first postnatal days.[28,88,89] In addition, lower levels of $PaCO_2$ are associated with slowing of EEG activity, likely induced by decreased cerebral oxygen delivery.[89] These effects are most significant in the first 24 postnatal hours, less evident on the second day, and gone by the third postnatal day. These findings support the notion that the first hours of postnatal life represent a period of heightened vulnerability to CBF fluctuations. Not surprisingly, severe hypocapnia in VLBW neonates during the immediate transitional period is associated with PWMI and cerebral palsy.[90] Importantly, it appears that hypercapnia also has an impact on cerebral hemodynamics, in that $PaCO_2$ values higher than 45 mm Hg during the first 2 postnatal days are associated with compromised CBF autoregulation (Fig. 2-8).[91] It is tempting to speculate that this effect may, at least in part, explain the findings of retrospective studies revealing a strong independent association between hypercapnia and P/IVH in very preterm neonates.[92-94] Accordingly, the use of permissive hypercapnia during the immediate postnatal period may put the VLBW neonate at higher risk for cerebral injury.[95]

Finally, high mean airway pressures in the immediate postnatal period have also been implicated in low systemic blood flow and thus low cerebral blood flow and a predilection for PV/IVH.[26] Beyond ventilatory maneuvers and interventions,

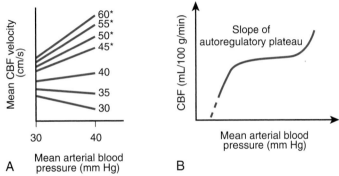

Figure 2-8 Effect of hypercapnia on cerebral blood flow (CBF) autoregulation in 43 ventilated very low-birth-weight neonates during the first 2 postnatal days. **A,** Lines represent the estimated mean slopes of the autoregulatory plateau from 30 to 60 mm Hg $PaCO_2$ with mean blood pressure values between 30 and 40 mm Hg. Horizontal line at slope zero indicates intact autoregulation, with lines at 30, 35, and 40 mm Hg being not significantly different from zero. **B,** The estimated means of the slope of the autoregulatory plateau (cm/s/mm Hg) increased as $PaCO_2$ increased from 40 mm Hg ($P = 0.004$).

commonly used medications such as midazolam and morphine have also been associated with potentially harmful changes in CBF,[96] and even umbilical arterial blood sampling could have an effect on cerebral hemodynamics in these tiny infants.[97]

The preceding paragraphs emphasize how changes in ventilatory management, administration of commonly used medications, or simple interventions in the VLBW infant, especially during the first postnatal days, can have negative and potentially devastating effects on CBF and cerebral oxygenation acutely and on neurodevelopmental outcome ultimately. The mainstays of treatment have been, and should remain at this point, maintenance of homeostasis and avoidance of potentially harmful interventions and abrupt hemodynamic changes in this most vulnerable patient population.

Summary and Recommendations

As discussed in this chapter, the management of hypotension, low systemic and cerebral blood flow, in the VLBW infant during the first postnatal days presents a significant challenge because immaturity, underlying pathology, and postnatal transition all affect the hemodynamic response to pathologic processes and interventions. Because of these factors and the lack of evidence on how treatment affect mortality and short- and long-term morbidity, straightforward recommendations on the treatment of cardiovascular compromise in the VLBW neonate during the period of transition to postnatal life cannot be given.

Therefore, the following approach to diagnosis and treatment represents our view and should be considered only as such, especially because, as discussed in this chapter, evidence on the effectiveness of the treatment of shock in the VLBW neonate during the first postnatal days is not available.

Diagnosis of Hypotension

1. We use the 5th or 10th percentile of the gestational and postnatal age-dependent population-based blood pressure values as the definition of hypotension but initiate treatment at this point only if signs of tissue hypoperfusion or echocardiographic evidence of decreased systemic perfusion or poor myocardial contractility are present. However, we attempt to maintain the mean blood pressure at 23 to 24 mm Hg even if signs of tissue hypoperfusion are not present in the most immature ELBW neonates during the first postnatal day, because cerebral electrical activity appears to be depressed at blood pressure values below this level.

2. Irrespective of the blood pressure value, whenever there is indirect or direct evidence of poor tissue perfusion, we monitor both systemic blood flow and

blood pressure closely and attempt to maintain appropriate systemic blood flow without much fluctuation in the blood pressure. Because a blood pressure breakpoint of the CBF autoregulatory curve may exist at 28 to 30 mm Hg and because more than 90% of even ELBW neonates not receiving vasopressor support maintain their mean blood pressure at 30 mm Hg or higher by the third postnatal day, we carefully attempt to slowly increase mean blood pressure during the first three postnatal days and maintain it in the 28- to 30-mm Hg range by the third postnatal day. However, it must be kept in mind that an increase in blood pressure during this period does not necessarily ensure rapid normalization of systemic and cerebral blood flow and that there are no data that this approach improves long-term neurodevelopmental outcome. Finally, the presence of a hemodynamically significant PDA affects our approach to maintaining and focusing on mean arterial blood pressure primarily and, in these cases, we carefully consider diastolic blood pressure and interrogate the cardiovascular system for evidence of systemic steal during diastole.

3. Although most neonatologists would agree with the approach described here, there is another, less frequently practiced approach that needs to be mentioned. Neonatologists using this approach initiate cardiovascular support only if there is clear evidence of poor systemic perfusion as long as mean blood pressure is at or higher than 20 mm Hg in the ELBW neonate during the first postnatal day. Because within the first 24 hours it is hard to define poor perfusion, especially without the use of functional echocardiography, and because lactic acidosis heralds the presence of (ongoing or previously present) tissue ischemia, we do not practice this diagnostic and treatment philosophy and do not allow mean arterial blood pressure to be around 20 mm Hg during the first postnatal day. However, there is no direct evidence at present that the use of permissive hypotension as an approach to diagnosis and management of cardiovascular compromise in VLBW neonates during the immediate postnatal period affects outcomes.

Treatment of Hypotension

With regard to the kind of treatment utilized, the most appropriate strategy requires identification of the underlying pathogenesis of hypotension. As described earlier, the most common etiologic factors are inappropriate peripheral vasoregulation and dysfunction of the myocardium complicated by the presence of a large PDA in VLBW neonates during the first postnatal days. Although the following approach may be recommended and we practice it, we must emphasize again that there is no evidence that treatment of hypotension in this patient population improves mortality, morbidity, or long-term neurodevelopmental outcome:

1. In the case of hypotension, because low to moderate doses of dopamine (or epinephrine) improve both blood pressure and CBF, we carefully titrate dopamine in a stepwise manner using 3- to 5-minute cycles and make every effort to avoid inducing significant rapid changes in blood pressure. If low systemic blood flow is detected with low-normal to normal blood pressure during the first postnatal day, we add dobutamine to low-dose dopamine and monitor for indirect (CRT, urine output, base deficit) and direct (functional echocardiography) signs of improvement in systemic perfusion.

2. In the presence of a hemodynamically significant PDA, we attempt to close the ductus arteriosus with a cyclooxygenase inhibitor (we use indomethacin) along with providing appropriate supportive care. If pharmacologic closure fails in the patient with a hemodynamically significant PDA, and we have evidence of ongoing or worsening systemic tissue hypoperfusion, we surgically ligate the ductus arteriosus. During the wait for surgical closure to take place, our goal is to decrease the left-to-right shunting across the ductus. As briefly described earlier, we attempt to achieve this goal by carefully increasing pulmonary resistance in a stepwise manner. Using this approach, we frequently are successful at increasing pulmonary vascular resistance,

and the associated decrease in left-to-right shunting results in improvement of systemic blood flow and blood pressure. We also use dopamine in babies with a hemodynamically significant PDA, because it has been shown that, in patients with increased pulmonary blood flow, dopamine increases pulmonary vascular resistance and systemic perfusion.[98] Interestingly, there is no evidence that dopamine preferentially increases pulmonary vascular resistance in neonates without preexisting pulmonary overcirculation. It is tempting to speculate that the increased pulmonary blood flow–associated protective upregulation of vasoconstrictive mechanisms (enhanced α-adrenergic and endothelin-1 receptor expression) and downregulation of the vasodilatory mechanisms (endogenous nitric oxide and vasodilatory prostaglandin production) in the pulmonary arteries are responsible for this observation. We add dobutamine only in the presence of impaired myocardial function, because most VLBW neonates with hemodynamically significant PDA after the first postnatal day usually have normal or hyperdynamic cardiac function. Indeed, the indiscriminate use of dobutamine in these patients may compromise myocardial filling and diastolic function. Finally, administration of fluids to increase blood volume must be restricted because excessive (or even liberal) use of volume is associated with greater mortality and morbidity in this patient population.

3. Finally, because $PaCO_2$ is a much more potent mediator of cerebral vascular tone than blood pressure, we make every effort to keep $PaCO_2$ within the

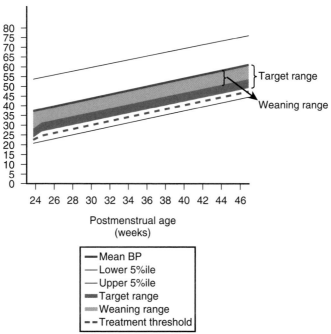

Figure 2-9 Postmenstrual age-dependent definition of hypotension and the target and weaning blood pressure ranges. *Hypotension* is defined as the treatment threshold, which is 1 to 3 points above the 5th percentile (5%ile) for postmenstrual age.[14-16] Below the treatment threshold, we usually initiate treatment of hypotension. The target range is defined as where mean blood pressure is intended to be kept. The target range is between 2 and 3 mm Hg above the treatment threshold and the 50th percentile of the mean blood pressure.[14-16] Finally, the weaning range is defined as the mean blood pressure range where careful weaning of vasopressors and/or inotropic agents is commenced. This range is between 5 mm Hg above the lower limits of target range and the 50th percentile of the mean blood pressure. Note that the upper limit of the target range does not exceed the 50th percentile of the mean blood pressure in order to decrease the risk of achieving an increase in blood pressure by causing significant increases in systemic vascular resistance and thus, potentially, decreases in cardiac output when vasopressors/inotropic agents are being administered. This graph was developed in collaboration with the Under Pressure hemodynamic group created as part of a Vermont-Oxford Network (VON) initiative for 2004 to 2006. One of us (IS) served as the VON expert on hemodynamics for this initiative.

45- to 50-mm Hg range. We hope that by keeping $PaCO_2$ relatively constant we minimize the incidence of hypocapnia-associated white matter injury and cerebral palsy and the hypercapnia-associated increased risk of P/IVH. In addition, in the presence of constant $PaCO_2$ levels, the integrity of CBF autoregulation is likely to be maximized.

Figure 2-9 illustrates our postmenstrual age–dependent approach to the diagnosis and treatment of hypotension in preterm and term neonates. It is important to note that our definition of hypotension (*dotted line*) and the target and weaning ranges have all been arbitrarily defined with the use of epidemiologic data and extrapolation of hemodynamic findings and the data on the association between blood pressure and systemic and cerebral blood flow. Because this approach, just like any other approach to manage the cardiovascular compromise in the neonatal patient population, is not evidence-based, it cannot be recommended in general and only illustrates one of the many options in the diagnosis and treatment of neonatal hypotension. We use these numbers only as guidance, carefully assess the indirect clinical signs of tissue perfusion, and perform targeted echocardiographic evaluations when more information is needed. In the future and after completion of the ongoing investigations, we plan to utilize the real-time information our comprehensive cardiovascular monitoring and data acquisition system provides.

References

1. Perlman JM, McMenamin JB, Volpe JJ. Fluctuating cerebral blood flow velocity in respiratory distress syndrome. Relation to the development of intraventricular hemorrhage. *N Engl J Med*. 1983;309: 204-209.
2. Van Bel F, Van de Bor M, Stijnen T, et al. Aetiological role of cerebral blood flow alterations in development and extension of peri-intraventricular hemorrhage. *Dev Med Child Neurol*. 1987;29: 601-614.
3. Miall-Allen VM, de Vries LS, Whitelaw AG. Mean arterial pressure and neonatal cerebral lesions. *Arch Dis Child*. 1987;62:1068-1069.
4. Bada HS, Korones SB, Perry EH, et al. Mean arterial blood pressure changes in premature infants and those at risk for intraventricular hemorrhage. *J Pediatr*. 1990;117:607-614.
5. Tsuji M, Saul PJ, duPlessis A, et al. Cerebral intravascular oxygenation correlates with mean arterial pressure in critically ill premature infants. *Pediatrics*. 2000;106:625.
6. Hunt R, Evans N, Rieger I, et al. Low superior vena cava flow and neurodevelopment at 3 years in very preterm infants. *J Pediatr*. 2004;145:588-592.
7. Goldstein RF, Thompson Jr RJ, Oehler JM, et al. Influence of acidosis, hypoxemia, and hypotension on neurodevelopmental outcome in very low birth weight infants. *Pediatrics*. 1995;95:238-243.
8. Damman O, Allred EN, Kuban KCK, et al. Systemic hypotension and white matter damage in preterm infants. *Dev Med Child Neurol*. 2002;44:82-90.
9. Fanaroff JM, Wilson-Costello DE, Newman NS, et al. Treated hypotension is associated with neonatal morbidity and hearing loss in extremely low birth weight infants. *Pediatrics*. 2006;117:1131-1135.
10. Dempsey EM, Alhazzani Dr F, Barrington KJ. Permissive hypotension in the extremely low birth weight infant with signs of good perfusion. *Arch Dis Child Fetal Neonatal Ed.*. 2009;94:F241-F244.
11. Pellicer A, del Carmen Bravo M, Madero R, et al. Early systemic hypotension and vasopressor support in low birth weight infants: impact on neurodevelopment. *Pediatrics*. 2009;123:1369-1376.
12. Pellicer A, Valverde E, Elorza MD, et al. Cardiovascular support for low birth weight infants and cerebral hemodynamics: a randomized blinded clinical trial. *Pediatrics*. 2005;115:1501.
13. Batton B, Zhu X, Fanaroff J. Blood pressure, anti-hypotensive therapy, and neurodevelopment in extremely preterm infants. *J Pediatr*. 2009;154:351-357.
14. Nuntnarumit P, Yang W, Bada-Ellzey HS. Blood pressure measurements in the newborn. *Clin Perinatol*. 1999;26:981-996.
15. Development of audit measure sand guidelines for good practice in the management of neonatal respiratory distress syndrome. Report of a Joint Working Group of the British Association of Perinatal Medicine and the Research Unit of the Royal College of Physicians. *Arch Dis Child*. 1992;67:1221-1227.
16. Engle WD. Blood pressure in the very low birth weight neonate. *Early Hum Dev*. 2001;62: 97-130.
17. Seri I. Circulatory support of the sick newborn infant. *Semin Neonatol*. 2001;6:85-95.
18. Greisen G. Autoregulation of cerebral blood flow in newborn babies. *Early Hum Dev*. 2005;81: 423-428.
19. Milligan DWA. Failure of autoregulation and intraventricular haemorrhage in preterm infants. *Lancet*. 1980;1(8174):896-899.
20. Munro MJ, Wong FY, Walker AM, Barfield CP. Hypotensive extremely low birth weight infants have reduced cerebral blood flow. *Pediatrics*. 2004;114:1591.
21. Kissack CM, Garr R, Wardle SP, Weindling AM. Cerebral fractional oxygen extraction is inversely correlated with oxygen delivery in the sick, newborn preterm infant. *J Cerebr Blood Flow Metab*. 2005;25:545-553.

22. Weindling AM, Victor NM. Definition of hypotension in very low birth weight infants during the immediate neonatal period. *NeoReviews*. 2007;8:c32-c43.

23. Victor S, Marson AG, Appleton RE, et al. Relationship between blood pressure, cerebral electrical activity, cerebral fractional oxygen extraction and peripheral blood flow in very low birth weight newborn infants. *Pediatr Res*. 2006;59:314-319.

24. Victor S, Appleton RE, Beirne M, et al. The relationship between cardiac output, cerebral electrical activity, cerebral fractional oxygen extraction and peripheral blood flow in premature newborn infants. *Pediatr Res*. 2006;60:1-5.

25. Kluckow M, Evans N. Low superior vena cava flow and intraventricular haemorrhage in preterm infants. *Arch Dis Child*. 2000;82:188-194.

26. Kluckow M, Evans N. Relationship between blood pressure and cardiac output in preterm infants requiring mechanical ventilation. *J Pediatr*. 1996;129:506.

27. Kluckow M, Evans N. Superior vena cava flow in newborn infant: a novel marker of systemic blood flow. *Arch Dis Child Fetal Neonatal Ed*. 2000;82:182-187.

28. Kissack CM, Garr R, Wardle SP, et al. Cerebral fractional oxygen extraction in very low birth weight infants is high when there is low left ventricular output and hypocarbia but is unaffected by hypotension. *Pediatr Res*. 2004;55:400-405.

29. Seri I. Hemodynamics during the first two postnatal days and neurodevelopment in preterm neonates. *J Pediatr*. 2004;145:573-575.

30. Noori S, Stavroudis TA, Seri I. Systemic and cerebral hemodynamics during the transitional period after premature birth. *Clin Perinatol*. 2009;36:723-736.

31. Tsuji M, Saul JP, du Plessis A, et al. Cerebral intravascular oxygenation correlates with mean arterial pressure in critically ill premature infants. *Pediatrics*. 2000;106:625-632.

32. O'Leary H, Gregas M, Limperopoulos C. Elevated cerebral pressure passivity is associated with prematurity-related intracranial hemorrhage. *Pediatrics*. 2009;124:302-309.

33. Greisen G. Cerebral blood flow in preterm infants during the first week of life. *Acta Paediatr Scand*. 1986;75:43-51.

34. Pryds O, Andersen E, Hansen BF. Cerebral blood flow reactivity in spontaneously breathing infants shortly after birth. *Acta Paediatr Scand*. 1990;79:391-396.

35. Pryds O, Greisen P. Effect of PaCO$_2$ and haemoglobin concentration on day to day variation of CBF in preterm neonates. *Acta Paediatr Scand*. 1989;360:33-36.

36. Greisen G, Trojaborg W. Cerebral blood flow, PaCO$_2$ changes and visual evoked potentials in mechanically ventilated preterm infants. *Acta Paediatr Scand*. 1987;76:394-400.

37. Altman DI, Powers WJ, Perlman JM, et al. Cerebral blood flow requirement for brain viability in newborn infants is lower than in adults. *Ann Neurol*. 1988;24:218-226.

38. Kluckow M, Evans N. Low systemic blood flow and hyperkalemia in preterm infants. *J Pediatr*. 2001;139:227-232.

39. Osborn D, Evans N, Kluckow M. Randomised trial of dopamine and dobutamine in preterm infants with low systemic blood flow. *J Pediatr*. 2002;140:183-191.

40. Hernandez MJ, Hawkins RA, Brennan RW. Sympathetic control of regional cerebral blood flow in the asphyxiated newborn dog. In: Heistad DD, Marcus ML, eds. *Cerebral Blood Flow, effects of nerves and neurotransmitters*. New York: Elsevier; 1982:359-366.

41. Ashwal S, Dale PS, Longo LD. Regional cerebral blood flow: studies in the fetal lamb during hypoxia, hypercapnia, acidosis, and hypotension. *Pediatr Res*. 1984;18:1309-1316.

42. Noori S, McCoy M, Gottipati V, et al. Temporal relationship of cerebral hemorrhage with changes in cerebral fractional oxygen extraction and cardiac function in extremely preterm infants. Presented at Perinatal brain injury: mechanisms and risk factors. Colorado Convention Center, Denver, May 3, 2011.

43. Kehrer M, Blumenstock G, Ehehalt S, et al. Development of cerebral blood flow volume in preterm neonates during the first two weeks of life. *Pediatr Res*. 2005;58:927-930.

44. Takami T, Sunohara D, Kondo A, et al. Changes in cerebral perfusion in extremely LBW infants during the first 72 h after birth. *Pediatr Res*. 2010;68:435-439.

45. Osborn D, Evans N, Kluckow M. Clinical detection of low upper body blood flow in very premature infants using blood pressure, capillary refill time and central-peripheral temperature difference. *Arch Dis Child Fetal Neonatal Ed*. 2004;89:168.

46. Evans N, Iyer P. Longitudinal changes in the diameter of the ductus arteriosus in ventilated preterm infants: correlation with respiratory outcomes. *Arch Dis Child Fetal Neonatal Ed*. 1995;72:F156-F161.

47. West CR, Groves AM, Williams CE, et al. Early low cardiac output is associated with compromised electroencephalographic activity in very preterm infants. *Pediatr Res*. 2006;59:610-615.

48. Kluckow M, Seri I, Evans N. Functional echocardiography—an emerging clinical tool for the neonatologist. *J Pediatr*. 2007;150:125-130.

49. Gilbert RD, Pearce WJ, Ashwal S, Longo LD. Effects of hypoxia on contractility of isolated fetal lamb cerebral arteries. *J Dev Physiol*. 1990;13:199-203.

50. Hansen NB, Stonestreet BS, Rosenkrantz TS, Oh W. Validity of Doppler measurements of anterior cerebral artery blood flow velocity: correlation with brain blood flow in piglets. *Pediatrics*. 1983;72: 526-531.

51. Greisen G, Johansen K, Ellison PH, et al. Cerebral blood flow in the newborn: comparison of Doppler ultrasound and [133]xenon clearance. *J Pediatr*. 1984;104:411-418.

52. Raju TN. Cerebral Doppler studies in the fetus and the newborn infant. *J Pediatr*. 1991;119:165-174.

53. Suttner S, Schollhorn T, Boldt J, et al. Noninvasive assessment of cardiac output using thoracic electrical bioimpedance in hemodynamically stable and unstable patients after cardiac surgery: a comparison with pulmonary artery thermodilution. *Intensive Care Med*. 2006;32:2053-2058.

54. Norozi K, Beck C, Osthaus WA, et al. Electrical velocimetry for measuring cardiac output in children with congenital heart disease. *Br J Anaesth*. 2008;100:88-94.
55. Noori S, Drabu B, Seri I. Continuous non-invasive cardiac output measurements in the neonate by electrical cardiometry: a comparison with echocardiography. Presented at the Pediatric Academic Societies (PAS) Conference, Vancouver, May 2010.
56. Brazy JE, Lewis DV, Mitnisk MH, et al. Noninvasive monitoring of cerebral oxygenation in preterm infants: preliminary observation. *Pediatrics*. 1985;75:217-225.
57. Patel J, Marks K, Roberts I, et al. Measurement of cerebral blood flow in newborn infants using near infrared spectroscopy with indocyanine green. *Pediatr Res*. 1998;43:34-39.
58. Dullenkopf A, Kolarova A, Schulz G, et al. Reproducibility of cerebral oxygenation measurement in neonates and infants in the clinical setting using the NIRO 300 oximeter. *Pediatr Crit Care Med*. 2005;6:344-347.
59. Bucher HU, Edwards AD, Lipp AE, et al. Comparison between near-infrared spectroscopy and ^{133}xenon clearance for estimation of cerebral blood flow in critically ill preterm infants. *Pediatr Res*. 1993;33:56-60.
60. Dujovny M, Ausman JI, Stoddart H, et al. Somanetics INVOS 3100 cerebral oximeter. *Neurosurgery*. 1995 37:160.
61. Toet MC, Lemmers PM. Brain monitoring in neonates. *Early Hum Dev*. 2009;85:77-84.
62. Toet MC, Hellstrom-Westas L, Groenendaal F, et al. Amplitude integrated EEG 3 and 6 hours after birth in full term neonates with hypoxic-ischaemic encephalopathy. *Arch Dis Child Fetal Neonatal Ed*. 1999;81:F19-F23.
63. Toet MC, van der Mei W, de Vries LS, et al. Comparison between simultaneously recorded amplitude-integrated electroencephalogram (cerebral function monitor) and standard electroencephalogram in neonates. *Pediatrics*. 2002;109:772-779.
64. Ter Horst HJ, Sommer C. Bergman KA, et al. Prognostic significance of amplitude-integrated EEG during the first 72 hours after birth in severely asphyxiated neonates. *Pediatr Res*. 2004;55: 1026-1033.
65. Shalak LF, Laptook AR, Velaphi SC, et al. Amplitude-integrated electroencephalography coupled with an early neurologic examination enhances prediction of term infants at risk for persistent encephalopathy. *Pediatrics*. 2003;111:351-357.
66. Hellstrom-Westas L, Klette H, Thorngren-Jerneck K, et al. Early prediction of outcome with aEEG in preterm infants with large intraventricular hemorrhages. *Neuropediatrics*. 2001;32:319-324.
67. Olischar M, Klebermass K, Kuhle S, et al. Reference values for amplitude-integrated electroencephalographic activity in preterm infants younger than 30 weeks' gestational age. *Pediatrics*. 2004;113: e61-e66.
68. Klebermass K, Kuhle S, Olischar M, et al. Intra-and extrauterine maturation of amplitude-integrated electroencephalographic activity in preterm infants younger than 30 weeks of gestation. *Biol Neonate*. 2006;89:120-125.
69. Seri I, Rudas G, Bors Z, et al. Effects of low dose dopamine infusion on cardiovascular and renal functions, cerebral blood flow and plasma catecholamine levels in sick preterm neonates. *Pediatr Res*. 1993;34:742-749.
70. Evans N, Moorcraft J. Effect of patency of the ductus arteriosus on blood pressure in very preterm infants. *Arch Dis Child*. 1992;67:1169.
71. Kluckow M, Evans N. Early echocardiographic prediction of symptomatic patent ductus arteriosus in preterm infants undergoing mechanical ventilation. *J Pediatr*. 1995;127:774-779.
72. Osborn DA, Evans N, Kluckow M. Effect of early, targeted indomethacin on the ductus arteriosus and blood flow to the upper body and brain in the preterm infant. *Arch Dis Child Fetal Neonatal Ed*. 2003;88:477-482.
73. Yanowitz TD, Yao AC, Werner JC, et al. Effects of prophylactic low-dose indomethacin on hemodynamics in very low birth weight infants. *J Pediatr*. 1998;132:28-34.
74. Thomas RL, Parker GC, Van Overmeire B, et al. A meta-analysis of ibuprofen versus indomethacin for closure of patent ductus arteriosus. *Eur J Pediatr*. 2005;164:135-140.
75. Seri I. Cardiovascular, renal and endocrine actions of dopamine in neonates and children. *J Pediatr*. 1995;126:333-344.
76. Seri I, Abbasi S, Wood DC, et al. Regional hemodynamic effects of dopamine in the sick preterm neonate. *J Pediatr*. 1998;133:728-734.
77. Lundstrom K, Pryds O, Greisen G. The haemodynamic effects of dopamine and volume expansion in sick preterm infants. *Early Hum Dev*. 2000;57:157-163.
78. Chang AC, Atz A, Wernovsky G, et al. Milrinone: systemic and pulmonary hemodynamic effects in neonates after cardiac surgery. *Crit Care Med*. 1995;23:1907-1911.
79. Hoffman TM, Wernovsky G, Atz AM, et al. Efficacy and safety of milrinone in preventing low cardiac output syndrome in infants and children after corrective surgery for congenital heart disease. *Circulation*. 2003;107:996-1002.
80. Paradisis M, Evans N, Kluckow M, et al. Pilot study of milrinone for low systemic blood flow in very preterm infants. *J Pediatr*. 2006;148:306-313.
81. Paradisis M, Evans N, Kluckow M, Osborn D. Randomized trial of milrinone versus placebo for prevention of low systemic blood flow in very preterm infants. *J Pediatr*. 2009;154:189-195.
82. Noori S, Friedlich P, Seri I. Cardiovascular and renal effects of dobutamine in the neonate. *NeoReviews*. 2004;5:E22-E26.
83. Ng PC, Lee CH, Lam CWK, et al. Transient adrenocortical insufficiency of prematurity and systemic hypotension in very low birth weight infants. *Arch Dis Child Fetal Neonatal Ed*. 2004;89:F119-F126.

84. Fernandez E, Schrader R, Watterberg K. Prevalence of low cortisol values in term and near-term infants with vasopressor-resistant hypotension. *J Perinatol*. 2005;25:114-118.
85. Seri I, Tan R, Evans J. The effect of hydrocortisone on blood pressure in preterm neonates with pressor-resistant hypotension. *Pediatrics*. 2001;107:1070-1074.
86. Noori S, Friedlich P, Wong P, et al. Hemodynamic changes after low-dose hydrocortisone administration in vasopressor-treated preterm and term neonates. *Pediatrics*. 2006;118:1456-1466.
87. Niijima S, Shortland DB, Levene MI, et al. Transient hyperoxia and cerebral blood flow velocity in infants born prematurely and at full term. *Arch Dis Child*. 1988;63:1126-1130.
88. Tyszczuk L, Meek J, Elwell C, et al. Cerebral blood flow is independent of mean arterial blood pressure in preterm infants undergoing intensive care. *Pediatrics*. 1998;102:337-341.
89. Victor S, Appleton RE, Beirne M, et al. Effect of carbon dioxide on background cerebral electrical activity and fractional oxygen extraction in very low birth weight infants just after birth. *Pediatr Res*. 2005;58:579-585.
90. Murase M, Ishida A. Early hypocarbia of preterm infants: its relationship to periventricular leukomalacia and cerebral palsy, and its perinatal risk factors. *Acta Paediatr*. 2005;94:85-91.
91. Kaiser JR, Gauss CH, Williams DK. The effects of hypercapnia on cerebral autoregulation in ventilated very low birth weight infants. *Pediatr Res*. 2005;58:931-935.
92. Kaiser JR, Gauss CH, Pont MM, Williams DK. Hypercapnia during the first 3 days of life is associated with severe intraventricular hemorrhage in very low birth weight infants. *J Perinatol*. 2006;26:279-285.
93. Fabres J, Carlo WA, Phillips V, et al. Both extremes of arterial carbon dioxide pressure and the magnitude of fluctuations in arterial carbon dioxide pressure are associated with severe intraventricular hemorrhage in preterm infants. *Pediatrics*. 2007;119:299-305.
94. Vela-Huerta MM, Amador-Licona M, Medina-Ovando N, Aldana-Valenzuela C. Factors associated with early severe intraventricular haemorrhage in very low birth weight infants. *Neuropediatrics*. 2009;40:224-227.
95. McKee LA, Fabres J, Howard G, et al. PaCO2 and neurodevelopment in extremely low birth weight infants. *J Pediatr*. 2009;155:217-221.
96. van Alfen-van der Velden AAEM, Hopman JCW, Klaessens JHGM, et al. Effects of midazolam and morphine on cerebral oxygenation and hemodynamics in ventilated premature infants. *Biol Neonate*. 2006;90:197-202.
97. Roll C, Huning B, Kaunicke M, et al. Umbilical artery catheter blood sampling volume and velocity: impact on cerebral blood volume and oxygenation in very-low-birthweight infants. *Acta Paediatr*. 2006;95:68-73.
98. Bouissou A, Rakza T, Klosowski S, et al. Hypotension in preterm infants with significant patent ductus arteriosus: effects of dopamine. *J Pediatr*. 2008;153:790-794.

CHAPTER 3

Intraventricular Hemorrhage and White Matter Injury in the Preterm Infant

Toshiki Takenouchi, MD, and Jeffrey M. Perlman, MB, ChB

- Periventricular-Intraventricular Hemorrhage
- Periventricular White Matter Injury Associated with IVH
- White Matter Injury in the Absence of Hemorrhage
- Outcome
- Gaps in Knowledge

CASE HISTORY

HW was a 700-g 24-week premature twin B male infant born to a 29-year-old G1P0 (gravida 1, para 0) mother whose pregnancy was complicated by the onset of premature labor. The mother received a dose of betamethasone approximately 6 hours prior to a vaginal delivery. She also was started on antibiotics and given magnesium sulfate. The infant was delivered with minimal respiratory effort and a heart rate of 70. Resuscitation included bag-mask ventilation with room air and intubation, with a rapid improvement in heart rate. The infant was admitted to the intensive care unit and was given one dose of a surfactant preparation for respiratory distress syndrome (RDS). The early course was complicated by a pneumothorax that required chest tube drainage on day of life (DOL) 1. On DOL 2 there was an acute deterioration in the respiratory status with evidence of pulmonary hemorrhage, associated hypoxic respiratory failure, and significant metabolic acidosis. A head ultrasound scan showed a grade III intraventricular hemorrhage on the left with dilation of the ventricle and an associated ipsilateral intraparenchymal echodensity involving frontoparietal white matter. In addition, the infant developed a patent ductus arteriosus (PDA) diagnosed by echocardiogram on DOL 3, initially treated with indomethacin. The infant was weaned to continuous positive airway pressure by DOL 14, and was briefly reintubated for the surgical ligation of the PDA and on the second occasion for a nosocomial infection. Other issues included recurrent apnea and bradycardia and frequent unprovoked desaturation episodes. He required supplemental oxygen through the 35th week of postconceptual age. He required parenteral nutrition for 3 weeks and subsequently received enteral breast milk. Repeat head ultrasound scans on DOLs 7, 14, 28, 42, and 56 revealed progressive communicating hydrocephalus involving the lateral third and fourth ventricles that peaked in dilation by DOL 28 and then gradually decreased in size by DOL 56. The parenchymal lesion evolved into a small left porencephalic cyst. The infant underwent a magnetic resonance imaging (MRI) evaluation on DOL 92 that revealed mild ventriculomegaly and the left cystic lesion and some periventricular white matter loss. The infant was discharged on DOL 100. He was seen and evaluated at 18 months. At that time the clinical findings indicated mild right hemiparesis. He recently started walking, was very active, and had minimal speech. Evaluation using the Bayley battery of tests found that he had a mental developmental index of 75 and a psycho-motor developmental index of 82.

This case illustrates a typical course of a premature infant who is at greatest risk for severe periventricular-intraventricular hemorrhage (PV-IVH) even when managed in the later era of neonatology. Thus, at this time, although the overall incidence of PV-IVH in the premature infant has decreased, hemorrhage remains an important problem in the very low-birth-weight infant (<1000 g), particularly in cases of rapid delivery when the potential for full dosing of peridelivery glucocorticoids is not possible.[1,2] This chapter focuses on a brief review of the pathogenesis of PV-IVH as well as white matter injury, and discusses various approaches or strategies to the diagnosis and treatment as well as outcomes, and highlights gaps in knowledge.

Periventricular-Intraventricular Hemorrhage

Background

The overall occurrence of PV-IVH has declined with time, although severe hemor-rhage remains a significant clinical problem in the tiniest of the very low-birth-weight population.[1,3,4] Thus, 21% of infants born at 23 weeks of gestation and 13% to 14% in infants born at 24-25 weeks still have the most severe forms of hemor-rhage.[3] This observation is highly relevant because survival of the infants born at the cutting edge of viability continues to increase, and long-term neurocognitive deficits are more likely with severe hemorrhage. However, evidence now points to neurocognitive deficits even with lesser grades of hemorrhage—grades II and III IVH and even when the cranial sonogram is interpreted as being normal (see later discus-sion).[5,6] These observations are important because they point to the limitations of cranial sonography in identifying subtle white matter injury as well as injury to cortical or deep gray matter. The latter are more readily identified by MRI studies performed closer to term.[7,8]

Neuropathology: Relevance to Clinical Findings

The primary lesion in PV-IVH is bleeding from small vessels in the subependymal germinal matrix (GM), a transitional gelatinous region that provides limited support for the luxurious but very immature capillary bed that courses through it.[9] With maturation, this matrix region becomes less prominent, and by term it is essentially absent. The hemorrhage, when it evolves, may be confined to the GM region (grade I IVH), or it may extend and rupture into the adjacent ventricular system (grade II or III IVH, depending on the extent of hemorrhage), or extend into the white matter (termed a grade IV or intraparenchymal echogenicity [IPE]) (Fig. 3-1A).[2,10] IPE, which is invariably unilateral, represents an area of hemorrhagic necrosis of varying size within periventricular white matter, dorsal and lateral to the external angle of the lateral ventricle (Fig. 3-1B).[2,11,12]

Pathogenesis

The genesis of bleeding from capillaries within the GM is complex, multifactorial, and influenced in part by intravascular, vascular, and extravascular factors. Several factors point to a critical role for intravascular factors and specifically perturbations in blood pressure as a principal mechanism of capillary rupture and hemorrhage (see also Chapter 2). Thus, it has been shown, through the use of different methods to assess cerebral blood flow (CBF), including Doppler ultrasonography, near-infrared spectroscopy, and xenon-enhanced computed tomography (CT), that the cerebral circulation of the sick infant is pressure passive—that is, CBF varies directly

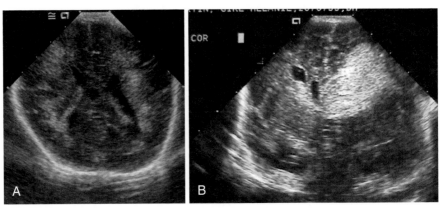

Figure 3-1   Coronal ultrasound scans. **A,** Note a bilateral germinal matrix and intraventricular hemorrhage (grade III). **B,** Note the large left-sided germinal matrix and intraventricular hemorrhage. There is a large ipsilateral intraparenchymal echodensity involving periventricular white matter.

with changes in systemic blood pressure.[13-15] Clearly this state would be expected to increase the vulnerability of the GM capillaries to periods of both hypotension and hypertension. Indeed, experimental studies and clinical observations support this hypothesis. Thus in a beagle puppy model, GM hemorrhage can be produced by systemic hypertension with or without prior hypotension.[16,17] Moreover, clinical temporal associations have been demonstrated between fluctuations in systemic blood pressure and simultaneous fluctuations in CBF velocity as may occur in the ventilated premature infant with RDS, increases in CBF as may occur with rapid volume expansion or a pneumothorax, and the subsequent development of PV-IVH.[18-20] Conversely, decreases in CBF secondary to systemic hypotension, which may occur in utero or postnatally, may also play a prominent role in the genesis of PV-IVH in certain infants.[21] Hypercarbia produced by potential modulation of autoregulation increases the risk for severe IVH.[22,23] A presumed mechanism in this context is that of rupture upon reperfusion.[1,14] Finally, elevations in venous pressure may be an important additional intravascular mechanism of hemorrhage and may reflect the peculiarity of the anatomy of the venous drainage of GM and the white matter.[2] Thus, at the level of the head of the caudate nucleus and the foramen of Monro, the terminal, choroidal, and thalamostriate veins course anteriorly to a point of confluence to form the internal cerebral vein. The blood flow then makes a U turn at the usual site of hemorrhage, raising the possibility that an elevation in venous pressure increases the potential for venous distention with obstruction of the terminal and medullary veins and hemorrhagic infarction. Indeed, simultaneous increases in venous pressure have been observed in infants who exhibit variability in arterial blood pressure, such as occurs with RDS and associated complications, such as pneumothorax and pulmonary interstitial emphysema, or with mechanical or high-frequency ventilation.[24] To summarize, it is likely that both arterial and venous perturbations contribute to the genesis of IVH. However, later evidence suggests that these intravascular responses may be modulated by inflammation or the administration of medications to the mother, such as glucocorticoids (see later discussion).[25-27] For example, in one series, infants with fetal inflammation had a significantly higher incidence of severe IVH than infants with no fetal inflammation (49% vs. 17%) ($P = 0.04$). Infants with fetal inflammation had significantly higher heart rate ($P = 0.005$), catecholamine index ($P = 0.02$), and volume load ($P = 0.02$) in the first 24 hours of life.[28]

   In addition to the intravascular factors, vascular and extravascular influences—the poorly supported blood vessels, excessive fibrinolytic activity noted within the matrix region, and a prominent postnatal decrease in tissue pressure—may all contribute to hemorrhage.[2,29,30]

Periventricular White Matter Injury Associated with IVH

The pathogenesis of white matter injury associated with hemorrhage remains unclear but appears to be closely linked to the adjacent bleed. Two potential pathways have been proposed to explain this intricate relationship. The first suggests a direct relationship to the PV-IVH, on the basis of several clinical observations, as follows: (1) the white matter lesion is always noted concurrent with or following a large GM and/or IVH and is rarely if ever observed prior to the hemorrhage; and (2) the white matter injury is always observed ipsilateral to the side of the larger hemorrhage when there is bilateral involvement of the ventricular system.[1,2,12] This consistent relationship between the GM and the white matter injury may in part be explained by the venous drainage of the deep white matter (see earlier discussion). A second explanation is a de novo evolution of white matter injury. Thus it is proposed that the PV-IVH and the white matter injury occur concurrently. Because both the GM and the periventricular white matter are border-zone regions, the risk for ischemic injury is increased during periods of systemic hypotension, particularly in the presence of a pressure-passive cerebral circulation.[1,2,14] Hemorrhage in these regions may then occur as a secondary phenomenon, or reperfusion injury. In support of this theory is the fairly consistent observation of the simultaneous detection of PV-IVH and white matter injury on cranial ultrasonography. Moreover, elevated hypoxanthine and uric acid levels (perhaps as markers of reperfusion injury) have been observed on the first postnatal day in infants in whom white matter injury subsequently developed.[31,32]

Identification of the mechanisms contributing to periventricular white matter injury is crucial to prevention of this lesion. Thus if the white matter injury is directly related to PV-IVH, then prevention of the latter should reduce the occurrence of the white matter injury. However if the PV-IVH and the white matter injury occur simultaneously as a result of a primary ischemic event with the hemorrhage occurring as a secondary phenomenon, then prevention of the secondary hemorrhage may not affect the primary ischemic lesion. Indeed, the two follow-up studies on indomethacin treatment to prevent IVH in the neonatal period are supportive of this latter concern. Thus, although the incidence of severe IVH was reduced in infants treated with indomethacin in both studies, neurodevelopmental outcomes at 18-month follow-up, including cerebral palsy, were comparable in the indomethacin-treated group the controls (Table 3-1).[33,34]

Clinical Features

In most cases (up to 70% of less severe IVH cases), the diagnosis is made with a screening sonogram.[2] In the earlier descriptions of PV-IVH, the majority of cases, about 90%, evolved within the first 72 hours of postnatal life.[35] However, the time to initial diagnosis of hemorrhage has shifted to a later onset in recent years.[10] Thus, for neonates weighing less than 1000 g, the IVH diagnosis is made early, within the first 24 hours in approximately 80% of infants. However some cases are now noted after the 10th postnatal day. This changing pattern may reflect the complexity of

Table 3-1 SHORT- AND LONG-TERM NEUROLOGIC OUTCOME IN INFANTS WHO RECEIVED INDOMETHACIN AND INFANTS WHO RECEIVED A PLACEBO

Outcome	Indomethacin Group (n = 574)	Placebo Group (n = 569)	Adjusted Odds Ratio (95% Confidence Interval)	P value
Severe intraventricular hemorrhage	9%	13%	0.6 (0.4-0.9)	0.02
Cerebral palsy	12%	12%	1.1 (0.7-1.6)	0.64
Cognitive delay (Mental Development Index < 70)	27%	26%	1.0 (0.8-1.4)	0.86

Adapted from Schmidt B, Davis P, Moddemann D, et al. Trial of Indomethacin Prophylaxis in Preterms Investigators. Long-term effects of indomethacin prophylaxis in extremely-low-birth-weight infants. *N Engl J Med.* 2001;344:1966-1972.

disease in the tiniest infants and the extent of supportive medical care, especially the prolonged use of high-frequency ventilation. Infants with the more severe IVH frequently exhibit clinical signs such as a bulging fontanel, seizures, a drop in hematocrit, hyperglycemia, metabolic acidosis, and pulmonary hemorrhage.[1]

Complications

The two most significant complications of IVH are extension into adjacent white matter (see earlier discussion) and the development of post-hemorrhagic hydrocephalus (see Chapter 4).

Prevention

Perinatal Strategies

Prevention of PV-IVH and its complications continues to focus on both perinatal and postnatal strategies. Perinatal pharmacologic interventions have included the administration of phenobarbital and vitamin K without any beneficial effect.[36-38] More recently, a combination of aminophylline, magnesium with steroids, and ritodrine has been studied in a relatively small sample (n = 128) and has resulted in an apparent reduction in rates of all IVH and severe IVH.[39] The antenatal administration of a single short course of glucocorticoids to augment pulmonary maturation has had the positive, unanticipated benefit of a significant reduction in the incidence of severe IVH.[26,40-46] From a review of several large observational databases, the unadjusted odds ratio for severe IVH following any antenatal glucocorticoid exposure has ranged from 0.43 to 0.69.[26] The mechanisms whereby glucocorticoids reduce severe IVH remain unclear but may relate to less severe RDS, higher resting blood pressures, or accelerated maturation of the germinal matrix region.[30,47,48] The value of repeated doses of antenatal steroids has come into question with regard to potential adverse effects on the developing brain. Thus, infants who were exposed to several doses of antenatal steroids had a higher incidence of cerebral palsy than a placebo group, although the difference was not statistically significant (6/206 vs. 1/195; $P = 0.12$).[49] Further, multiple courses of antenatal corticosteroids, every 14 days, did not improve preterm birth outcomes and were associated with decreased weight, length, and head circumference at birth.[50] Therefore, repeated doses of antenatal corticosteroids are not routinely recommended.

One maternal medical condition associated with a lower incidence of IVH is pregnancy-induced hypertension (PIH). Thus, a lower incidence of severe PV-IVH in infants born to mothers with PIH (8.2%) than to those without PIH (14%), with an odds ratio (OR) estimate of 0.43 (95% confidence interval [CI] 0.30-0.61) was noted in one report,[51] a finding consistent with other reports.[52,53] The mechanisms through which the chance of IVH may be reduced by the presence of PIH are not clear, but accelerated brain maturation in such infants, or the use of medications, specifically magnesium sulfate, to treat the mother are possible.[53-55] Later retrospective data suggest that magnesium sulfate is not associated with a reduction in PV-IVH.[56-58] Moreover, tocolytic agents in general, including magnesium sulfate, are associated with an increased risk for IVH.[59-61] However, a large prospective randomized controlled trial of magnesium sulfate administered to mothers at 24 to 31 weeks of gestation demonstrated a reduced rate of cerebral palsy among infant survivors.[62] A meta-analysis of antenatal magnesium sulfate therapy given to women at risk for preterm birth concluded that it substantially reduced the risk of cerebral palsy in the child (relative risk [RR] 0.68; 95% CI 0.54 to 0.87; in five trials involving 6145 infants). The number of women needed to be treated to benefit one baby by avoiding cerebral palsy is 63 (95% CI 43 to 87).[63]

Route of Delivery

There are conflicting data regarding the route of delivery and subsequent IVH.[52,64-66] Interpretation of the data is difficult because most are retrospective. This problem does not exclude the possibility that under certain circumstances, intrapartum events may contribute to the pathogenesis of severe IVH. Thus, in some studies there is a higher risk for IVH with increasing duration of the active phase of labor, and a lower risk in infants delivered via cesarean section prior to the active phase of labor.[52,64] Many of these studies were analyzed prior to the more frequent use of antenatal glucocorticoids.[67] In a study in infants of birth weight less than 751 g whose mothers were given steroids, vaginal delivery was a predictor for severe IVH.[68] By contrast, in a retrospective cohort study of extremely low-birth-weight (LBW) infants (401-1000 g), the influence of labor on extremely LBW infants who were born by cesarean delivery was examined with reference to neonatal and neurodevelopmental outcomes. The analysis revealed that labor does not appear to play a significant role in the genesis of IVH.[69] Similarly, in a later retrospective analysis, severe IVH was not influenced by mode of delivery in vertex-presenting, singleton, very LBW infants after data were controlled for gestational age.[70]

Importantly, any analysis that evaluates the impact of labor or route of delivery must account for an important role of placental inflammation, and in particular fetal vasculitis, in the genesis of IVH, a role that may supersede the influence of the route of delivery.[71] Thus in one study, although vaginal delivery was associated with an increased risk of IVH by univariate analysis, the risks attributable to vaginal delivery were no longer increased when adjustments were made in multivariate analysis for fetal vasculitis and other potential confounding factors.[71] This issue clearly warrants further prospective study and analysis.

Postnatal Strategies

Any approach to intervention should at the least consider the following: (1) the target population should be those infants in whom severe IVH is most likely to develop, that is, with birth weights less than 1000 g³; and (2) the condition of the infant at delivery, which appears to be an important mediator of subsequent IVH (Box 3-1). The latter appears to be strongly influenced in part by perinatal events and in particular the administration of antenatal glucocorticoids[26] or the presence or absence of fetal vasculitis.[71] The type of glucocorticoid administered to the mother may also be important. Thus antenatal exposure to dexamethasone, but not betamethasone, was associated with an increased risk of IVH as well as white matter injury in premature infants.[72,73] However, a meta-analysis concluded that dexamethasone may have greater benefits than betamethasone, such as less IVH and possibly some improved biophysical parameters, although a higher rate of neonatal

---

Box 3-1   FACTORS ASSOCIATED WITH RISK FOR THE DEVELOPMENT OF SEVERE INTRAVENTRICULAR HEMORRHAGE

High Risk
Minimal intrapartum care
No glucocorticoid exposure
Chorioamnionitis/funisitis
Fetal distress
Lower gestational age
Lower birth weight
Respiratory distress syndrome
Respiratory morbidity (i.e., pneumothorax)
Fluctuations or rapid elevations in systemic blood pressure and/or cerebral blood flow
Hypotension
Sudden and repeated increases in venous pressure

Lower Risk
Antenatal glucocorticoids (short course)
Medical condition (e.g., pregnancy-induced hypertension)
Intrauterine growth restriction
Higher gestational age
Higher birth weight
Postnatal medications (e.g., indomethacin)

intensive care unit (NICU) admission was seen with dexamethasone administration in one study.[74]

Postnatal Factors Associated with an Increased Risk

Postnatal factors associated with a higher risk for IVH include decreasing gestational age, lower birth weight (<1000 g), male sex, intubation, and RDS (see Box 3-1).[2,75] By contrast, the risk for severe IVH in the nonintubated infant is low(<10%).[76] For infants with RDS, the risk for IVH is even greater with associated perturbations in arterial and venous pressures as well as with hypercarbia.[18,19,22-24] These vascular perturbations are in part related to the infant's breathing patterns, which are usually out of synchrony with the ventilator breath.[77] The perturbations can be minimized with careful ventilator management, including the use of synchronized mechanical ventilation, assist/control ventilation, sedation, or, in more difficult cases, paralysis.[2,78] Interestingly enough, although surfactant administration improved respiratory ventilation, the improvement was not accompanied by a significant reduction in the incidence of IVH.[79]

Postnatal Administration of Medications to Reduce Severe IVH

Medications administered postnatally to reduce or prevent IVH have included phenobarbital,[80-82] vitamin E,[83] ethamsylate,[84] and indomethacin.[34,85-87] Although there was initial enthusiasm for the use of each of these medications in the prevention of IVH, the effect has not been borne out over time. In one noteworthy study, infants who received phenobarbital exhibited a higher incidence of severe IVH than controls.[82] Currently, the early postnatal administration of indomethacin is believed to be of benefit in the prevention of severe hemorrhage.[34,86] Two studies demonstrated a significant reduction in the incidence of severe IVH in infants who received indomethacin in comparison with control infants. However, at long-term follow-up, the incidence of cerebral palsy was comparable in the two groups (see Table 3-1).[34,86] This observation, coupled with the known reduction in CBF that accompanies indomethacin administration, warrants cautious use of this agent.[87,88] Perhaps it should be reserved for those infants at greatest risk—those delivered precipitously without the benefit of perinatal glucocorticoids (see Fig. 3-3).

White Matter Injury in the Absence of Hemorrhage

CASE HISTORY

BS was a 28-week AGA female infant born to a 42-year-old primigravida whose pregnancy was complicated by cervical shortening with funneling. The mother was started on bed rest, given a course of betamethasone, treated with antibiotics, and received magnesium sulfate. However after 3 days, fetal distress was noted and the infant was delivered vaginally. Resuscitation in the delivery room included brief bag-mask ventilation, and the infant was started on CPAP and assigned to the neonatal intensive care unit. The Apgar scores were 6 (1 minute) and 8 (5 minutes). The infant was rapidly weaned to room air while receiving CPAP. She was treated with antibiotics for 7 days, in part because of the perinatal history as well as abnormal blood count indices (initial immature-to-total neutrophil ratio 0.39, which normalized within 24 hours). The culture results remained negative. The clinical course was characterized by recurrent apnea and bradycardia, for which caffeine was administered. A cranial sonogram performed on DOL 5 revealed increased bilateral periventricular echodensities (Fig. 3-2A). Sonograms done on DOL 28 showed the evolution of bilateral diffuse cystic encephalomalacia (see Fig. 3-2B). An MRI performed at 36 weeks postconceptual age revealed extensive cystic PVL with mild diffuse parenchymal volume loss and diffuse thinning of the corpus callosum (see Fig. 3-2C). Placental pathology demonstrated an immature placenta with evidence of acute chorioamnionitis and funisitis.

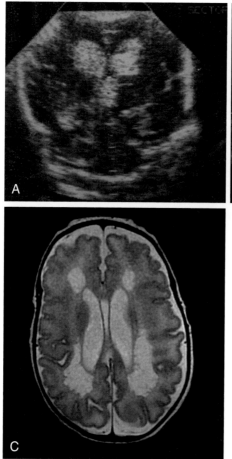

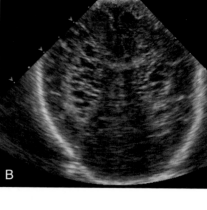

Figure 3-2 **A,** Coronal ultrasound scan from an infant in the first week showing increased periventricular echogenicity. **B,** Coronal scan from the same infant at 4 weeks showing bilateral cystic formation in the areas of prior hyperechogenicity. **C,** Magnetic resonance image (axial view) prior to discharge showing T2-hyperintense periventricular signal abnormality bilaterally that is consistent with cystic periventricular leukomalacia.

This case illustrates the more typical ultrasonographic expression of white matter injury in the premature infant, characterized by hyperechogenicity, followed by the evolution of cystic changes in the absence of overt postnatal provocative clinical factors.[2,10,89,90] Although cysts usually became apparent within the first 2 to 3 weeks of life, data have now shown the evolution of cysts beyond the first month in an increasing numbers of cases.[10,91] Moreover, progressive nonhemorrhagic dilation of the lateral ventricles, which in some cases is consistent with diffuse white matter injury, is also becoming more common. The extent of injury to white matter in the premature infant when evaluated by cranial ultrasonography ranges from 4% to 15%.[2,75,92,93] However, MRI indicates that white matter injury is more prevalent than is apparent from cranial ultrasonography.[7]

Periventricular Leukomalacia

Periventricular leukomalacia (PVL) refers to necrosis of white matter adjacent to the external angles of the lateral ventricles, and it has long been regarded as the principal ischemic lesion of the premature infant.[2] However, later evidence suggests that the evolution of injury is much more complex (see later discussion). The pathologic features of PVL include focal as well as more diffuse cerebral white matter involvement.[89,94-96] The focal periventricular necrosis is distributed commonly at the level of the occipital radiation at the trigone of the lateral ventricles and at the level of the cerebral white matter around the foramen of Monro.[2] The typical histologic changes are characterized by coagulation necrosis, microglial infiltration, astrocytic proliferation, and eventual cyst formation. These cavities usually diminish in size over time secondary to gliosis (see Fig. 3-2). The diffuse cerebral white matter necrosis less frequently undergoes cystic change, and ventricular dilation is also more prominent. PVL is more commonly noted in the smaller premature infant requiring prolonged ventilator support (see earlier discussion).[93]

Pathogenesis

Experimental and clinical observations suggest two basic pathogenetic mechanisms, vascular factors and the intrinsic vulnerability of the differentiating oligodendrocyte.[96-98]

Vascular Factors

Several features peculiar to the premature infant are important in the vascular mechanism of PVL. The first relates to the vascular development and supply. Specifically, the penetrating branches of the anterior, middle, and posterior cerebral arteries end in border zones, which are most vulnerable to decreases in CBF. It is within these border zones that the focal necrosis of PVL (as described previously) typically occurs.[98,99] Furthermore, the penetrating cerebral vessels, which include long branches that terminate in the deep periventricular white matter and short branches that terminate in the subcortical white matter, vary as a function of gestational age.[100] Thus, early on, at approximately 24 to 30 weeks of gestation, the long penetrators have few side branches and limited intraparenchymal anastomosis with the short branches, resulting in border zones in white matter beyond the periventricular region. This feature may account for the more diffuse lesion noted in the smaller premature infant.[90] From 32 weeks on, there is a marked increase in vascular supply as a result of increase in vessel length and anastomoses. It is this vascular maturation that likely accounts for the uncommon presentation of this lesion in the larger infant. A second feature relates to the limited vasodilatory response of the blood vessels supplying the white matter to increases in $PaCO_2$ in comparison with the vasodilatory responses of the blood vessels supplying other regions of brain, such as medulla and gray matter,[101] as well as a persistent decrease in CBF to white matter during the phase of reperfusion following ischemia, despite recovery in all other brain areas.[102] Finally, impairment of CBF autoregulation, as may occur in the sick premature infant (see earlier discussion), increases the risk for ischemia to the border-zone regions of white matter during episodes of systemic hypotension.[14,95,103] Clinically, loss of CBF autoregulation and/or decreases in CBF may occur in the sick infant secondary to events such as hypotension, acidosis, septic shock, hypocarbia, PDA, recurrent apnea, and bradycardia and may in part explain the association of such events with PVL.[22,104-112]

Intrinsic Vulnerability of the Differentiating Oligodendrocyte

It has been established that the early differentiating oligodendrocyte is most vulnerable to injury secondary to release of numerous factors, including free radicals, excitotoxins, and cytokines, as well as a lack of growth factors. The mechanism of cell death due to these factors appears to be mediated via apoptosis.[113] Moreover, studies in newborn animal models subjected to hypoxia-ischemia and/or infection have demonstrated apoptotic cell death in immature cerebral white matter.[114,115] In a neuropathologic study, apoptotic cell death was observed significantly more often in infants dying of white matter injury than in infants without white matter injury.[116] In the diffuse white matter injury, a marked prominence of activated microglia, identified by a specific immunocytochemical marker, and astrocytosis have been observed. The presence of the activated microglia raises the possibility of a role for these cells in the causation of the diffuse injury to the preoligodendrocytes (see later discussion).[117]

Free Radical Injury

The prominence of activated microglia in the diffuse component of PVL suggests that these cells may be involved in the generation of reactive oxygen species (ROS) and reactive nitrogen species (RNS) found in the human lesion. Microglia have been shown to be activated by ischemia and to remain activated for weeks following the insult. When activated microglia have been shown to release ROS and RNS, which then cause cell death. Experimental studies have demonstrated vulnerability of the early differentiating preoligodendrocyte to injury by free radicals, such as hydrogen peroxide and hydroxyl radical.[117-119] This maturation-dependent vulnerability of preoligodendrocytes to ROS and RNS appears to be related to such factors as deficient antioxidant defenses and acquisition of iron for differentiation. Indeed, specific markers have identified evidence in preoligodendrocytes for lipid peroxidation and protein nitration in diffuse white matter injury. The role of free radical–induced damage in triggering the death of the early differentiating oligodendrocyte is supported by the cryoprotection provided by free radical scavengers, such as superoxide dismutase, deferoxamine, and vitamin E.[2,117] In an extension of these observations, it was shown that hyperoxia triggers maturation-dependent apoptosis in preoligodendrocytes when cultured cells were exposed to 80% oxygen for varying times up to 24 hours.[120] Accumulation of superoxide and generation of ROS were detected after 2 hours of oxygen exposure. Cell death was mediated by a caspase-dependent apoptotic pathway and could be blocked by a specific pan-caspase inhibitor zVAD-fmk. Rats studied on postnatal day 3 (P3) and P6 showed bilateral reduction in myelin basic protein expression with 24 hours of exposure to 80% oxygen, an effect not noted when they were studied on P10. Hyperoxia caused oxidative stress and triggered maturation-dependent apoptosis in preoligodendrocytes, which involved the generation of ROS and caspase activation, and led to white matter injury in the neonatal rat brain.[120] This effect could be blocked by estradiol, which produced significant dose-dependent protection by preventing hyperoxia-induced proapoptotic Fas upregulation and caspase-3 activation.[121]

Excitotoxic Injury (Glutamate)

Glutamate can lead to the death of oligodendroglial precursors via both receptor and nonreceptor mechanisms . The nonreceptor mechanism involves intracellular entry of glutamate in exchange for cystine via activation of a glutamine-cystine exchange transporter, resulting in a decrease in intracellular cystine and thereby glutathione synthesis.[117] The result is glutathione depletion and free radical–mediated cell death. The latter can be totally prevented by the addition of free radical scavengers such as vitamin E.[117] The receptor-mediated injury appears to be mediated via activation of AMPA (2-amino-3-[5-methyl-3-oxo-1,2- oxazol-4-yl]propanoic acid)/kainate–type glutamate receptors. Data now suggest that this form of cell death occurs only in developing and not mature oligodendroglia.[122] It has also been shown, in an immature animal model of diffuse white matter injury, that non–N-methyl-D-aspartate (NMDA) receptors are present on preoligodendrocytes that cause free radical–mediated death of these cells when activated in vitro, and that in vivo cause death of preoligodendrocytes when activated by hypoxia-ischemia.[123] The relevance of this mechanism to hypoxia-ischemia–induced white matter injury has been demonstrated in an immature rat model, in which such injury is prevented by the systemic administration of the non–NMDA receptor antagonist 6-nitro-7-sulfamoylbenzo[f] quinoxaline-2,3-dione (NBQX) following termination of the insult.[124]

Cytokines

Cytokines appear to participate in an important mechanism for preoligodendroglial cell death. That a paradigm of ischemia/reperfusion is accompanied by a rapid activation of microglia, secretion of cytokines, and migration of inflammatory cells has been well established in animals.[125] Moreover, cytokines and inflammatory cells are also consistent features of the response to infection. Within the central nervous system, microglia release tumor necrosis factor α (TNFα), interleukin-1 (IL-I), and IL-6. Cell culture studies suggest that TNFα is toxic to oligodendroglia.[126] Fairly new evidence suggests that interferon-γ is also toxic to oligodendroglia, an effect that is potentiated by TNFα.[127] However, numerous additional cytokines, microglia, or white blood cells may be involved in this process.[128] Indeed, in one study, increased levels of circulating proinflammatory cytokines during the first 72 hours of life were associated with arterial hypotension and with the development of brain damage as detected by ultrasonography.[129] Increases in IL-6, IL-8, and IL-10 were associated with arterial hypotension, and increases in IL-6 and IL-8 with severe IVH. Prolonged rupture of membranes was associated with increased postnatal levels of interferon-γ, which in turn were associated with white matter injury.[129] The potential deleterious effects of cytokines may be mediated via other mechanisms, including increased permeability of the blood-brain barrier,[130] vascular endothelial damage,[131] and decreased CBF to white matter after endotoxin exposure.[132]

Maternal Fetal Infection and/or Inflammation and White Matter Injury

There are both experimental data and clinical evidence demonstrating an association between maternal infection/inflammation of the chorion and amnion ± fetal vascular involvement (i.e., funisitis) and white matter injury. Thus, intraperitoneal injection of lipopolysaccharides into kittens and exposing pregnant rabbits to intrauterine infection induce white matter injury similar to that observed in humans.[114,133] Several clinical studies have demonstrated an association between chorioamnionitis and PVL.[104,134] As in IVH, this association appears to be accentuated in the presence of funisitis.[135] The link between chorioamnionitis may be mediated via cytokines. Thus high levels of cytokines (IL-6 and IL-1β) have been found in the amniotic fluid,[136-138] of IL-6 in cord blood,[139] and of IL-1, IL-6, and interferon in neonatal blood of preterm infants in whom PVL or cerebral palsy develops.[129,140-142] Microglial expression of TNF-α and IL-6 immunoreactivity is found twice as commonly in the white matter of infants with PVL as in infants without injury to the region.[143,144] Additionally, in one series, TNFα expression was significantly higher in the plasma ($P < 0.001$) and supernatants of lipopolysaccharide-stimulated peripheral blood mononuclear cells ($P < 0.003$) in a group with PVL-associated cerebral palsy than in a control group.[145]

In contrast to these potential deleterious effects, focal cerebral ischemia was found to be exacerbated in a mouse model of hypoxia-ischemia lacking TNFα.[146] Injury-induced microglial activation was suppressed in the TNFα-knockout mice. These latter observations point to the complex interrelationships between cytokines and white matter injury.

Clinical Factors Associated with PVL

Perinatal events associated with postnatal cystic PVL and/or progressive white matter injury include a history of chorioamnionitis (see earlier discussion), prolonged rupture of membranes, peripartum hemorrhage, severe fetal acidemia, hypovolemia, sepsis, hypocarbia, symptomatic PDA, postnatal infection/sepsis, and recurrent apnea and bradycardia.[22,104-112,134,147] A common feature of many of these conditions is a reduction in systemic blood pressure. Indeed, in one study, chorioamnionitis was associated with increased IL-6 and IL-1β concentrations in cord blood, elevated newborn heart rate, and decreased mean and diastolic blood pressures, and the cord blood IL-6 concentration correlated inversely with newborn systolic, mean, and diastolic blood pressures.[25] By contrast, in a study of 14 infants in whom PVL developed, only 4 (30%) had overt evidence of postnatal systemic hypotension, and asphyxia was an uncommon finding.[104] Other studies have also been unable to demonstrate a consistent association between hypotension and PVL.[148-150]

Prevention

From the preceding discussion, it is likely that prevention of PVL will be difficult. First, it is relatively uncommon; second, as noted previously, the pathogenesis of PVL is complex (Fig. 3-3); and third, the presentation is often subtle and detected only with neuroimaging. Although there is evidence pointing to an association between perinatal infection (chorioamnionitis) and PVL,[2,104,134] the precise mechanisms linking the two remain unclear; the positive predictive value of a history of chorioamnionitis and subsequent PVL is low, approximating 10%, and many cases of infection are asymptomatic with the diagnosis established only on histologic examination of the placenta.[3,71] More specific potential strategies are as follows: (1) the appropriate treatment of infants with low blood pressure for a given gestational

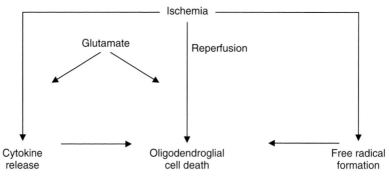

Figure 3-3   Potential pathways leading to white matter injury.

age (see Chapter 2) with volume replacement therapy or inotropic support as clinically indicated; and (2) the careful ventilatory management of infants with respiratory distress so as to avoid hypocarbia. However, it is important to note that the mechanisms of white matter injury with hypocarbia also remain unclear. Thus ventilation-induced hypocarbia is often associated with higher mean airway pressures. Rises in mean airway pressure are associated with impairment of venous return, a fall in cardiac output, as well as increases in sagittal sinus pressure.[24,151] The increase in venous coupled with a concomitant decrease in CBF, as may occur with hypocarbia, would be expected to reduce cerebral perfusion pressure, including flow to white matter. The use of antioxidant therapy to counter the free radical injury demonstrated in the experimental model is another therapeutic possibility. However, antioxidant therapy has not been uniformly successful in the treatment of other neonatal conditions presumed to be related in part to free radical injury.[152]

Outcome

Intraventricular Hemorrhage

The infant with severe IVH is at highest risk for adverse neurodevelopmental outcome (both motor and cognitive) (see Chapter 13). This risk is related in part to the extent of the white matter involvement noted on cranial ultrasonography. Thus, with a large IPE (>1 cm in diameter) (see Fig. 3-1B) the outcome is invariably poor, with major motor and cognitive defects consistently noted at follow-up.[2,12,153] With smaller lesions (<1 cm in diameter), the outcome is less precise, and a small percentage of patients (approximately 20%) may even have a normal outcome.[12]

However, as noted previously, the issue is much more complicated, and even infants with normal ultrasonography findings as well as those with lesser grades of hemorrhage are at risk for motor and cognitive deficits. Thus in the first of these studies with normal cranial sonogram findings, major neurologic disability was noted in 5% to 10% of infants, and a mental developmental index (MDI) less than 70 in 25% of cases.[5] In the second study of infants with lesser grades of hemorrhage (grades 1 and 2 IVH), major neurologic disabilities were noted in 13%, and a MDI less than 70 in 45% of cases.[6] Moreover, the comparable neurodevelopmental outcomes for infants with and without IVH in the indomethacin study (see Box 3-1) clearly indicates that the genesis of brain injury in the sick premature infant is much more complex than can be deduced from the neonatal neurologic ultrasonographic appearance (see Chapter 15).

PVL

Although the ultrasonographic diagnosis of cystic PVL affects only a small percentage of preterm infants (approximately 3%), MRI performed at term shows that diffuse noncystic injury to white matter is much more common. This finding poses a significant burden, in that the majority of affected infants has major long-term neurodevelopmental problems.[104,154-157] The most commonly described long-term motor sequela of PVL is spastic diplegia.[2] Later reports, however, describe a more severe deficit with involvement of all four extremities as well as visual and cognitive deficits.[158-162] This more severe outcome is consistent with the diffuse white matter injury noted on neuropathology in preterm infants who die with PVL as well as on MRI.[90,155] The genesis of the cognitive deficits in infants with PVL remains unclear. It has been speculated that the injury may secondarily affect neuronal cortical organization as a result of injury to subplate neurons or late migrating astrocytes.[2,163] Later data indicate substantial diffuse white matter injury identified by MRI including volumetric imaging coupled with reduced gray matter volumes in very LBW infants imaged at term.[164] The latter findings may explain the substantial cognitive deficits noted at follow-up. A similar observation has been made in adults with severe cognitive injury.[165]

Gaps in Knowledge

1. The mechanisms contributing to the motor deficits in up to 10% to 15% of infants and to the cognitive deficits in up to one third of infants with normal sonogram findings and/or lesser grades of IVH remain unclear but critical to delineate.[5,6] Also, although prophylactic administration of indomethacin has been shown to result in a reduction in incidence of severe hemorrhage, it remains unclear why the incidence of cerebral palsy at 18 months in treated infants was comparable to that observed in control infants.[34] Furthermore, incidences of moderate to severe cognitive deficits were comparable in the two groups and were substantially higher than incidences of motor deficits.

2. Does delayed cord clamping (30-45 seconds vs. 10-15 seconds) confer neuroprotection? In a randomized study of 72 mother/infant pairs of relatively later gestational age (around 28 weeks), IVH developed in 2 of 23 male infants in the delayed group, compared with 8 of 19 in the early group. Will these observations hold true in premature infants of lesser gestational age? In addition, why is it only the male infant who appears to be protected?[166]

3. Can low cord blood levels of the chemokine be used as a marker to predict IVH? In a series of 163 infants, low cord blood level of chemokine ligand 18 (CCL18) was an independent risk factor for IVH.[167]

4. The genesis of cognitive deficits remains unclear but critical to elucidate. Approximately 25,000 infants are born weighing less than 1000 g in the United States annually. If one assumes a 30% occurrence of moderate to severe deficits, then approximately 8000 very LBW infants will progress to have moderate to severe mental retardation each year. Factors predisposing to such deficits include additional vulnerable regions (basal ganglia, hippocampus, subplate neurons, and cortical gray matter),[168] medical complications of prematurity, such as chronic lung disease, necrotizing enterocolitis, nosocomial infections, hypoglycemia, and hyperbilirubinemia, as well as medications used to treat the infants, including glucocorticoids and xanthine derivatives.[168] The impact of the stressful environment of the neonatal intensive care unit on the developing brain and in particular the hippocampus is likely to be considerable (see Chapter 13). In addition, the influence of the post-discharge environment likely also plays a critical role.

5. Severe IVH is much more common in infants without perinatal glucocorticoid exposure, identifying them as a target group for future interventions. Indomethacin remains the best intervention to use in this high-risk target population.

6. Is there a role for erythropoietin as a potential neuroprotectant? In one report of extremely premature infants given erythropoietin to stimulate erythropoiesis, those who had received erythropoietin scored significantly better

than untreated children (i.e., 55% vs. 39% normally developed) at long-term follow-up ranging from 10 to 13 years ($P < 0.05$). Interestingly, these changes were ascribable to the associated IVH only.[169] However, these findings have not been consistent.[170]

7. Although an association between placental inflammation and white matter injury has been demonstrated, it still remains unclear why the majority of infants born under such circumstances do not demonstrate overt white matter injury.

8. Although many inherent factors increase the vulnerability of the white matter to reductions in blood pressure and, as a secondary consequence, a reduction in CBF, we do not know why the majority of infants with cystic leukomalacia do not demonstrate overt evidence of postnatal hypotension. One could argue that the period of vulnerability occurs during the labor process. However, the increasing observation of late development of cystic PVL and the identification of many cases of noncystic PVL upon routine MRI points to a critical role for postnatal influences—free radicals, excitotoxic injury, as well as cytokines—in the genesis of preoligodendrocyte injury.

Conclusions

PV-IVH and adjacent white matter injury remain a significant problem in the premature infant. The potential mechanisms contributing to injury are complex and involve factors related to blood flow and its regulation as well as cellular mediators, including cytokines, free radical formation, and excitotoxic release. Although a reduction in the occurrence of severe IVH can be achieved with indomethacin, the reduction has not translated into long-term neurodevelopmental benefit. This fact reinforces the concept of a more diffuse insidious injury to brain in sick premature infants, a concept reinforced by MRI changes identified at follow-up.

References

1. Shalak L, Perlman JM. Hemorrhagic-ischemic cerebral injury in the preterm infant: Current Concepts. *Clin Perinatol.* 2002;29:745-763.
2. Volpe JJ. *Neurology of the Newborn.* 4th ed. Philadelphia: WB Saunders Co; 2008.
3. Stoll BJ, Hansen NE, Bell EF, et al. Neonatal outcomes of extremely premature infants from the NICHD neonatal research network. *Pediatrics.* 2010;126:443-456.
4. Philips AGS, Allen WC, Tito AM, et al. Intraventricular hemorrhage in preterm infants: declining incidence in the 1980's. *Pediatrics.* 1989;84:797-800.
5. Laptook AR, O'Shea TM, Shankaran S, Bhaskar B. Adverse neurodevelopmental outcomes among extremely low birth weight infants with a normal head ultrasound: prevalence and antecedents. *Pediatrics.* 2005;115:673-680.
6. Patra K, Wilson-Costello D, Taylor HG. Grades I-II intraventricular hemorrhage in extremely low birth weight infants: effects on neurodevelopment. *J Pediatrics.* 2006;149:169-173.
7. Inder TE, Anderson NJ, Spencer C, et al. White matter injury in the premature infant: a comparison between serial cranial sonographic and MR findings at term. *Am J Neuroradiol.* 2003;24:805-809.
8. Dyet LE, Kennea N, Counsell SJ. Natural history of brain lesions in extremely preterm infants studied with serial magnetic resonance imaging from birth and neurodevelopmental assessment. *Pediatrics.* 2006;118:536-548.
9. Hambleton G, Wigglesworth JS. Origin of intraventricular hemorrhage in the preterm infant. *Arch Dis Child.* 1976;57:651-655.
10. Perlman JM, Rollins N. Surveillance protocol for the detection of intracranial abnormalities in premature neonates. *Arch Pediatr Adolesc Med.* 2000;154:822-826.
11. Gould SJ, Howard S, Hope PL, Reynold EO. Periventricular intraparenchymal cerebral hemorrhage in preterm infants: the role of venous infarction. *J Pathol.* 1987;151:197-202.
12. Guzzetta F, Schackelford GD, Volpe S, et al. Periventricular intraparenchymal echodensities in the premature newborn: critical determinant of neurologic outcome. *Pediatrics.* 1986;78:945-1006.
13. Lou CH, Lassen NA, Friis-Hansen B. Impaired autoregulation of cerebral blood flow in the distressed newborn infant. *J Pediatr.* 1979;94:118-125.
14. Pryds O, Griesen G, Lou H, et al. Heterogeneity of cerebral vasoreactivity in preterm infants supported by mechanical ventilation. *J Pediatr.* 1989;115:638-645.
15. Tsuji M, Saul JP, du Plessis A, et al. Cerebral intravascular oxygenation correlates with mean arterial pressure in critically ill premature infants. *Pediatrics.* 2000;106:625-632.

16. Goddard-Finegold J, Armstrong D, Zeller RS. Intraventricular hemorrhage following volume expansion after hypovolemic hypotension in the newborn beagle. *J Pediatr.* 1982;100:796-799.
17. Ment LR, Stewart WB, Duncan CC, et al. Beagle puppy model of intraventricular hemorrhage. *J Neurosurg.* 1982;57:219-223.
18. Goldberg RN, Chung D, Goldman SL, et al. The associations of rapid volume expansion and intraventricular hemorrhage in the preterm infant. *J Pediatr.* 1980;96:1060-1063.
19. Hill A, Perlman JM, Volpe JJ. Relationship of pneumothorax to the occurrence of intraventricular hemorrhage in the premature newborn. *Pediatrics.* 1982;69:144-149.
20. Perlman JM, McMenamin JB, Volpe JJ. Fluctuating cerebral blood flow velocity in respiratory distress syndrome. Relation to the development of intraventricular hemorrhage. *N Engl J Med.* 1983;309:204-209.
21. Bada HS, Korones SB, Perry EH, et al. Mean arterial blood pressure changes in premature infants and those at risk for intraventricular hemorrhage. *J Pediatr.* 1990;117:607-614.
22. Kaiser JR, Gauss CH, Poot MM, Williams DK. Hypercapnia in the first 3 days of life is associated with severe intraventricular hemorrhage in very low birth weight infants *J Perinatol.* 2006;26:279-285.
23. Fabres J, Carlo WA, Philips V, Howard G, Ambalavan N. Both extremes of arterial carbon dioxide pressure and the magnitude of fluctuation in arterial carbon dioxide pressure are associated with severe intraventricular hemorrhage in very low birth weight infant. *Pediatrics.* 2007;119:299-305.
24. Perlman JM, Volpe JJ. Are venous circulatory changes important in the pathogenesis of hemorrhagic and/or ischemic cerebral injury? *Pediatrics.* 1987;80:705-711.
25. Yanowitz TD, Potter DM, Bowen A, et al. Variability in cerebral oxygen delivery is reduced in premature neonates exposed to chorioamnionitis. *Pediatr Res.* 2006;59:299-304.
26. Roberts D, Dalziel S. Antenatal corticosteroids for accelerating fetal lung maturation for women at risk of preterm birth. *Cochrane Database Syst Rev.* 2006;(3):CD004454.
27. Salhab W, Hyman L, Perlman JM. Partial or complete antenatal steroids treatment and neonatal outcome in extremely low birth weight infants less than or equal to 1000 grams: is there a dose dependent effect? *J Perinatol.* 2004;23:668-672.
28. Furukawa S, Sameshima H, Ikenoue T. Circulatory disturbances during the first postnatal 24 hours in extremely premature infants 25 weeks or less of gestation with histological fetal inflammation. *J Obstet Gynecol Res.* 2008;34:27-33.
29. Takashima S, Tanaka K. Microangiography and fibrinolytic activity in the matrix of the premature brain. *Brain Dev.* 1972;4:222-228.
30. Georgiadis P XH, Chua C, Hu F, et al. Characterization of acute brain injuries and neurobehavioral profiles in a rabbit model of germinal matrix hemorrhage. *Stroke.* 2008;39: 3378-3388.
31. Perlman JM, Risser R. Relationship of uric acid concentrations and severe intraventricular hemorrhage/leukomalacia in the premature infant. *J Pediatr.* 1998;132:436-439.
32. Russell GAB, Jeffers G, Cook RWI. Plasma hypoxanthine: a marker for hypoxic-ischemic induced periventricular leukomalacia? *Arch Dis Child.* 1992;67:388-392.
33. Allen WC, Vohr B, Makuch RW. Antecedents of cerebral palsy in a multicenter trial of indomethacin for intraventricular hemorrhage. *Arch Pediatr Adolesc Med.* 1997;151:581-585.
34. Schmidt B, Davis P, Moddemann D, et al. Trial of indomethacin prophylaxis in preterms investigators: Long-term effects of indomethacin prophylaxis in extremely-low-birth-weight infants. *N Engl J Med.* 2001;344:1966-1972.
35. Perlman JM, Volpe JJ. Intraventricular hemorrhage in the extremely small premature infant. *Am J Dis Child.* 1986;140:1122-1124.
36. Kazzi N, Llagan NB, Liang KC, et al. Maternal administration of vitamin K does not improve the coagulation profile of preterm infants. *Pediatrics.* 1989;84:1045-1050.
37. Pomerance JJ, Teal JG, Gogolok JF, et al. Maternally administered antenatal vitamin K: effect on neonatal prothrombin activity, partial prothrombin time and intraventricular hemorrhage. *Obstet Gynecol.* 1987;70:235-241.
38. Shankaran S, Papile LA, Wright LL, et al. The effect of antenatal phenobarbital therapy on neonatal intracranial hemorrhage in preterm infants. *N Engl J Med.* 1997;337:466-471.
39. Di Renzo G, Mignosa M, Gerli S,et al. The combined maternal administration of magnesium sulfate and aminophylline reduces intraventricular hemorrhage in very preterm neonates. *Am J Obstet Gynecol.* 2005;192:433-438.
40. Crowley P, Chalmers I, Keirse MJ. The effects of corticosteroid administration before preterm delivery: an overview of the evidence from clinical trials. *Br J Obstet Gynecol.* 1990;97:11-25.
41. Garite TJ, Rumney PJ, Briggs GC, et al. A randomized placebo controlled trial of betamethasone for the prevention of respiratory distress syndrome at 24-28 weeks gestation. *Am J Obstet Gynecol.* 1992;166:646-651.
42. Jobe AH, Mitchell BR, Gunkel JH. Beneficial effects of combined use of prenatal steroids and postnatal surfactant on preterm infants. *Am J Obstet Gynecol.* 1993;168:508-513.
43. Kari MA, Hallman M, Gronen M, et al. Prenatal dexamethasone treatment in conjunction with rescue therapy of human surfactant: a randomized placebo-controlled multicenter study. *Pediatrics.* 1994;93:730-736.
44. Leviton A, Dammann O, Allred EN, et al. Antenatal corticosteroids and cranial ultrasonographic abnormalities. *Am J Obstet Gynecol.* 1999;181:1007-1017.
45. Maher JE, Cliver SP, Goldenberg RL, et al. March of Dimes Multicenter Study Group: the effect of glucocorticoid therapy in the very premature infant. *Am J Obstet Gynecol.* 1994;170:869-873.

46. Wright LL, Homar JD, Gunkel H. Evidence from multicenter networks on the current use and effectiveness of antenatal corticosteroids in low birthweight infants. *Am J Obstet Gynecol*. 1995;173:263-269.
47. Demarini S, Dollberg S, Hoath SB, et al. Effects of antenatal corticosteroids on blood pressure in very low birth weight infants during the first 24 hours of life. *Journal of Perinatology*. 1999;19:419-425.
48. Garland JS, Buck R, Leviton A. Effect of maternal glucocorticoid exposure on risk of severe intraventricular hemorrhage in surfactant-treated preterm infants. *J Pediatr*. 1995;126:272-279.
49. Wapner RJ, Sorokin Y, Mele L, et al. Long-term outcomes after repeat doses of antenatal corticosteroids. *N Engl J Med*. 2007;357:1190-1198.
50. Murphy KE, Hannah ME, Willan AR, et al. Multiple courses of antenatal corticosteroids for preterm birth (MACS): a randomised controlled trial. *Lancet*. 2008;372:2143-2151.
51. Perlman JM, Risser RC, Gee JB. Pregnancy induced hypertension and reduced intraventricular hemorrhage in preterm infants. *Pediatr Neurol*. 1997;17:29-33.
52. Kuban KCK, Leviton A, Pagano M, et al. Maternal toxemia is associated with a reduced incidence of germinal matrix hemorrhage in premature babies. *J Child Neurol*. 1992;7:70-76.
53. Leviton A, Pagano M, Kuban KCK, et al. The epidemiology of germinal matrix hemorrhage during the first half-day of life. *Dev Med Child Neurol*. 1988;33:138-145.
54. Gould JB, Gluck L, Kulovich MV. The relationship between accelerated pulmonary maturity and accelerated neurologic maturity in certain chronically stressed pregnancies. *Am J Obstet Gynecol*. 1997;127:181-186.
55. Hadi HA. Fetal cerebral maturation in hypertension disorder in pregnancy. *Obstet Gynecol*. 1984;63:214-219.
56. Nelson KB, Grether JK. Can magnesium sulfate reduce the risk of cerebral palsy in very low birth-weight infants? *Pediatrics*. 1995;95:263-269.
57. Leviton A, Paneth N, Susser MW, et al. Magnesium receipt does not appear to reduce the risk of neonatal white matter damage. *Pediatrics*. 1997;99:4.E2.
58. Paneth N, Jettan J, Pinto-Martron J, et al. Magnesium sulfate and risk of neonatal brain lesions and cerebral palsy in low birthweight infants. *Pediatrics*. 1997;99:5.1-5.7.
59. Canterino JC, Verma UL, Visintainer PF, et al. Maternal magnesium sulfate and the development of neonatal periventricular leucomalacia and intraventricular hemorrhage. *Obstet Gynecol*. 1999;93:396-402.
60. Atkinson MW, Goldenberg RL, Gaudier FL, et al. Maternal corticosteroid and tocolytic treatment and morbidity and mortality in very low birthweight infants. *Am J Obstet Gynecol*. 1995;173:299-304.
61. Groome LJ, Goldenberg RL, Cliver SP, et al. March of Dimes Multicenter Study Group: neonatal periventricular-intraventricular hemorrhage after maternal β-sympathomimetic tocolysis. *Am J Obstet Gynecol*. 1992;167:873-879.
62. Rouse DJ, Hirtz DJ, Thom E, et al. A randomized, controlled trial of magnesium sulfate for the prevention of cerebral palsy. *N Engl J Med*. 2008;359;895-905.
63. Doyle LW, Crowther CA, Middleton P, et al. Magnesium sulphate for women at risk of preterm birth for neuroprotection of the fetus. *Cochrane Database Syst Rev*. 2007;(3):CD004661.
64. Anderson GD, Bada HS, Shaver BM, et al. The effect of Cesarean section on intraventricular hemorrhage in the premature infant. *Am J Obstet Gynecol*. 1992;166:1091-1101.
65. Low JA, Galbraith RS, Sauerbrei EE, et al. Maternal fetal and newborn complications associated with newborn intracranial hemorrhage. *Am J Obstet Gynecol*. 1986;154:345-352.
66. Strauss A, Kirz D, Mandalou HD, et al. Perinatal events and intraventricular/ependymal hemorrhage in the very low birthweight infant. *Am J Obstet Gynecol*. 1985;151:1022-1027.
67. Ment LR, Oh W, Ehrenkrantz R, et al. Antenatal steroids, delivery mode and intraventricular hemorrhage in preterm infants. *Am J Obstet Gynecol*. 1995;172:795-800.
68. Deulofeut R, Sola A, Lee B, et al. The impact of vaginal delivery in premature infants weighing less than 1,251 grams. *Obstet Gynecol*. 2005;105:525-531.
69. Wadhawan R, Vohr BR, Fanaroff AA, et al. Does labor influence neonatal and neurodevelopmental outcomes of extremely-low-birth-weight infants who are born by cesarean delivery? *Am J Obstet Gynecol*. 2003;189:501-506.
70. Riskin A, Riskin-Mashiah S, Bader D, et al. Delivery Mode and Severe Intraventricular Hemorrhage in Single, Very Low Birth Weight, Vertex Infants. *Obstet Gynecol*. 2008;112:21-28.
71. Hansen A, Leviton A. Labor and delivery characteristics and risks of cranial ultrasonographic abnormalities among very-low-birth-weight infants. The Developmental Epidemiology Network Investigators. *Am J Obstet & Gynecol*. 1999;181:997-1006.
72. Baud O, Foix-L'Helias L, Kaminski M, et al. Antenatal glucocorticoid treatment and cystic periventricular leukomalacia in very premature infants. *N Engl J Med*. 1999;341:1190-1196.
73. Lee BH, Stoll BJ, McDonald SA, et al. Adverse neonatal outcomes associated with antenatal dexamethasone versus antenatal betamethasone. *Pediatrics*. 2006. 117:1503-1510.
74. Brownfoot FC, Crowther CA, Middleton P. Different corticosteroids and regimens for accelerating fetal lung maturation for women at risk of preterm birth. *Cochrane Database System Rev*. 2008;(4):CD006764.
75. Perlman JM. White matter injury in the preterm infant: an important determinant of abnormal neurodevelopmental outcome. *Early Human Dev*. 1998;53:99-120.
76. Perlman JM. Intraventricular hemorrhage. *Pediatrics*. 1989;84;913-914.
77. Perlman JM, Thach BT. Respiratory origin of fluctuations in arterial blood pressure in premature infants with respiratory distress syndrome. *Pediatrics*. 1988;81:399-403.

78. Perlman JM, Goodman S, Kreusser KL, et al. Reduction of intraventricular hemorrhage by elimination of fluctuating cerebral blood flow velocity in preterm infants with respiratory distress syndrome. N Engl J Med. 1985;312:1253-1257.

79. Jobe AH. Pulmonary surfactant therapy. N Engl J Med. 1993;328:861-868.

80. Bedard MP, Shankaran S, Slovis TL, et al. Effect of prophylactic phenobarbital on intraventricular hemorrhage in high risk infants. Pediatrics. 1984;73:435-439.

81. Donn S, Roloff DW, Goldstein GW. Prevention of intraventricular hemorrhage in preterm infants by phenobarbitone: a controlled trial. Lancet. 1981;ii(8240):215-217.

82. Kuban KC, Leviton A, Krishnamoorthy KS, et al. Neonatal intracranial hemorrhage and phenobarbital. Pediatrics. 1986;77:443-450.

83. Sinha S, Davis J, Tonger N, et al. Vitamin E supplementation reduces frequency of periventricular hemorrhage in very preterm infants. Lancet. 1987;1(8531):466-471.

84. Morgan ME, Benson JT, Cooke RW. Ethamsylate reduces the incidence of periventricular haemorrhage in very low birthweight babies. Lancet. 1981;2(8251):830-831.

85. Bada HS, Green RS, Pourcyrous M, et al. Indomethacin reduces the risk of severe intraventricular hemorrhage. J Pediatr. 1990;115:631-637.

86. Ment LR, Oh W, Ehrenkranz RA, et al. Low-dose indomethacin and prevention of intraventricular hemorrhage: A multicenter randomized trial. Pediatrics. 1994;94:543-550.

87. Edwards AD, Wyatt JS, Richardson C, et al. Effects of indomethacin on cerebral hemodynamics in very preterm infants. Lancet. 1990;335:491-495.

88. Pryds O, Griesen G, Johansen KH. Indomethacin and cerebral blood flow in preterm infants treated for patent ductus arteriosus. J Pediatrics. 1988;147:315-316.

89. De Vries L, Wiggelsworth JS, Regev R, Dubowitz LM. Evaluation of periventricular leukomalacia during the neonatal period and infancy: correlation of imaging and postmortem findings. Early Hum Dev. 1988;17:205-219.

90. Paneth N, Rudelli R, Monte W, et al. White matter necrosis in the very low birth weight infants: neuropathologic and ultrasonographic findings in infants surviving six days or longer. J Pediatr. 1990;116:975-984.

91. De Vries LS, Regev R, Dubowitz LMS. Late onset cystic leukomalacia. Arch Dis Child. 1986; 61-298-299.

92. De Vries LS, Regev R, Dubowitz LMS, et al. Perinatal risk factors for the development of extensive cystic leukomalacia. Am J Dis Child. 1988;142:732-735.

93. Leviton A, Paneth N. White matter damage in preterm newborns— an epidemiologic perspective. Early Hum Dev. 1990;24:1-22.

94. Armstrong D, Norman MG. Periventricular leukomalacia in neonates: complications and sequelae. Arch Dis Child. 1974;49:367-375.

95. Banker BQ, Larroche JC. Periventricular leukomalacia of infancy: a form of neonatal anoxic encephalopathy. Arch Neurol. 1962;7:386-410.

96. De Reuck J, Chatta AS, Richardson EP Jr. Pathogenesis and evolution of periventricular leukomalacia in infancy. Arch Neurol. 1972;27:229-236.

97. De Reuck J. The human periventricular arterial blood supply and the anatomy of cerebral infarctions. Eur Neurol. 1971;5:321-334.

98. Takashima S, Tanaka K. Development of cerebrovascular architecture and its relationship to periventricular leukomalacia. Arch Neurol. 1978;35:11-16.

99. De Reuck J. Cerebral angioarchitecture and perinatal brain lesions in premature and full term infants. Acta Neurol Scand. 1984;70:391-395.

100. Rorke LB. Anatomic features of the developing brain implicated to hypoxic-ischemic injury. Brain Pathol. 1992;2:211-221.

101. Cavazzutti M, Duffy TE. Regulation of local cerebral blood flow in normal and hypoxic newborn dogs. Ann Neurol. 1982;11:247-257.

102. Szymonowicz W, Walker AM, Yu YH, et al. Regional cerebral blood flow after hemorrhagic hypotension in the preterm, near term and term lamb. Pediatr Res. 1990;28:361-370.

103. Young RSK, Hernandez MJ, Yagel SK. Selective reduction of blood flow to white matter during hypotension in newborn dogs: a possible mechanism of periventricular leukomalacia. Ann Neurol. 1982;12:445-448.

104. Perlman JM, Risser R, Broyles RS. Bilateral cystic periventricular leukomalacia in the premature infant: associated risk factors. Pediatrics. 1996;97:822-827.

105. Faix RG, Donn SM. Association of septic shock caused by early onset group B streptococcal sepsis and periventricular leukomalacia in the preterm infant. Pediatrics. 1985;76:415-419.

106. Fujimoto S, Togari H, Yamaguchi N, et al. Hypocarbia and cystic periventricular leukomalacia in premature infants. Arch Dis Child. 1994;71:F107-F110.

107. Griesen G, Munck H, Lou H. Severe hypocarbia in preterm infants and neurodevelopmental deficit. Acta Paediatr Scand. 1986;76:401-404.

108. Sharakaran S, Langer JC, Kazzi SN, et al. Cumulative index of exposure to hypocarbia and hyperoxia as risk factors for periventricular leukomalacia in low birth weight infants. Pediatrics. 2006;118; 1654-1659.

109. Low JA, Froese AF, Galbraith RS, et al. The association of fetal and newborn acidosis with severe periventricular leukomalacia in the preterm infant. Am J Obstet Gynecol. 1990;162:977-982.

110. Perlman JM, Hill A, Volpe JJ. The effect of patent ductus arteriosus on flow velocity in the anterior cerebral arteries: ductal steal in the premature newborn infant. J Pediatr. 1981;99:767-771.

111. Perlman JM, Volpe JJ. Episodes of apnea and bradycardia in the preterm newborn: impact on cerebral circulation. Pediatrics. 1985;76:333-338.

3

112. Wiswell TE, Graziani LJ, Kornhauser MS. Effects of hypocarbia on the development of cystic peri-ventricular leukomalacia in premature infants treated with high frequency jet ventilation. *Pediatrics.* 1996;98:918-924.
113. Back SA, Volpe JJ. Cellular and molecular pathogenesis of periventricular white matter injury. *Ment Retard Dev Disabil Res Rev.* 1997;3:96-107.
114. Yoon BH, Kim CJ, Romero CJ. Experimentally induced intrauterine infection causes fetal brain white matter lesions in rabbits. *Am J Obstet Gynecol.* 1997;177:797-802.
115. Yue X, Mehmet H, Penrie J, et al. Apoptosis and necrosis in the newborn piglet brain following transient cerebral hypoxia ischemia. *Neuropathol Appl Neurobiol.* 1997;23:16-25.
116. Chamnanvanakij S, Margraf LR, Burns D, Perlman JM. Apoptosis and white matter injury in preterm infants. *Pediatr Dev Pathol.* 2002;5.
117. Volpe JJ. Brain injury in premature infants. *Lancet Neurol.* 2009;8:1474-1422.
118. Oka A, Belliveau MJ, Rosenberg PA, et al. Vulnerability of oligodendroglia to glutamate pharmacol-ogy, mechanisms and prevention. *J Neurosci.* 1993;13:1331-1453.
119. Yonezawa M, Back SA, Gan X, et al. Cystine deprivation induces oligodendroglial death. Rescue by free radical scavengers and by a diffusible glial factor. *J Neurochem.* 1996;67:566-573.
120. Gerstner B, De Silva TM, Gentz K, et al. Hyperoxia causes maturation-dependent cell death in the developing white matter. *J Neurosci.* 2008;28;1236-1245.
121. Gerstner B, Sifringer B, Dzietko M, et al. Estradiol attenuates hyperoxia-induced cell death in the developing white matter. *Ann Neurol.* 2007;61:562-571.
122. Gan XD, Back SA, Rosenberg PA, Volpe JJ. State-specific vulnerability of rat oligodendrocytes in culture to non-NMDA receptors mediated toxicity. *Soc Neurosci.* 1997;2:17420.
123. Yoshioka A, Bacskai B, Pleasure D. Pathophysiology of oligodendroglial excitotoxicity. *J Neurosci Res.* 1996;46:427.
124. Follett PL, Rosenberg RA, Volpe JJ, Jensen FG. NBQX attenuates excitotoxic injury in developing white matter. *J Neurosci.* 2000;20:9235-9241.
125. Bona E, Andersson AL, Blomgren K, et al. Chemokines and inflammatory cell response to hypoxia ischemia in immature rats. *Pediatr Res.* 1999;45:500-549.
126. Selmaj K, Raine CS, Farooq M. Cytokine cytotoxicity against oligodendrocytes: apoptosis induced by lymphotoxin. *J Immunol.* 1991;147:1522-1529.
127. Andrews T, Zhang P, Bhat NR. TNFα potentiates IFNγ-induced cell death in oligodendrocyte pre-cursor. *Neurosci Res.* 1998;54:574-583.
128. Dommergues MA, Patkai J, Renauld JC, et al. Proinflammatory cytokines and interleukin 9 exac-erbate excitotoxic lesions of the newborn murine neopallium. *Ann Neurol.* 2000;4:154-156.
129. Hansen-Pupp I, Harling S, Berg A, et al. Circulating interferon-gamma and white matter brain damage in preterm infants. *Pediatr Res.* 2005;58:946-952.
130. Saija A, Princi P, Lanza M, et al. Systemic cytokine administration can affect blood-brain permeabil-ity in the rat. *Life Sci.* 1995;56:775-784.
131. Nestlin WF, Gimbrone MA Jr. Neutrophil mediated damage to human vascular endothelium: role of cytokine activation. *Am J Pathol.* 1993;142:117-128.
132. Ando M, Takashima S, Mito T. Endotoxin, cerebral blood flow, amino acids and brain damage in young rabbits. *Brain Dev.* 1988;10:365-370.
133. Gilles FH, Leviton A, Kerr CS. Endotoxin leukoencephalopathy in the telencephalon of the newborn kitten. *J Neurol Sci.* 1976;27:183-191.
134. Zusban V, Gonzalez P, Lacaze Masmontiel T, et al. Periventricular leukomalacia: risk factors revisited. *Dev Med Child Neurol.* 1996;38:1066-1070.
135. Leviton A, Pareth N, Reuss L et al. Maternal infection, fetal inflammatory response and brain damage in very low birth weight infants. *Pediatr. Res.* 1999;46:566-575.
136. Baud O, Emilie D, Pelletier E, et al. Amniotic fluid concentrations of interleukin-1beta, interleukin-6 and TNF-alpha in chorioamnionitis before 32 weeks of gestation: histological associations and neonatal outcome. *Br J Obstet Gyn.* 1999;106:72-77.
137. Hillier SL, Witkin SS, Krohn MA, et al. The relationship of amniotic fluid cytokines and preterm delivery, amniotic fluid infection, histologic chorioamnionitis and chorioamnion infection. *Obstet Gynecol.* 1996;174:330-334.
138. Saito S, Kasahara T, Kato Y, et al. Elevation of amniotic fluid interleukin 6- (IL-6), IL-8, and granu-locyte stimulating factor (G-CSF) in term and preterm parturition. *Cytokines.* 1993;5:81-88.
139. Yoon BH, Jun JK, Romero R, et al. Interleukin-6 concentrations in umbilical cord plasma are elevated in neonates with white matter lesions associated with periventricular leukomalacia. *Am J Obstet Gynecol.* 1996;174:1433-1440.
140. Grether JK, Nelson KD. Maternal infection and cerebral palsy in infants at normal birth weight. *JAMA.* 1997;278:207-211.
141. Grether JK, Nelson KB, Dambrosia JM, Philips TM. Interferons and cerebral palsy. *J Pediatr.* 1999;134:324-332.
142. Wu YW, Colford JM Jr. Chorioamnionitis as a risk factor of cerebral palsy: a meta-analysis. *JAMA.* 2000;284:1417-1424.
143. Deguchi K, Mizoguchi M, Takashima S. Immunohistochemical expression of tumor necrosis factor α in neonatal leukomalacia. *Pediatr Neurol.* 1996;14:6-13.
144. Yoon BH, Romero R, Kim CJ, et al. High expression of tumor necrosis factor α and interleukin 6 in periventricular leukomalacia. *Am J Obstet Gynecol.* 1997;177:406-411.
145. Lin CY, Chang YC, Wang ST, et al. Altered inflammatory responses in preterm children with cerebral palsy. *Ann Neurol.* 2010;68:204-212.

146. Bonce AJ, Boling W, Kindy MS, et al. Altered neuronal and microglial response to excitotoxic and ischemic brain injury in mice lacking TNF receptor. *Nat Med.* 1996;2:788-794.
147. Glass HC, Bonifacio SL, Chau V, et al. Recurrent postnatal infections are associated with progressive white matter injury in premature infants. *Pediatrics.* 2008;122:299-305.
148. Graziani LJ, Spitzer AR, Mitchell DG, et al. Mechanical ventilation in preterm infants: neurosonographic and developmental studies. *Pediatrics.* 1992;90:515-522.
149. Trounce JQ, Shaw DE, Levene MI, Rutter N. Clinical risk factors and periventricular leukomalacia. *Arch Dis Child.* 1988;63:17-22.
150. Weindling AM, Wilkinson AR, Cook F, et al. Perinatal events, which precede periventricular hemorrhage and leukomalacia in the newborn. *Br J Obstet Gynecol.* 1985;92:1218-1223.
151. Mirro R, Buslta D, Green R, et al. Relationship between mean airway pressure, cardiac output and organ blood flow with normal and decreased respiratory compliance. *J Pediatr.* 1987;111:101-106.
152. Phelps DL, Rosenbaum AL, Isenberg SJ, et al. Tocopherol efficacy and safety for preventing retinopathy of prematurity: a randomized controlled, boule-masked trial. *Pediatrics.* 1987;79:489-500.
153. Stewart AL, Reynolds EOR, Hope RL, et al. Probability of neurodevelopmental disorders estimated from ultrasound appearance of brains of very preterm infants. *Dev Med Child Neurol.* 1987;29:3-11.
154. Fazzi E, Lanzi G, Gerardo A, et al. Neurodevelopmental outcome in very low birth weight infants with or without periventricular hemorrhage and/or leukomalacia. *Acta Paediatr.* 1992;81:808-811.
155. Roger B, Msall M, Owens T, et al. Cystic periventricular leukomalacia and type of cerebral palsy in preterm infants. *J Pediatr.* 1994;125:51-58.
156. Inder TE, Anderson NJ, Spencer C, et al. White matter injury in the premature infant: a comparison between serial cranial sonographic and MR findings at term. *Am J Neuroradiol.* 2003;24:805-809.
157. Woodward LJ, Anderson PJ, Austin NC, et al. Neonatal MRI to predict neurodevelopment outcome in preterm infants. *N Engl J Med.* 2006;355:685-694.
158. De Vries LS, Connell JA, Dubowitz LMS, et al. Neurological electrophysiological and MRI abnormalities in infants with extensive cystic leukomalacia. *Neuropediatrics.* 1987;18:61-66.
159. De Vries LS, Eken P, Groenendaal F, et al. Correlation between the degree of periventricular leukomalacia using cranial ultrasound and MRI in infancy, in children with cerebral palsy. *Neuropediatrics.* 1993;24:263-268.
160. Jacobson LK, Dutton GN. Periventricular leukomalacia: an important cause of visual and ocular motility dysfunction in children. *Surv Ophthalmol.* 2000;45:1-13.
161. Melhem ER, Hoon AH, Ferrucci JT, et al. Periventricular leukomalacia: relationship between lateral ventricular volume on brain MR images and severity of cognitive and motor impairment. *Radiology.* 2000;214:199-204.
162. Scher MS, Dobson V, Carpenter NA, Guthrie RD. Visual and neurological outcome of infants with periventricular leukomalacia. *Dev Med Child Neurol.* 1989;31:353-365.
163. Volpe JJ. Encephalopathy of Prematurity Includes Neuronal Abnormalities. *Pediatrics.* 2005;116:221-225.
164. Inder TE, Huppi PS, Warfield S, et al. Periventricular white matter injury in the premature infant is followed by reduced cerebral cortical gray matter volume at term. *Ann Neurol.* 1999;46:755-760.
165. de Groot JC, de Leeuw FE, Oudkerk M, et al. Periventricular white matter lesions predict rate of cognitive decline. *Ann Neurol.* 2002;52:335-341.
166. Mercer JS, Vohr BR, McGrath M, et al. Delayed cord clamping in very preterm infants reduces the incidence of intraventricular hemorrhage and late-onset sepsis: a randomized, controlled trial. *Pediatrics.* 2006;117:1235-1242.
167. Kallankari H, Kaukola T, Ojaniemi M, et al. Chemokine CCL18 predicts intraventricular hemorrhage in very preterm infants. *Ann Med.* 2010;42:416-425.
168. Perlman JM. Neurobehavioral deficits in premature graduates of intensive care. Potential medical and environmental risk factors. *Pediatrics.* 2001;108:1339-1348.
169. Neubauer AP, Voss W, Wachtendorf D, Jungman T. Erythropoietin improves neurodevelopmental outcome of extremely preterm infants *Ann Neurol.* 2010;67:657-666.
170. Ohls RK, Ehrenkranz RA, Das A, et al. Neurodevelopmental outcome and growth at 18 to 22 months' corrected age in extremely low birth weight infants treated with early erythropoietin and iron. *Pediatrics.* 2004;114:1287-1291.

CHAPTER 4

Posthemorrhagic Hydrocephalus Management Strategies

Andrew Whitelaw, MD, FRCPCH

4

- Question 1: What Measurements of Ventricular Size Are Used in Diagnosis of PHVD?
- Question 2: How Can I Distinguish Ventricular Dilation Driven by Cerebrospinal Fluid under Pressure from Ventricular Dilation Due to Loss of Periventricular White Matter?
- Question 3: How Do We Define Excessive Head Enlargement?
- Question 4: How Is Raised Intracranial Pressure Recognized?
- Question 5: What Is Infant A's Prognosis?
- Question 6: What Is the Mechanism of PHVD?
- Question 7: How Can PHVD Injure White Matter?
- Question 8: What Interventions Have Been Used in PHVD, and Is There Any Evidence That They Improve Outcome?
- Gaps in Knowledge

Hemorrhage into the ventricles of the brain is one of the most serious complications of premature birth despite improvements in the survival of premature infants. Large intraventricular hemorrhage (IVH) has a high risk of neurologic disability, and more than 50% of children with IVH go on to have progressive ventricular dilation.[1] Increasing survival of extremely premature infants is associated with posthemorrhagic ventricular dilation (PHVD) with high morbidity and considerable mortality.[2] Overall, approximately two thirds of these children have cerebral palsy and about one third have multiple impairments.[3,4] The term posthemorrhagic hydrocephalus is generally reserved for cases in which PHVD is persistent and associated with excessive head enlargement. This condition still does not have a safe and effective "cure" but advances in our understanding of the pathophysiology and experience from clinical trials allow us to suggest some guidelines on assessment and management and to identify gaps in knowledge where further advances are needed.

CASE HISTORY: INFANT A

A mother in her third pregnancy suffered a placental abruption at 28 weeks and delivered a male infant weighing 877 g at delivery. He was intubated at birth and received surfactant prophylactically. He was ventilated at low pressures and had a low oxygen requirement until, on day 2, he suffered a pulmonary hemorrhage with a period of hypotension (mean arterial pressure below 25 mm Hg for 2 hours), which was corrected with the use of dopamine and blood transfusion. His respiratory status stabilized within hours. On day 3 a cranial ultrasound scan showed bilateral intraventricular hemorrhage (Fig. 4-1A). He progressed from minimal ventilation settings to nasal

Figure 4-1 Cranial ultrasound scans from Infant A (Case History). **A,** Midcoronal view obtained on day 3, showing hemorrhage in both lateral ventricles. **B,** Left parasagittal view, obtained on day 3, showing extensive blood clot within the left lateral ventricle. **C,** Midcoronal view, obtained on day 18, showing enlargement of both lateral ventricles and the third ventricle.

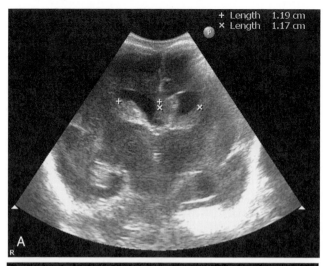

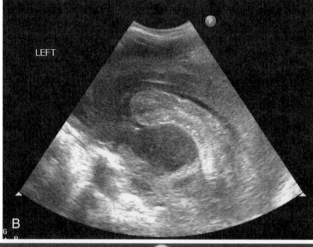

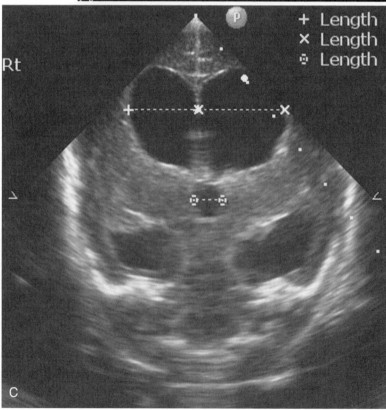

continuous positive airway pressure. He was then scanned twice a week. Ventricular dimensions progressively enlarged until day 18 (see Fig. 4-1B). Head circumference had increased by 1.5 cm over 7 days. A lumbar puncture (LP) produced 12 mL (10 mL/kg) of port wine–colored cerebrospinal fluid (CSF). This procedure reduced head circumference by 0.3 cm. Two days later, head circumference had increased by 0.5 cm from the post-puncture measurement. A second LP was carried out, which again produced 12 mL (10 mL/kg) of CSF. Head circumference decreased by 0.3 cm but then increased by 0.5 cm from the post-puncture measurement 2 days later. A third LP produced only 6 mL of CSF before flow stopped. Head circumference did not decrease, the fontanelle remained full, and ultrasonography confirmed that the ventricles were still "ballooned."

As there was a need for repeated tapping of CSF and repeated LP was becoming impractical, an Ommaya reservoir (ventricular access device) was inserted frontally in the right ventricle with the patient under general anesthesia. At the time of its insertion, 13 mL (10 mL/kg) of CSF was removed. In order to avoid raised pressure and resultant CSF leak with a risk of infection, the reservoir was tapped daily, at 10 mL/kg/day for 5 days. Thereafter, the reservoir was tapped as required to control excessive expansion or suspected pressure symptoms. Head circumference enlargement necessitated tapping 10 mL/kg every 1 to 2 days. Pressure measurement at the start of tapping typically showed a pressure of 6 to 7 mm Hg. After 10 mL/kg had been removed, pressure had fallen to 3 mm Hg. Clinically, apnea increased at the time of head expansion and decreased after tapping.

This regimen of tapping as required was reviewed every 7 days to confirm that head enlargement in 1 week had not been excessive. CSF protein was initially 4.1 g/L. Tapping the reservoir continued to be necessary for 6 weeks, and on a few days, it was obvious that 10 mL/kg had been insufficient to control head enlargement and the subsequent tap had been increased to 15 mL/kg. CSF protein continued to remain high (1.8-2.0 g/L), and tapping was continued for a further 2 weeks, by which time CSF protein had decreased to 1.45 g/L and the baby's weight had risen to nearly 2500 g. Nasal catheter oxygen was no longer required. A ventriculoperitoneal low-pressure shunt was inserted when Infant A reached full-term gestational age. Postoperatively there was no pulmonary problem, CSF leak, or infection but Infant A initially needed to be on a considerable head-up tilt to facilitate adequate shunt function and control of head circumference. Although control of head circumference and suspected pressure had been maintained, magnetic resonance imaging (MRI) at term showed considerable ventricular dilation with some loss of periventricular white matter.

Question 1: What Measurements of Ventricular Size Are Used in Diagnosis of PHVD?

The chances of progressive ventricular dilation increase with the amount of blood visible in the ventricles. With a small intraventricular hemorrhage (grade 2 on Papile scale[5] or 2a on De Vries grading[6]), measurement of ventricular size once a week for 4 weeks and then at discharge is appropriate; with a large IVH (grade 3 on Papile scale[5] or 2b on De Vries grading[6]), twice-weekly ultrasonography is needed because dilation is likely and may be rapid. Although large, balloon-shaped ventricles are obvious without formal measurements, quantitative documentation is essential if serial scans are being done by different ultrasonographers as well as in epidemiologic studies and clinical trials. Reference ranges for measurement of the width (midline to lateral border) of the lateral ventricles at the midcoronal level were first published in 1981.[7] Since 1984, an "action line," defined as width 4 mm higher than the 97th centile width for age, has been used as a definition of serious PHVD in therapeutic trials[3,4] and as a secondary outcome in randomized trials of neonatal intensive care interventions (Fig. 4-2A). This measurement has the advantage that it is highly reproducible among observers because it is relatively unaffected by anterior or posterior angulation of the scan head as the lateral wall of the ventricle in this orientation runs fairly parallel to the midline. The frequency of PHVD using this definition is 1 in 3000 births among residents of Bristol, United Kingdom. However, ventricular enlargement is not always sideways, and sometimes the most marked change is posterior enlargement or a change from thin slit to round balloon. With this in mind, Davies and colleagues[8] published reference ranges for anterior horn width (to capture the change in shape to balloon) (95th centile approximately 3 mm), thalamo-occipital width (to capture posterior enlargement) (95th centile approximately 25 mm) (Fig. 4-2B), and third ventricle width (95th centile approximately 2 mm). My colleagues and I have found the anterior horn, thalamo-occipital, and third ventricle widths to be practical and useful but with greater interobserver variation. We have used all three measurements since 2003, requiring all three measurements (bilaterally) to be 1 mm over the 95th centile as a criterion for PHVD.

Question 2: How Can Ventricular Dilation Driven by Cerebrospinal Fluid Under Pressure Be Distinguished from Ventricular Dilation Due to Loss of Periventricular White Matter?

The distinction CSF under pressure and loss of periventricular white matter as the cause of ventricular dilation is important because removing fluid that has accumulated as a replacement for dead brain is unlikely to improve outcome.

CSF-driven ventricular enlargement can be slow or rapid, it is characterized by balloon-shaped lateral ventricles, and if CSF pressure is measured, it is found to be raised or near the upper limit of normal (mean 3 mm Hg, upper limit 6 mm Hg[9]). Furthermore, head circumference growth over time is accelerated, although it may lag behind ventricular enlargement by 1 to 2 weeks. In contrast, ventricular enlargement from atrophy is always slow, it is more irregular in outline rather than balloon shaped, and if CSF pressure is measured, it is found not to be raised. Head circumference velocity is either normal or slow but is not accelerated. Nonprogressive mild ventricular dilation at term is widely recognized as a marker of periventricular leukomalacia.

Question 3: How Is Excessive Head Enlargement Defined?

Head circumference normally enlarges by approximately 1 mm per day between 26 weeks of gestation and 32 weeks, and about 0.7 mm per day between 32 and 40 weeks.[10] We regard a persistent increase of 2 mm per day as excessive. Measuring head circumference accurately, although "low-tech," is not as easy as it sounds. The relevant measurement is the maximum fronto-occipital circumference. Detecting a difference of 1 mm from day to day is difficult, and we do not react to a difference of 2 mm from one day to the next unless there is other evidence of raised intracranial pressure. However, an increase of 4 mm over 2 days is more likely to be real, and an increase of 14 mm over 7 days is definitely excessive.

Question 4: How Is Raised Intracranial Pressure Recognized?

It is possible to detect a change in palpation of the fontanelle from concave to bulging and, as described previously, to document excessive head enlargement. The preterm skull is very compliant and can easily accommodate an increase in CSF by expanding with separation of the sutures. When CSF pressure was measured with an electronic transducer in infants in whom ventricles were expanding after IVH, the

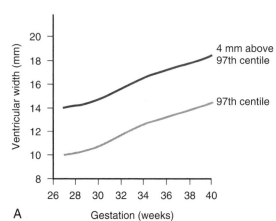

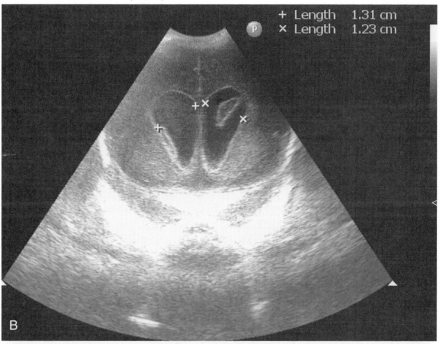

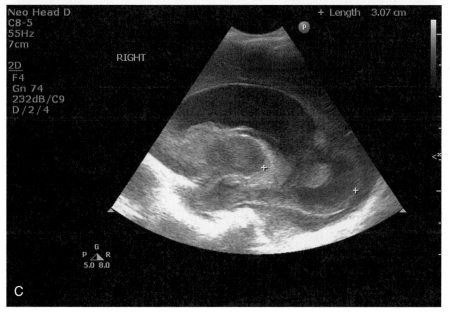

Figure 4-2 A, 97th centile for ventricular width with the 97th centile + 4-mm line ("action line") as the criterion for diagnosis of PHVD. B and C, Cranial ultrasound scans from Infant A (Case History) obtained on day 18. Frontal coronal view (B) showing the anterior horn width marked with calipers (×). Right parasagittal view (C) showing the thalamo-occipital dimension with calipers (×). (A modified from Levene M. Measurement of the growth of the lateral ventricles in preterm infants with real-time ultrasound. *Arch Dis Child* 1981;56:900-904.)

4

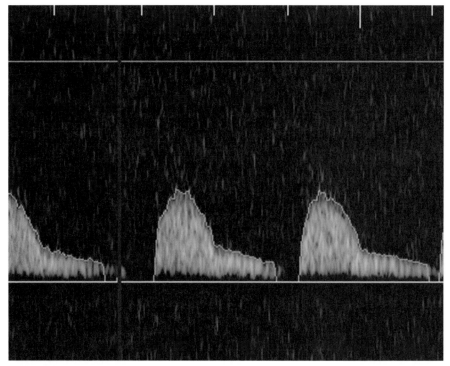

Figure 4-3 Cerebral blood flow velocity Doppler spectra from an infant with posthemorrhagic ventricular dilation and an intracranial pressure of 15 mm Hg. There is loss of end-diastolic velocities. When the pressure was reduced to 6 mm Hg, end-diastolic velocities returned.

mean CSF pressure was approximately 9 mm Hg, three times the mean in normal infants.[10] There was a considerable range, with ventricle and head expansion in some infants at a pressure of 5 to 6 mm Hg, and in a small number with CSF pressure around 15 mm Hg. A CSF pressure of 9 mm Hg does not necessarily produce clinical signs but may be associated with an increase in apnea or vomiting, hypotonia, hypertonia, or decreased alertness.

Obtaining serial calculations of the Doppler flow-velocity resistance index (RI) on the anterior cerebral artery is a useful and practical way of detecting impairment of cerebral perfusion by raised intracranial pressure and can easily be done during ultrasound imaging. The resistance index is calculated as follows: (systolic velocity – diastolic velocity)/systolic velocity. This measurement is independent of the angle of insonation. If intracranial pressure rises to a level exceeding the infant's compensation, end-diastolic velocity tends to decrease, eventually becoming zero (RI is then 1.0) (Fig. 4-3). Serial increases in RI above 0.85 while the ventricles are rapidly expanding would be evidence that pressure is rising.[11] This statement assumes that the infant does not have a significant left-to-right shunt at the ductal level and that Pco_2 has not decreased recently, because both of these physiologic changes could increase RI. Severe intracranial hypertension may cause reversed end-diastolic velocities. The sensitivity of resistance index can be increased by applying pressure to the fontanelle during the examination. An infant who is close to the limit of cranial compliance responds with a large decrease in end-diastolic velocities—that is, an increase in RI.[12] Amplitude-integrated electroencephalography (EEG) may show a deterioration, with electroencephalographic activity becoming less frequent as dilation increases and improving with effective CSF drainage.[13]

Question 5: What Is Infant A's Prognosis?

The prognosis at diagnosis of PHVD using the preceding criteria is influenced by the presence of identifiable parenchymal lesions. The Ventriculomegaly and PHVD Drug Trial used the 4 mm + 97th centile definition of PHVD and had standardized follow-up. Of children in whom careful ultrasonographic examination shows no persistent echodensities or echolucencies (cysts), approximately 40% will have cerebral palsy and about 25% will have multiple impairments.[3,4] Cerebral magnetic rsonance imaging at term is increasingly used to assess infants with PHVD because this technique can reveal parenchymal injury that cannot be easily demonstrated with ultrasonography.[14] Lesions detected by magnetic resonance imaging include abnormal signal in the white matter without cyst formation, gray matter abnormality, and cerebellar secondary atrophy. In Infant A's case, there were no ultrasonographic abnormalities in the parenchyma, and thus, the risk of some level of cerebral palsy would be no higher than 40%.

Question 6: What Is the Mechanism of PHVD?

Following a large IVH, multiple blood clots can obstruct the ventricular system or channels of reabsorption, initially leading to a phase of CSF accumulation.[15] Although tissue plasminogen activator can be demonstrated in posthemorrhagic CSF, fibrinolysis is very inefficient in the CSF, which has low levels of plasminogen and high levels of plasminogen activator inhibitor.[16,17] This potentially reversible obstruction by thrombi may lead to a chronic obliterative, fibrosing arachnoiditis, and subependymal gliosis[18] involving deposition of extracellular matrix proteins in the foramina of the fourth ventricle and the subarachnoid space. Figure 4-4A shows the brainstem and cerebellum of an infant with PHVD who died at age 2 months. A layer of collagenous connective tissue surrounds the brainstem. Figure 4-4B shows perivascular deposition of the extracellular matrix protein, laminin, in the subependymal region in another infant with PHVD who also died at age 2 months.

Transforming growth factor-β (TGF-β) is likely to be a key mediator of this process because TGF-β is involved in the initiation of wound healing and fibrosis.[19] TGF-β elevates the expression of genes encoding fibronectin, various types of collagen,[20,21] and other extracellular matrix components,[22] and is involved in a number of serious diseases in which there is excessive deposition of collagen, including diabetic nephropathy and cirrhosis.[23] TGF-β has three isoforms, β1, β2, and β3. TGF-β1 is stored in platelets. Thus IVH, by definition, provides a store of TGF-β1 for many weeks in the CSF. TGF-β is elevated in the CSF of adults with hydrocephalus after subarachnoid hemorrhage, and intrathecal administration of TGF-β to mice resulted in hydrocephalus.[24,25] My colleagues and I have demonstrated that TGF-β1 and TGF-β2 concentrations in CSF from infants with posthemorrhagic ventricular dilation are 10 to 20 times those in nonhemorrhagic CSF and that the concentration of TGF-β in CSF is predictive of later shunt surgery.[26] Heep and colleagues[27] have confirmed elevations of TGF-β1 in posthemorrhagic hydrocephalus CSF as well as a product of TGF-β, aminoterminal propeptide of type 1 collagen.[27] Chow and associates[28] have demonstrated elevation of TGF-β2 and nitrated chondroitin sulfate proteoglycans (an extracellular matrix protein) in CSF from preterm infants with posthemorrhagic hydrocephalus.[28]

A rat pup model of PHVD has also provided evidence of the involvement of TGF-β and its downstream products, fibronectin, laminin, and vitronectin.[29,30] Transgenic mice that overexpress TGF-β1 in the central nervous system are born with hydrocephalus.[31] Thus there is a strong possibility of a role for the TGF-βs in the development and/or maintenance of hydrocephalus after ventricular hemorrhage. However, two drugs that inhibit TGF-β, pirfenidone and losartan, did not reduce ventricular size or improve neuromotor performance in a rat pup model of PHVD.[32]

Question 7: How Can PHVD Injure White Matter?

Damage to periventricular white matter is probably exacerbated by ischemia due to raised intracranial pressure and parenchymal compression, by oxidative stress due to the generation of free radicals, and by the actions of inflammatory cytokines.

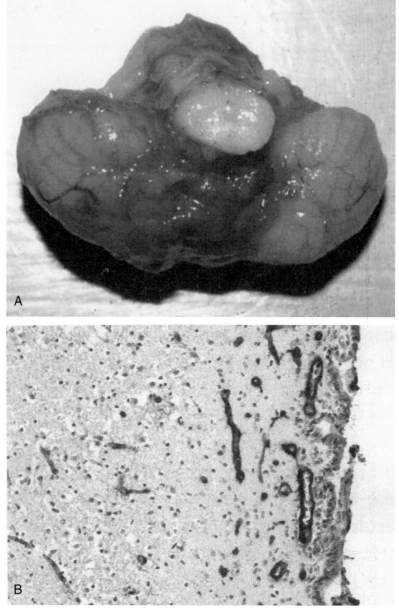

Figure 4-4 **A,** Brainstem and cerebellum of an infant with posthemorrhagic ventricular dila-tion (PHVD) who died at age 2 months. In addition to the staining from old blood, there are gray strands of connective tissue wrapped around the brainstem. **B,** Histologic section from the subependymal region of the brain of another infant with PHVD who also died at age 2 months. Immunostaining shows increased perivascular deposition of the extracellular matrix protein laminin.

Raised Intracranial Pressure, Parenchymal Compression, and Ischemia

PHVD raises CSF pressure to, on average, three times normal.[9] Figure 4-3 shows that in an infant with PVHD, an intracranial pressure of 15 mm Hg was high enough to prevent cerebral blood flow during diastole; cerebral perfusion was restored when the pressure was reduced to 6 mm Hg. Clearly, a reduction of perfusion of this magnitude substantially raises the risk of ischemic injury. There is also evidence that distortion of periventricular axons due to ventricular dilation may cause injury independently of ischemia.[33]

Free Radical–Mediated Injury

Non–protein-bound iron is readily detectable in the CSF of neonates with PHVD.[34] Hemoglobin that enters the CSF as a result of IVH releases large amounts of iron, which is likely to exceed the protein-binding capacity of the CSF and lead to the generation of hydroxyl free radicals from hydrogen peroxide via the Fenton reaction. Inder and coworkers[35] demonstrated products of lipid peroxidation in the CSF of infants with periventricular leukomalacia. Whether these products are also present in PHVD has not yet been investigated. Further evidence of potential oxidative stress comes from the finding of raised concentrations of hypoxanthine in the CSF of infants with PHVD.[36] Under conditions of ischemia, xanthine dehydrogenase is modified to form xanthine oxidase, which uses oxygen as the electron acceptor.[37] On restoration of cerebral perfusion, xanthine oxidase–mediated oxidation of xanthine and hypoxanthine generates superoxide and hydrogen peroxide, which cause oxidative damage. Oligodendrocyte progenitors, abundant in the periventricular white matter of premature infants, are highly susceptibility to oxidative damage.[38]

Proinflammatory Cytokines

Clinical evidence suggests that inflammation causes damage to immature white matter.[39] The concentration of tumor necrosis factor α, interleukin-1β, interleukin-6, interleukin-8, and interferon-γ are significantly elevated in the CSF of infants with PHVD.[40] Tumor necrosis factor α and interleukin-1β have both been implicated in the development of periventricular leukomalacia,[41] and it seems likely that these proinflammatory cytokines also contribute to white matter damage in PHVD.

Loss of White Matter and Gray Matter

In the rat model of PHVD, there is a significant negative correlation between the extent of ventricular dilation and the thickness of both the corpus callosum and the frontal cortex.[42] The development of hydrocephalus is associated with a mean reduction in the thickness of the corpus callosum of 48%, and of the frontal cortex of 31%. Loss of white matter is also marked in the lateral periventricular region, where my colleagues and I have shown that loss of myelin and axons is associated with a reduced density of oligodendrocytes.[42]

Question 8: What Interventions Have Been Used in PHVD, and Is There Any Evidence That They Improve Outcome?

Box 4-1 lists therapeutic interventions that have been used in infants with PHVD.

Ventriculoperitoneal Shunt Surgery

Ventriculoperitoneal (VP) shunt surgery is the conventional approach to other types of established hydrocephalus. Treatment of PHVD is more difficult than of other

---

Box 4-1   THERAPEUTIC INTERVENTIONS THAT HAVE BEEN USED IN INFANTS WITH POSTHEMORRHAGIC HYDROCEPHALUS

- Repeated early lumbar punctures/ventricular taps
- Diuretic drugs to reduce cerebrospinal fluid (CSF) production
- Intraventricular fibrinolytic therapy
- External ventricular drain
- Ventricular reservoir and repeated taps
- Third ventriculostomy
- Choroid plexus coagulation
- Ventriculoperitoneal shunt after CSF clears and CSF protein level <1.5 g/L
   NONE IS BOTH SAFE AND EFFECTIVE

types of hydrocephalus because the large amount of blood in the ventricles combined with the small size and instability of the patient make an early VP shunt operation impossible. In one series of 19 infants with PHVD requiring shunt surgery, there were 29 shunt blockages and 12 infections.[43] The risk of shunt blockage was increased if the CSF protein concentration was more than 1.5 g/L at the time of shunt insertion. In a series of 36 infants who underwent shunt placement for PHVD, shunt blockage and infection occurred only in those operated on before 35 days of age.[44] There is a considerable complication rate throughout a child's life from VP shunt surgery, and the child is permanently dependent on the shunt system. A VP shunt is a treatment but not a cure, and the child is vulnerable to shunt dysfunction. Shunt blockage after the cranial sutures have fused can rapidly raise intracranial pressure, resulting in permanent cerebral damage. Cases of sudden blindness and death have been recorded in such circumstances. Repeated shunt revisions are associated with a worsening of neurologic outcome.[45] Shunt infection is another complication that can further injure the developing brain.

Objectives in Treating PHVD

The objectives of treatment for PHVD are as follows:
1. To reduce secondary injury to the brain from pressure, distortion, free radicals, and inflammation.
2. To minimize iatrogenic injury from interventions, especially in those infants in whom PHVD resolves after a period of weeks.
3. To minimize the need for a VP shunt.

Repeated Lumbar Punctures or Ventricular Taps

Repeated lumbar punctures (LPs) were suggested as a way of controlling pressure, preventing progressive ventricular enlargement, and removing some of the red cells and protein from the CSF. Kressuer and associates[46] showed that a minimum of 10 mL/kg needed to be removed for the removal to have a significant effect on ventricular size. In our experience, only a minority of infants with PHVD have consistently communicating PHVD with a sufficient yield of CSF. Tapping of ventricular CSF must therefore be considered. A policy of repeated early tapping of lumbar or ventricular CSF for PHVD has been tested in four controlled clinical trials.[47] Overall, there was no evidence that this approach reduced the rate of VP shunt surgery or disability, and there was a 7% infection rate among the infants who underwent repeated tapping in the Ventriculomegaly Trial.[4]

Drug Treatment to Reduce CSF Production

Faced with this lack of effect and risk of infection from invasive procedures, investigators turned to pharmacologic treatment to reduce CSF production, which seemed an excellent approach. Acetazolamide had been in clinical use for benign intracranial hypertension and appeared to have acceptable adverse effects as long as electrolyte and acid-base balances were monitored. Uncontrolled reports were positive about the effect of acetazolamide in PHVD. Further work showed that acetazolamide produced an initial increase in cerebral blood flow mediated by an increase in tissue CO_2 and inhibition of respiratory elimination of CO_2.[48] Clinical investigation of infants with chronic lung disease of prematurity showed that acetazolamide produced an increase in P_{CO_2}.[49] Eventually a large multicenter randomized trial of acetazolamide combined with furosemide (which also reduces CSF production) was carried out. Not only was there no clinical benefit, but the group receiving the combined drug treatment had significantly worse outcome in terms of shunt surgery and death or disability.[50]

Intraventricular Fibrinolytic Therapy

The idea of injecting a fibrinolytic agent intraventricularly grew out of Pang's experimental PHVD model, in which blood was injected intraventricularly into dogs. In this model, hydrocephalus developed in 80% of subjects, but if urokinase was injected intraventricularly, only 10% demonstrated hydrocephalus.[51] The idea was supported by our own laboratory work showing that there was weak endogenous fibrinolytic activity in posthemorrhagic CSF[16,17] and by the relative safety and effectiveness of low-dose fibrinolytic therapy administered locally. A number of small nonrandomized trials of intraventricular streptokinase, urokinase, and tissue plasminogen activator, as well as two small randomized trials, have collectively shown that there is no reduction in VP shunt surgery and there is a risk of secondary intraventricular bleeding in infants receiving these agents.[52]

External Ventricular Drain

The insertion of an external ventricular drain is a logical way of providing continuous relief from raised pressure, preventing distortion from ventricular enlargement and removing protein and red blood cells. This approach has certainly been used in a small number of centers, but to our knowledge it has not been tested in a randomized trial.[53] The concern among neurosurgeons has been the risk of infection from prolonged presence of a ventricular drain.

Tapping via an Ommaya Reservoir

The most widely used approach we have encountered in neonatal units that treat a considerable number of infants with PHVD is the insertion of ventricular access device—that is, an Ommaya reservoir (Fig. 4-5)—in those cases in which repeated tapping is necessary to control excessive head enlargement and suspected raised pressure. This approach approximates that used in the conservative "arm" of the ventriculomegaly and PHVD drug trials and, in our view, should be regarded as standard treatment now. Not all infants with PHVD demonstrate excessive head enlargement or signs of raised pressure, so this is a selective approach. Once it becomes obvious that repeated CSF tapping is necessary, the surgically inserted reservoir enables it to be done whenever the need arises and in a small peripheral neonatal unit without neurosurgical or tertiary care neonatologists. This approach has been published but not yet tested in a randomized trial.[54] It is clear that in a unit with a sufficient volume of patients, a ventricular access device can be inserted into any extremely small infant (e.g., 700 g) with a very low complication rate. In

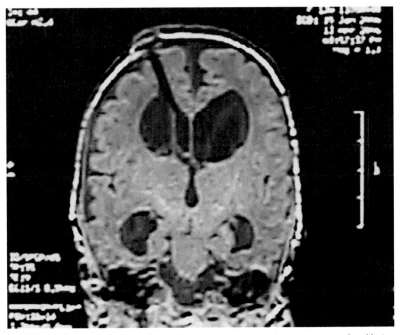

Figure 4-5   T1-weighted coronal magnetic resonance image showing ventricular dilation with a subcutaneous Ommaya reservoir and catheter to the right lateral ventricle.

Bristol a total of 100 such procedures have been carried out in preterm infants over 10 years with no cases of perioperative mortality and only one infection. There is currently a trial of this approach in the Netherlands comparing low-threshold intervention (ventricular width over the 97th centile and frontal horn 6 mm) with high-threshold intervention (ventricular width 4 mm over the 97th centile and frontal horn 10 mm).

Third Ventriculostomy

Third ventriculostomy is carried out endoscopically and can be a good treatment for other types of hydrocephalus, especially aqueduct stenosis. The endoscope is inserted into the ventricular system and then into the third ventricle. A hole is made in the midline of the floor of the third ventricle, with care to avoid the arteries on either side. This communication between the third ventricle and the subarachnoid space allows CSF to bypass obstruction in the aqueduct and foramina of the fourth ventricle. However, in PHVD, the problem is reabsorption of CSF and is not usually restricted to the aqueduct and fourth ventricle. Experience with third ventriculostomy in PHVD has been limited, and the results disappointing.[55]

Choroid Plexus Coagulation

Choroid plexus coagulation is carried out endoscopically and is based on the fact that most CSF production comes from the choroid plexus within the lateral ventricles and third ventricle. Because the problem with PHVD is primarily failed reabsorption and not overproduction of CSF, it would seem unlikely that this approach would be successful in PHVD. Choroid plexus coagulation has never been subjected to a controlled trial in PHVD.[56]

Drainage, Irrigation and Fibrinolytic Therapy

Drainage, irrigation, and fibrinolytic therapy (DRIFT), also known as ventricular lavage, is an approach that grew out of the unsatisfactory results of the preceding treatments and the emerging evidence that free radical injury and inflammation result from intraventricular blood and injure the brain over many weeks (Fig. 4-6). The objectives are to remove as much as possible of the intraventricular blood and to gently decompress the ventricles earlier.

The procedure involves insertion of right frontal and left occipital ventricular catheters. Tissue plasminogen activator (TPA) is injected intraventricularly at a dose 0.5 mg/kg that is insufficient to produce a systemic effect, and it is left for approximately 8 hours. Artificial Cerebrospinal Fluid (Torbay Pharmaceutical Manufacturing Unit) is then pumped into the frontal ventricular catheter at 20 mL/hr with continuous intracranial pressure monitoring. The occipital ventricular catheter is connected to a sterile close ventricular drainage system, and the height of the drainage reservoir is adjusted to keep intracranial pressure below 7 mm Hg. The drainage fluid initially looks like cola but gradually clears to look like white wine, at which point irrigation is stopped and the catheters are removed. This process commonly takes 72 hours but can require up to 7 days.

Ventricular lavage has been tested in a randomized trial that recruited 77 preterm infants with PHVD; 39 received DRIFT and 38 received standard treatment (LP followed by ventricular reservoir to be tapped to control expansion and pressure). There was no reduction in the proportion of either group who underwent surgical shunt placement or died.[57] All survivors were followed up at 2 years corrected age. Of the 39 (54%) patients in the DRIFT group, 21 (54%) were severely disabled or dead, compared with 27 of the 38 (71%) in the standard treatment group. Eleven of 35 survivors assessed with the Bayley scale (31%) in the DRIFT group had severe cognitive disability, compared with 19 of 32 (59%) in the standard group.[58] There was significantly more secondary intraventricular bleeding in the DRIFT group, but the bleeding was not associated with increased disability. Ventricular lavage is the only intervention for PHVD that has been objectively shown to improve any outcome, but it is a demanding and invasive procedure requiring close collaboration among the neonatologist, neuroimaging service, and

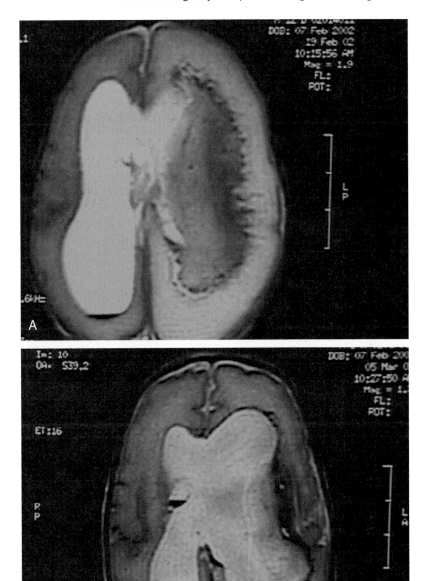

Figure 4-6 T2-weighted magnetic resonance images of an infant with posthemorrhagic ventricular dilation. **A,** This image shows extensive intraventricular debris, parenchymal injury and edema of the left ventricle, and gravitation of blood to the occipital pole of the right ventricle. **B,** Image in the same infant after DRIFT (drainage, irrigation, and fibrinolytic therapy), showing that the intraventricular debris has been removed, and the hemispheric edema reduced.

neurosurgeon. Work is under way to make ventricular lavage simpler and safer so that it can be tested in a larger multicenter randomized trial.

Conclusions

1. Posthemorrhagic hydrocephalus is characterized by deposition of extracellular matrix proteins weeks after intraventricular hemorrhage.

2. Raised intracranial pressure, distortion, inflammation, and free radical injury from iron are mechanisms by which periventricular white matter can be progressively injured.
3. Eight different therapeutic approaches have been used without objective evidence of efficacy and safety.
4. Although ventricular lavage, in a small randomized trial, reduced cognitive disability, this is still an experimental treatment requiring more evidence.

Gaps in Knowledge

Gaps in knowledge about PVHD can be summarized in the following questions:
1. How important is injury from free radicals, and can chelation improve neurologic outcome or reduce shunt dependence?
2. Does very early drainage of CSF to prevent distortion and pressure improve neurologic outcome or reduce shunt dependence?
3. Can ventricular lavage be made more efficient, easier, and safer so that it can be tested in more centers?

References

1. Volpe JJ. *Neurology of the Newborn.* 5th ed. Philadelphia: WB Saunders; 2008:428-493.
2. Murphy BP, Inder TE, Rooks V, et al. Posthemorrhagic ventricular dilatation in the premature infant: natural history and predictors of outcome. *Arch Dis Child.* 2002;87:F37-F41.
3. Ventriculomegaly Trial Group. Randomised trial of early tapping in neonatal posthaemorrhagic ventricular dilatation. *Arch Dis Child.* 1990;65:3-10.
4. International PHVD Drug Trial Group. International randomised trial of acetazolamide and furosemide in posthaemorrhagic ventricular dilatation. *Lancet.* 1998;352:433-440.
5. Papile LA, Burstein J, Burstein R, Koffler H. Incidence and evolution of subependymal and intraventricular hemorrhage: a study of infants with birth weights less than 1,500 gm. *J Pediatr.* 1978;92: 529-534.
6. De Vries LS, Dubowitz LM, Dubowitz V, et al. Predictive value of cranial ultrasound in the newborn baby: a reappraisal. *Lancet.* 1985;20;2(8447):137-140.
7. Levene M. Measurement of the growth of the lateral ventricle in preterm infants with real-time ultrasound. *Arch Dis Child.* 1981;56:900-904.
8. Davies MW, Swaminathan M, Chuang SL, et al. Reference ranges for linear dimensions of intracranial ventricles in preterm neonates. *Arch Dis Child.* 2000;82:F218-F223.
9. Kaiser A, Whitelaw A. Cerebrospinal fluid pressure during posthemorrhagic ventricular dilatation in newborn infants. *Arch Dis Child.* 1985;60:920-923.
10. Fenton TR. A new growth chart for preterm babies: Babson and Benda's chart updated with recent data and a new format. *BMC Pediatrics.* 2003;3:13.
11. Quinn MW, Ando Y, Levene MI. Cerebral arterial and venous flow-velocity measurements in posthaemorrhagic ventricular dilatation. *Dev Med Child Neurol.* 1992;34:863-869.
12. Taylor GA, Madsen JR. Neonatal hydrocephalus: hemodynamic response to fontanelle compression: correlation with intracranial pressure and need for shunt placement. *Radiology.* 1996;201: 685-689.
13. Olischar M, Klebermass K, Hengl B, et al. Cerebrospinal fluid drainage in posthaemorrhagic ventricular dilatation leads to improvement in amplitude-integrated electroencephalographic activity. *Acta Paediatr.* 2009;98:1002-1009.
14. Inder TE, Wells SJ, Mogridge NB, et al. Defining the nature of the cerebral abnormalities in the premature infant: a qualitative magnetic resonance imaging study. *J Pediatr.* 2003;143: 171-179.
15. Hill A, Shackelford GD, Volpe JJ. A potential mechanism of pathogenesis for early post-hemorrhagic hydrocephalus in the premature newborn. *Pediatrics.* 1984;73:19-21.
16. Whitelaw A, Mowinckel MC, Abildgaard U. Low levels of plasminogen in cerebrospinal fluid after intraventricular haemorrhage: a limiting factor for clot lysis? *Acta Paediatr.* 1995;84:933-936.
17. Hansen A, Whitelaw A, Lapp C, Brugnara C. Cerebrospinal fluid plasminogen activator inhibitor-1: a prognostic factor in posthaemorrhagic hydrocephalus. *Acta Paediatr.* 1997;86:995-998.
18. Larroche JC. Posthemorrhagic hydrocephalus in infancy. *BioNeonate.* 1972;20:287-299.
19. Beck LS, Chen TL, Amman AJ et al. Accelerated healing of ulcer wounds in the rabbit ear by recombinant human transforming growth factor beta-1. *Growth Factors.* 1990;2:273-282.
20. Ignotz RA, Massague J. Transforming growth factor beta stimulates the expression of fibronectin and collagen and their incorporation into the extracellular matrix. *J Biol Chem.* 1986;261:4337-4345.
21. Roberts AB, Sporn MB, Assoian RK et al. Transforming growth factor type β: rapid induction of fibrosis and angiogenesis in vivo and stimulation of collagen formation in vitro. *Proc Natl Acad Sci USA.* 1986;83:4167-4171.
22. Border WA, Ruoslahti E. Transforming growth factor-beta 1 induces extracellular matrix formation in glomerulonephritis. *Cell Differ Dev.* 1990;32:425-431.
23. Castilla A, Prieto J, Fausto N. Transforming growth factors beta 1 and alpha in chronic liver disease. Effects of interferon alfa therapy. *N Engl J Med.* 1991;324:933-940.

4

24. Kitazawa K, Tada T. Elevation of transforming growth factor beta-1 level in cerebrospinal fluid of patients with communicating hydrocephalus after subarachnoid hemorrhage. *Stroke.* 1994;25: 1400-1404.

25. Tada T, Kanaji M, Kobayashi S. Induction of communicating hydrocephalus in mice by intrathecal injection of human recombinant transforming growth factor beta-1. *J Neuroimmunol.* 1994;50: 153-158.

26. Whitelaw A, Christie S, Pople I. Transforming growth factor β-1: a possible signal molecule for post-hemorrhagic hydrocephalus? *Pediatr Res.* 1999;46:576-580.

27. Heep A, Bartmann P, Stoffel-Wagner B, et al. Cerebrospinal fluid obstruction and malabsorption in human neonatal hydrocephaly. *Childs Nerv Syst.* 2006;22:1249-1255.

28. Chow LC, Soliman A, Zandian M, et al. Accumulation of transforming growth factor-beta2 and nitrated chondroitin sulfate proteoglycans in cerebrospinal fluid correlates with poor neurologic outcome in preterm hydrocephalus. *Biol Neonate.* 2005;88:1-11.

29. Cherian SS, Love S, Silver IA, et al. Posthemorrhagic ventricular dilation in the neonate: development and characterization of a rat model. *J Neuropathol Exp Neurol.* 2003;62:292-303.

30. Cherian S, Thoresen M, Silver IA, et al. Transforming growth factor-betas in a rat model of neonatal posthaemorrhagic hydrocephalus. *Neuropathol Appl Neurobiol.* 2004;30:585-600.

31. Wyss-Coray T, Feng L, Masliah E, et al. Increased central nervous system production of extracellular matrix components and development of hydrocephalus in transgenic mice overexpressing transforming growth factor-beta 1. *Am J Pathol.* 1995;147:53-67.

32. Aquilina K, Hobbs C, Tucker A, et al. Do drugs that block transforming growth factor beta reduce posthaemorrhagic ventricular dilatation in a neonatal rat model? *Acta Paediatr.* 2008;97:1181-1186.

33. Del Bigio MR. Neuropathological changes caused by hydrocephalus. *Acta Neuropathol.* 1993;85: 573-585.

34. Savman K, Nilsson UA, Blennow M, et al. Non-protein-bound iron is elevated in cerebrospinal fluid from preterm infants with posthemorrhagic ventricular dilatation. *Pediatr Research.* 2001;49: 208-212.

35. Inder T, Mocatta T, Darlow B, et al. Elevated free radical products in the cerebrospinal fluid of VLBW infants with cerebral white matter injury. *Pediatr Res.* 2002;52:213-218.

36. Bejar R, Saugstad OD, James H, Gluck L. Increased hypoxanthine concentrations in cerebrospinal fluid of infants with hydrocephalus. *J Pediatr.* 1983;103:44-48.

37. Nishino T, Tamura I. The mechanism of conversion of xanthine dehydrogenase to oxidase and the role of the enzyme in reperfusion injury. *Adv Exp Med Biol.* 1991;309A:327-333.

38. Back SA, Luo NL, Borenstein NS, et al. Late oligodendrocyte progenitors coincide with the developmental window of vulnerability for human perinatal white matter injury. *J Neurosci.* 2001;21: 1302-1312.

39. Leviton A, Paneth N, Reuss ML, et al. Maternal infection, fetal inflammatory response, and brain damage in very low birth weight infants. *Pediatr Res.* 1999;46:566-575.

40. Savman K, Blennow M, Hagberg H, et al. Cytokine responses in cerebrospinal fluid from preterm infants with posthaemorrhagic ventricular dilatation. *Acta Paediatr.* 2002;91:1357-1363.

41. Kadhim H, Tabarki B, Verellen G, et al. Inflammatory cytokines in the pathogenesis of periventricular leukomalacia. *Neurology.* 2001;56:1278-1284.

42. Cherian S, Whitelaw A, Thoresen M, Love S. The pathogenesis of neonatal post-hemorrhagic hydrocephalus. *Brain Pathol.* 2004;14:305-311.

43. Hislop JE, Dubowitz LM, Kaiser AM, et al. Outcome of infants shunted for post-haemorrhagic ventricular dilatation. *Dev Med Child Neurol.* 1988;30:451-456.

44. Taylor AG, Peter JC. Advantages of delayed VP shunting in post-haemorrhagic hydrocephalus seen in low-birth-weight infants. *Childs Nerv Syst.* 2001;17:328-333.

45. Tuli S. Risk factors for repeated cerebrospinal shunt failures in pediatric patients with hydrocephalus. *J Neurosurg.* 2000;92:31-38.

46. Kreusser KL, Tarby TJ, Kovnar E, et al. Serial lumbar punctures for at least temporary amelioration of neonatal posthemorrhagic hydrocephalus. *Pediatrics.* 1985;75:719-724.

47. Whitelaw A. Repeated lumbar or ventricular punctures in newborns with intraventricular hemorrhage. *Cochrane Database Syst Rev.* 2001;(1):CD000216.

48. Thoresen M, Whitelaw A. Effect of acetazolamide on cerebral blood flow velocity and CO_2 elimination in normotensive and hypotensive newborn piglets. *Biol Neonate.* 1990;58:200-207.

49. Cowan F, Whitelaw A. Acute effects of acetazolamide on cerebral blood flow velocity and pCO_2 in the newborn infant. *Acta Paediatr Scand.* 1991;80:22-27.

50. Whitelaw A, Kennedy CR, Brion LP. Diuretic therapy for newborn infants with posthemorrhagic ventricular dilatation. *Cochrane Database Syst Rev.* 2001;(2):CD002270.

51. Pang D, Sclabassi RJ, Horton JA. Lysis of intraventricular blood clot with urokinase in a canine model: Part 3. Effects of intraventricular urokinase on clot lysis and posthemorrhagic hydrocephalus. *Neurosurgery.* 1986;19:553-572.

52. Whitelaw A, Odd DE. Intraventricular streptokinase after intraventricular hemorrhage in newborn infants. *Cochrane Database Syst Rev.* 2007;(4):CD000498.

53. Berger A, Weninger M, Reinprecht A, et al. Long-term experience with subcutaneously tunneled external ventricular drainage in preterm infants. *Childs Nerv Syst.* 2000;16:103-109.

54. de Vries LS, Liem KD, van Dijk K, et al.; Dutch Working Group of Neonatal Neurology. Early versus late treatment of posthaemorrhagic ventricular dilatation: results of a retrospective study from five neonatal intensive care units in The Netherlands. *Acta Paediatr.* 2002;91:212-217.

55. Buxton N, Macarthur D, Mallucci C, et al. Neuroendoscopic third ventriculostomy in patients less than 1 year old. *Pediatr Neurosurg.* 1998;29:73-76.

56. Pople IK, Edwards RJ, Aquilina K. Endoscopic methods of hydrocephalus treatment. *Neurosurg Clin N Am.* 2001;12:719-735.
57. Whitelaw A, Evans D, Carter M, et al. Randomized clinical trial of prevention of hydrocephalus after intraventricular hemorrhage in preterm infants: brain-washing versus tapping fluid. *Pediatrics.* 2007; 119:e1071-e1078.
58. Whitelaw A, Jary S, Kmita G, et al. Randomized trial of drainage, irrigation and fibrinolytic therapy for premature infants with posthemorrhagic ventricular dilatation: developmental outcome at 2 years. *Pediatrics.* 2010;125:e852-e858.

4

CHAPTER 5

The Use of Hypothermia to Provide Neuroprotection for Neonatal Hypoxic-Ischemic Brain Injury

Abbot R. Laptook, MD

- ● Case History
- ● Experimental Evidence for the Use of Therapeutic Hypothermia
- ● Implementation of a New Therapy
- ● Temperature Control Before and After Therapeutic Hypothermia
- ● Assessment of Encephalopathy
- ● Is an Amplitude-Integrated Electroencephalography Necessary?
- ● Cooling on Transport
- ● Selective Use of Therapeutic Hypothermia
- ● Future of Therapeutic Hypothermia

Hypoxic-ischemic encephalopathy (HIE) represents a clinical condition characterized by an altered sensorium, abnormalities of muscle tone, activity, and primitive reflexes, and difficulty initiating and/or sustaining respiratory efforts at birth.[1] With more severe involvement, seizures may accompany these abnormal findings of the neurologic examination. A specific test does not exist to establish a diagnosis of HIE; rather a sequence of events is usually linked together across the in utero, intrapartum, and neonatal environments that support a role for hypoxia-ischemia as the etiology of or strong contributor to the pathogenesis of the encephalopathy.[2] Neonatal encephalopathy is a relatively infrequent condition, with estimates of 3 to 4 per 1000 live births based on geographic populations. Hypoxia-ischemia represents the etiology for neonatal encephalopathy in up to 30% of infants with this condition.[3] The importance of determining the presence of acute hypoxia-ischemia is that it represents a modifiable condition for which a therapy can alter outcome.[4] For the majority of other causes of neonatal encephalopathy (e.g., congenital infections, brain malformations, chromosomal abnormalities, teratogen exposure), no specific therapy exists.

Starting in 2005 and increasing up until the present, targeted reductions in temperature have become incorporated into the management approach for infants of a gestational age of 36 weeks or greater in whom encephalopathy is believed to be due to hypoxia-ischemia. The following case history illustrates how alterations in temperature have become part of the armamentarium of the clinician.

CASE HISTORY

The mother was a 26-year-old gravida 3 now para 1 who was at 37^1 weeks of gestation when she noted a decrease in fetal movement. Prior obstetric history included a spontaneous abortion and an ectopic pregnancy. The current pregnancy was notable for gestational diabetes, which was diet controlled, and otherwise routine prenatal care. A nonstress test in the obstetrician's office was nonreactive and prompted immediate referral to the hospital. In the emergency department, a biophysical profile indicated a score of 2 of 10 (for amniotic fluid volume), and the mother was sent for immediate delivery via cesarean section. At delivery the infant required intubation, positive-pressure ventilation, and chest compressions, and extreme pallor was noted. By 7 minutes of age the heart rate was greater than 100 beats per minute. An umbilical venous catheter was placed but fluid volume was not administered in the operating room. Apgar scores were 0 (1 min), 1 (5 min), 2 (10 min), 3 (15 min) and 5 (20 min) and the infant was moved to the neonatal intensive care unit (NICU).

In the NICU the infant was noted to be appropriate for gestational age (birth weight 3.11 kg), to have modestly low blood pressure, to be hypoglycemic (blood glucose 6 mg/dL), to have a metabolic acidosis with a base excess of -15.2 mmol/L, and to be profoundly anemic (hemoglobin 2.8 g/dL). There was no evidence of hydrops, hepatosplenomegaly, skin lesions, or microcephaly. Spontaneous respiratory efforts were noted upon admission to the unit, but the infant was maintained on ventilator support. The infant was stabilized with dextrose boluses, colloid volume expansion, and transfusions of packed red blood cells. An umbilical artery catheter was placed for monitoring blood pressure. A Kleihauer-Betke test on the mother confirmed a large fetal-maternal hemorrhage. At 2.5 hours of age a neurologic evaluation indicated a severe encephalopathy with stupor, absence of spontaneous activity, flaccid muscle tone, extension of all extremities, weak suck, and a weak respiratory effort. A decision was made to initiate therapeutic hypothermia, and by 3 hours of age an esophageal temperature probe had been inserted and the infant was placed on a cooling blanket with initiation of whole body cooling.

This case is typical of the current use of therapeutic hypothermia for an infant with encephalopathy in whom supporting data indicate a role for hypoxia-ischemia. Initiation of therapeutic hypothermia was relatively rapid and was accomplished within 15 to 20 minutes. However, this time frame is achievable only in NICUs that are prepared, have the equipment readily available, and have trained personnel to facilitate the setup process. There was reasonable confidence that hypoxia-ischemia contributed to the clinical condition of the fetus/newborn because there had been an in utero event that compromised fetal oxygenation (fetal-maternal hemorrhage) and was associated with cardiopulmonary depression at birth that necessitated cardiopulmonary resuscitation (CPR). The metabolic acidosis evident on the first postnatal blood gas analysis supported a hypoxic state, which in this case was anemic hypoxia. The neurologic finding of a severe encephalopathy completed the sequence of events from in utero through the delivery room to the NICU and puts the infant at high risk of long-term neurodevelopmental impairment. The intent of criteria for therapeutic hypothermia is to identify infants with acute hypoxia-ischemia proximate to the time of birth and to mimic experimental laboratory conditions in which hypothermia was tested.[5-7] This case also illustrates that there is some uncertainty about the details of the hypoxic-ischemic event; specifically, precise timing of the insult is difficult, and complete certainty that this infant experienced acute hypoxia-ischemia proximate to birth, as opposed to low-grade anemic hypoxia for hours prior to delivery, is unclear.

Important questions therefore still remain regarding therapeutic hypothermia even though it represents the sole proven therapy for neonatal hypoxic-ischemia. Dissemination of the therapy has led to new questions that have not been resolved by randomized clinical trials. The objective of this chapter is to provide an overview of the following three areas pertinent to therapeutic hypothermia: (1) review of the data that support use of hypothermia for hypoxic-ischemic encephalopathy;

(2) delineation of important issues encountered during dissemination of this relatively new therapy; and (3) summary of future directions for treatment of hypoxic-ischemic encephalopathy.

Experimental Evidence for the Use of Therapeutic Hypothermia

Animal Work

The temporal profile of hypoxic-ischemic brain injury is one of a primary phase of injury followed by a secondary phase at a time remote from the inciting hypoxia-ischemia.[8] The *primary phase* refers to processes that are triggered as a direct result of failed cellular energetics and includes excitotoxicity, free radical and peroxidative injury, and disordered osmoregulation, much of which is linked to disturbed intracellular calcium homeostasis.[9] The severity of hypoxia-ischemia can be so extreme that injury or death occurs during the primary phase irrespective of interventions. If hypoxia-ischemia can be reversed by resuscitation or other timely and effective interventions, then there is the possibility of a secondary phase of injury. The interval between the primary and secondary insult is known as a *latent phase* or *therapeutic window* because therapies initiated during this interval can attenuate the extent of injury. Progression to the *secondary phase* signifies that brain injury will almost certainly follow. Prominent pathologic processes of the secondary phase of injury include inflammation, apoptosis, and suppression of growth factors and protein synthesis.[10] It has long been thought that the latent phase is a quiescent interval between primary and secondary insults because phosphorylated metabolites and intracellular acid-base balance largely return to baseline during this time. There is growing evidence that triggers for events during the secondary phase of injury are initiated during the latent phase in spite of recovery of the energy state.[9,11]

Hypothermia represents a nonspecific neuroprotective therapy that favorably alters processes of both the primary and secondary phases of injury. Under laboratory conditions reduction in brain temperature is effective even when initiated up to 5.5 hours following hypoxia-ischemia.[12] This characteristic makes it a potentially clinically applicable therapy because time is needed after birth to assess and stabilize sick neonates. Furthermore, therapeutic hypothermia is effective across the maturational range from fetus to adult and has provided neuroprotection in many different animal species.[12,13]

Clinical Trials

The first two randomized clinical trials of therapeutic hypothermia for infants with hypoxic-ischemic encephalopathy were published in 2005[14,15] and were reviewed in detail in the first edition of this book.[16] Since that time four other large clinical trials have been completed, and three of them have been published.[17-20] Although there are other published studies on therapeutic hypothermia, these six are presented because they all have follow-up for the primary outcome at 18 months of age. Salient characteristics of each trial are listed in Table 5-1.

These trials, with a combined enrollment of 1371 infants, have many similarities but also some important differences. Four of the trials enrolled infants at 36 weeks of gestation or later; Zhou and colleagues[20] enrolled infants at 37 weeks of gestation or later, and Jacobs and associates, enrolled infants at 35 weeks or later. Inclusion criteria all involved a tiered approach with fulfillment of specific clinical and/or biochemical variables, followed by determination of moderate or severe encephalopathy. A third tier of criteria, evidence of electrophysiologic abnormality, was used in three of the trials. Hypothermia regimens entailed either combined head and body cooling or body cooling alone, with the latter using a lower core target temperature. In all of the trials therapeutic hypothermia was initiated prior to 6 hours of age, was continued for 72 hours, and was followed by active rewarming at a rate of no more than 0.5° C per hour. Exceptions to the latter were the trial by Zhou and colleagues,[18] which allowed for spontaneous rewarming, and

Table 5-1 CLINICAL TRIALS OF THERAPEUTIC HYPOTHERMIA THAT HAVE NEURODEVELOPMENTAL OUTCOME AT OR BEYOND 18 MONTHS OF AGE

Author(s)	Year Published	Infants Treated with Hypothermia (n)	Control Infants* (n)	aEEG for Inclusion?	Mode of Hypothermia[†]	Core Temperature (° C)[‡]
Gluckman et al[14]	2005	116	118	Yes	Head/body	34-35
Shankaran et al[15]	2005	102	106	No	Body	33.5
Azzopardi et al[17]	2009	163	162	Yes	Body	33-34
Zhou et al[18]	2010	138	118	No	Head/body	34-35
Simbruner et al[19]	2010	62	65	Yes	Body	33.5
Jacobs et al[20]	2010	110	111	No	Body	33.5

aEEG, Amplitude-integrated electroencephalography.
*Control infants fulfilled the criteria for hypothermia but were randomly allocated to maintenance of their core body temperatures at approximately 37° C.
[†]Mode of hypothermia was either the use of a cooling cap combined with cooling the body or solely cooling the body.
[‡]Core temperature was recorded from either rectal or esophageal sites.

that by Jacobs and associates,[20] which warmed infants at no more than 0.5° C every 2 hours. Cooling on transport was a part of the protocols for the trials by Azzopardi and coworkers[17] and Jacobs and associates.[20] The primary outcome in each trial was the combined end point of death or neurodevelopmental disability by 18 to 24 months of age. In all trials the extent of neurodevelopmental disability criterion was severe, except for the trial of Shankaran and colleagues,[15] in which it was moderate or severe. In that trial, one in three infants had a moderate disability, and thus the outcome variable was similar to that in other trials. Results for the primary outcome are shown in Table 5-2.

Table 5-2 OUTCOMES OF DEATH OR DISABILITY AT 18-24 MONTHS FOR CLINICAL TRIALS OF THERAPEUTIC HYPOTHERMIA

Author(s)	Primary Outcome* Hypothermia n	%	Follow-Up Rate (%)	Primary Outcome* Control n	%	Follow-Up Rate (%)	Relative Risk	95% Confidence Interval
Gluckman et al[14]	59/108	54.6	93.1	73/110	66.4	93.2	0.82	0.66-1.02
Shankaran et al[15]	45/102	44.1	100	64/103	62.1	97.2	0.72	0.54-0.95
Azzopardi et al[17]	74/162	45.7	99.4	86/161	53.4	99.4	0.86	0.69-1.07
Zhou et al[18]	31/100	31.0	72.5	46/94	48.9	80.0	0.63	0.44-0.91
Simbruner et al[19]	27/53	50.9	85.5	48/58	82.8	90.5	0.62	0.46-0.82
Jacobs et al[20]	55/107	51.4	97.3	67/101	66.3	92.7	0.77	0.62-0.98

*Primary outcome is death or neurodevelopmental disability.

The relative risk (RR) of death or disability was reduced with therapeutic hypothermia in each study, and the reduction was statistically significant in four trials.[15,18-20] The point estimate for the risk of death or disability was lowest for the trials conducted by Zhou and colleagues[18] and Simbruner and associates,[19] which have the lowest follow-up rates among the trials. The higher loss to follow-up among the latter two studies may result in the absence of results on the sickest, most impaired infants and lead to an unrealistic effect size. The four studies with follow-up rates greater than 90% have point estimates for the relative risk of the primary outcome that are relatively tight (0.72-0.86) and suggest a less prominent effect than the Zhou and Simbruner trials. In addition, in spite of the inclusion criteria of moderate or severe encephalopathy in the trial by Zhou and colleagues,[18] 20% of enrolled infants were characterized as having mild encephalopathy.

An important secondary outcome from the trials reported by Azzopardi and coworkers[17] and Jacobs and associates[20] was that therapeutic hypothermia was associated with an increased survival without neurologic abnormalities (RR 1.57 and 1.75; 95% confidence interval [CI], 1.16-2.12 and 1.13-2.70, respectively). A similar direction of effect was present in other trials but not was significant (Shankaran et al[21]: RR 1.40, 95% CI 0.88-2.22; Gluckman et al[14]: RR 1.48, 95% CI 0.89-2.45). These studies also suggest that the mode of cooling is not a major determinant of benefit from therapeutic hypothermia, although there will probably never be a comparison of body cooling with head plus body cooling to determine this issue.

There are other interesting differences between these trials (e.g., sedation/analgesia, other supportive care) that may ultimately contribute to the observed outcomes. However, when taken collectively, these six trials provide strong evidence that initiation of reduced brain temperature within 6 hours of birth with continuation for 72 hours for infants with HIE imparts neuroprotection. Meta-analyses will be forthcoming that will further define the benefit of therapeutic hypothermia using data from all of these trials. A meta-analysis by Edwards and colleagues[4] analyzed the combined results of the 767 infants in the Gluckman,[14] Shankaran,[15] and Azzopardi[17] trials. In subjects at 18 months of age, having received therapeutic hypothermia was associated with a reduction in death or disability (RR 0.81; 95% CI 0.71-0.93) and an increase in survival without any neurodevelopmental abnormality (RR, 1.53, 95% CI 1.22-1.93). Both components of the primary outcome were reduced with therapeutic hypothermia (mortality: RR 0.78; 95% CI 0.66-0.93; severe disability among survivors: RR 0.71; 95% CI 0.56-0.91). Each component of a severe disability was favorably affected by therapeutic hypothermia (cerebral palsy, neuromotor delay, neurodevelopmental delay, and blindness) except for deafness.[4] Importantly, the benefit of therapeutic hypothermia was achieved without appreciable toxicity, although low-frequency serious adverse events have not been excluded. An important question from all of the therapeutic hypothermia trials is whether neuroprotection persists beyond 18 to 24 months. Shankaran and colleagues[22] followed up infants from their trial and compared the composite outcome of death or an IQ less than 70 at 6 or 7 years of age, which was available for 91% of infants in the original trial. Death or IQ less than 70 was 47% and 62% for hypothermia and control groups, respectively (RR 0.76; 95% CI 0.58-0.99). When the results were adjusted for center effects, the RR was 0.78 with 95% CI 0.61-1.01. The results provide support that the beneficial effects of hypothermia persist into childhood.

Implementation of a New Therapy

Therapeutic hypothermia appears to have completed many of the hurdles of evaluation of a novel therapy, including laboratory observations, efficacy in animals, pilot studies in humans, and finally, completion of clinical trials demonstrating benefit. Therapeutic hypothermia is currently moving through a phase of dissemination and implementation as the treatment is adopted by centers that did not participate in clinical trials. Dissemination of new therapies often uncovers challenges evident in everyday practice that were not addressed in clinical trials even if the latter were

5

rigorously conducted. The following sections review important issues encountered as therapeutic hypothermia was disseminated throughout the neonatal community.

Temperature Control Before and After Therapeutic Hypothermia

An unanticipated observation of most randomized trials is that elevated temperatures occurred in the control group who were cared for under "normothermic" conditions. The percentages of infants with at least one core temperature value above 38.0° C were 39% in the study by Shankaran and colleagues,[15] 31% in the study by Gluckman and associates,[14] and 23% in the study by Azzopardi and coworkers.[17] Elevation of temperature in the setting of prior hypoxia-ischemia is of concern because it exacerbated the extent of injury following hypoxia-ischemia in 7-day-old rat pups.[23] Similarly, preventing hyperthermia reduced the extent of hypoxic-ischemic brain injury and seizures in 10-day-old rat pups.[24] Spontaneous hyperthermia is a well-recognized entity that occurs after hypoxia-ischemia or ischemia in animals[25] and after stroke in adult humans,[26] although the mechanism remains speculative. The elevated temperatures may be secondary to damage to the hypothalamic thermo-regulatory centers, endogenous pyrogens, or cytokine release.[27,28] It remains unclear whether the elevations in temperature found among infants in clinical trials of therapeutic hypothermia for neonatal HIE reflect existing brain injury as noted in experimental models[29] or lack of meticulous temperature control by the bedside provider.

Irrespective of the reason for the elevated temperature, there was an association between elevated temperature and poor outcome at follow-up among infants in the control arms of therapeutic hypothermia trials.[30,31] Results for such associations for the study by Shankaran and colleagues[15] are listed in Table 5-3. Logistic regressions were used to explore associations between temperature and outcome (death or neurodevelopmental disability) at 18 to 22 months of age.[31] The results indicate that there were relationships between elevated temperatures and outcome. Specifically, the average of the highest quartile of esophageal temperature for control infants was associated with a fourfold increase in the odds of death or disability for each degree increase in esophageal temperature. The odds of death alone were increased more than sixfold. Even the median esophageal temperature was associated with a 5.9-fold increase in the odds of death for each degree increase in esophageal temperature. There were no associations between the lowest quartile of esophageal temperature and death or disability.

These observations are pertinent to the care of infants at risk for or with evolving HIE prior to and after hypothermia therapy. Hyperthermia is to be avoided, and the goal should be stabilization with achievement and maintenance of normothermic temperatures. The latter principal has been embraced by the Neonatal Resuscitation Chapter Collaborators.[32] The implications for bedside providers are that monitoring of core body temperature needs to be frequent, a goal temperature range must be defined, and recognition by providers that temperatures exceeding the upper target

Table 5-3 ASSOCIATIONS BETWEEN ELEVATED ESOPHAGEAL TEMPERATURE AND DEATH OR DISABILITY AT 18-22 MONTHS*

Esophageal Temperature[†]	Death or Disability (n = 99)	Death (n = 99)	Disability (n = 65)
Highest quartile	4.0 (1.5-11.2)[‡]	6.2 (2.1-17.9)	1.8 (0.4-8.2)
Median	3.3 (0.9-11.2)	5.9 (1.5-22.7)	1.0 (0.2-5.1)

*Associations were determined by logistic regressions to relate esophageal temperature to death or disability with adjustment for race, gender, level of encephalopathy, and gestational age.
†Serial esophageal temperatures of each control infant during the 72-hour intervention were ranked, and the average of the highest quartile and the median temperature for each infant were used in the logistic regressions.
‡Results represent the odds ratio per degree centigrade change in temperature and the 95% confidence interval (in parentheses).

range merit prompt action. Confirmation of temperatures exceeding the upper limits should lead to preplanned interventions to rapidly reduce temperature into the goal target temperature range.

Assessment of Encephalopathy

All hypothermia regimens include a neurologic examination to determine whether infants are moderately or severely encephalopathic. As therapeutic hypothermia becomes disseminated, the issue of experience of medical providers who perform neurologic assessments will become more important. Newborn encephalopathy is not a common condition, and population studies indicate an incidence of 3.8 per 1000 term live births for moderate and severe involvement.[33] Unless medical providers work in high-volume patient centers, it may be difficult to maintain expertise in performing careful neurologic examinations. The extremes of abnormality—that is, no encephalopathy compared with severe encephalopathy—are straightforward to distinguish. The challenge is the infant who has some features of both mild and moderate encephalopathy. Programs that offer therapeutic hypothermia need to develop educational programs for such high-risk, low-frequency events to ensure accurate identification of encephalopathic infants and avoid subjecting infants to an unnecessary therapy.

Adding to the challenges of the neurologic status is the fact that the examination is not static and can improve or worsen, especially during the early hours following birth. It can be difficult to distinguish infants who have a poor respiratory drive and hypotonia at birth as a result of transient effects related to delivery (maternal analgesia, anesthesia, stress of delivery) from those with clinically important hypoxia-ischemia. Objective markers of impaired gas exchange (e.g., fetal acidemia based on cord blood or blood samples collected within an hour of birth) can help distinguish these possibilities, but such markers may not be available especially for infants born at outlying hospitals. In some animal models (fetal sheep) there was a clear relationship between time of initiation and efficacy of the therapy; greater neuroprotection was associated with earlier initiation of hypothermia.[6,34,35] Such experimental data support initiation of therapeutic hypothermia as fast as feasible after birth. In practice there are realistic limitations in the ability to initiate therapy in the first hour or two following birth. Often, hypoxic-ischemic events are unexpected, infants have undergone cardiopulmonary resuscitation, and an interval of stabilization (ventilator support, blood pressure, vascular access, acid-base correction as described in the case history) is needed before a careful neurologic examination can be performed. Time is also needed following birth to ensure that other etiologies do not account for the encephalopathy. Finally, not all animal models indicate that initiating hypothermia sooner is better.[36] Thus efforts should be made to avoid delay in the start of therapeutic hypothermia, but there are practical issues in stabilizing critically ill neonates that can limit achievement of this goal. Given these considerations, the neurologic examinations may end up being performed a few hours after birth, when the findings are less likely to be transient in nature.

Is an Amplitude-Integrated Electroencephalography Necessary?

As noted previously, it may be difficult to distinguish infants with mild encephalopathy from those with moderate encephalopathy because infants may have a mix of neurologic findings encountered in both levels of encephalopathy. The concept of using an objective measure of neurophysiologic function is therefore attractive. Three of the six randomized controlled trials of hypothermia for HIE presented used abnormalities on amplitude-integrated electroencephalography (aEEG) as an inclusion criterion to ensure that this new therapy was evaluated in infants with a high risk of brain injury and to avoid its use in infants with a favorable prognosis and little likelihood of benefit.[14,17,19] The aEEG inclusion criterion was part of a stepwise

5

approach in which potential study candidates needed to demonstrate biochemical/clinical abnormalities, followed by encephalopathy (modified Sarnat score) and moderate or severe abnormalities on aEEG. The data to justify aEEG as an inclusion criterion for enrollment into clinical trials were based upon multiple investigations that indicated that an abnormal aEEG pattern between 3 and 6 hours following birth is an accurate predictor of neurodevelopmental outcome at 1 year or beyond.[37-39] A meta-analysis of aEEG use in full-term infants with HIE indicated that aEEG had an overall sensitivity of 91% (95% CI 87%-95%) and a negative likelihood ratio of 0.09 (95% CI 0.06-0.15) for prediction of poor outcome.[40] These investigations are supported by those of the Cool Cap trial reported by Wyatt and colleagues, in which the aEEG amplitude pattern was independently associated with an unfavorable outcome (Gross Motor Functional Scores of 3-5, Bayley II Mental Developmental Index <70 or bilateral cortical visual impairment).[30] Subsequent reports comparing the prediction of outcome based on an aEEG acquired before 6 hours of age for infants kept normothermic compared with those undergoing hypothermia reflected the impact of cooling on neurodevelopmental outcome. Specifically, the positive predictive value of an abnormal aEEG pattern was 84% for normothermic infants and 59% for infants undergoing hypothermia.[41]

As use of aEEG has increased in NICUs, artifacts have been reported in the recordings that may alter the interpretation of the tracings.[42,43] Artifacts in EEG recordings may reflect muscle activity, electrode positioning, and application technique. Current devices allow inspection of the raw EEG signal that the aEEG is derived from and help determine whether artifacts are present. However, interpretation of the raw EEG signal is moving away from the original intent of the aEEG device, which was to provide a tool in which pattern recognition could be used by personnel without training in EEG. Of greater concern is the report from a single site in which the negative predictive value of the aEEG for adverse short-term outcomes (abnormal magnetic resonance imaging findings or death) was less than 50% and resulted in withholding of therapeutic hypothermia from infants with encephalopathy.[44] The latter observations raise the question of what is the added value of an aEEG recording for infants who fulfilled the criteria of biochemical/clinical abnormalities and have moderate or severe encephalopathy. A study initiated as part of the Shankaran trial continued after its end evaluated the predictive value of a 30-minute aEEG obtained at less than 9 hours of age for death or disability at 18 to 22 months of age among patients meeting criteria for therapeutic hypothermia.[45] Patients were enrolled from both the control and hypothermic groups of the Shankaran trial (n = 46) and were combined with infants enrolled after the study and before publication of results (n = 62). The results indicated that the positive predictive value of severe encephalopathy prior to 6 hours of age was higher than that of an abnormal aEEG pattern, but the positive predictive value of moderate encephalopathy was lower than of an abnormal aEEG pattern. Logistic regression was used to examine associations between the aEEG pattern, stage of encephalopathy, and hypothermia treatment with the outcome of death or disability. The odds of death or disability were higher with severe than with moderate encephalopathy (odds ratio [OR] 9.2; 95% CI 3.2-26.5). Hypothermia decreased the odds of death or disability (OR 0.3; 95% CI 0.1-0.8). There was no association between the aEEG pattern and death or disability, and no interactions between the aEEG pattern and either hypothermia or stage of encephalopathy.

The clinician is thus faced with conflicting results to discern whether an aEEG adds informative data that will alter the application of therapeutic hypothermia for individual patients. It has been speculated that an abnormal aEEG pattern in an infant who is encephalopathic may identify an infant who has either sustained a more severe insult or is manifesting greater injury than an encephalopathic infant who does not undergo aEEG. Available data cannot confirm this assertion. Given the favorable results of multiple clinical trials, adoption and application of therapeutic hypothermia should conform to guidelines established as part of protocols used in clinical trials and may have aEEG as an inclusion criterion. Providers using aEEG should be aware of potential caveats regarding aEEG technology.

Cooling on Transport

Among studies reporting outborn status, 45% to 82% of patients enrolled in clinical trials of therapeutic hypothermia had such status.[15,18-20] For clinicians outside of tertiary care centers, an important issue is temperature regulation following resuscitation and stabilization at birth until an infant is either enrolled in a trial or evaluations justify initiation of targeted temperature reduction. There is enthusiasm to initiate cooling at referral hospitals and during transport, given concerns over the duration of the therapeutic window. The duration of the therapeutic window for newborn infants is unknown but the best available data are from studies of fetal sheep undergoing brain ischemia with initiation of therapeutic hypothermia at different intervals following resolution of the ischemia. On the basis of this work the therapeutic window appears to be approximately 6 hours.[6,34,35]

Although cooling on transport has been used in some trials,[17,20,46] a systematic approach has not been developed. Specifically, biomedical devices that are designed for clinical use to monitor and control core temperature of neonates and be compatible with transport equipment do not exist. Clinical efforts to date to initiate hypothermia on transport have either stopped provision of exogenous heat and/or applied refrigerated gel packs over selected portions of the body.[47] The challenge of cooling on transport is underscored by observations that the metabolic response to a fall in ambient temperature (chemical regulation, increases in oxygen consumption) differs during normoxia and hypoxia and that it affects the rate of fall in temperature.[48] Whether alterations in chemical regulation persist following hypoxia-ischemia or such changes are proportionate to the extent of hypoxia-ischemia is unknown. Such gaps in knowledge underscore the potential for harm when cooling is initiated with the use of methods that cannot be controlled (e.g., removal of exogenous heat, local application of ice or cool gel packs to infants) even though temperature is being monitored. Later observations indicate that 34% of infants undergoing cooling on transport have rectal temperatures lower than 32° C, and infants with severe encephalopathy have greater falls in temperature than those with moderate encephalopathy.[49] Conversely, a fall in temperature following hypoxia-ischemia may be an adaptation to reduce metabolic demands and therefore may be potentially desirable.[50] However, the ideal or target temperature for an infant's temperature to fall to is unclear. Firm data to guide thermoregulatory practices for late preterm and term infants are lacking, and so the data used have largely been extrapolated from preterm infants studied in nurseries and without preceding hypoxia-ischemia. Given that brain temperature tracks systemic temperature with body cooling,[51] it is unclear how much vacillation in brain temperature occurs when uncontrolled cooling is undertaken because overshoot of target temperature prompts rewarming[52]; whether such temperature profiles are therapeutic or detrimental is unclear. Understanding the metabolic response to cooling among infants with HIE may help guide the induction of hypothermia in as safe a manner as possible.

There are attempts to develop consensus guidelines for "passive" cooling.[49,53] In the United Kingdom, a 9-month experience has been collated using such an approach.[53] The latter involved removal of exogenous heat combined with continuous monitoring of skin temperatures and intermittent monitoring of rectal temperature among referring centers after discussion with the retrieving center. Upon arrival of the transport team, continuous rectal temperature monitoring was initiated in combination with an algorithm of adjusting the air temperature of the transport isolette (by 0.5° C, starting value 25° C) and use of blankets if the temperature was too low. Results of this approach are plotted in Figure 5-1. The data demonstrated a convergence of rectal temperatures toward the target temperature range and at first glance suggest that this approach is acceptable. However, convergence to the target temperature is enhanced by the very wide temperature range upon leaving the referral hospital ($\approx$31° to >36° C). This range raises concerns regarding the efficacy of initiating cooling at referring hospitals by personnel who do not perform this function frequently. In addition many of the transports were of short duration (30 minutes) and maintenance of temperature over longer intervals needs to be studied further.

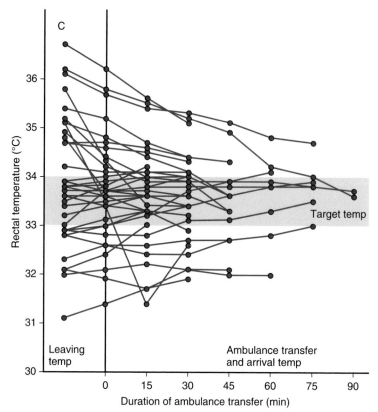

Figure 5-1 Rectal temperatures are plotted for each infant transported to a center for therapeutic hypothermia. Final temperatures at the referring hospital prior to transport are plotted on the left side of the figure (Leaving temp). Target temperature range (Target temp) is demarcated by the *shaded horizontal band* (33°-34° C). Temperatures on transport are plotted every 15 minutes for infants until their arrival at the retrieving center. (Data from Kendall GS, Kapetanakis A, Ratnavel N, et al. Passive cooling for initiation of therapeutic hypothermia in neonatal encephalopathy. *Arch Dis Child Fetal Neonatal Ed.* 2010;95:F408-F412.)

These observations emphasize that what is needed to properly initiate cooling on transport are biomedical devices that interface with existing transport equipment, allow continuous monitoring of core temperature, and provide an efficient mechanism to keep temperature within a narrow range. Existing devices have limited abilities in this regard,[54] although there are newer devices that may be better suited.[55,56]

Selective Use of Therapeutic Hypothermia

Should therapeutic hypothermia be initiated in all encephalopathic infants, assuming there is reasonable certainty that hypoxia-ischemia is the etiology? The issue arises from follow-up results of encephalopathic infants in which the outcome of infants with severe encephalopathy was almost uniformly death or severe neurodevelopmental disability.[57,58] Importantly, these follow-up results reflect associations between the maximal stage of encephalopathy (mild, moderate, or severe) during the first week of life and early childhood outcome. This situation differs from that in all clinical trials of therapeutic hypothermia, in which stage of encephalopathy was determined prior to 6 hours of age.[14,15,17-20] In all of the published trials listed in Table 5-1, the primary outcome was assessed as a function of stage of encephalopathy at randomization. Meta-analysis of the Gluckman,[14] Shankaran,[14] and Azzopardi[17] trials by Edwards and associates[4] indicated that death or disability was reduced by hypothermia among infants with moderate encephalopathy (RR 0.73; 95% CI 0.58-0.92) but not for severe encephalopathy (RR 0.87; 95% CI 0.75-.1.01). Similar results were reported in the meta-analysis by Shah,[59] who analyzed six studies, but the confidence intervals were wider for severe encephalopathy (RR 0.62; 95% CI 0.33-1.18) relative to the Edwards analysis. The results of both meta-analyses suggest that initiating hypothermia for infants with severe encephalopathy is doing no harm and the direction of effect is toward benefit for the studies analyzed by Edwards and associates.[4]

Future of Therapeutic Hypothermia

The currently available data provide a strong evidence base that therapeutic hypothermia reduces death or disability among infants born at 36 weeks of gestation or later with encephalopathy due to hypoxia-ischemia. Although only selected studies demonstrated a significant reduction in the outcome, meta-analyses indicates a relatively homogenous effect among major trials and a significant decrease in death or disability.[4,59] Therapeutic hypothermia represents the only proven therapy to change the outcome of infants with HIE. Yet, it is striking that 40% to 50% of infants treated with therapeutic hypothermia still have an outcome of death or disability. When the current status is viewed from this perspective, there is a pressing need for improvements in therapy for this condition.

One future direction for investigation would be improvements in the efficacy of current therapeutic hypothermia regimens. Current regimens (head or body cooling, time to initiate therapy, target temperature, duration of cooling, and rate of rewarming) were arrived at on the basis of best extrapolation from prior animal studies. Whether these parameters are optimal and result in the best possible outcomes from therapeutic hypothermia was not evaluated in any of the trials to date and remains a knowledge gap. There is now ample evidence in newborn models of brain injury that the cascade of events (e.g., inflammation, apoptosis) contributing to injury extends over days to even weeks.[10] A randomized trial is ongoing to determine whether a lower target temperature or a longer duration of therapeutic hypothermia improve outcome relative to current regimens.[60] At present there is no proven therapy for infants with encephalopathy who meet criteria for therapeutic hypothermia after 6 hours of age. A randomized trial is ongoing to address this issue because the duration of the therapeutic window is unknown for human infants and may be modified by many clinical variables.[61]

Another research strategy following neonatal hypoxia-ischemia is to combine therapeutic hypothermia with other potential neuroprotective therapies. This approach may provide benefit by creating a synergistic effect or incrementally adding improvement to the outcome achieved with hypothermia. Hypothermia functions to stop the cascade of potentially injurious events and is not known to promote repair; it may serve to widen the therapeutic window and provide time for initiation of other therapies. Candidate therapies that have shown promise in the laboratory include erythropoietin,[62,63] xenon,[64] topiramate,[65] N-acetylcysteine,[66] and melatonin.[67] A number of these therapies have been combined with hypothermia and have enhanced the neuroprotective effect of temperature reductions.[66,68,69] Therapies used in combination with hypothermia require close scrutiny for intrinsic toxicity to brain as well as modification of drug/metabolite excretion by hypothermia and/or hypoxic-ischemic hepatic and renal injury.[70]

The importance of therapeutic hypothermia goes beyond the trials conducted to date. The experience with this therapy confirms that encephalopathy secondary to hypoxia-ischemia is a modifiable condition and has accelerated the focus of research to both improve hypothermia regimens and find other interventions to supplement hypothermia.

References

1. American College of Obstetricians and Gynecologists, American Academy of Pediatrics. Background. In: *Neonatal encephalopathy and cerebral palsy: Defining the pathogenesis and pathophysiology*. Washington, DC: American College of Obstetricians and Gynecologists Distribution Center; 2003:1-11.
2. Freeman JM, Nelson KB. Intrapartum asphyxia and cerebral palsy. *Pediatrics*. 1988;82:240-249.
3. Badawi N, Kurinczuk JJ, Keogh JM, et al. Intrapartum risk factors for newborn encephalopathy: the Western Australian case-control study. *BMJ*. 1998;317:1554-1558.

5

4. Edwards AD, Brocklehurst P, Gunn AJ, et al. Neurological outcomes at 18 months of age after moderate hypothermia for perinatal hypoxic ischaemic encephalopathy: synthesis and meta-analysis of trial data. *BMJ*. 2010;340:c363.

5. Thoresen M, Penrice J, Lorek A, et al. Mild hypothermia after severe transient hypoxia-ischemia ameliorates delayed cerebral energy failure in the newborn piglet. *Pediatr Res*. 1995;37:667-670.

6. Gunn AJ, Gunn TR, de Haan HH, et al. Dramatic neuronal rescue with prolonged selective head cooling after ischemia in fetal lambs. *J Clin Invest*. 1997;99:248-256.

7. Laptook AR, Corbett RJ, Sterett R, et al. Modest hypothermia provides partial neuroprotection for ischemic neonatal brain. *Pediatr Res*. 1994;35:436-442.

8. Lorek A, Takei Y, Cady EB, et al. Delayed ("secondary") cerebral energy failure after acute hypoxia-ischemia in the newborn piglet: continuous 48-hour studies by phosphorus magnetic resonance spectroscopy. *Pediatr Res*. 1994;36:699-706.

9. Johnston MV, Trescher WH, Ishida A, Nakajima W. Neurobiology of hypoxic-ischemic injury in the developing brain. *Pediatr Res*. 2001;49:735-741.

10. Ferriero DM. Neonatal brain injury. *N Engl J Med*. 2004;351:1985-1995.

11. Vannucci RC, Towfighi J, Vannucci SJ. Secondary energy failure after cerebral hypoxia-ischemia in the immature rat. *J Cereb Blood Flow Metab*. 2004;24:1090-1097.

12. Gunn AJ, Thoresen M. Hypothermic neuroprotection. *NeuroRx*. 2006;3:154-169.

13. Laptook AR, Corbett RJ. The effects of temperature on hypoxic-ischemic brain injury. *Clin Perinatol*. 2002;29:623-649.

14. Gluckman PD, Wyatt JS, Azzopardi D, et al. Selective head cooling with mild systemic hypothermia after neonatal encephalopathy: multicentre randomised trial. *Lancet*. 2005;365:663-670.

15. Shankaran S, Laptook AR, Ehrenkranz RA, et al. Whole-body hypothermia for neonates with hypoxic-ischemic encephalopathy. *N Engl J Med*. 2005;353:1574-1584.

16. Laptook A. Brain cooling for neonatal encephalopathy: Potential indications for use. In: Perlman JM, ed. *Neurology: Neonatology questions and controversies*. Philadelphia: Saunders Elsevier; 2008: 66-78.

17. Azzopardi DV, Strohm B, Edwards AD, et al. Moderate hypothermia to treat perinatal asphyxial encephalopathy. *N Engl J Med*. 2009;361:1349-1358.

18. Zhou WH, Cheng GQ, Shao XM, et al. Selective head cooling with mild systemic hypothermia after neonatal hypoxic-ischemic encephalopathy: a multicenter randomized controlled trial in China. *J Pediatr*. 2010;157:367-372.

19. Simbruner G, Mittal RA, Rohlmann F, Muche R. Systemic hypothermia after neonatal encephalopathy: outcomes of neo.nEURO.network RCT. *Pediatrics*. 2010;126:e771-e778.

20. Jacobs SE, Morley CJ, Inder TE, et al. Whole body hypothermia for term and near term newborns with hypoxic-ischemic encephalopathy. *Arch Pediatr Adolesc Med*. 2011;165:692-700.

21. Shankaran S, Pappas A, Laptook AR, et al. Outcomes of safety and effectiveness in a multicenter randomized, controlled trial of whole-body hypothermia for neonatal hypoxic-ischemic encephalopathy. *Pediatrics*. 2008;122:e791-e798.

22. Shankaran S. Does neuroprotective effect of whole body hypothermia for neonatal hypoxic-ischemic encephalopathy persist to childhood? E-PAS2011:16608.

23. Fukuda H, Tomimatsu T, Kanagawa T, et al. Postischemic hyperthermia induced caspase-3 activation in the newborn rat brain after hypoxia-ischemia and exacerbated the brain damage. *Biol Neonate*. 2003;84:164-171.

24. Yager JY, Armstrong EA, Jaharus C, et al. Preventing hyperthermia decreases brain damage following neonatal hypoxic-ischemic seizures. *Brain Res*. 2004;1011:48-57.

25. Reglodi D, Somogyvari-Vigh A, Maderdrut JL, et al. Postischemic spontaneous hyperthermia and its effects in middle cerebral artery occlusion in the rat. *Exp Neurol*. 2000;163:399-407.

26. Boysen G, Christensen H. Stroke severity determines body temperature in acute stroke. *Stroke*. 2001;32:413-417.

27. Chai Z, Gatti S, Toniatti C, et al. Interleukin (IL)-6 gene expression in the central nervous system is necessary for fever response to lipopolysaccharide or IL-1 beta: a study on IL-6-deficient mice. *J Exp Med*. 1996;183:311-316.

28. Lesnikov VA, Efremov OM, Korneva EA, et al. Fever produced by intrahypothalamic injection of interleukin-1 and interleukin-6. *Cytokine*. 1991;3:195-198.

29. Dietrich WD, Bramlett HM. Hyperthermia and central nervous system injury. *Prog Brain Res*. 2007;162:201-217.

30. Wyatt JS, Gluckman PD, Liu PY, et al. Determinants of outcomes after head cooling for neonatal encephalopathy. *Pediatrics*. 2007;119:912-921.

31. Laptook A, Tyson J, Shankaran S, et al. Elevated temperature after hypoxic-ischemic encephalopathy: risk factor for adverse outcomes. *Pediatrics*. 2008;122:491-499.

32. Perlman JM, Wyllie J, Kattwinkel J, et al; Neonatal Resuscitation Chapter Collaborators. Part 11: neonatal resuscitation: 2010 International Consensus on Cardiopulmonary Resuscitation and Emergency Cardiovascular Care Science With Treatment Recommendations. *Circulation*. 2010;122(Suppl 2):S516-S538.

33. Badawi N, Kurinczuk JJ, Keogh JM, et al. Antepartum risk factors for newborn encephalopathy: the Western Australian case-control study. *BMJ*. 1998;317:1549-1553.

34. Gunn AJ, Gunn TR, Gunning MI, et al. Neuroprotection with prolonged head cooling started before postischemic seizures in fetal sheep. *Pediatrics*. 1998;102:1098-1106.

35. Gunn AJ, Bennet L, Gunning MI, et al. Cerebral hypothermia is not neuroprotective when started after postischemic seizures in fetal sheep. *Pediatr Res*. 1999;46:274-280.

36. Taylor DL, Mehmet H, Cady EB, Edwards AD. Improved neuroprotection with hypothermia delayed by 6 hours following cerebral hypoxia-ischemia in the 14-day-old rat. *Pediatr Res.* 2002; 51:13-19.
37. Hellstrom-Westas L, Rosen I, Svenningsen NW. Predictive value of early continuous amplitude integrated EEG recordings on outcome after severe birth asphyxia in full term infants. *Arch Dis Child Fetal Neonatal Ed.* 1995;72:F34-F38.
38. Toet MC, Hellstrom-Westas L, Groenendaal F, et al. Amplitude integrated EEG 3 and 6 hours after birth in full term neonates with hypoxic-ischaemic encephalopathy. *Arch Dis Child Fetal Neonatal Ed.* 1999;81:F19-F23.
39. Shany E, Goldstein E, Khvatskin S, et al. Predictive value of amplitude-integrated electroencephalography pattern and voltage in asphyxiated term infants. *Pediatr Neurol.* 2006;35:335-342.
40. Spitzmiller RE, Phillips T, Meinzen-Derr J, Hoath SB. Amplitude-integrated EEG is useful in predicting neurodevelopmental outcome in full-term infants with hypoxic-ischemic encephalopathy: a meta-analysis. *J Child Neurol.* 2007;22:1069-1078.
41. Thoresen M, Hellstrom-Westas L, Liu X, de Vries LS. Effect of hypothermia on amplitude-integrated electroencephalogram in infants with asphyxia. *Pediatrics.* 2010;126:e131-e139.
42. Hagmann CF, Robertson NJ, Azzopardi D. Artifacts on electroencephalograms may influence the amplitude-integrated EEG classification: a qualitative analysis in neonatal encephalopathy. *Pediatrics.* 2006;118:2552-2554.
43. Suk D, Krauss AN, Engel M, Perlman JM. Amplitude-integrated electroencephalography in the NICU: frequent artifacts in premature infants may limit its utility as a monitoring device. *Pediatrics.* 2009; 123:e328-e332.
44. Sarkar S, Barks JD, Donn SM. Should amplitude-integrated electroencephalography be used to identify infants suitable for hypothermic neuroprotection? *J Perinatol.* 2008;28:117-122.
45. Shankaran S, Pappas A, McDonald SA, et al. Predictive value of an early amplitude integrated electroencephalogram and neurologic examination. *Pediatrics.* 2011;128:e112-e120.
46. Eicher DJ, Wagner CL, Katikaneni LP, et al. Moderate hypothermia in neonatal encephalopathy: efficacy outcomes. *Pediatr Neurol.* 2005;32:11-17.
47. Zanelli SA, Naylor M, Dobbins N, et al. Implementation of a 'Hypothermia for HIE' program: 2-year experience in a single NICU. *J Perinatol.* 2008;28:171-175.
48. Mortola JP, Dotta A. Effects of hypoxia and ambient temperature on gaseous metabolism of newborn rats. *Am J Physiol.* 1992;263:R267-R272.
49. Fairchild K, Sokora D, Scott J, Zanelli S. Therapeutic hypothermia on neonatal transport: 4-year experience in a single NICU. *J Perinatol.* 2010;30:324-329.
50. Wood SC, Gonzales R. Hypothermia in hypoxic animals: mechanisms, mediators, and functional significance. *Comp Biochem Physiol B Biochem Mol Biol.* 1996;113:37-43.
51. Laptook AR, Shalak L, Corbett RJ. Differences in brain temperature and cerebral blood flow during selective head versus whole-body cooling. *Pediatrics.* 2001;108:1103-1110.
52. Hallberg B, Olson L, Bartocci M, et al. Passive induction of hypothermia during transport of asphyxiated infants: a risk of excessive cooling. *Acta Paediatr.* 2009;98:942-946.
53. Kendall GS, Kapetanakis A, Ratnavel N, et al. Passive cooling for initiation of therapeutic hypothermia in neonatal encephalopathy. *Arch Dis Child Fetal Neonatal Ed.* 2010;95:F408-F412.
54. Rabenstein E, Tyree M, Dirnberger D, DiGeronimo R. Whole body hypothermia using a portable cooling unit in a neonatal pig model: Implications for transport. *J Neonatal-Perinatal Med.* 2010;3: 15-20.
55. Strohm B, Azzopardi D. Temperature control during therapeutic moderate whole-body hypothermia for neonatal encephalopathy. *Arch Dis Child Fetal Neonatal Ed.* 2010;95:F373-F375.
56. Hoque N, Chakkarapani E, Liu X, Thoresen M. A comparison of cooling methods used in therapeutic hypothermia for perinatal asphyxia. *Pediatrics.* 2010;126:e124-e130.
57. Robertson C, Finer N. Term infants with hypoxic-ischemic encephalopathy: outcome at 3.5 years. *Dev Med Child Neurol.* 1985;27:473-484.
58. Robertson CM, Finer NN, Grace MG. School performance of survivors of neonatal encephalopathy associated with birth asphyxia at term. *J Pediatr.* 1989;114:753-760.
59. Shah PS. Hypothermia: a systematic review and meta-analysis of clinical trials. *Semin Fetal Neonatal Med.* 2010;15:238-246.
60. U.S. National Institutes of Health. ClinicalTrials.gov: Optimizing (longer, deeper) cooling for neonatal hypoxic-ischemic encephalopathy. http://clinicaltrials.gov/ct2/show/NCT01192776?term=hypothermia+AND+neonatal+hypoxic+ischemic.
61. U.S. National Institutes of Health. ClinicalTrials.gov: Late hypothermia for hypoxic-ischemic encephalopathy. http://clinicaltrials.gov/ct2/show/NCT00614744?term=hypothermia+AND+neonatal+hypoxic+ischemic.
62. Gonzalez FF, Abel R, Almli CR, et al. Erythropoietin sustains cognitive function and brain volume after neonatal stroke. *Developmental neuroscience.* 2009;31:403-411.
63. Gonzalez FF, McQuillen P, Mu D, et al. Erythropoietin enhances long-term neuroprotection and neurogenesis in neonatal stroke. *Dev Neurosci.* 2007;29:321-330.
64. David HN, Haelewyn B, Rouillon C, et al. Neuroprotective effects of xenon: a therapeutic window of opportunity in rats subjected to transient cerebral ischemia. *FASEB J.* 2008;22:1275-1286.
65. Schubert S, Brandl U, Brodhun M, et al. Neuroprotective effects of topiramate after hypoxia-ischemia in newborn piglets. *Brain Res.* 2005;1058:129-136.
66. Jatana M, Singh I, Singh AK, Jenkins D. Combination of systemic hypothermia and N-acetylcysteine attenuates hypoxic-ischemic brain injury in neonatal rats. *Pediatr Res.* 2006;59:684-689.

67. Carloni S, Perrone S, Buonocore G, et al. Melatonin protects from the long-term consequences of a neonatal hypoxic-ischemic brain injury in rats. *J Pineal Res.* 2008;44:157-164.
68. Thoresen M, Hobbs CE, Wood T, et al. Cooling combined with immediate or delayed xenon inhalation provides equivalent long-term neuroprotection after neonatal hypoxia-ischemia. *J Cereb Blood Flow Metab.* 2009;29:707-714.
69. Liu Y, Barks JD, Xu G, Silverstein FS. Topiramate extends the therapeutic window for hypothermia-mediated neuroprotection after stroke in neonatal rats. *Stroke.* 2004;35:1460-1465.
70. Roka A, Melinda KT, Vasarhelyi B, et al. Elevated morphine concentrations in neonates treated with morphine and prolonged hypothermia for hypoxic ischemic encephalopathy. *Pediatrics.* 2008; 121:e844-e849.

5

General Supportive Management of the Term Infant with Neonatal Encephalopathy Following Intrapartum Hypoxia-Ischemia

Ericalyn Kasdorf, MD, and Jeffrey M. Perlman, MB, ChB

6

- Delivery Room Management
- Early Identification of Infants at Highest Risk for Development of Hypoxic-Ischemic Brain Injury
- Supportive Care
- Potential Neuroprotective Strategies Aimed at Ameliorating Secondary Brain Injury
- Gaps on Knowledge

CASE HISTORY

HI was a 3200-g, 38-week male infant born to a 28-year-old G2P1 (gravida 2, para 1) mother following an uncomplicated pregnancy. Labor was complicated by a maternal temperature of 38.5° C (mother was treated with antibiotics), prolonged second stage associated with variable decelerations, and a bradycardic episode that resulted in an emergency cesarean section. Meconium staining of the amniotic fluid was noted. The infant was delivered floppy and with no respiratory effort. Resuscitation included intubation for meconium that was negative, reintubation, and positive-pressure ventilation (PPV). The initial heart rate was 50 beats per minute (bpm) but increased rapidly to >100 bpm within 30 seconds of the start of PPV. The infant's color improved, and he took a first gasp at 4 minutes and made a first respiratory effort at 8 minutes. A rectal temperature in the delivery room was 38.2° C. The Apgar scores were 1 (1), 4 (5), and 7 (10). The infant was transferred to the neonatal intensive care unit (NICU) for further management. The cord arterial blood gas analysis revealed a PCO_2 of 101 mm Hg, pH of 6.78, and base deficit of −23 mEq/L. The initial arterial blood gas analysis at 30 minutes revealed a PaO_2 of 146 mm Hg (on 50% oxygen), PCO_2 of 30 mm Hg, and pH of 7.12. Initial blood glucose was 32 mg/dL. This was treated with a 2-mL/kg bolus of $D_{10}W$, and subsequent glucose was 84 mg/dL. The initial clinical assessment revealed a lethargic infant with a low-level sensory response. The anterior fontanel was soft. The capillary refill time was approximately 2 seconds. Pertinent cardiovascular findings were heart rate 134 bpm and blood pressure 44/24 mm Hg with a mean of 34 mm Hg. He was intubated and on modest ventilator support with equal but coarse breath sounds. The abdomen was soft and without masses. The central nervous examination revealed pupils that were 3 mm and reactive. There were weak gag and suck reflexes, along with central hypotonia with proximal weakness. The reflexes were present and symmetric. The encephalopathy at this stage was categorized as Sarnat stage 2. Because of the history and clinical findings, the infant underwent an amplitude-integrated electroencephalography (aEEG) examination that revealed a moderately suppressed pattern without seizure activity.

The infant met criteria for cooling, which was initiated at approximately 4 hours of age. At 12 hours of age the infant began to exhibit subtle seizure activity with blinking of the eyes, mouth smacking, and horizontal eye deviation associated with desaturation episodes. A clinical diagnosis of seizures was made, and the infant was loaded with phenobarbital (40 mg/kg). The seizures, including the evolution of aEEG seizures, persisted over the next 12 hours and the infant was given phosphenytoin and additional phenobarbital and was started on a midazolam drip before control of the clinical as well as the electrographic seizures was achieved. The encephalopathy peaked on day of life (DOL) 2, and the infant remained in Sarnat stage 2 encephalopathy. The supportive management included fluid restriction; the initial urine output was less than 1 mL/kg/hour for the first 24 hours but increased thereafter, and by DOL 3 the infant was in a diuretic phase. Sodium was initially 136 mEq/L, reached a nadir of 128 mEq/L on DOL 3, but corrected over the next 36 hours. The initial serum bicarbonate level was 18 mEq/L with an anion gap of 16. Both resolved spontaneously by DOL 3. The infant received assisted ventilation until DOL 3, and the P_{CO_2} values ranged between 40 and 50 mm Hg. Additional abnormalities included low calcium and magnesium (DOL 2) and mildly elevated liver enzymes. The infant was started on low-dose dopamine for approximately 24 hours for a low mean blood pressure. He was treated with antibiotics for 7 days for presumed sepsis, although the blood culture results remained negative. Parenteral nutrition was initiated on DOL 3, tube feedings were started on DOL 4, and the infant was able to achieve full nipple feedings on DOL 14. The neurologic findings improved although were still abnormal—central hypotonia and increased deep tendon reflexes at the time of discharge. Magnetic resonance imaging (MRI) on DOL 7 revealed marked hyperintensity on the diffusion-weighted images within the putamen and thalamus bilaterally. Findings of repeat EEG were pertinent for mild background slowing. Finally, the placental pathology was consistent with acute chorioamnionitis. The infant was discharged on DOL 16.

This case illustrates typical evolving neonatal encephalopathy following intrapartum hypoxia-ischemia against the background of placental infection/inflammation. The brain injury that develops is an evolving process that is initiated during the insult and extends into a recovery period, the latter referred to as the "reperfusion phase" of injury.[1-3] Management of such an infant should be initiated in the delivery room with effective resuscitation and continued through the evolving process. It comprises identification of the infant at high risk for developing evolving brain injury, supportive therapy to facilitate adequate perfusion and nutrients to the brain, and neuroprotective strategies, including therapeutic hypothermia as well as therapy targeted at the cellular level to ameliorate the processes of ongoing brain injury (see Chapter 5). These management components are briefly discussed in this chapter.

Hypoxic-ischemic encephalopathy (HIE) is an infrequent event with a range of reported incidences but likely occurring in less than 1 of 1000 live term deliveries in the developed world. HIE secondary to intrapartum asphyxia is a widely recognized cause of long-term neurologic sequelae, including cerebral palsy.[4] Severe and prolonged interruption of placental blood flow will ultimately lead to asphyxia, the biochemical process characterized by worsening hypoxia, hypercarbia, and acidosis (in the more severe cases defined as an umbilical arterial cord pH $\leq$ 7.00).[5] During the acute phase of asphyxia, the ability to autoregulate cerebral blood flow (CBF) in order to maintain cerebral perfusion is lost. When this state occurs, CBF becomes entirely dependent on blood pressure to maintain perfusion pressure, a term known as a *pressure-passive cerebral circulation*.[1] With interruption of placental blood flow the fetus will attempt to maintain CBF by redistributing cardiac output not only to the brain but also to the adrenal glands and myocardium. This redistribution occurs at the expense of blood flow to kidneys, intestine, and skin.[5] Even a moderate decrease in blood pressure at this stage could lead to severely compromised CBF. With ongoing hypoxia-ischemia, CBF declines, leading to deleterious cellular effects. With oxygen depletion a number of cellular alterations occur, including replacement of oxidative phosphorylation with anaerobic metabolism, diminution of adenosine triphosphate (ATP), intracellular acidosis, and accumulation particularly of calcium. The ultimate deleterious effects include the release of excitatory neurotransmitters, such as glutamate, free radical production from fatty acid peroxidation, and nitric oxide (NO)–mediated neurotoxicity, all resulting in cell death.[4,5] Following resuscitation and the reestablishment of CBF and oxygenation, a phase of secondary energy failure occurs. In the experimental paradigm this phase transpires from 6 to 48 hours after the initial insult and is thought to be related to extension of the preceding mechanisms, leading to mitochondrial dysfunction.[2] It is clear that during asphyxia, not only the brain but also many other vital organs are at risk for injury. For this reason, postresuscitation management of the infant who has suffered intrapartum hypoxia-ischemia must also focus on supporting those systemic organs that may have been injured. Future therapies must also target the cellular injury that occurs following asphyxia.

Delivery Room Management

The use of room air or oxygen in the delivery room has been previously identified as a gap in knowledge that is crucial to resolve. Resuscitation of the depressed neonate is aimed at restoring blood flow and oxygen delivery to the tissues. In the past it was recommended to initiate resuscitation with 100% oxygen at the time of delivery. However, the most current international guidelines recommend beginning resuscitation with room air or blended oxygen, with the goal of achieving oxygen saturations in the interquartile range of preductal saturations measured in healthy term babies born vaginally at sea level (Table 6-1).[6] This concept is based in part on three meta-analyses. The first pooled analysis from 2004 demonstrated decreased mortality when room air was used in place of 100% oxygen for resuscitation, although no individual trial demonstrated a difference in mortality.[7] A 2005 Cochrane meta-analysis showed a significant reduction in the rate of death in infants resuscitated with room air in comparison with 100% oxygen (relative risk [RR] 0.71; 95% confidence interval [CI] 0.54-0.94). Of note, there was no significant difference in incidence of grade 2 or 3 hypoxic-ischemic encephalopathy (based on Sarnat staging) between groups.[8] The third meta-analysis, performed by Rabi and colleagues,[8] included two additional studies and demonstrated similar findings—a lower mortality in the room air group than in the 100% oxygen resuscitation group in the first week of life (odds ratio [OR] 0.7; 95% CI 0.5-0.98), and at 1 month (OR 0.63; 95% CI 0.42-0.94). Again, there was no difference between groups in incidence of grade 2 or 3 HIE.[9] It remains unclear why this discordance exists, because one might have

Table 6-1 TARGETED PREDUCTUAL SpO$_2$ AFTER BIRTH

Time after Birth (min)	SpO$_2$ Level (%)
1	60-70
2	65-70
3	70-75
4	75-80
5	80-85
10	85-95

Adapted from Kattwinkel J, Perlman JM, Aziz K, et al. Neonatal resuscitation: 2010 American Heart Association Guidelines for Cardiopulmonary Resuscitation and Emergency Cardiovascular Care. *Pediatrics.* 2010;126:e1400-e1413.

anticipated more severe encephalopathy in the oxygen-treated group if brain injury and mortality are linked. Clearly the mechanisms contributing to death in the oxygen group are important to determine. An additional potentially important observation in another study is the finding of biochemical markers indicative of oxidative stress, present even after 4 weeks of life, in infants resuscitated at birth with 100% oxygen compared with room air.[10] Finally, in the context of resuscitation, there was a delay to both first cry and sustained pattern of respirations in this study in infants resuscitated with 100% oxygen.[10]

There have been few studies comparing room air with 100% oxygen during resuscitation that assessed long-term follow-up. One study demonstrated increased risk of adverse outcome, defined as death or severe neurodevelopmental disability, by 24 months of age in infants diagnosed with asphyxia and exposed to severe hyperoxemia in the first 2 hours of life (defined as PaO_2 >200 mm Hg).[11] A second study with follow-up at 18 to 24 months (albeit with a high dropout rate) showed no difference in neurologic handicap between the group resuscitated with room air and that resuscitated with 100% oxygen.[12]

Some experimental studies do suggest of oxygen over room air as it relates to the brain and systemic circulation. Thus resuscitation with 100% oxygen is associated with significantly more rapid restoration of hypoxia-depressed CBF, improved cerebral perfusion, and significantly lower levels of excitatory amino acid levels in striatum as well as more favorable short- and long-term outcomes in surviving adult mice.[13,14] Additionally, in mice exposed to hypoxia-ischemia associated with circulatory arrest, resuscitation with 100% oxygen resulted in significantly greater rates of return of spontaneous circulation than that with room air.[15] These observations may be akin to the neonate with sustained bradycardia in the delivery room that is reflective of circulatory hypoperfusion. Currently the international consensus is to begin with room air for those infants requiring positive-pressure ventilation at the time of birth. However the oxygen concentration should be increased in those infants with depressed heart rate despite effective ventilation or with oxygen saturation not reaching the desired range.[6,16]

There is a critical need for ongoing studies assessing the use of room air versus supplemental oxygen, because three of the largest studies that have driven the meta-analyses and the international guidelines were conducted in developing countries where antenatal and peripartum care, as well as neonatal mortality rates, differ from those in the developed world.[8]

Early Identification of Infants at Highest Risk for Development of Hypoxic-Ischemic Brain Injury

The initial step in management is early identification of those infants at greatest risk for going on to have the syndrome of HIE. This is a highly relevant issue because the therapeutic window—that is, the interval following hypoxia-ischemia during which interventions might be efficacious in reducing the severity of ultimate brain injury—is likely to be short. It is estimated on the basis of experimental studies to vary from soon following the insult to approximately 6 hours. Given this presumed short window of opportunity, infants must be identified as soon as possible following delivery in order to facilitate the implementation of early interventions as described in the case history. What put the infant at high risk? There was clinical evidence to suggest chorioamnionitis, there was fetal bradycardia prior to delivery, the infant was severely depressed, there was the need for resuscitation in the delivery room (i.e., intubation and positive-pressure ventilation), and there was evidence of severe fetal acidemia,[17] followed by evidence of early abnormal neurologic findings and abnormal cerebral function as demonstrated by amplitude-integrated EEG.[18-20] Indeed the infant progressed to stage 2 encephalopathy with seizures.

Supportive Care

A summary of supportive management is given in Box 6-1.

> **Box 6-1   SUMMARY OF SUPPORTIVE MANAGEMENT FOR NEONATAL ENCEPHALOPATHY AFTER HYPOXIA-ISCHEMIA**
>
> Delivery room:
> - Resuscitation beginning with room air ± supplemental oxygen if needed
>
> Temperature:
> - Avoid hyperthermia
>
> Ventilation:
> - Maintain $PaCO_2$ in normal range
>
> Perfusion:
> - Promptly treat hypotension
> - Avoid hypertension
>
> Fluid status:
> - Initial fluid restriction
> - Follow serum sodium concentration and daily weights

Ventilation

Assessment of adequate respiratory function is critical in the infant with HIE. Inadequate ventilation and frequent apneic episodes are not uncommon in severely affected infants, necessitating assisted ventilation. Changes in $PaCO_2$ can affect CBF such that hypercarbia increases and hypocarbia decreases blood flow.[21] Thus careful monitoring of the arterial blood gases and level of $PaCO_2$ is of particular importance. Some experimental studies suggest that modest elevation in $PaCO_2$ (50-55 mm Hg) at the time of hypoxia-ischemia is associated with better outcome than when the $PaCO_2$ is within the normal (mid-30s) range.[22] However, this is a complex issue, in that progressive hypercarbia in ventilated premature infants is associated with loss of autoregulation.[23] In patients with head trauma, hyperventilation has been used as a strategy to lower intracranial pressure. However, when hyperventilation with subsequent hypocarbia has been used for the treatment of term infants with pulmonary hypertension, there has been associated hearing loss. In a study of term infants diagnosed with intrapartum asphyxia, severe hypocapnia (defined as $PaCO_2$ <20 mm Hg) led to increased risk of adverse outcome defined as death or severe neurodevelopmental disability at 12 months of age.[11] Moreover in the management of preterm infants with respiratory distress syndrome (RDS), the presence of hypocarbia has been associated with periventricular leukomalacia (PVL) (see Chapter 3). Because of the divergent experimental and clinical data, it is recommended that the $PaCO_2$ be maintained in the normal range in mechanically ventilated infants at risk for HIE. This process is more complicated in clinical practice, because these infants often compensate for the underlying metabolic acidosis present via hyperventilation with resultant hypocarbia. In a study assessing carbon dioxide levels and adverse outcomes in infants with HIE, only 11.5% of infants demonstrated normocapnia through the first 3 days of life; moderate hypocapnia was seen in 29% of infants, and severe hypocapnia in 5.8%.[24] These observations illustrate the difficulty in maintaining carbon dioxide levels within a target range.

Maintenance of Adequate Perfusion

Given the presence of a pressure-passive circulation as discussed earlier, the management strategy should be to maintain the arterial blood pressure within a normal range for age and gestation. It is not uncommon for infants with hypoxia-ischemia to exhibit hypotension, as in our case. The hypotension may be related to myocardial dysfunction, to endothelial cell damage, or rarely to volume loss. The treatment should be directed toward the cause—that is, inotropic support should be given for myocardial dysfunction, and volume replacement for intravascular depletion.[25] On rare occasions infants may be hypertensive, though this is usually observed in association with seizures.

Fluid Status

Hypoxic-ischemic infants often progress to a fluid overload state. Delivery room management may contribute to this problem, because many infants may receive fluid volume as part of the resuscitation process. Animal studies have suggested that fluid volume infusion at time of resuscitation may be detrimental in some cases. Thus in the asphyxiated neonatal piglet model, animals who received volume infusion during resuscitation demonstrated increased pulmonary edema and decreased lung compliance 2 hours after resuscitation.[26] The fluid overload seen following delivery may be related to renal failure secondary to acute tubular necrosis or to the syndrome of inappropriate antidiuretic hormone release (SIADH). Clinically such infants present with an increase in weight, low urine output, and hyponatremia. The management is fluid restriction. Indeed, in our case, all these findings were present. The treatment comprised fluid restriction and the gradual introduction of sodium supplementation on day of life 2. Others have taken a different approach, treating the oliguria on the basis of the following presumed mechanism. After hypoxia-ischemia, adenosine acts as a vasoconstrictive metabolite that contributes to a decreased glomerular filtration rate. This vasoconstriction can be blocked by theophylline. In two randomized controlled studies, "asphyxiated" infants received a single dose of theophylline (8 mg/kg) within the first hour. Theophylline was associated with a decrease in serum creatinine and urinary β_2-microglobulin concentrations as well as enhancement of creatinine clearance.[27,28]

Control of Blood Glucose Concentration

In the context of cerebral hypoxia-ischemia, experimental studies suggest that both hyperglycemia and hypoglycemia may accentuate brain damage. In adult experimental models as well as in humans, hyperglycemia accentuates brain damage, whereas in immature animals subjected to cerebral hypoxia-ischemia, significant hyperglycemia to a blood glucose concentration of 600 mg/dL entirely prevents the occurrence of brain damage.[29,30] Conversely the effects of hypoglycemia in experimental neonatal models vary, as do the mechanisms of the hypoglycemia. Thus, insulin-induced hypoglycemia is detrimental to immature rat brain subjected to hypoxia-ischemia. However, if fasting induces hypoglycemia, a high degree of protection is noted.[30] This protective effect is thought to be secondary to the increased concentrations of ketone bodies, which presumably serve as alternative substrates to the immature brain. In the clinical setting, hypoglycemia when associated with hypoxia-ischemia is detrimental to the brain. Thus term infants delivered in the presence of severe fetal acidemia (umbilical arterial pH <7.0) who presented with an initial blood glucose concentration lower than 40 mg/dL were 18 times more likely to progress to moderate or severe encephalopathy as compared to infants with a level higher than 40 mg/dL.[31] This was another risk factor in our case because the infant presented with an initial blood glucose concentration of 32 mg/dL. In the ongoing management of hypoxia-ischemia, a glucose level should be screened shortly after birth and monitored closely. If the blood glucose concentration is low it should be promptly corrected.

Temperature

In both animal and human studies, ischemic brain injury has been shown to be influenced by temperature, in that elevation either during or following the insult exacerbates brain injury, whereas a modest reduction in temperature reduces the extent of injury (see Chapter 5).[32] The potential risks associated with an elevated temperature were highlighted in an observational secondary study of whole-body cooling by the National Institute of Child Health and Human Development.[33] The study found that an increased temperature in the control group following hypoxia-ischemia was associated with a higher risk of adverse outcome. The odds ratio of death or disability at 18 to 22 months of age was increased 3.6- to 4-fold for each 1-degree Celsius increase in the highest quartile of skin or esophageal temperatures (see also Chapter 5).[33] Therefore, it is important for the clinician to pay close attention to temperature in the infant who has suffered a hypoxic-ischemic event. At the time of delivery the infant's temperature may be in the normal range or may be elevated in the context of clinical chorioamnionitis with maternal fever, making temperature a highly relevant issue. This raises the important question of how to manage temperature immediately following resuscitation of a near-term or term infant. Should the goal be to maintain the temperature in a normal range until it is evident that the neonate is a potential candidate for therapeutic hypothermia? On the other hand, the clinician could consider initiating passive cooling even at the time of delivery, with discontinuation of use of the radiant warmer in the delivery room. In a study of passive cooling initiated prior to and during transport to a referral center for possible therapeutic hypothermia, passive cooling resulted in initiation of therapy 4.6 hours earlier than if therapy had been started at the cooling center.[34] This concept is especially relevant because most infants who may be treated with therapeutic hypothermia are born at referring centers. Thus, in a study of 45 term infants with moderate or severe HIE treated at a single center with selective head cooling, 96% were outborn, and the time to initiate cooling was 4.69 ± 0.79 hours.[35] Clearly the important and still unanswered question of the role of passive cooling in those infants who are likely to undergo therapeutic hypothermia is an important gap in knowledge (see Chapter 5).

Seizures

Hypoxic-ischemic cerebral injury is the most common cause of early-onset neonatal seizures. Although seizures are a consequence of the underlying brain injury, seizure activity in itself may contribute to ongoing injury. Experimental evidence strongly suggests that repetitive seizures disturb brain growth and development as well as increase the risk for subsequent epilepsy.[36,37] Despite the potential adverse effects of seizures, the question of which infants should be treated remains controversial. This situation is in part related to the observation that not all clinical seizures have an electrographic correlate (see also Chapter 8).[38,39] Clinical seizures are treated with an anticonvulsant, usually phenobarbital, and treatment is continued if seizures persist until the anticonvulsant therapy (e.g., phenobarbital, phosphenytoin, or midazolam) has been maximized, particularly when the seizures are associated with systemic signs—that is, hypertension, bradycardia, and/or desaturations. The optimal management of electrographic seizures in the absence of clinical seizures in the nonparalyzed infant remains unclear. Most of these types of seizures are left untreated because they are generally brief in nature and require excessive anticonvulsants for controlling the electrographic activity. However, some clinicians prefer to eliminate all seizure activity.

Prophylactic Phenobarbital

Experimental data indicate that barbiturate pretreatment and even early post-treatment in adult animals subjected to cerebral hypoxia-ischemia reduces the severity of ultimate brain damage. The prophylactic administration of "high-dose" barbiturates to infants at highest risk for going on to have HIE has been evaluated in small studies with conflicting results. In one randomized study, the administration of thiopental initiated within 2 hours and infused for 24 hours did not alter the frequency of seizures, intracranial pressure, or short-term neurodevelopmental outcome at 12 months.[40] Of importance was the observation that systemic hypotension occurred significantly more often in the treated group. In another randomized study, 40 mg/kg body weight of phenobarbital administered intravenously between 1 and 6 hours to asphyxiated infants, was associated with subsequent neuroprotection. Although there was no difference in the frequency of seizures between the two groups in the neonatal period, 73% of the pretreated infants compared with 18% of the control group (P <0.05) demonstrated normal neurodevelopmental outcome at 3-year follow-up. No adverse effect of phenobarbital administration was observed in this study.[41] There have been additional studies, however, that have demonstrated a decrease in seizures in infants treated with prophylactic phenobarbital. In one small study evaluating phenobarbital administration within 6 hours of life to term and near-term asphyxiated infants, 8% in the treatment group versus 40% in the control group had seizures ($P = 0.01$). Mortality and neurologic outcome at discharge were not statistically different between the two groups.[42] Similarly, in a second study, infants who were given 40 mg/kg of prophylactic phenobarbital during whole-body cooling had fewer clinical seizures than a control group of infants (15% vs. 82%, $P < 0.0001$). There was, however, no reduction in neurodevelopmental impairment.[43]

Animal studies lend support to the potential role of prophylactic phenobarbital in combination with hypothermia. In the neonatal rat model of HIE, those rats treated with both 40 mg/kg phenobarbital and hypothermia had better early and late outcomes than hypothermia-only treatment. Early outcomes included better sensorimotor performance and less cortical damage in the phenobarbital-treated group. Late beneficial outcomes included better sensorimotor performance and lower neuropathology scores.[44] It is clear more studies are needed to assess the potential protective effect of prophylactic phenobarbital when used in combination with hypothermia.

Potential Neuroprotective Strategies Aimed at Ameliorating Secondary Brain Injury

In addition to hypothermia (see Chapter 5), the following potential neuroprotective strategies have been considered.

Oxygen Free Radical Inhibitors and Scavengers

One therapeutic approach for the elimination of oxygen free radicals generated during and following hypoxia-ischemia is the administration of specific enzymes known to degrade highly reactive radicals to a nonreactive component. Superoxide dismutase and catalase are antioxidant enzymes conjugated to polyethylene glycol, a process that prolongs their circulatory half-life and facilitates penetration across the blood-brain barrier.[1] Because of their large molecular size, they are restricted to the vascular space. Thus, the positive effects of these conjugated compounds occur presumably from within cerebral vasculature by improving CBF.[1] In newborn animals, neuroprotection has been shown only when these agents have been administered several hours prior to the hypoxic-ischemic insult.[45]

A second group of free radical inhibitors that have been shown to be effective in experimental animals are agents that inhibit specific reactions in the production of xanthines. Thus, both allopurinol and oxypurinol, which are xanthine oxidase inhibitors, protected immature rats from hypoxic-ischemic brain damage when the drugs were administered early during the recovery phase following resuscitation.[1] In experiments and a clinical study, asphyxiated infants who received allopurinol demonstrated lower blood concentrations of oxygen free radicals than control infants.[46,47] However, translating this finding into clinical practice seems less hopeful at this time. In a 2008 Cochrane review examining three trials, involving 114 infants with encephalopathy treated with allopurinol, there was no significant difference between treated and control groups in the risk of death during infancy or of neonatal seizures.[48] Clearly, with such a small number of patients in these studies, larger studies may be needed to determine whether there is truly no benefit.

A third group of free radical inhibitors has targeted blocking the formation of free radicals, specifically hydroxyl radical, from free iron during reperfusion.[1] Deferoxamine, a chelating agent, prevents the formation of free radicals from iron, reduces the severity of brain injury, and improves cerebral metabolism in animal models of hypoxia-ischemia when given during reperfusion.[47] Other studies have shown less benefit from deferoxamine treatment, including a study investigating the combination of the antioxidant effect of deferoxamine with the antiapoptotic effect of erythropoietin. In this study using the neonatal rat model of HIE, neuronal protection following HIE was not seen with deferoxamine nor when used in combination with erythropoietin.[49]

Excitatory Amino Acid Antagonists

Given the important role of excessive stimulation of neuronal surface receptors by glutamate in promoting a cascade of events leading to cellular death,[1] it has been logical to identify pharmacologic agents that would either inhibit glutamate release or block its postsynaptic action. Glutamate receptor antagonists (i.e., N-methyl-D-aspartate [NMDA] subtypes) have been extensively investigated in experimental animals. Noncompetitive antagonists provided a reduction in brain damage in adult animals even when administered up to 24 hours after the insult. The available NMDA antagonists include dizocilpine (MK-801), magnesium, xenon, phencyclidine (PCP), dextrometrophan, and ketamine.[1] Most of the previously mentioned NMDA antagonists are not widely used. However, the benefits of magnesium, which is commonly used, and xenon, which shows potential benefit, are discussed in the following sections.

Potential Role of Magnesium

Magnesium is an NMDA antagonist, blocking neuronal influx of Ca^{2+} within the ion channel. The effect of magnesium also appears to be dependent on the maturation of the glutamate receptor system. Thus, in a developmental study in mice, excitotoxic neuronal death was limited by magnesium, but only after development of several aspects of the excitotoxic cascade. These aspects included the coupling of calcium influx following NMDA overstimulation and the presence of magnesium-dependent calcium channels.[50] Magnesium sulfate is an appealing agent because of its frequent use in mothers for tocolysis or to prevent seizures in women with pregnancy-induced hypertension. One large multicenter trial assessed outcomes of infants born to women treated with magnesium sulfate when at imminent risk for delivery between 24 and 31 weeks of gestation.[51] Moderate or severe cerebral palsy occurred significantly less frequently in the magnesium-treated group (1.9% vs. 3.5%; RR 0.55; 95% CI 0.32-0.95).[52] A 2009 meta-analysis of five trials (n = 6145 infants), including the preceding study, confirmed the considerably reduced risk of cerebral palsy, and the number needed to treat would be 63 women to avoid cerebral palsy in 1 infant.[53]

With this promise of neuroprotection in preterm infants, there has been speculation about potential benefit in term asphyxiated infants. In a piglet model of asphyxia, magnesium sulfate administered 1 hour after resuscitation did not decrease the severity of delayed cerebral energy failure.[54] In addition, in a near-term fetal lamb model, magnesium sulfate administered before and during umbilical cord occlusion did not influence electrophysiologic responses or neuronal loss.[55] Results of human studies of term or near-term infants to investigate the potential neuroprotective effect of magnesium had conflicted with those of the animal studies. There are properties of magnesium that could provide benefit in the setting of perinatal asphyxia by the following mechanisms; impaired excitotoxic amino acid release, NMDA receptor blockade, antioxidant, anticytokine, and antiplatelet effects, as well as vasodilatory properties that could potentially preserve uteroplacental blood flow.[1] Potential benefit was demonstrated in a study of term infants with severe perinatal asphyxia who received three doses of magnesium (250-mg/kg/dose) within 6 hours of birth and at 24-hour intervals. An abnormal neurologic examination at discharge, performed by a clinician blinded to group assignment, was found in 22% of the treatment group compared with 56% of the placebo group (P = 0.04). Although not statistically significant, a trend towards fewer abnormal findings on head computed tomography performed at 14 days of life in the treatment group was also reported.[56] Clearly more human studies are needed, as well as studies assessing the combined effect of magnesium with hypothermia.

Xenon

Xenon appears to have a synergistic neuroprotective effect when combined with hypothermia at doses that are likely to be well tolerated.[1] In the past xenon has been used as an inhaled anesthetic, with rapid induction and recovery secondary to poor blood solubility. It does, however, rapidly cross the blood-brain barrier, and in the

6

brain acts as a noncompetitive antagonist of the NMDA subtype of the glutamate receptor.[1,51] Xenon also exhibits antiapoptotic effects by decreasing expression of Bax, a proapoptotic protein factor, and enhancing Bcl-x$_L$, which acts to counteract Bax.[57] There have been several studies investigating the use of xenon with hypothermia in the setting of asphyxia. In the newborn pig model, animals subjected to 45 minutes of global hypoxia-ischemia demonstrated 75% histologic (averaged regional neuropathology scores) global neuroprotection when 18 hours of 50% xenon inhalation was combined with 24 hours of hypothermia. Although regional neuroprotection was evident in all seven brain regions assessed, it was most prominent in the basal ganglia and thalamus. Protection was seen as an additive, not synergistic, effect.[58] One of the first animal studies to assess long-term functional and pathologic protection of the combination of xenon and hypothermia after HIE found almost complete restoration of long-term functional outcomes as well as improved regional histopathology.[59] As in the previously mentioned study, the effect of xenon with hypothermia was additive and not synergistic. In the former study, hypothermia was initiated within 40 minutes and xenon 30 minutes after the hypoxic-ischemic insult, and in the latter, both hypothermia and xenon were administered during recovery from hypoxia. This leaves the unanswered question of whether xenon would be neuroprotective if administered later, but still before 6 hours following injury, the time window in which clinicians can institute hypothermia for asphyxiated newborns. In a study evaluating the protective effect of xenon with hypothermia both in vivo and in vitro, when xenon was administered concurrently with hypoxia in vivo, a dose-dependent decrease in brain injury was present at concentrations of 40% and more. Xenon was also found to be protective up to 6 hours after the insult at concentrations of 70% administered for 90 minutes.[57] This well-tolerated anesthetic, which lacks major side effects, is, however, expensive. With the concentration needed, a specialized ventilator that can scavenge exhaled xenon is needed.[60] Further studies are still needed to determine the time window in which xenon could be administered with hypothermia, as well as the duration of treatment needed.

Erythropoietin

Erythropoietin (Epo) is a glycoprotein hormone most recognized for its role in erythropoiesis. However, it has also been shown to naturally increase during hypoxia-ischemia, along with an increase in Epo receptors. Erythropoietin is thought to provide a neuroprotective adaptive response during hypoxia-ischemia because of this effect.[1] Suggested protective mechanisms of action include antioxidant and anti-inflammatory responses, induction of antiapoptotic factors, as well as decreased nitric oxide–mediated injury and susceptibility to glutamate toxicity.[51] Both stroke and hypoxic-ischemic animal models have demonstrated histologic protection with recombinant human Epo (rEpo) treatment. In the neonatal rat stroke model, animals treated with 1000 U/kg at 0 hours, 24 hours, and 7 days after injury did not differ from sham animals (those without stroke) and performed better in most components of spatial learning and memory performance. Animals treated with three doses of erythropoietin also demonstrated higher volumes of striatum, hippocampus, and neocortex than animals subjected to middle cerebral artery occlusion and treated with placebo.[61] Similar beneficial effects of erythropoietin have been demonstrated in hypoxic-ischemic animals. In a small study of hypoxic-ischemic neonatal rats, a single intracerebroventricular injection of rEpo immediately following hypoxia-ischemia significantly decreased mean infarct volume at 7 days.[62] Obviously, translating this treatment into clinical practice may be difficult, and a less invasive mode of delivery would be more practical for the clinical setting. In a study of 7-day-old rat pups exposed to hypoxia-ischemia and subsequently treated with one, three, or seven subcutaneous doses of 2500, 5000, or 30,000 U/kg of rEpo, those treated with three doses of 5000 or one dose of 30,000 U/kg were conferred the most neuroprotection. There was no sex-specific difference in injury in this study.[63] A study assessing short- and long-term sensorimotor function and histologic outcome in the hypoxic-ischemic neonatal mouse model treated with three doses of erythropoietin, however, did

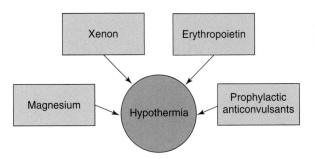

Figure 6-1 Potential strategies to evaluate in high-risk infants treated with therapeutic hypothermia.

demonstrate a gender difference. In this study, the administration of 5000 U/kg, and not 20,000 U/kg, improved sensorimotor function and protected against hippocampal injury, striatum atrophy, and white matter loss in female mice only.[64] The greater neuroprotective effect for females than males was also seen in a study of term infants with moderate/severe HIE. In this study infants were randomly assigned to receive rEpo at either 300 U/kg or 500 U/kg every other day for 2 weeks beginning at less than 48 hours after birth. The rate of death or moderate/severe disability at 18 months was significantly reduced, with 43.8% in the control group versus 24.6% in the rEpo group (RR 0.62; 95% CI 0.41-0.94). Benefit was seen in infants with moderate ($P = 0.001$) but not severe HIE ($P = 0.227$). Overall, disability was also significantly reduced for females, but not males. However, it is important to note that significantly fewer females were enrolled in this study than males. There was no difference in primary outcome between doses used in this study.[65] It would be important to study this effect of rEpo in combination with therapeutic hypothermia in term infants.

Other Therapies

Calcium channel blockers have been studied in the past, but any possible benefit from these agents is counteracted by their adverse hemodynamic effects, so they remain contraindicated in neonates.[66] Other avenues of potential neuroprotection that have been studied in animals, but have not yet proved benefit in clinical practice, are platelet-activating factor antagonists, adenosinergic agents, monosialoganglioside GM_1, growth factors (e.g., nerve growth factor [NGF], insulin growth factor-1), melatonin, and minocycline.

Gaps in Knowledge

1. Is it possible to perform more trials comparing 21% with higher concentrations of supplemental oxygen during intensive resuscitation using a uniform definition of HIE and performed in the developed world?
2. Is there a critical mean blood pressure below which cerebral perfusion becomes compromised?
3. Is there a benefit to prophylactic anticonvulsant therapy in the high-risk infant, given that around 50% of infants enrolled in the hypothermia studies presented with early seizures[67-69]?
4. Would xenon be protective beyond 4 but within 6 hours, the time window within which cooling is often initiated?
5. What are the possible implications of the use of rEpo, magnesium, xenon, or prophylactic anticonvulsants along with therapeutic hypothermia (Fig. 6-1)?
6. What is the optimal dose of rEpo to confer neuroprotection?

References

1. Volpe JJ. *Neurology of the newborn*. 5th ed. Philadelphia: Saunders/Elsevier; 2008.
2. Perlman JM. Intervention strategies for neonatal hypoxic-ischemic cerebral injury. *Clin Ther*. 2006;28: 1353-1365.
3. Shalak L, Perlman JM. Hypoxic-ischemic brain injury in the term infant-current concepts. *Early Hum Dev*. 2004;80:125-141.

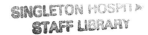

4. Perlman JM. Summary proceedings from the neurology group on hypoxic-ischemic encephalopathy. *Pediatrics*. 2006;117:S28-S33.
5. Stola A, Perlman J. Post-resuscitation strategies to avoid ongoing injury following intrapartum hypoxia-ischemia. *Semin Fetal Neonatal Med*. 2008;13:424-431.
6. Kattwinkel J, Perlman JM, Aziz K, et al. Neonatal resuscitation: 2010 American Heart Association Guidelines for Cardiopulmonary Resuscitation and Emergency Cardiovascular Care. *Pediatrics*. 2010;126:e1400-e1413.
7. Davis PG, Tan A, O'Donnell CP, Schulze A. Resuscitation of newborn infants with 100% oxygen or air: a systematic review and meta-analysis. *Lancet*. 2004;364:1329-1333.
8. Tan A, Schulze A, O'Donnell CP, Davis PG. Air versus oxygen for resuscitation of infants at birth. *Cochrane Database Syst Rev*. 2005;(2):CD002273.
9. Rabi Y, Rabi D, Yee W. Room air resuscitation of the depressed newborn: a systematic review and meta-analysis. *Resuscitation*. 2007;72:353-363.
10. Vento M, Asensi M, Sastre J, et al. Resuscitation with room air instead of 100% oxygen prevents oxidative stress in moderately asphyxiated term neonates. *Pediatrics*. 2001;107:642-647.
11. Klinger G, Beyene J, Shah P, Perlman M. Do hyperoxaemia and hypocapnia add to the risk of brain injury after intrapartum asphyxia? *Arch Dis Child Fetal Neonatal Ed*. 2005;90:F49-F52.
12. Saugstad OD, Ramji S, Irani SF, et al. Resuscitation of newborn infants with 21% or 100% oxygen: follow-up at 18 to 24 months. *Pediatrics*. 2003;112:296-300.
13. Presti AL, Kishkurno SV, Slinko SK, et al. Reoxygenation with 100% oxygen versus room air: late neuroanatomical and neurofunctional outcome in neonatal mice with hypoxic-ischemic brain injury. *Pediatr Res*. 2006;60:55-59.
14. Solas AB, Kutzsche S, Vinje M, Saugstad OD. Cerebral hypoxemia-ischemia and reoxygenation with 21% or 100% oxygen in newborn piglets: effects on extracellular levels of excitatory amino acids and microcirculation. *Pediatr Crit Care Med*. 2001;2:340-345.
15. Matsiukevich D, Randis TM, Utkina-Sosunova I, et al. The state of systemic circulation, collapsed or preserved defines the need for hyperoxic or normoxic resuscitation in neonatal mice with hypoxia-ischemia. *Resuscitation*. 2010;81:224-229.
16. Perlman JM, Wyllie J, Kattwinkel J, et al. Neonatal resuscitation: 2010 International Consensus on Cardiopulmonary Resuscitation and Emergency Cardiovascular Care Science with Treatment Recommendations. *Pediatrics*. 2010;126:e1319-e1344.
17. Perlman JM, Risser R. Can asphyxiated infants at risk for neonatal seizures be rapidly identified by current high-risk markers? *Pediatrics*. 1996;97:456-462.
18. Hellstrom-Westas L, Rosen I, Svenningsen NW. Predictive value of early continuous amplitude integrated EEG recordings on outcome after severe birth asphyxia in full term infants. *Arch Dis Child Fetal Neonatal Ed*. 1995;72:F34-F38.
19. al Naqeeb N, Edwards AD, Cowan FM, Azzopardi D. Assessment of neonatal encephalopathy by amplitude-integrated electroencephalography. *Pediatrics*. 1999;103:1263-1271.
20. Shalak LF, Laptook AR, Velaphi SC, Perlman JM. Amplitude-integrated electroencephalography coupled with an early neurologic examination enhances prediction of term infants at risk for persistent encephalopathy. *Pediatrics*. 2003;111:351-357.
21. Rosenberg AA, Jones Jr MD, Traystman RJ, et al. Response of cerebral blood flow to changes in PCO2 in fetal, newborn, and adult sheep. *Am J Physiol*. 1982;242:H862-H866.
22. Vannucci RC, Brucklacher RM, Vannucci SJ. Effect of carbon dioxide on cerebral metabolism during hypoxia-ischemia in the immature rat. *Pediatr Res*. 1997;42:24-29.
23. Kaiser JR, Gauss CH, Williams DK. The effects of hypercapnia on cerebral autoregulation in ventilated very low birth weight infants. *Pediatr Res*. 2005;58:931-935.
24. Nadeem M, Murray D, Boylan G, et al. Blood carbon dioxide levels and adverse outcome in neonatal hypoxic-ischemic encephalopathy. *Am J Perinatol*. 2010;27:361-365.
25. Wyckoff MH, Perlman JM, Laptook AR. Use of volume expansion during delivery room resuscitation in near-term and term infants. *Pediatrics*. 2005;115:950-955.
26. Wyckoff M, Garcia D, Margraf L, et al. Randomized trial of volume infusion during resuscitation of asphyxiated neonatal piglets. *Pediatr Res*. 2007;61:415-420.
27. Jenik AG, Ceriani Cernadas JM, Gorenstein A, et al. A randomized, double-blind, placebo-controlled trial of the effects of prophylactic theophylline on renal function in term neonates with perinatal asphyxia. *Pediatrics*. 2000;105(4):E45.
28. Bhat MA, Shah ZA, Makhdoomi MS, Mufti MH. Theophylline for renal function in term neonates with perinatal asphyxia: a randomized, placebo-controlled trial. *J Pediatr*. 2006;149:180-184.
29. Vannucci RC, Mujsce DJ. Effect of glucose on perinatal hypoxic-ischemic brain damage. *Biol Neonate*. 1992;62:215-224.
30. Yager JY. Hypoglycemic injury to the immature brain. *Clin Perinatol*. 2002;29:651-674, vi.
31. Salhab WA, Wyckoff MH, Laptook AR, Perlman JM. Initial hypoglycemia and neonatal brain injury in term infants with severe fetal acidemia. *Pediatrics*. 2004;114:361-366.
32. Laptook AR, Corbett RJ. The effects of temperature on hypoxic-ischemic brain injury. *Clin Perinatol*. 2002;29:623-649, vi.
33. Laptook A, Tyson J, Shankaran S, et al; National Institute of Child Health and Human Development Neonatal Research Network. Elevated temperature after hypoxic-ischemic encephalopathy: risk factor for adverse outcomes. *Pediatrics*. 2008;122:491-499.
34. Kendall GS, Kapetanakis A, Ratnavel N, et al. Passive cooling for initiation of therapeutic hypothermia in neonatal encephalopathy. *Arch Dis Child Fetal Neonatal Ed*. 2010;95:F408-F412.

35. Takenouchi T, Cuaycong M, Ross G, et al. Chain of Brain Preservation—a concept to facilitate early identification and initiation of hypothermia to infants at high risk for brain injury. *Resuscitation.* 2010;81:1637-1641.
36. Dzhala V, Ben-Ari Y, Khazipov R. Seizures accelerate anoxia-induced neuronal death in the neonatal rat hippocampus. *Ann Neurol.* 2000;48:632-640.
37. Holmes GL, Gairsa JL, Chevassus-Au-Louis N, Ben-Ari Y. Consequences of neonatal seizures in the rat: morphological and behavioral effects. *Ann Neurol.* 1998;44:845-857.
38. Mizrahi EM. Consensus and controversy in the clinical management of neonatal seizures. *Clin Perinatol.* 1989;16:485-500.
39. Scher MS, Aso K, Beggarly ME, et al. Electrographic seizures in preterm and full-term neonates: clinical correlates, associated brain lesions, and risk for neurologic sequelae. *Pediatrics.* 1993;91: 128-134.
40. Goldberg RN, Moscoso P, Bauer CR, et al. Use of barbiturate therapy in severe perinatal asphyxia: a randomized controlled trial. *J Pediatr.* 1986;109:851-856.
41. Hall RT, Hall FK, Daily DK. High-dose phenobarbital therapy in term newborn infants with severe perinatal asphyxia: a randomized, prospective study with three-year follow-up. *J Pediatr.* 1998;132: 345-348.
42. Singh D, Kumar P, Narang A. A randomized controlled trial of phenobarbital in neonates with hypoxic ischemic encephalopathy. *J Matern Fetal Neonatal Med.* 2005;18:391-395.
43. Meyn Jr DF, Ness J, Ambalavanan N, Carlo WA. Prophylactic phenobarbital and whole-body cooling for neonatal hypoxic-ischemic encephalopathy. *J Pediatr.* 2010;157:334-336.
44. Barks JD, Liu YQ, Shangguan Y, Silverstein FS. Phenobarbital augments hypothermic neuroprotection. *Pediatr Res.* 2010;67:532-537.
45. Shimizu K, Rajapakse N, Horiguchi T, et al. Neuroprotection against hypoxia-ischemia in neonatal rat brain by novel superoxide dismutase mimetics. *Neurosci Lett.* 2003;346:41-44.
46. Van Bel F, Shadid M, Moison RM, et al. Effect of allopurinol on postasphyxial free radical formation, cerebral hemodynamics, and electrical brain activity. *Pediatrics.* 1998;101:185-193.
47. Peeters-Scholte C, Braun K, Koster J, et al. Effects of allopurinol and deferoxamine on reperfusion injury of the brain in newborn piglets after neonatal hypoxia-ischemia. *Pediatr Res.* 2003;54: 516-522.
48. Chaudhari T, McGuire W. Allopurinol for preventing mortality and morbidity in newborn infants with suspected hypoxic-ischaemic encephalopathy. *Cochrane Database Syst Rev.* 2008;(2):CD006817.
49. van der Kooij MA, Groenendaal F, Kavelaars A, et al. Combination of deferoxamine and erythropoietin: therapy for hypoxia-ischemia-induced brain injury in the neonatal rat? *Neurosci Lett.* 2009;451: 109-113.
50. Marret S, Gressens P, Gadisseux JF, Evrard P. Prevention by magnesium of excitotoxic neuronal death in the developing brain: an animal model for clinical intervention studies. *Dev Med Child Neurol.* 1995;37(6):473-484.
51. Kelen D, Robertson NJ. Experimental treatments for hypoxic ischaemic encephalopathy. *Early Hum Dev.* 2010;86:369-377.
52. Rouse DJ, Hirtz DG, Thom E, et al. A randomized, controlled trial of magnesium sulfate for the prevention of cerebral palsy. *N Engl J Med.* 2008;359:895-905.
53. Doyle LW, Crowther CA, Middleton P, et al. Magnesium sulphate for women at risk of preterm birth for neuroprotection of the fetus. *Cochrane Database Syst Rev.* 2009;(1):CD004661.
54. Penrice J, Amess PN, Punwani S, et al. Magnesium sulfate after transient hypoxia-ischemia fails to prevent delayed cerebral energy failure in the newborn piglet. *Pediatr Res.* 1997;41:443-447.
55. de Haan HH, Gunn AJ, Williams CE, et al. Magnesium sulfate therapy during asphyxia in near-term fetal lambs does not compromise the fetus but does not reduce cerebral injury. *Am J Obstet Gynecol.* 1997;176:18-27.
56. Bhat MA, Charoo BA, Bhat JI, et al. Magnesium sulfate in severe perinatal asphyxia: a randomized, placebo-controlled trial. *Pediatrics.* 2009;123:e764-e769.
57. Ma D, Hossain M, Chow A, et al. Xenon and hypothermia combine to provide neuroprotection from neonatal asphyxia. *Ann Neurol.* 2005;58:182-193.
58. Chakkarapani E, Dingley J, Liu X, et al. Xenon enhances hypothermic neuroprotection in asphyxiated newborn pigs. *Ann Neurol.* 2010;68:330-341.
59. Hobbs C, Thoresen M, Tucker A, et al. Xenon and hypothermia combine additively, offering long-term functional and histopathologic neuroprotection after neonatal hypoxia/ischemia. *Stroke.* 2008; 39:1307-1313.
60. Cilio MR, Ferriero DM. Synergistic neuroprotective therapies with hypothermia. *Semin Fetal Neonatal Med.* 2010;15:293-298.
61. Gonzalez FF, Abel R, Almli CR, et al. Erythropoietin sustains cognitive function and brain volume after neonatal stroke. *Dev Neurosci.* 2009;31:403-411.
62. Aydin A, Genc K, Akhisaroglu M, et al. Erythropoietin exerts neuroprotective effect in neonatal rat model of hypoxic-ischemic brain injury. *Brain Dev.* 2003;25:494-498.
63. Kellert BA, McPherson RJ, Juul SE. A comparison of high-dose recombinant erythropoietin treatment regimens in brain-injured neonatal rats. *Pediatr Res.* 2007;61:451-455.
64. Fan X, Heijnen CJ, van der KM, et al. Beneficial effect of erythropoietin on sensorimotor function and white matter after hypoxia-ischemia in neonatal mice. *Pediatr Res.* 2011;69:56-61.
65. Zhu C, Kang W, Xu F, et al. Erythropoietin improved neurologic outcomes in newborns with hypoxic-ischemic encephalopathy. *Pediatrics.* 2009;124:e218-e226.

66. Levene MI, Gibson NA, Fenton AC, et al. The use of a calcium-channel blocker, nicardipine, for severely asphyxiated newborn infants. *Dev Med Child Neurol*. 1990;32:567-574.
67. Gluckman PD, Wyatt JS, Azzopardi D, et al. Selective head cooling with mild systemic hypothermia after neonatal encephalopathy: multicentre randomised trial. *Lancet*. 2005;365:663-670.
68. Shankaran S, Laptook AR, Ehrenkranz RA, et al. Whole-body hypothermia for neonates with hypoxic-ischemic encephalopathy. *N Engl J Med*. 2005;353:1574-1584.
69. Azzopardi DV, Strohm B, Edwards AD, et al. Moderate hypothermia to treat perinatal asphyxial encephalopathy. *N Engl J Med*. 2009;361:1349-1358.

CHAPTER 7

Perinatal Stroke

Eliza H. Myers, MD, and Laura R. Ment, MD

The emergence of sophisticated neuroimaging techniques has permitted the diagnosis of stroke in the developing brain. Ischemic perinatal stroke (IPS) may occur prenatally, antenatally, or postnatally, and the ischemia may be due to venous thrombosis, arterial embolism, or primary or secondary hemorrhage. When the ischemic event occurs from the 20th week of gestation through delivery, it is termed *fetal stroke*; when the event occurs in the course of delivery through the 28th day of life, it is classified as *neonatal stroke*. Stroke in the fetus is likely a rare event (the true incidence is unknown), although the incidence of neonatal stroke is reported to range from 17 to 93 per 100,000 live births. A new term, *presumed perinatal ischemic stroke* (PPIS), is used to describe stroke diagnosed in infants older than 28 postnatal days in whom it is presumed that an ischemic event occurred some time between the 20th week of fetal life through the 28th postnatal day, but in whom the timing of the insult is otherwise unknown.

Review of risk factor and genetic studies suggests that, like many other human diseases, stroke in the developing brain is a complex disorder. Differences in clinical presentation and outcome are found to be reported when one evaluates those cases occurring in utero (fetal stroke), those that happen during or after birth, and those in which infants incidentally present with hemiparesis. Stroke is a common cause of seizures in the neonatal period, and ischemic perinatal stroke is now thought to be an important cause not only of hemiplegic cerebral palsy but also of epilepsy and cognitive disorders. Pregnancy is a naturally thrombotic state, and although the role of genetic and acquired thrombophilias remains incompletely understood, laboratory advances have not only suggested a difference between infants who experience stroke in the fetal and neonatal time periods but also posited an interaction between neonatal and maternal thrombophilias. Defining the timing, environmental risk factors, and genetic susceptibilities of ischemic perinatal stroke will aid in the diagnosis, prevention, and treatment of this important injury to the developing brain.

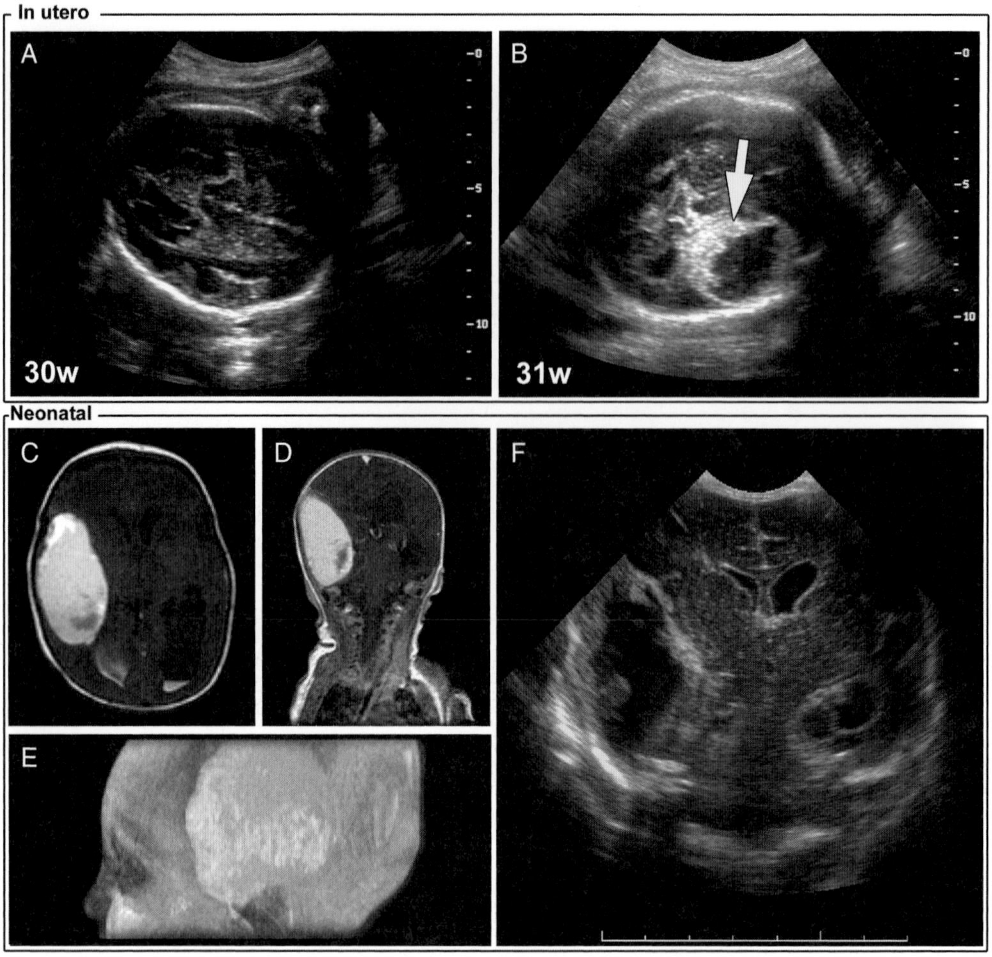

Figure 7-1 Prenatal and postnatal imaging findings in the patient with alloimmune thrombocytopenia and resultant fetal stroke (Patient 1). **A** and **B,** Uterine ultrasound scans show the hemorrhage in the temporal lobe at 31 weeks (*arrow*). Axial **(C)** and coronal **(D)** T1-weighted magnetic resonance (MR) images show the intraparenchymal hematoma in the right temporal lobe as well as ventriculomegaly and intraventricular blood. **E,** Three-dimensional reconstruction of the MR images. **F,** A postnatal ultrasound scan in the coronal plane.

Case Histories

PATIENT 1

The patient was the 1.57-kg product of a 32-week gestation born by cesarean section to a G2P1 (gravida 1, para 1) 31-year-old. The gestation was significant for alloimmune thrombocytopenia, class A1 gestational diabetes, fetal intracranial hemorrhage at 31 weeks (Fig. 7-1A and B), and the onset of preterm labor. Apgar scores were 9 at 1 minute and 9 at 5 minutes, and the infant's platelet count was 13,000. She was treated with fresh-frozen plasma, intravenous immunoglobulin (IVIG), and platelet transfusions, which resulted in resolution of the thrombocytopenia.

Computed tomography (CT) and subsequent magnetic resonance imaging (MRI) demonstrated a large right frontotemporoparietal hemorrhagic stroke with shift of the midline and ventriculomegaly (Fig. 7-1C to F). Subsequent hospital course was complicated by the development of obstructive hydrocephalus, surgery for clot removal, hyperbilirubinemia treated with phototherapy, sepsis treated with antibiotics, and neonatal seizures well controlled by phenobarbital. Phenobarbital was discontinued prior to hospital discharge, and seizures did not recur.

The child was evaluated at age 12 months and was found to have nonfocal neurologic findings and developmental milestones appropriate for age.

PATIENT 2

The patient was the 3.25-kg product of a 39-week gestation complicated by systemic lupus erythematosus (SLE) to a G2P0AB1 (1 abortion) 39-year-old. The patient's mother was blood type A positive, antibody screen negative, rubella immune, and group B streptococcus negative; she was treated briefly with prednisone for her SLE during the first trimester.

On the day prior to delivery, she presented for a routine obstetric visit in labor; findings on routine fetal ultrasound scan from the previous week were unremarkable. Labor was augmented by pitocin, but delivery was accomplished by cesarean section secondary to failure to progress. Apgar scores were 5 at 1 minute and 9 at 5 minutes, and the child was noted to have petechiae on her abdomen.

In the newborn intensive care unit (NICU), the infant was noted to have a platelet count of 28,000; her initial course was otherwise unremarkable. Later on the first day of life, the infant demonstrated focal seizures and was treated with phenobarbital. Findings of a cranial ultrasound scan performed on the first day of life were unremarkable, but a CT scan the following day and subsequent MRI study demonstrated left frontal, parietal, and occipital as well as right parietal hemorrhage with subarachnoid hemorrhage (Fig. 7-2A to E). Electroencephalography (EEG) findings were unremarkable.

Evaluation for hemorrhagic neonatal stroke demonstrated platelet-specific maternal antibodies with incompatibility at the HPA-1A locus. Results of all other testing, including that for protein C, protein S, antithrombin III, factor V Leiden, prothrombin mutation, MTHFRC mutation, total homocysteine level, and lipoprotein (a), were normal.

At age 6 months, neurodevelopmental examination results were unremarkable, and follow-up MRI demonstrated resolution of hemorrhage with focal encephalomalacia (Fig. 7-2F and G).

PATIENT 3

The patient was the 3.5-kg product of a full-term pregnancy complicated by recurrent migraine headaches to a G1P0 25-year-old. Labor and delivery were unremarkable at an outlying hospital, but the patient was said to be floppy and fed poorly during the first several days of life. He was discharged to home at age 5 days but was noted to be a somewhat quiet baby who did not feed well.

He gradually became more alert with improved feeding and activity level but delay in acquisition of early milestones. At age 5 to 6 months, the child was noted to be batting at objects with his right hand but not his left. Subsequent neurologic examination demonstrated a mild left hemiparesis, and an MRI demonstrated ex vacuo dilation of the frontal horn of the right lateral ventricle (Fig. 7-3).

Evaluation for PPIS demonstrated heterozygosity for factor V Leiden deficiency. Results of all other testing, including that for protein C, protein S, antithrombin III, prothrombin mutation, MTHFRC mutation, total homocysteine level, and lipoprotein (a), were normal.

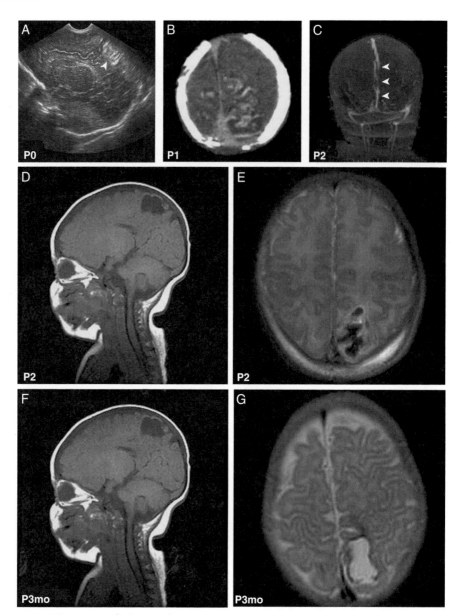

Figure 7-2   Imaging findings in the patient with neonatal stroke secondary to maternal anti-platelet antibodies (Patient 2). Early neonatal imaging with ultrasound study **(A)** at the day of birth, computed tomography study on day 1 **(B)**, and magnetic resonance imaging (MRI) study on day 2 of life **(C to E)**. Note the parenchymal hemorrhagic stroke in the parasagittal location. MRI confirms the findings, and showing intact venous flow in the sinuses (*arrows* in **C**) excludes the diagnosis of a venous sinus thrombosis. Follow-up MRI, with T1-weighted image in the sagittal plane **(F)** and T2-weighted image **(G)** in the axial plane, shows resolution of the hemorrhage with focal encephalomalacia.

Definitions

A 2006 workshop sponsored by the National Institute of Child Health and Human Development and the National Institute of Neurological Disorders defined *ischemic perinatal stroke* (IPS) as stroke that occurs between 20 weeks of gestation and 28 days of life.[1] Although older series of neonates with stroke frequently grouped perinatal, peripartum, and neonatal events and suggested common pathophysiologies for stroke at different points in time, the participants of the IPS workshop strongly recommended adherence to a consistent nomenclature and definition scheme. IPS

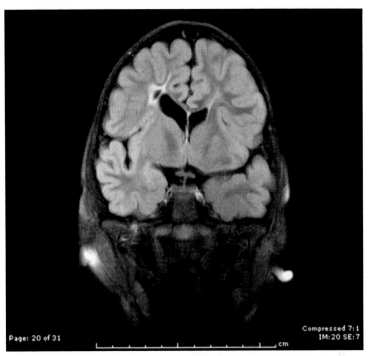

Figure 7-3 Follow-up magnetic resonance imaging (MRI) scan, in coronal view, at 6 years in a child with presumed perinatal ischemic stroke (Patient 3). The patient was the 3.5-kg product of a full-term pregnancy complicated by recurrent migraine headaches to a G1P0 woman. Labor and delivery were unremarkable, but the infant was floppy and fed poorly. He gradually improved but was noted to have a right-hand preference at age 5 to 6 months. MRI at 6 months and this follow-up image both demonstrate ex vacuo dilation of the right frontal horn of the lateral ventricle and periventricular ischemic lesion.

was defined as "a group of heterogeneous conditions in which there is focal disruption of cerebral blood flow secondary to arterial or cerebral venous thrombosis or embolization, between 20 weeks of fetal life through the 28th postnatal day, confirmed by neuroimaging or neuropathologic studies."[1] Because the timing of the precipitating event is almost never known, it was further suggested that the classification of IPS be based on gestational age at diagnosis, as shown in Table 7-1.

For the purposes of this review, fetal stroke is defined as a focal ischemic, thrombotic, and/or hemorrhagic event occurring between 20 weeks of gestation and the onset of labor resulting in delivery. For those patients without labor the period is between 20 weeks and the start of cesarean delivery. Ischemic events that occur earlier in pregnancy (before 20 weeks) may manifest in the form of other pathologic

Table 7-1   CLASSIFICATION OF ISCHEMIC PERINATAL STROKE

Term	Definition
Fetal stroke	Focal ischemic, thrombotic, and/or hemorrhagic event occurring between 20 weeks of gestation and the onset of labor (or beginning of the cesarean section for patients without labor) resulting in delivery.
Neonatal stroke	Focal ischemic, thrombotic, and/or hemorrhagic event occurring between labor resulting in delivery and 28 days of life. For those patients without labor, between delivery and 28 days
Presumed perinatal ischemic stroke (PPIS)	Chronic, focal infarction on neuroimaging of infants > 28 days of age in whom it is presumed (but not certain) that either an ischemic event or a periventricular venous infarction occurred some time between the 20th week of fetal life and the 28th postnatal day

pictures, such as hydranancephaly[2] and other destructive lesions. These pathologies of uncertain cause are excluded from the definition of fetal stroke. The clinical manifestations of fetal stroke are variably manifest, and many fetal strokes are not diagnosed until after the newborn period.

Neonatal stroke is defined as a focal ischemic, thrombotic and/or hemorrhagic event occurring between labor resulting in delivery and 28 days of life. For those patients without labor, this period is between delivery and 28 days (including preterm neonates). Stroke in the term newborn brain may manifest in the form of arterial ischemic infarction, cerebral sinovenous thrombosis, primary hemorrhage, or hemorrhage due to underlying vascular disruptions or neoplastic lesions. Term infants with these lesions are commonly symptomatic in the neonatal period; symptomatology may be more difficult to discern in the preterm infant.

Finally, PPIS is diagnosed in infants older than 28 days in whom it is presumed that the inciting event occurred some time between the 20th week of fetal life and the 28th postnatal day.

Etiology

The etiologies of fetal and neonatal stroke are summarized in Figure 7-4.

Etiology and Risk Factors for Fetal Stroke

In approximately half of cases of fetal stroke, a possible predisposing condition is identified or suspected. Most cases of fetal stroke thus identified are attributed to hematologic disorders and maternal trauma. Only a small proportion of fetal stroke cases have undergone a comprehensive investigation to identify possible genetic or environmental etiologies.[3-5]

For descriptive purposes, the etiologies of fetal stroke may be grouped into maternal conditions, pregnancy disorders, and fetal conditions. In our previous review of the literature, the most common causes of fetal stroke were complicated twin pregnancies and alloimmune thrombocytopenia followed by maternal trauma, maternal diabetes and in utero growth retardation.[6]

Maternal medical conditions such as diabetes, epilepsy, and juvenile rheumatoid arthritis are significant causes of fetal stroke and are present in 20% of fetal

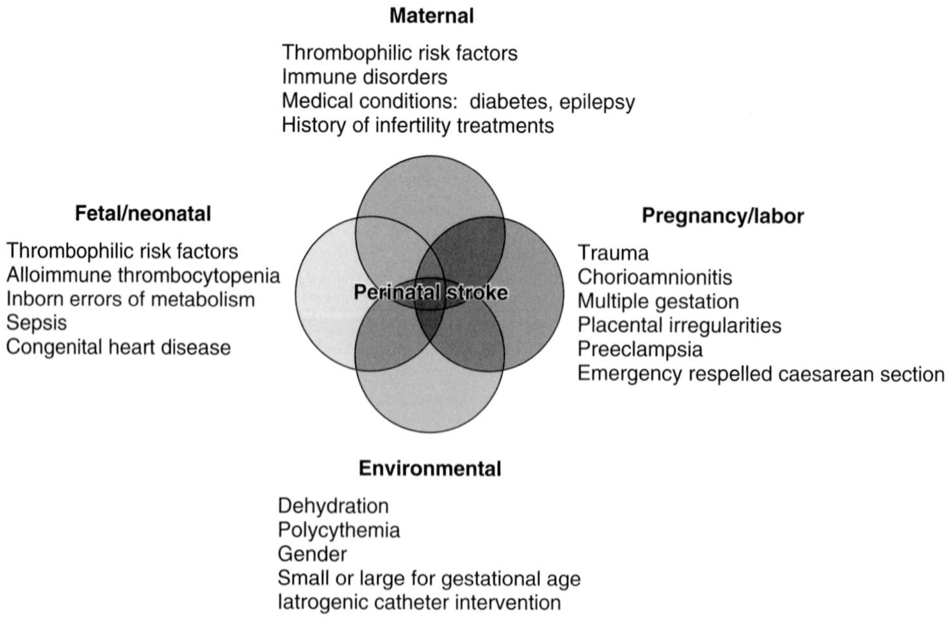

Maternal
Thrombophilic risk factors
Immune disorders
Medical conditions: diabetes, epilepsy
History of infertility treatments

Fetal/neonatal
Thrombophilic risk factors
Alloimmune thrombocytopenia
Inborn errors of metabolism
Sepsis
Congenital heart disease

Perinatal stroke

Pregnancy/labor
Trauma
Chorioamnionitis
Multiple gestation
Placental irregularities
Preeclampsia
Emergency respelled caesarean section

Environmental
Dehydration
Polycythemia
Gender
Small or large for gestational age
Iatrogenic catheter intervention

Figure 7-4 Etiologies for perinatal stroke include maternal, fetal/neonatal, pregnancy/labor, and environmental risk factors.

cases with an identifiable cause.[6] Maternal *coagulation disorders*—both hereditary and acquired—have also been reported as a significant etiology of fetal stroke. These include maternal hypercoagulability, anticoagulation with warfarin, and immune thrombocytopenic purpura (ITP).[7-10] The role of maternal *thrombophilias* in fetal stroke remains unclear, although investigations into maternal and neonatal thrombophilias suggest a link to neonatal stroke.

The most commonly encountered pregnancy-related condition is a complicated multiple gestation. Incidence of ischemic brain injury in multiple gestations is reported to be relatively high and is estimated to be 30% for monochorionic twins and 3% for dichorionic twins.[11,12] The risk is particularly increased upon death of a twin, which may create an indication for fetal MRI. It should be kept in mind, however, that neither ultrasound nor MRI can exclude brain damage in the surviving twin with absolute certainty.[13] Ischemic injury has been postulated as a major mechanism in cases of significant maternal trauma, placental hemorrhage, or placental abruption. Maternal trauma can affect the fetus through multiple mechanisms, including direct fetal brain trauma, maternal hypotension, and placental injury. In our investigation of trauma associated with fetal stroke, evidence for placental hemorrhage was observed in one pregnancy, and in two other cases placental abruption was documented before fetal stroke was noted.[6]

Fetal conditions are thought to be causative in about a third of fetal stroke cases. Among cases with an identifiable cause, alloimmune thrombocytopenia was the most common etiology (about 10% in our review). Alloimmune thrombocytopenia is estimated to occur 1 in 2000 to 5000 pregnancies.[14] Stroke is the most significant complication and is reported to occur in 10% to 30% of cases, and one fourth to one half of these hemorrhages are known to occur in utero.[15]

Inborn errors of metabolism have also been identified as causative factors. Although it is very uncommon for an inborn error of metabolism to become manifest in the form of fetal stroke, the incidence of such errors among cases with an identifiable cause was about 5% in our previous analysis.[6] Pyruvate carboxylase and carnitine palmitoyltransferase deficiencies are thought to act through different mechanisms, but both conditions were associated with fetal hemorrhagic lesions.[16-20] It has been postulated that chronic ischemia secondary to metabolic depletion in the germinal matrix tissues may be the cause of stroke in patients with pyruvate-carboxylase deficiency because the germinal matrix has been demonstrated to have a high metabolic rate during the period of neurogenesis/gliogenesis.[18-20] Of note, both cases of carnitine palmitoyltransferase deficiency were associated with intraparenchymal calcifications.[16,17]

Etiology and Risk Factors for Neonatal Stroke

Etiologic risk factors for stroke in the neonate can also be grouped into maternal, pregnancy/labor-related, and fetal or neonatal conditions (Table 7-2).

Maternal thrombophilias, particularly those involving factor V Leiden and antiphospholipid antibodies, have been implicated in perinatal stroke.[21] Simchen and colleagues[21] describe a retrospective analysis of mother-infant pairs in which the infants suffered IPS. These investigators found increased incidences of both maternal and neonatal thrombophilias, suggesting a potential relationship of susceptibility and insult. In 78% of the mother-infant pairs, either the mother or the infant was found to have a thrombophilic risk factor, and in 13% the mother-infant pair had the same thrombophilic risk factor.[21]

Among further maternal causes, Lee and associates[22] found infertility as an independent risk factor for perinatal stroke, and an association with maternal diabetes has been found for both fetal and neonatal stroke.[23]

Pregnancy/labor complications are reported in more than half of cases with neonatal stroke.[22,24] Normal pregnancy results in a prothrombotic state, with increased incidence of clot formation even in women without genetic thrombophilias; thrombotic events in the placenta can lead to embolism or ischemia in the fetus. In addition, preeclampsia is associated with endothelial disruption, which may further predispose to prothrombotic tendencies.[1]

Table 7-2   REPORTED PATHOLOGIES ASSOCIATED WITH FETAL AND NEONATAL STROKE*

	Fetal Stroke	Neonatal Stroke
Maternal conditions	Immune thrombocytopenic purpura Warfarin use Diabetes Trauma[76] Maternal fever with gastroenteritis Antiepileptic medication[77] History of infertility[22] Salicylate ingestion[78]	Diabetes Factor V Leiden, antiphospholipid antibodies (anticardiolipin antibodies, lupus anticoagulant)
Pregnancy- or labor-related disorders	Placental hemorrhage[9] Placental thromboses Abruptio placentae Complicated multiple gestations Chorioamnionitis Oligohydramnios	Hypoxic ischemic encephalopathy[22,23,42] Birth trauma Preeclampsia Prolonged rupture of membranes Prolonged second stage of labor[22] Cord abnormalities[22] Vacuum assistance Emergency cesarean delivery Chorioamnionitis
Fetal-neonatal conditions	Pyruvate decarboxylase deficiency[20] Carnitine palmitoyltransferase deficiency Fetal alloimmune thrombocytopenia CMV infection[79] Non-A, non-B hepatitis[80] Von Willebrand's disease[81] Protein C deficiency Fetal anemia[42]	Septicemia Bacterial meningitis Intrauterine growth retardation and fetal distress Thrombophilic risk factors: antithrombin deficiency, protein C or S deficiency, lipoprotein (a), factor V, factor II, methylene tetrahydrofolate reductase mutations Antiphospholipid antibodies Vitamin K deficiency[82] Alpha$_1$-antitrypsin deficiency[83-86] Catheterization Extracorporeal membrane oxygenation

*Superscript numbers indicate chapter references.

Prolonged rupture of membranes and prolonged second stage of labor are also associated with an increased risk of neonatal stroke, and birth trauma may result in thrombosis of the middle cerebral artery (MCA).[1] Finally, maternal chorioamnionitis is implicated in neonatal stroke[25]; a 2009 case report documented umbilical venous thrombosis in a neonate with left MCA territory stroke.[26] The mechanism of stroke secondary to intrauterine infection has been attributed to thrombosis with embolization as noted in the previous case versus an increased fetal inflammatory response in a procoagulant cytokine milieu.[25,26]

Among fetal and neonatal causes of neonatal stroke, fetal thrombophilias deserve a special consideration. Several groups have reported a high incidence of thrombophilias in cases of neonatal stroke, but their role was thought to be more likely permissive and requiring a triggering environmental event. New to the body of perinatal stroke literature is a meta-analysis suggesting that all recognized thrombophilias may serve as risk factors for perinatal stroke.[27] Neonatal prothrombotic risk factors reported in the literature in patients with perinatal stroke are mutations of factor V (G1691A),[27,28] factor V Leiden (R506Q),[1] factor II (G20210A),[27,28] methylene tetrahydrofolate reductase (MTHFR) mutations (T667T),[27,28] particularly when associated with hyperhomocysteinemia,[28] elevated factor VIIIc,[28] lipoprotein (a),[27] and deficiencies of antithrombin III[27] and protein C or protein S.[27,28] A multicenter case-control study found that term neonates with a symptomatic ischemic stroke were 6.7 times more likely to have at least one prothrombotic disorder than age- and sex-matched controls.[23] The mechanism for arterial thromboembolic disease is most likely multifactorial.[23,28] Kurnik and associates[28] reported a triggering condition, such as cardiac malformation and immobilization, diarrhea, mastoiditis, or moyamoya syndrome, in 71% of patients with a prothrombotic condition and a recurrent thrombotic event, suggesting that both the genome and the environment contribute to this complex disorder.

Also of special note when one is considering the hypercoagulable state of the neonate are cerebral sinovenous thromboses (SVTs); these thrombotic events likely account for a significant proportion of neonatal strokes. One large population-based study in the Netherlands found a yearly incidence of 1.4 to 12 sinovenous thromboses per 100,000 term newborns.[29] In this study by Berfelo and colleagues,[29] which examined risk factors specific to cerebral sinovenous thrombosis, complicated delivery was the most common risk factor identified.[29] Dehydration and polycythemia are also implicated in hypercoagulable states in the newborn.[1]

Cardiac abnormalities are a common cause of stroke in the childhood years, and both congenital cardiac defects and corrective surgery may result in neonatal stroke.[30,31] In some reports, stroke is the most common white matter injury noted preoperatively in neonates with congenital heart disease, particularly dextro-transposition of the great arteries.[32] Presumably this predisposition to stroke relates partly to anatomic anomalies and perhaps also to altered organogenesis; this hypothesis provides another example of the multifactorial nature of neonatal stroke.

Sepsis or bacterial meningitis in the neonatal period may also result in neonatal stroke.[1] Hypoglycemia in late preterm (<37 weeks) infants has been associated with IPS.[33] Finally, iatrogenic causes of neonatal stroke have also been reported, which include catheterization of the umbilical vein or the temporal vein,[1] the use of extracorporeal membrane oxygenation (ECMO),[34] and the use of balloon atrial septostomy.[32]

Pathology

Fetal Stroke

Tissue reaction to a hemorrhagic or ischemic insult is dependent on fetal brain maturity. In the second trimester the damaged tissue undergoes pure liquefaction necrosis with subsequent resorption without scar formation, resulting in cavities. *Porencephaly, multicystic encephalomalacia,* and *hydranencephaly* are terms used for different patterns of cavities. More mature fetal brain reacts to injury with gliosis. The majority of fetal strokes are hemorrhagic. Classification of intracranial hemorrhage includes five groups: intraventricular, intraparenchymal, infratentorial (cerebellar), subdural, and subarachnoid hemorrhages. Most fetal strokes are intraventricular or intraparenchymal.

Neonatal Stroke

The majority of neonatal strokes are ischemic. In the term neonate, arterial ischemic stroke is most likely related to a focal ischemic lesion in the distribution of a specific cerebral artery. Miller[35] reported that 83% of the arterial ischemic strokes occurred in the MCA territory. As previously noted, Lee and associates[22] reported a similar incidence (70%). Lesions of the anterior or posterior cerebral artery territories are much less commonly reported.[35] Lesions are left-sided in 53% to 75% of perinatal stroke cases.[22,35] The predominance of MCA lesions, and particularly left MCA lesions, is likely related to fact that the patent foramen ovale of the fetal and early neonatal circulation directs blood flow toward the left MCA. Infarcts are hemorrhagic in 20% of these cases.[36] In slightly more mature preterm infants (>33 weeks' gestational age [GA]) the left MCA is the most predominantly affected vessel; in more premature infants (28-32 weeks GA) with neonatal stroke, the lenticulostriate branches are also commonly affected.[37]

Incidence

The true incidence and prevalence of stroke in the fetal and neonatal periods remain poorly defined. There is no unbiased, evidence-based study on the incidence of fetal or neonatal stroke. There are few studies on the incidence of antenatal cases and thus the true incidence of fetal stroke is unknown.[5,38] This situation is due to both deficiencies in diagnosis and a lack of understanding of the etiologies of this injury.[4]

7

A report from a tertiary referral center indicated an incidence of 0.46 per 1000 deliveries.[16] It should be kept in mind, however, that a considerable fraction of fetal stroke cases results in intrauterine death or stillbirth, and another group likely goes undiagnosed in utero but manifests later in infancy or childhood; these factors are likely concealing a much higher incidence of fetal stroke.

An analysis of several studies reveals a very broad range of numbers for the incidence of neonatal stroke, ranging from 17 to 93 per 100,000 live births and as high as 5.4% in neonatal autopsies. The incidence varies according to the methods used, which include national registries, autopsy studies, and studies analyzing neonatal seizures. Fullerton and coworkers[39] noted that this incidence is 17 times higher than the incidence of large-vessel ischemic stroke in patients older than 18 years. According to results of the Canadian Childhood Stroke Registry, the incidence of perinatal stroke is 93 per 100,000.[3] In this registry the neonates accounted for 25% of acute ischemic strokes in childhood. In the National Hospital Discharge Survey, the rate of stroke was 26.4 per 100,000 live births per year in infants younger than 30 days.[38] Barmada and associates[40] reported a 5.4% incidence of arterial stroke in neonatal autopsies. Most of the infants were term neonates and presented with embolic lesions.

Stroke is a common cause of seizure, particularly focal seizure, in the term infant.[41] Statistics obtained from studies on neonatal seizures therefore have been one of the early resources on incidence of fetal-neonatal stroke. In these studies the incidence has been estimated at between 25 and 35 per 10,000. Govaert and associates,[42] in a retrospective study of routinely performed ultrasounds in their neonatal intensive care unit over a 10-year period, found the incidence to be 0.35 per 1000 live births. Estan and Hope[43] found a slightly lower incidence in newborns with seizures. It should be kept in mind, however, that information derived from these studies likely underestimates the incidence. An unknown proportion of fetal and neonatal strokes remain undiagnosed in the fetal and neonatal periods, and some are completely silent. Furthermore, seizures are not the only mode of presentation, and incidence of seizures varies considerably among studies, adding another level of bias. Additionally a significant proportion of stroke cases may be missed by routine ultrasound studies.[43-45]

Gender Effect in the Incidence of Stroke

The true effect of gender in the incidence of stroke remains under investigation, with multiple studies suggesting that male gender is a risk factor for perinatal strokes of all types. In one retrospective study of 66 term children with neonatal arterial stroke and 32 term children with neonatal cerebral sinovenous thrombosis, all confirmed by CT or MRI, Golomb and colleagues[46] reported that both entities were more commonly diagnosed in boys (62.1% and 78.1%, respectively). In a later large, multicenter analysis of confirmed stroke cases, the same investigators found the incidence in boys to be 60%.[47] In another prospective study of 100 term neonates with symptomatic stroke, 62% were boys.[48]

Clinical Manifestations

Seizures

Although seizures are a frequent manifestations of perinatal stroke, the clinical picture in both the fetal and neonatal periods may be very subtle,[2,4] and focal signs are uncommon in the early neonatal period.[43,49]

Arterial ischemic stroke is a common identifiable cause of focal neonatal seizures.[41] In an otherwise healthy neonate presenting with seizures, the reported probability of a cerebral infarct ranges from 12% to 30%.[42,43,50] Conversely, the incidence reported for a seizure presentation ranges from 85% to 92% in infants with stroke.[43,51]

Lee and associates,[22] in their analysis of 40 cases of neonatal and fetal stroke, concluded that 70% presented with neonatal seizures. In the cohort reported by Perlman and associates,[52] 75% presented with seizures. Of these, 50% were focal motor, 33% were generalized motor, and 17% were subtle seizures. Of 12 infants who presented with seizures in the series reported by Estan and Hope,[43] 67% had focal motor, 25% had generalized motor, and the remaining had 8% subtle seizures. In these infants, seizures usually occurred within the first 72 hours after birth.[43,53]

Neonatal Encephalopathy

Patients with fetal or neonatal stroke may present with nonspecific clinical signs, such as hypotonia, which will require differential diagnosis from hypoxic, metabolic, and infectious disorders. In one study of stroke, 25% of patients presented with apnea and hypotonia.[52] Similarly, Kurnik and associates[28] reported that 13% of their patients presented with apneas, and 10% with hypotonia.

Spastic Hemiplegic Cerebral Palsy

It is estimated that 20% to 30% of cases of hemiplegic cerebral palsy (CP) are related to fetal or neonatal stroke. In infants with spastic hemiplegic CP who are born at term, stroke is reported to be responsible for 50% to 70% of cases.[54] Similarly, data from Sweden also suggest that congenital hemiplegia due to prenatal or perinatal brain damage is the most common form of CP among children born at term and the second most common form of CP among prematurely born children.[55] Two thirds of these children are of normal intelligence.[55]

The spasticity is more marked in the upper extremities, and transitory hemiparesis or generalized tone anomalies may be seen in the neonatal period for a course of days.[10,49,56] In some cases this spastic paresis is preceded by a transient hypotonia contralateral to the affected side.[10]

Diagnosis

A number of patients remain undiagnosed during the fetal and neonatal periods and their strokes become manifest only in late infancy; these children had previously been described as having "delayed presentation" but now fit the criteria for the new entity PPIS, in which the timing of the insult is otherwise unknown. This presumptive fetal or neonatal event usually manifests as an asymmetry of reach and grasp at a median of 6 months.[24,53] Seizures and language delay are also seen.[53] An interesting observation is that internal capsule damage is significantly more common among those children who presented later in childhood, suggesting that this injury may be relatively silent in the fetal and neonatal periods.[53] A suggested diagnostic workup is presented in Table 7-3.

Role of Ultrasound

The diagnosis of fetal intraventricular hemorrhage (IVH) and stroke first became possible with the use of fetal cranial ultrasonography (US).[57] Considering that a significant percentage of fetal stroke cases remain asymptomatic, in utero ultrasound,

Table 7-3 SUGGESTED DIAGNOSTIC WORKUP OF NEONATAL STROKE

History	Factors Noted in Table 7-2
Radiologic examination	Cranial ultrasound, magnetic resonance imaging/angiography/venography with diffusion-weighted imaging If appropriate, echocardiography, ultrasound of neck vessels or indwelling catheters
Laboratory examination*	Coagulopathy workup: protein C and S, antithrombin III, factor V Leiden, anticardiolipin Ab, lupus anticoagulant/antiphospholipid Ab, fasting homocysteine, methylene tetrahydrofolate reductase C 677T mutation, prothrombin 20210 variant, lipoprotein (a), fibrinogen, plasminogen, factor VIIIC
Placental evaluation	Complete pathologic examination of placenta

*There is no consensus on how many of these tests are to be performed in cases of ischemic perinatal stroke.

with its wide availability and low cost, is a practical screening tool. Screening fetal US is usually performed during the early portion of the second trimester, a time before stroke typically occurs.[58,59] When US is performed during the late second or third trimester, however, it is an effective screening tool because both cerebral cavitary lesions and hemorrhage are easily diagnosed by this modality. If one is practical, however, ultrasound scans lack the sensitivity of computed tomography and MRI for the detection of either acute or small ischemic lesions. In a study of fetal strokes, MRI enabled a more accurate diagnosis of injury than either other modality in 21% of the cases.[16]

Role of Magnetic Resonance Imaging

Fetal MRI now permits excellent definition of anatomic and functional injury to the fetal cerebrum and the extent of ongoing plasticity. Even early and small ischemic lesions can by identified by MRI. The modalities of choice for clinical diagnosis include T2-weighted imaging, magnetic resonance angiography, and diffusion-weighted imaging.

The use of diffusion-weighted imaging for diagnosis of cerebral infarction in the neonate was first reported in 1994.[60] Further reports established this modality as the most sensitive imaging modality for the detection of acute stroke in the fetus or the newborn.[61] Diffusion-weighted imaging is most specific within days of injury, and diffusion-weighted abnormalities may appear to normalize within a week, whereas T2-weighted MRI becomes more sensitive over time.[62] Use of both modalities together should be considered in order to best determine extent of injury.

A newer technique, functional MRI (fMRI), although not yet used clinically in neonates, presents an appealing strategy to study the functional consequences of the insult.

Role of Placental Pathology

As described by Raju and colleagues,[1] examination of placental pathology may elucidate the source of thromboemboli.

Treatment

Today there is no definitive treatment for fetal or neonatal stroke. Late diagnosis of the entity further limits potential therapies, and current efforts are directed at understanding the underlying pathology. Maternal thrombocyte infusion via cordocentesis is used in fetal alloimmune thrombocytopenia.[63,64] Pooled immunoglobulins may be administered to the mother with maternal immune thrombocytopenic purpura.[8] The only potential therapy to treat maternal warfarin use is fresh-frozen plasma transfusion through cordocentesis, because fetal bioavailability of maternally administered vitamin K is only 5% of maternal levels.[7] Cerebral sinovenous thrombosis may be treated with unfractionated or low-molecular-weight heparin, although no clinical consensus yet exists to support this therapy.[29]

Prognosis

Fetal Stroke

Mortality and Long-Term Outcome

There is limited information on the outcome of fetal stroke. In an earlier publication of 54 cases of fetal stroke cases, we found 46 cases with a reported outcome; approximately half resulted in fetal or neonatal death, and 55% of the survivors were handicapped at follow-up ages of 3 months to 6 years.[4] Ghi and colleagues[65] published the findings of 109 cases of fetal intracranial hemorrhages, which included 16 of their cases and 93 cases from the literature. They reported that 40% of the infants in their cases died in utero or within the first month after birth. Only 53% of the reported newborns who survived were without sequelae at a median follow-up of 11.6 months.

Indicators of Long-Term Prognosis

Several studies have shown that fetal stroke with ventriculomegaly is associated with a poor outcome. In our analysis ventriculomegaly was present in more than half of the cases, and only a small number of these patients were alive and neurodevelopmentally appropriate at last follow-up.[4]

Two studies commenting on the association of the ultrasound findings with postnatal outcome stated that the complete disappearance of the hemorrhage on follow-up scanning was associated with a better postnatal neurologic outcome than hemorrhages that progressed to more extensive bleeding over time.[16,65]

Neonatal Stroke

Mortality

The infant mortality rate in the United States related to stroke during 1995 through 1998 was 5.33 per 100,000. According to the National Hospital Discharge Survey[1] from 1980 through 1998, the neonatal inhospital mortality related to stroke was 10.1%. Similarly the Canadian Pediatric Stroke registry[3] reported mortality less than 10% following neonatal stroke. When comparing term and premature cases with cerebral arterial infarction, Govaert and colleagues[42] found that the likelihood of neonatal death was over six times higher in the premature group.[42]

Recurrence

There are no conclusive studies on the risk of recurrence of neonatal stroke. However, reported risk is well below that of childhood or adult stroke. Lee and colleagues reported no recurrence in the follow-up of 176 patients for a median of 41 months. In a recent prospective follow-up study, Kurnik and associates[28] found a 1.86% risk of recurrent cerebral arterial stroke and a total of 3.3% risk of arterial or venous thrombosis with a median follow-up of 3.5 years. The highest incidence of recurrence, which was reported by the Canadian Pediatric Stroke Registry, ranged from 3% to 5%.[3,66] A higher incidence of prothrombotic disorders in this cohort may be responsible for the higher incidence of stroke recurrence, which at the same time supports the notion that the risk of recurrence is determined by the underlying pathology.[3,28,66]

Long-Term Prognosis

Much of the information on long-term prognosis following neonatal stroke is based on retrospective analysis. This problem is further complicated by the variance in stroke types, follow-up duration, methods of assessment, and populations studied.[67] Westmacott and coworkers[68] reported emerging cognitive deficits in their population of neonatal stroke patients studied longitudinally at ages 3 and 6 years, suggesting that timing of follow-up testing may influence long-term prognosis. Several other investigators indicated a relatively poor outcome.[69,70] Lynch and colleagues,[38] in their literature review of 415 cases over a 30-year period, reported that only 40% of the patients had a normal development and that 3% had died. In the Canadian Pediatric Stroke Registry, outcome was normal in a third of patients with neonatal stroke.[66] Sreenan and associates[49] reported that two thirds of the children in their cases were affected by some mental-motor deficit. Lee and colleagues[53] found that only 19% of patients had a normal outcome. Estan and Hope,[43] on the contrary, reported a better outcome, indicating that 11 of 12 children with unilateral cortical infarction at birth were entirely normal at the age of 12 to 18 months. In their analysis, de Vries and Levene[36] found that when the neonatal thromboembolic event involved the main branch of the MCA, the patient had significant morbidity but that the involvement of other branches had a more favorable outcome. In a study by Berfelo and coworkers[29] examining stroke exclusively attributed to neonatal cerebral sinovenous thrombosis, approximately half of survivors had persistent neurologic deficits, and 16% exhibited persistent epilepsy.[29] For all strokes, motor deficits are generally diagnosed during infancy or early childhood, but cognitive and behavioral deficits usually become manifest at later ages. As discussed previously, spastic hemiplegia is the most common sequela of neonatal stroke.

Indicators of Long-Term Prognosis

Certain symptomatology, EEG, and imaging findings may be indicative of late outcome.[67] Although Sreenan and colleagues[49] found an association between abnormal neurologic findings at discharge from the neonatal intensive care unit and long-term disability,[49] this finding has not been supported by other studies.[71] Several investigators have also suggested that cases presenting beyond the neonatal period had a higher incidence of permanent neurologic problems[24] and CP.[53]

Diffuse or multifocal injury, as demonstrated by diffuse background abnormality on neonatal EEG, is suggestive of increased risk for epilepsy. In a study by Mercuri and associates,[71] an abnormal back ground in an EEG study within the first week after stroke correlated with future hemiplegia in 83% of cases. Sreenan and colleagues,[49] in their study of 47 term neonates with cerebral infarction as diagnosed on computed tomography, interestingly reported that the absence of seizures in the neonatal period was associated with the absence of long-term disability.

Localization or the extent of findings on computed tomography are not correlated with long-term outcome.[49] This finding may be explained in part by the inability of the modality to differentiate between a truncal and a complete form of MCA stroke.[42]

MRI may be of practical importance in predicting long-term outcome. Hemiplegia was reported in only a small proportion of cases with cerebral infarction on neonatal MRI and was present only in children who had concomitant involvement of hemisphere, internal capsule, and basal ganglia.[72] The same study concluded that involvement of the internal capsule is always associated with motor disturbance to some degree when assessed at school age.[72] De Vries and colleagues[73] confirmed that the involvement of cortex, basal ganglia, and internal capsule invariably resulted in hemiplegia. A prospective study of MRI findings obtained within the first few weeks of life and correlated with motor outcome at age 2 years demonstrated that involvement of the corticospinal tract (CST) resulted in hemiplegia in more than half of cases, and absence of involvement of the corticospinal tract was associated with nearly 100% normal motor outcome.[74]

Several studies have indicated a normal intelligence in children with neonatal stroke.[70] However, lower IQs have been documented in children with epilepsy and children with more widespread infarcts.[75] A study of children with fetal and neonatal strokes and unilateral brain damage found no evidence of clinically significant behavioral or emotional problems between affected individuals and control individuals, even when the frontal lobe was involved.[70]

Finally, a 2009 study suggested a trend toward higher incidence of residual neurologic deficit in perinatal patients with stroke who were found to have thrombophilic risk factors than in those without such factors.[21]

In summary, accurate outcome data are difficult to interpret because of the heterogeneity of both the disease process and the spectrum of outcomes. In general, early neonatal diagnosis is generally a result of early clinical seizures, so early diagnosis is often associated with epilepsy. Later diagnosis is often a result of emerging hemiplegia presentation, so later diagnosis is associated with motor delays. One survey suggested that in children in whom diagnosis is made in the newborn period, 37% of cases progress to hemiplegic cerebral palsy, compared with 82% in children in whom diagnosis is made later in infancy.[53] Both early and late diagnosed IPS or PPIS may also be associated with visual, behavioral, cognitive, and language deficits.[1]

Conclusions

For the developing brain, stroke is most certainly a complex disorder. Although the true incidence of fetal stroke remains largely unexplored, stroke occurs in 17 to 93 per 100,000 live term births. Stroke in the fetus is almost always hemorrhagic, but stroke in the term neonate is more commonly caused by embolic or thromboembolic events. The most common causes of stroke in the fetus are twin gestation, alloimmune thrombocytopenia, and maternal trauma, whereas prothrombotic disorders, cardiac disorders, polycythemia, preeclampsia, prolonged rupture of membranes and chorioamnionitis are most commonly diagnosed in series of neonatal stroke.

Finally, stroke—whether fetal or neonatal—results in significant disability in childhood and beyond. For this reason, better definitions of injury and targeted population, genetic analysis, and environmental risk factor studies are needed to prevent this injury to the developing brain.

Acknowledgment

This work was supported by NS 27116, NS 053865 and NICHD T32 07094.

References

1. Raju TN, Nelson KB, Ferriero D, Lynch JK. Ischemic perinatal stroke. Summary of a workshop sponsored by the National Institute of Child Health and Human Development and the National Institute of Neurological Disorders and Stroke. *Pediatrics.* 2007;120:609-616.
2. Chalmers EA. Perinatal stroke—risk factors and management. *Br J Haematol.* 2005;130:333-343.
3. DeVeber G. Canadian pediatric ischemic stroke registry. *Pediatr Child Health.* 2000;A17:5-14.
4. Ozduman K, Pober BR, Barnes P, et al. Fetal stroke. *Pediatr Neurol.* 2004;30:1511-1562.
5. deVeber G. Stroke and the child's brain: an overview of epidemiology, syndromes and risk factors. *Curr Opin Neurol.* 2002;15:133-138.
6. Ozduman K, de Veber G, Ment LR. Stroke in the fetus and neonate. In: Perlman JM, ed. *Neurology: Neonatology questions and controversies.* Philadelphia: Saunders/Elsevier; 2008:88-121.
7. Ville Y, Jenkins E, Shearer MJ, et al. Fetal intraventricular haemorrhage and maternal warfarin. *Lancet.* 1993;341:1211.
8. Tampakoudis P, Bili H, Lazaridis E, et al. Prenatal diagnosis of intracranial hemorrhage secondary to maternal idiopathic thrombocytopenic purpura: a case report. *Am J Perinatol.* 1995;12:268-270.
9. Scher MS, Belfar H, Martin J, Painter MJ. Destructive brain lesions of presumed fetal onset: antepartum causes of cerebral palsy. *Pediatrics.* 1991;88:898-906.
10. Scher MS, Wiznitzer M, Bangert BA. Cerebral infarctions in the fetus and neonate: maternal-placental-fetal considerations. *Clin Perinatol.* 2002;29:693-724.
11. Levine D. Case 46: encephalomalacia in surviving twin after death of monochorionic co-twin. *Radiology.* 2002;223:392-395.
12. Barkovich AJ. Brain and spine injuries in infancy and childhood. In: Barkovich AJ. *Pediatric Neuroimaging.* Philadelphia: Lippincott Williams and Wilkins; 2000:157-240.
13. Levine D. MR imaging of fetal central nervous system abnormalities. *Brain Cogn.* 2002;50:432-448.
14. Johnson JA, Ryan G, al-Musa A, et al. Prenatal diagnosis and management of neonatal alloimmune thrombocytopenia. *Semin Perinatol.* 1997;21:45-52.
15. Dale ST, Coleman LT. Neonatal alloimmune thrombocytopenia: antenatal and postnatal imaging findings in the pediatric brain. *AJNR: American Journal of Neuroradiology.* 2002;23:1457-1465.
16. Elchalal U, Yagel S, Gomori JM, et al. Fetal intracranial hemorrhage (fetal stroke): does grade matter? *Ultrasound Obstet Gynecol.* 2005;26:233-243.
17. Elpeleg ON, eHammerman C, Saada A, et al. Antenatal presentation of carnitine palmitoyltransferase II deficiency. *Am J Med Genet.* 2001;102:183-187.
18. Wong LT, Davidson AG, Applegarth DA, et al. Biochemical and histologic pathology in an infant with cross-reacting material (negative) pyruvate carboxylase deficiency. *Pediatr Res.* 1986;20:274-279.
19. Pineda M, Campistol J, Vilaseca MA, et al. An atypical French form of pyruvate carboxylase deficiency. *Brain Dev.* 1995;17:276-279.
20. Brun N, Robitaille Y, Grignon A, et al. Pyruvate carboxylase deficiency: prenatal onset of ischemia-like brain lesions in two sibs with the acute neonatal form. *Am J Med Genet.* 1999;84:94-101.
21. Simchen MJ, Goldstein G, Lubetsky A, et al. Factor V Leiden and antiphospholipid antibodies in either mothers or infants increase the risk for perinatal arterial ischemic stroke. *Stroke.* 2009;40:65-70.
22. Lee J, Croen LA, Backstrand KH, et al. Maternal and infant characteristics associated with perinatal arterial stroke in the infant. *JAMA.* 2005;293(6):723-729.
23. Gunther G, Junker R, Sträter R, et al; Childhood Stroke Study Group. Symptomatic ischemic stroke in full-term neonates: role of acquired and genetic prothrombotic risk factors. *Stroke.* 2000;31:2437-2441.
24. Golomb MR, MacGregor DL, Domi T, et al. Presumed pre- or perinatal arterial ischemic stroke: risk factors and outcomes. *Ann Neurol.* 2001;50:163-168.
25. Redline RW, Sagar P, King ME, et al. Case records of the Massachusetts General Hospital. Case 12-2008. A newborn infant with intermittent apnea and seizures. *N Engl J Med.* 2008;358:1713-1723.
26. Dueck CC, Grynspan D, Eisenstat DD, et al. Ischemic perinatal stroke secondary to chorioamnionitis: a histopathological case presentation. *J Child Neurol.* 2009;24:1557-1560.

7

27. Kenet G, Lütkhoff LK, Albisetti M, et al. Impact of thrombophilia on risk of arterial ischemic stroke or cerebral sinovenous thrombosis in neonates and children: a systematic review and meta-analysis of observational studies. *Circulation*. 2010;121:1838-1847.

28. Kurnik K, Kosch A, Sträter R, et al; Childhood Stroke Study Group. Recurrent thromboembolism in infants and children suffering from symptomatic neonatal arterial stroke: a prospective follow-up study. *Stroke*. 2003;34:2887-2892.

29. Berfelo FJ, Kersbergen KJ, van Ommen CH, et al. Neonatal cerebral sinovenous thrombosis from symptom to outcome. *Stroke*. 2010;41:1382-1388.

30. Kumar K. Neurological complications of congenital heart disease. *Ind J Pediatr*. 2000;67:287-291.

31. Miller G, Mamourian AC, Tesman JR, et al. Long-term MRI changes in brain after pediatric open heart surgery. *J Child Neurol*. 1994;9:390-397.

32. McQuillen PS, Miller SP. Congenital heart disease and brain development. *Ann N Y Acad Sci*. 2010;1184:68-86.

33. Benders MJ, Groenendaal F, Uiterwaal CS, et al. Maternal and infant characteristics associated with perinatal arterial stroke in the preterm infant. *Stroke*. 2007;38:1759-1765.

34. Watson JW, Brown DM, Lally KP, et al. Complications of extracorporeal membrane oxygenation in neonates. *South Med J*. 1990;83:1262-1265.

35. Miller V. Neonatal cerebral infarction. *Semin Pediatr Neurol*. 2000;7:278-288.

36. de Vries LS, Groenendaal F, Eken P, et al. Infarcts in the vascular distribution of the middle cerebral artery in preterm and fullterm infants. *Neuropediatrics*. 1997;28:88-96.

37. Benders MJ, Groenendaal F, De Vries LS. Preterm arterial ischemic stroke. *Semin Fetal Neonatal Med*. 2009;14:272-277.

38. Lynch JK, Nelson KB. Epidemiology of perinatal stroke. *Curr Opin Pediatr*. 2001;13:499-505.

39. Fullerton HJ, Wu YW, Zhao S, Johnston SC. Risk of stroke in children: ethnic and gender disparities. *Neurology*. 2003;61:189-194.

40. Barmada MA, Moossy J, Shuman RM. Cerebral infarcts with arterial occlusion in neonates. *Ann Neurol*. 1979;6:495-502.

41. Volpe JJ. *Neurology of the Newborn*. 4th ed. Philadelphia: Saunders; 2001:428-493.

42. Govaert P, Matthys E, Zecic A, et al. Perinatal cortical infarction within middle cerebral artery trunks. *Arch Dis Child Fetal Neonatal Ed*. 2000;82:F59-F63.

43. Estan J, Hope P. Unilateral neonatal cerebral infarction in full term infants. *Arch Dis Child Fetal Neonatal Ed*. 1997;76:F88-F93.

44. Krishnamoorthy KS, Soman TB, Takeoka M, Schaefer PW. Diffusion-weighted imaging in neonatal cerebral infarction: clinical utility and follow-up. *J Child Neurol*. 2000;15:592-602.

45. Mercuri E, Cowan F, Rutherford M, et al. Ischaemic and haemorrhagic brain lesions in newborns with seizures and normal Apgar scores. *Arch Dis Child Fetal Neonatal Ed*. 1995;73:F67-F74.

46. Golomb MR, Dick PT, MacGregor DL, et al. Neonatal arterial ischemic stroke and cerebral sinovenous thrombosis are more commonly diagnosed in boys. *J Child Neurol*. 2004;19:493-497.

47. Golomb MR, Fullerton HJ, Nowak-Gottl U, Deveber G; International Pediatric Stroke Study Group. Male predominance in childhood ischemic stroke: findings from the International Pediatric Stroke Study. *Stroke*. 2009;40:52-57.

48. Chabrier S, Saliba E, Nguyen The Tich S, et al. Obstetrical and neonatal characteristics vary with birthweight in a cohort of 100 term newborns with symptomatic arterial ischemic stroke. *Eur J Paediatr Neurol*. 2010;14:206-213.

49. Sreenan C, Bhargava R, Robertson CM. Cerebral infarction in the term newborn: clinical presentation and long-term outcome. *J Pediatr*. 2000;137:351-355.

50. Lien JM, Towers CV, Quilligan EJ, et al. Term early-onset neonatal seizures: obstetric characteristics, etiologic classifications, and perinatal care. *Obstet Gynecol*. 1995;85:163-169.

51. deVeber G, Monagle P, Chan A, et al. Prothrombotic disorders in infants and children with cerebral thromboembolism. *Arch Neurol*. 1998;55:1539-1543.

52. Perlman JM, Rollins NK, Evans D. Neonatal stroke: clinical characteristics and cerebral blood flow velocity measurements. *Pediatr Neurol*. 1994;11:281-284.

53. Lee J, Croen LA, Lindan C, et al. Predictors of outcome in perinatal arterial stroke: a population-based study. *Ann Neurol*. 2005;58:303-308.

54. Uvebrant P. Hemiplegic cerebral palsy. Aetiology and outcome. *Acta Paediatr Scand Suppl*. 1988; 345:1-100.

55. Hagberg B, Hagberg G, Beckung E, Uvebrant P. Changing panorama of cerebral palsy in Sweden. VIII. Prevalence and origin in the birth year period 1991-94. *Acta Paediatr*. 2001;90:271-277.

56. Mercuri E. Early diagnostic and prognostic indicators in full term infants with neonatal cerebral infarction: an integrated clinical, neuroradiological and EEG approach. *Minerva Pediatr*. 2001;53: 305-311.

57. Kim MS, Elyaderani MK. Sonographic diagnosis of cerebroventricular hemorrhage in utero. *Radiology*. 1982;142:479-480.

58. Catanzarite VA, Schrimmer DB, Maida C, Mendoza A. Prenatal sonographic diagnosis of intracranial haemorrhage: report of a case with a sinusoidal fetal heart rate tracing, and review of the literature. *Prenat Diagn*. 1995;15:229-235.

59. Groothuis AM, de Kleine MJ, Oei SG. Intraventricular haemorrhage in utero. A case-report and review of the literature. *Eur J Obstet Gynecol Reprod Biol*. 2000;89:207-211.

60. Cowan FM, Pennock JM, Hanrahan JD, et al. Early detection of cerebral infarction and hypoxic ischemic encephalopathy in neonates using diffusion-weighted magnetic resonance imaging. *Neuropediatrics*. 1994;25:172-175.

61. Venkataraman A, Kingsley PB, Kalina P, et al. Newborn brain infarction: clinical aspects and magnetic resonance imaging. *CNS Spectr*. 2004;9:436-444.
62. Rutherford M, Counsell S, Allsop J, et al. Diffusion-weighted magnetic resonance imaging in term perinatal brain injury: a comparison with site of lesion and time from birth. *Pediatrics*. 2004;114:1004-1014.
63. Dickinson JE, Marshall LR, Phillips JM, Barr AL. Antenatal diagnosis and management of fetomaternal alloimmune thrombocytopenia. *Am J Perinatol*. 1995;12:333-335.
64. de Vries LS, Connell J, Bydder GM, et al. Recurrent intracranial haemorrhages in utero in an infant with alloimmune thrombocytopenia. Case report. *Br J Obstet Gynaecol*. 1988;95:299-302.
65. Ghi T, Simonazzi G, Perolo A, et al. Outcome of antenatally diagnosed intracranial hemorrhage: case series and review of the literature. *Ultrasound Obstet Gynecol*. 2003;22:121-130.
66. deVeber GA, MacGregor D, Curtis R, Mayank S. Neurologic outcome in survivors of childhood arterial ischemic stroke and sinovenous thrombosis. *J Child Neurol*. 2000;15:316-324.
67. Lynch JK, Hirtz DG, DeVeber G, Nelson KB. Report of the National Institute of Neurological Disorders and Stroke workshop on perinatal and childhood stroke. *Pediatrics*. 2002;109:116-123.
68. Westmacott R, MacGregor D, Askalan R, deVeber G. Late emergence of cognitive deficits after unilateral neonatal stroke. *Stroke*. 2009;40:2012-2019.
69. Bates E, Thal D, Trauner D, et al. From first words to grammar in children with focal brain injury. *Dev Psychol*. 1997;13:275-343.
70. Trauner DA, Nass R, Ballantyne A. Behavioural profiles of children and adolescents after pre- or perinatal unilateral brain damage. *Brain*. 2001;124:995-1002.
71. Mercuri E, Rutherford M, Cowan F, et al. Early prognostic indicators of outcome in infants with neonatal cerebral infarction: a clinical, electroencephalogram, and magnetic resonance imaging study. *Pediatrics*. 1999;103:39-46.
72. Mercuri E, Barnett A, Rutherford M, et al. Neonatal cerebral infarction and neuromotor outcome at school age. *Pediatrics*. 2004;113:95-100.
73. De Vries LS, Van der Grond J, Van Haastert IC, Groenendaal F. Prediction of outcome in new-born infants with arterial ischaemic stroke using diffusion-weighted magnetic resonance imaging. *Neuropediatrics*. 2005;36:12-20.
74. Husson B, Hertz-Pannier L, Renaud C, et al; AVCnn Group. Motor outcomes after neonatal arterial ischemic stroke related to early MRI data in a prospective study. *Pediatrics*. 2010;126:912-918.
75. Vargha-Khadem F, Isaacs E, van der Werf S, et al. Development of intelligence and memory in children with hemiplegic cerebral palsy. The deleterious consequences of early seizures. *Brain*. 1992;115:315-329.
76. Strigini FA, Cioni G, Canapicchi R, et al. Fetal intracranial hemorrhage: is minor maternal trauma a possible pathogenetic factor? *Ultrasound Obstet Gynecol*. 2001;18:335-342.
77. Minkoff H, Schaffer RM, Delke I, Grunebaum AN. Diagnosis of intracranial hemorrhage in utero after a maternal seizure. *Obstet Gynecol*. 1985;65(suppl):22S-24S.
78. Govaert P, Staelens V, Vanhaesebrouch P. Perinatal intracranial hemorrhage due to maternal salicylate ingestion. *Clin Pediatr (Phila)*. 1995;34:174-175.
79. Anderson MW, McGahan JP. Sonographic detection of an in utero intracranial hemorrhage in the second trimester. *J Ultrasound Med*. 1994;13:315-318.
80. Leidig E, Dannecker G, Pfeiffer KH, et al. Intrauterine development of posthaemorrhagic hydrocephalus. *Eur J Pediatr*. 1988;147:26-29.
81. Mullaart RA, Van Dongen P, Gabreëls FJ, van Oostrom C. Fetal periventricular hemorrhage in von Willebrand's disease: short review and first case presentation. *Am J Perinatol*. 1991;8:190-192.
82. Aydinli N, Citak A, Caliskan M, et al. Vitamin K deficiency—late onset intracranial haemorrhage. *Eur J Paediatr Neurol*. 1998;2:199-203.
83. Jenkins HR, Leonard JV, Kay JD, et al. Alpha-1-antitrypsin deficiency, bleeding diathesis, and intracranial haemorrhage. *Arch Dis Child*. 1982;57:722-723.
84. Payne NR, Hasegawa DK. Vitamin K deficiency in newborns: a case report in alpha-1-antitrypsin deficiency and a review of factors predisposing to hemorrhage. *Pediatrics*. 1984;73:712-716.
85. Hope PL, Hall MA, Millward-Sadler GH, Normand IC. Alpha-1-antitrypsin deficiency presenting as a bleeding diathesis in the newborn. *Arch Dis Child*. 1982;57:68-70.
86. Bussel JB, Zabusky MR, Berkowitz RL, McFarland JG. Fetal alloimmune thrombocytopenia. *N Engl J Med*. 1997;337:22-26.

CHAPTER 8

Diagnosis and Treatment of Neonatal Seizures

Mark S. Scher, MD

Basic issues still remain regarding the recognition and treatment of neonatal seizures (Table 8-1). Which newborn with seizures to treat and how to treat him or her continues to occupy much discussion and controversy in written and oral presentations. Although clinical seizures remain a common occurrence in neonatal intensive care settings, with an incidence as high as 2.6 per 1000 live births for term infants and 30 to 130 per 1000 live preterm births, increasing use of bedside electrophysiologic monitoring has resulted in the growing recognition that the incidence of seizures may be even higher if the electrographic definition is applied. Yet the question of who in the algorithm to diagnose and treat neonatal seizures includes a heterogeneous cohort of newborns who may present throughout the neonatal period (i.e., through 30 days post-term). The manner of clinical presentation reflects alternative diagnostic explanations for seizure recurrence based on timing, etiology, or brain region of injury.[1] Presentation may imply part of a longstanding encephalopathic process prior to and/or during parturition in some newborns. Other infants present with isolated seizures or ictal events that herald the onset of new postnatal disease.

Seizure occurrence must be based on a reliance on both clinical sign recognition and coincident electrographic expression to define the exact duration (onset and offset) of seizures. This is also essential to more accurately define status epilepticus as well as the presence of nonepileptic movement disorders. The issue of seizure recognition highlights the controversy regarding the assessment of treatment efficacy, linking to the etiologic process as well as location and timing of injury. Unresolved questions also include the unknown duration of treatment for a neonate who experienced seizures after emergency treatment in the neonatal intensive care unit. Long-term treatment may be required for the child at an increased risk for childhood seizures and neurocognitive/neurobehavioral sequelae at an older age. Although issues of short- and long-term prognosis are not discussed in this review, the following caveat underscores the need for improved seizure recognition, diagnostic evaluation, and treatment: There remains a controversy as to whether electrical or clinical seizures are more detrimental to normal brain structure and function. Based on current epilepsy models in the immature and older populations, epilepsy-induced brain damage can occur as a direct result of the metabolic consequences of the

Table 8-1 QUESTIONS AND CONTROVERSIES CONCERNING NEONATAL
SEIZURES

Questions	Controversies
Who should be treated?	Timing of brain insult, age at presentation, presence or absence of an encephalopathy, underlying etiology
What constitutes a seizure?	Clinical versus electrical criteria for seizures, what constitutes status epilepticus
What is appropriate treatment?	Specific therapeutic choices Define the end points of treatment to assess efficacy on basis of etiology, timing, and location
How long to treat?	Ability to predict risk for sequelae (e.g., epilepsy, neurodevelopmental disorders)
Why treat?	To distinguish seizures as an epiphenomenon vs. a neuronal process that contributes to epilepsy-induced brain damage

seizures themselves and/or the underlying etiologies in which seizures are embedded.[2] Therefore the final section of this chapter discusses representative innovations that augment our understanding of seizures in the immature brain. Proposed and current research may lead to novel therapeutic approaches that are relevant to the pathophysiologic mechanisms responsible for both seizures and nonepileptic paroxysmal movement disorders in the context of the associated etiologies, location, and timing of injury in the immature brain. Both single and synergistic therapeutic protocols are now being proposed that address preventive, rescue, and repair phases after brain injury. Neonatal seizures constitute a complex phenotype that reflects past, present, and future risk. A developmental theory perspective underscores the importance of a life course approach to the neonate with seizures, given other challenges that confront the patient throughout childhood and into the adult years.

Recognition of Neonatal Seizures

There remains a fundamental controversy regarding seizure recognition,[3] assuming that the phenotype expression of seizures is defined as clinical or electrographic by description. Many clinicians continue to rely primarily on clinical criteria for the diagnosis of neonatal seizures while acknowledging that electrographic confirmation of seizures may also be necessary. This controversy has been fueled by the technologic advances in bedside evaluation using synchronized video-electroencephalographic monitoring. Simultaneous documentation of suspicious clinical behaviors with electrographic seizures is considered the neurophysiologic gold standard. With this technology, new classifications of neonatal seizures can draw a clearer distinction between epileptic and nonepileptic events, although some newborns can have both phenomena as independent or correlated occurrences. Failure to document electrographic seizures by scalp recordings suggests the possibility that clinical events may be either nonepileptic paroxysmal behaviors and/or subcortical seizure events without propagation to the surface to allow detection by scalp recordings. Although such seizures are commonly diagnosed in older childhood and adult populations, such explanations for neonates are less actively described. However, several authorities argue that traditionally described subtle seizures have no coincidental electrographic seizure occurrence on scalp recordings, underscoring the controversy. Electroencephalography (EEG) recordings are therefore helpful to avoid the giving of treatment with traditional antiepileptic drugs (AEDs) for paroxysmal nonepileptic events that ultimately may require alternative diagnostic and therapeutic choices.

The advocacy for electrographic confirmation should include the use of automated screening devices in concert with traditional EEG studies. First designed in the late 1960s to use only one channel of EEG, these devices usually rely on a single computerized algorithm to detect a pattern for neonatal seizures. A limited number of channels are inadequate to document the electrographic expression of seizures that may originate distant from the electrode site or may be of such low amplitude and/or duration to avoid definitive conclusions regarding the presence or duration of seizures.[4] There is as yet no consensus regarding the comparison of screening recordings with traditional EEG studies with respect to the detection of seizures with acceptable false-negative and false-positive results. A 2011 EMBASE and Medline reference search reviewed all relevant articles that compared the two technologies, with results favoring a combination of the approaches.[5] Two-tiered recording paradigms need to be incorporated in future studies to combine the results from screening devices with more traditional comprehensive neurophysiologic protocols, tailored to the diagnostic and therapeutic needs of the individual patient.

Clinical Seizure Criteria

Neonatal seizures are currently listed separately from the traditional classification of seizures and epilepsy during childhood. The International League Against Epilepsy (ILAE) classification adopted by the World Health Organization still considers neonatal seizures within an unclassified category.[6] A fairly new classification scheme now suggests a more strict distinction of clinical seizure (nonepileptic) events from electrographically confirmed (epileptic) seizures, with respect to possible treatment interventions.[7] Continued refinement of such novel classifications is needed to reconcile the variable agreement between clinical and EEG criteria for establishing a seizure diagnosis[8,9] in the context of nonepileptic movement disorders caused by acquired diseases, malformations, and/or medications.

Several caveats (Box 8-1) may be useful in the identification of suspected neonatal seizures and raise questions regarding the diagnostic acumen of using only clinical criteria.

The clinical criteria for neonatal seizure diagnosis were historically subdivided into five clinical categories: focal clonic, multifocal or migratory clonic, tonic, myoclonic, and subtle seizures.[10] A later classification expanded the clinical subtypes, adopting a strict temporal occurrence of specific clinical events with coincident electrographic seizures, to distinguish neonatal clinical nonepileptic seizures from epileptic seizures (Tables 8-2 and 8-3).[7]

Subtle Seizure Activity

Subtle seizure activity is the most frequently observed category of neonatal seizures and includes repetitive buccolingual movements, orbital-ocular movements, unusual bicycling or peddling, and autonomic findings (Fig. 8-1A). Subtle paroxysmal events that interrupt the expected behavioral repertoire of the neonatal state and that appear stereotypic or repetitive should heighten the clinician's level of suspicion for seizures. However, alterations in cardiorespiratory regularity, body movements, and other

---

Box 8-1 CAVEATS CONCERNING RECOGNITION OF NEONATAL SEIZURES

1. Specific stereotypic behaviors occur in association with normal neonatal sleep or waking states, medication effects, and gestational maturity.
2. Consider that any abnormal repetitive activity may be a clinical seizure if out of context for expected neonatal behavior.
3. Attempt to document coincident electrographic seizures with the suspected clinical event.
4. Abnormal behavioral phenomena may have inconsistent relationships with coincident electroencephalographic seizures, suggesting a subcortical seizure focus.
5. Nonepileptic pathologic movement disorders are events that are independent of the seizure state and may also be expressed by neonates.

Table 8-2   CLINICAL CHARACTERISTICS, CLASSIFICATION, AND PRESUMED
PATHOPHYSIOLOGY OF NEONATAL SEIZURES

Classification	Characterization
Focal clonic	Repetitive, rhythmic contractions of muscle groups of the limbs, face, or trunk May be unifocal or multifocal May occur synchronously or asynchronously in muscle groups on one side of the body May occur simultaneously but asynchronously on both sides Cannot be suppressed by restraint Pathophysiology: epileptic
Focal tonic	Sustained posturing of single limbs Sustained asymmetric posturing of the trunk Sustained eye deviation Cannot be provoked by stimulation or suppressed by restraint Pathophysiology: epileptic
Generalized tonic	Sustained symmetric posturing of limbs, trunk, and neck May be flexor, extensor, or mixed extensor/flexor May be provoked or intensified by stimulation May be suppressed by restraint or repositioning Presumed pathophysiology: nonepileptic
Myoclonic	Random, single, rapid contractions of muscle groups of the limbs, face, or trunk Typically not repetitive or may recur at a slow rate May be generalized, focal, or fragmentary May be provoked by stimulation Presumed pathophysiology: epileptic or nonepileptic
Spasms	May be flexor, extensor, or mixed extensor/flexor May occur in clusters Cannot be provoked by stimulation or suppressed by restraint Pathophysiology: epileptic
Motor Automatisms Ocular signs	Random and roving eye movements or nystagmus (distinct from tonic eye deviation) May be provoked or intensified by tactile stimulation Presumed pathophysiology: nonepileptic
Oral-buccal-lingual movements	Sucking, chewing, tongue protrusions May be provoked or intensified by stimulation Presumed pathophysiology: nonepileptic
Progression movements	Rowing or swimming movements Pedaling or bicycling movements of the legs May be provoked or intensified by stimulation May be suppressed by restraint or repositioning Presumed pathophysiology: nonepileptic
Complex purposeless movements	Sudden arousal with transient increased random activity of limbs May be provoked or intensified by stimulation Presumed pathophysiology: nonepileptic

From Mizrahi EM, Kellaway P. *Diagnosis and management of neonatal seizures.* Philadelphia: Lippincott-Raven; 1998.

behaviors during active (rapid eye movement [REM]) and quiet (non-REM [NREM]) sleep or waking segments also must be recognized before one proceeds to a seizure evaluation.[11,12] Within the subtle category of neonatal seizures are stereotypic changes in heart rate, blood pressure, oxygenation, or other autonomic signs, particularly during pharmacologic paralysis for ventilatory care. Other autonomic events include skin changes, salivation, and tearing. Autonomic expressions may be intermixed with motor findings. Isolated autonomic signs such as apnea, unless accompanied by other clinical findings, are rarely associated with coincident electrographic

Table 8-3 CLASSIFICATION OF NEONATAL SEIZURES BASED ON ELECTROCLINICAL FINDINGS

Clinical seizures with a consistent electrocortical signature (pathophysiology: epileptic)	
Focal clonic	Unifocal
	Multifocal
	Hemiconvulsive
	Axial
Focal tonic	Asymmetric truncal posturing
	Limb posturing
	Sustained eye deviation
Myoclonic	Generalized
	Focal
Spasms	Flexor
	Extensor
	Mixed extensor/flexor
Clinical seizures without a consistent electrocortical signature (pathophysiology: presumed nonepileptic)	
Myoclonic	Generalized
	Focal
	Fragmentary
Generalized tonic	Flexor
	Extensor
	Mixed extensor/flexor
Motor automatisms	Oral-buccal-lingual movements
	Ocular signs
	Progression movements
	Complex purposeless movements
Electrical seizures without clinical seizure activity	

From Mizrahi EM, Kellaway P. *Diagnosis and management of neonatal seizures.* Philadelphia: Lippincott-Raven; 1998.

seizures (see Fig. 8-1B).[13,14] Because subtle seizures are both clinically difficult to detect and only variably coincident with EEG seizures, synchronized video/EEG/polygraph recordings are recommended to document temporal relationships between clinical behaviors and coincident electrographic events.[7,15-17] Paroxysmal movements disorders, including specifically brainstem release movements, may best explain the clinical phenomena in the absence of electrographic expression by surface recordings. Despite the subtle expression of this seizure category, children with these features may still have suffered significant brain injury.

Clonic Seizures

Rhythmic movements of muscle groups in a focal distribution that consist of a rapid phase followed by a slow return movement are clonic seizures, to be distinguished from the symmetric to-and-fro movements of tremulousness or jitteriness.[1] Gentle flexion of the affected body part easily suppresses the tremor, but clonic seizures persist. Clonic movements can involve any body part, such as the face, arm, leg, and even diaphragmatic or pharyngeal muscles. Generalized clonic activities can occur in the newborn but rarely consist of a classic tonic phase followed by a clonic phase, which are characteristic of the generalized motor seizure noted in older children and adults. Focal clonic and hemiclonic seizures have been described with localized brain injury, usually from cerebrovascular lesions (Fig. 8-2A)[16,18-20] but can also be seen with generalized brain abnormalities. As in older patients, focal seizures

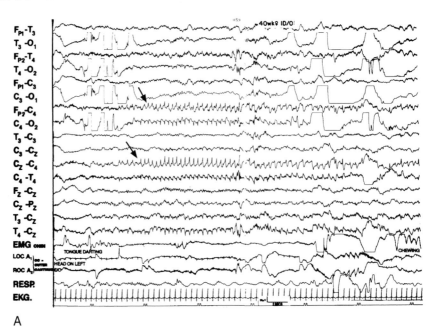

A

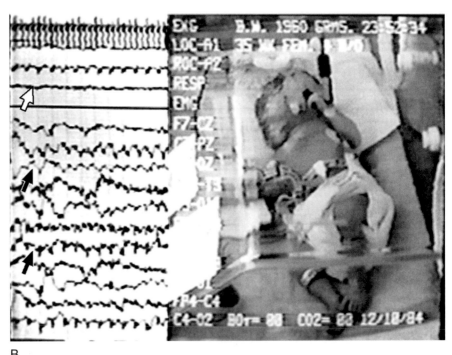

B

Figure 8-1 **A,** Electroencephalogram (EEG) segment for a 40-week-gestation, 1-day-old female following severe asphyxia resulting from rupture of velamentous insertion of the umbilical cord during delivery. An electrical seizure in the right central midline region is recorded *(arrows)*, coincident with buccolingual and eye movements (see comments and eye channels on recording). **B,** Synchronized video/EEG record of a 35-week gestation, 1-day-old female with *Escherichia coli* meningitis and cerebral abscesses. The *open arrow* denotes apnea coincident with prominent right hemispheric and midline electrographic seizures *(closed arrows).* In addition to apnea, other motoric signs coincident to EEG seizures were noted at other times during the recording. (**A** from Scher MS, Painter MJ. Electrographic diagnosis of neonatal seizures: Issues of diagnostic accuracy, clinical correlation and survival. In: Wasterlain CG, Vert P, eds. *Neonatal seizures.* New York: Raven Press; 1990; **B** from Scher MS, Painter MJ. Controversies concerning neonatal seizures. *Pediatr Clin North Am.* 1989;36:288.)

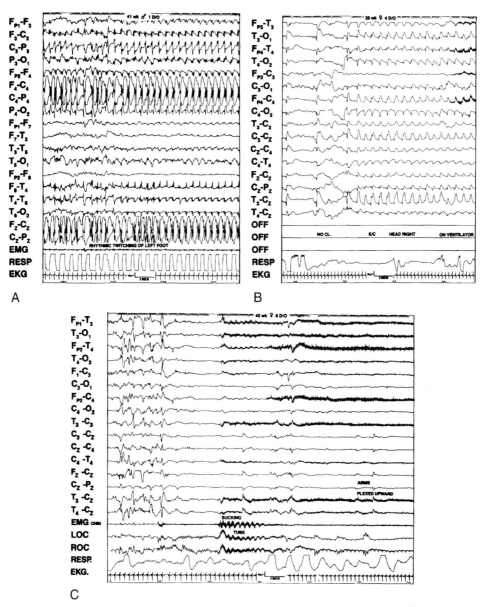

Figure 8-2 **A,** Segment of electroencephalogram (EEG) for a 41-week-gestation, 1-day-old male with an electroclinical seizure characterized by rhythmic clonic movements of the left foot coincident with bihemispheric electrographic discharges of higher amplitude in the right hemisphere. This seizure was documented prior to antiepileptic medication. **B,** Segment of EEG of a 25-week gestation, 4-day-old female with an electrographic seizure without clinical accompaniments. **C,** Segment of an EEG of a 40-week gestation, 6-day-old infant with stereotypic flexion posturing in the absence of electrographic seizures (note muscle artifact). (From Scher MS. Pediatric electroencephalography and evoked potentials. In: Swaiman KS, ed. *Pediatric neurology: principles and practice.* St. Louis: Mosby; 1999:164.)

in the neonate may be followed by transient motor weakness, historically referred to as a transient Todd's paresis or paralysis,[21] to be distinguished by a more persistent hemiparesis over multiple days to weeks. Clonic movements without EEG-confirmed seizures have been described in neonates with normal EEG backgrounds, and their neurodevelopment outcome will more likely be normal.[17] The less experienced clinician may misclassify myoclonic as clonic movements. Computational studies suggest strategies to extract quantitative information from video recordings of neonatal seizures as a method by which clinicians can differentiate myoclonic from focal clonic seizures as well as distinguish normal infant behaviors.[22]

Multifocal (Fragmentary) Clonic Seizures

Multifocal or migratory clonic activities spread over body parts in either a random or an anatomically appropriate fashion. Such seizure movements may alternate from side to side and appear asynchronously between the two halves of the child's body. The word *fragmentary* was historically applied to distinguish this event from the more classic generalized tonic-clonic seizure seen in the older child. Multifocal clonic seizures may also resemble myoclonic seizures, which alternatively consist of brief shocklike muscle twitching of the midline and/or extremity musculature. Neonates with this seizure description often die or have significant neurologic morbidity.[23]

Tonic Seizures

The term *tonic seizure* refers to a sustained flexion or extension of axial or appendicular muscle groups. Tonic movements of a limb or sustained head or eye turning may also be noted. Tonic activity with coincident EEG findings needs to be carefully documented, because 30% of such movements lack a temporal correlation with electrographic seizures (Fig. 8-3).[24] Brainstem release resulting from functional decortication after severe neocortical dysfunction or damage is one physiologic explanation for this nonepileptic activity, to be discussed later. Extensive neocortical damage or dysfunction permits the emergence of uninhibited subcortical expressions of extensor movements (see Fig. 8-6).[25] Tonic seizures may also be misidentified in patients in whom the nonepileptic movement disorder dystonia is the more appropriate behavioral description (see Figs. 8-2C and 8-3A). Both tonic movements and dystonic posturing may also simultaneously occur. Dystonia is one of three clinical presentations of hypertonicity, including rigidity and spasticity, that can imply specific subcortical anatomic sites as well as timing of brain insults.[26,27]

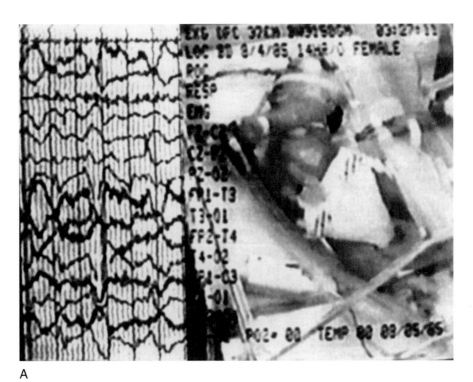

A

Figure 8-3 A, Segment of a synchronized video-electroencephalogram (EEG) record of a 37-week-gestation, 1-day-old female who suffered asphyxia, demonstrating prominent opisthotonos with left arm extension in the absence of coincident electrographic seizure activity.

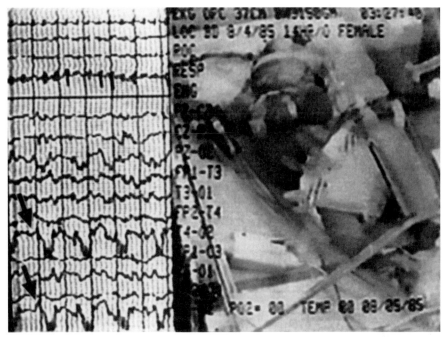

B

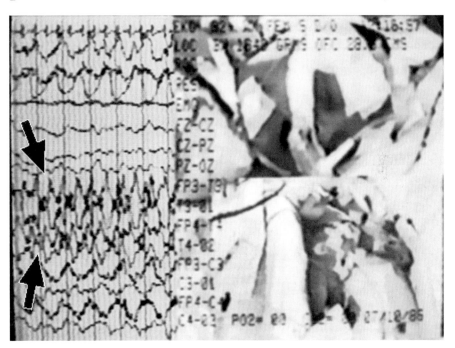

C

Figure 8-3, cont'd **B,** Synchronized video/EEG record of the same patient as in **A,** documenting electrographic seizure in the right posterior quadrant *(arrows)*, following cessation of left arm tonic movements and persistent opisthotonos. **C,** Segment of a video/EEG recording documenting a fixed tonic neck reflex with coincident electrographic seizures in the temporal regions *(arrows)*, described as a tonic seizure. (**A** from Scher MS. Neonatal seizures: an expression of fetal or neonatal brain disorders. In: Stevenson DK, ed. *Fetal and neonatal brain injury: mechanisms, management and the risks of practice.* 3rd ed. West Nyack, NY: Cambridge University Press; 2003:735; **C** from Scher MS, Painter MJ. Controversies concerning neonatal seizures. *Pediatr Clin North Am.* 1989;36:292.)

8

Myoclonic Seizures

Myoclonic movements are rapid, isolated jerks that can be generalized, multifocal, or focal in an axial or appendicular distribution. Myoclonus lacks the slow return phase of the clonic movement complex described previously. Healthy preterm infants commonly exhibit myoclonic movements without seizures or a brain disorder. EEG, therefore, is recommended to confirm the coincident appearance of electrographic discharges with these movements (Fig. 8-4A). Pathologic myoclonus in the absence of EEG seizures also can occur in severely ill preterm or full-term infants who have suffered severe brain dysfunction or damage.[28] As in older children and adults, myoclonus may reflect injury at multiple levels of the neuraxis from the spine and brainstem to cortical regions. Stimulus-evoked myoclonus with either coincident single coincident spike discharges or sustained electrographic seizures has been reported (see Fig. 8-4).[28] An extensive evaluation must be initiated to exclude metabolic, structural, and genetic causes. Healthy sleeping neonates can exhibit a parasomnia that subsides with arousal to the waking state[29,30]; this disorder, known as benign sleep myoclonus of the newborn, is diagnosed if an evaluation finds no pathologic explanations.

Nonepileptic Behaviors of Neonates

Specific nonepileptic neonatal movement repertoires continually challenge the physician's attempt to reach an accurate diagnosis of seizures and avoid the unnecessary use of AEDs for paroxysmal events that subserve different neuronal circuitry from neural networks assumed to express seizures. These nonepileptic events may occur along with seizures or as independent clinical phenomena independent of seizure occurrence. Coincident synchronized video/EEG/polygraph recordings are now the suggested diagnostic tools to confirm the temporal relationship between the suspicious clinical phenomena and electrographic expression of seizures.[31] The following three examples of nonepileptic movement disorders incorporate a new classification scheme based on the absence of coincident EEG seizures.[7]

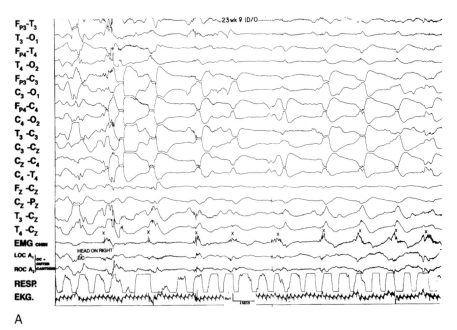

A

Figure 8-4 A, Electroencephalogram (EEG) segment of a 23-week-gestation, 1-day-old female with grade III intraventricular hemorrhage and progressive ventriculomegaly. An electroclinical seizure is noted with coincident myoclonic movements of the diaphragm (× *marks*).

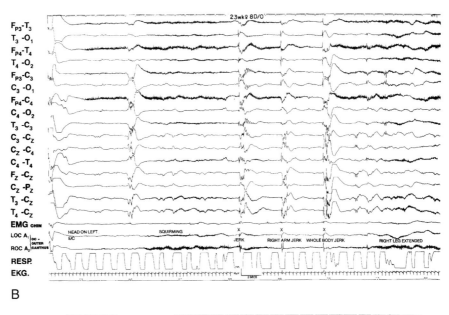

B

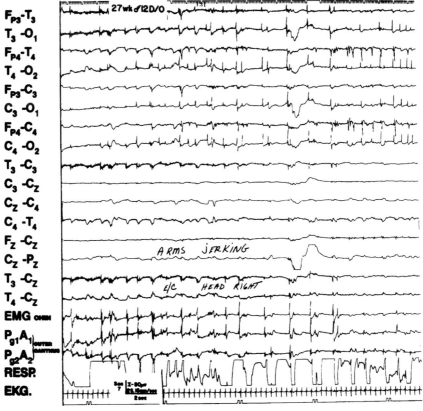

C

Figure 8-4, cont'd **B,** Segment of an EEG recording of an asymptomatic 23-week-gestation, 8-day-old female with spontaneous generalized focal myoclonus without electrographic discharges other than myogenic spike potentials. **C,** Segment of an EEG recording of an encephalopathic 27-week-gestation, 12-day-old male with herpes encephalitis who exhibits nonepileptic multifocal myoclonus (myogenic potentials as EEG artifacts). (From Scher MS. Pathological myoclonus of the newborn: electrographic and clinical correlations. *Pediatr Neurol.* 1985;1: 342-348.)

Tremulousness or Jitteriness with EEG Correlates

Tremors are frequently misidentified as clonic activity. Unlike the unequal phases of clonic movements described earlier, the flexion and extension phases of tremor are equal in amplitude. Children are generally alert or hyperalert but may also appear somnolent. Passive flexion and repositioning of the affected tremulous body part diminishes or eliminates the movement. Such movements are usually spontaneous but can be provoked by tactile stimulation. Metabolic or toxin-induced encephalopathies, including drug withdrawal, hypoglycemia, hypocalcemia, hypomagnesemia, intracranial hemorrhage, hypothermia, and growth restriction, are common clinical scenarios when such movements occur. Neonatal tremors generally decrease with age. For example, in 38 full-term infants, excessive tremulousness resolved spontaneously over a 6-week period, with 92% of the subjects found to be neurologically normal at 3 years of age.[32] Medications are rarely considered to treat this particular movement disorder.[33]

Neonatal Myoclonus without EEG Seizures

Myoclonic movements are either bilateral and synchronous or asymmetric and asynchronous in appearance. Clusters of myoclonic activity occur more predominantly during active (rapid eye movement) sleep, and are more predominant in the preterm infant (see Fig. 8-4B),[12,34] although they can occur in healthy full-term infants. Benign movements are not stimulus-sensitive, have no coincident electrographic seizure correlates, or are associated with EEG background abnormalities. When these movements occur in the healthy full-term neonate, the activity is suppressed during wakefulness. The clinical description of benign neonatal sleep myoclonus must be a diagnosis of exclusion made after a careful consideration of pathologic diagnoses.[29]

Infants with severe central nervous system dysfunction also may present with nonepileptic spontaneous or stimulus-evoked myoclonus. Different forms of metabolic encephalopathies (e.g., glycine encephalopathy), cerebrovascular lesions, brain infections, or congenital malformations may manifest as nonepileptic pathologic myoclonus (see Fig. 8-4C).[28] Encephalopathic neonates may respond to tactile or painful stimulation with isolated focal, segmental, or generalized myoclonic movements. Rarely, cortically generated spike or sharp wave discharges as well as seizures may also be noted on the EEG recordings that are coincident with these myoclonic movements (Fig. 8-5).[35] Medication-induced myoclonus as well as other stereotypic movements have also been described,[36] which resolve when the responsible drug is withdrawn.

A rare familial disorder in the neonatal and early infancy periods has been described and specifically termed *hyperekplexia*. The movements are usually misinterpreted as a hyperactive startle reflex. Infants are stiff, with severe hypertonia that may lead to apnea and bradycardia. Forced flexion of the neck or hips sometimes alleviates these events. EEG background rhythms are generally age-appropriate. The postulated defect for these individuals involve regulation of brainstem centers, which facilitate myoclonic movements.[37] Occasionally benzodiazepines or valproic acid lessens the startling, stiffening, or falling.[38] Neurologic prognosis is reported to be variable.

Neonatal Dystonia without EEG Seizures

Dystonia is a movement disorder that may be misinterpreted as tonic seizures. Dystonia can be associated with either acute or chronic disease states involving basal ganglia structures or the extrapyramidal pathways that innervate these regions. Antepartum or intrapartum adverse events commonly, such as severe asphyxia (i.e., status marmoratus),[10] or rarely, such as specific inherited metabolic diseases,[39,40] result in injury to these structures. Alternatively, posturing may reflect subcortical motor pathways that are functionally unopposed because of a diseased or malformed neocortex (Fig. 8-6; see Figs. 8-2C and 8-3A)[25] and are part of the clinical differential diagnosis of neonatal hypertonicity.[26,27] Documentation of EEG seizures with

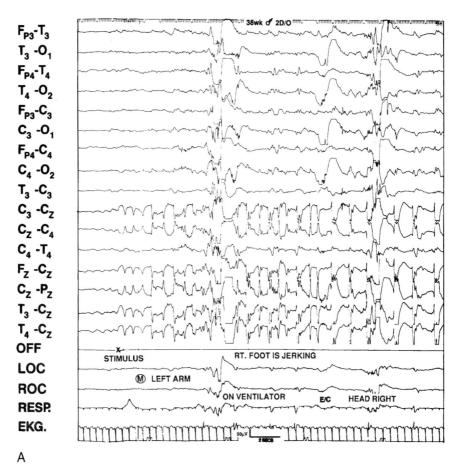

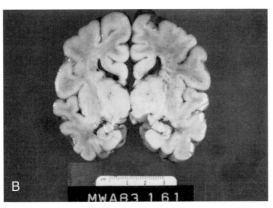

Figure 8-5 **A,** Segment of an electroencephalogram (EEG) recording of a 38-week-gestation, 2-day-old male with glycine encephalopathy who has stimulus-sensitive generalized and multifocal myoclonus. Note the onset of a midline (C$_z$ onset) electrographic seizure with a painful stimulus, followed by right foot myoclonus. **B,** Coronal section of the brain for the patient described in **A,** showing agenesis of the corpus callosum and batwing shape of lateral ventricles. Spongy myelinosis was noted on microscopic examination. (**A** from Scher MS. Neonatal seizures: an expression of fetal or neonatal brain disorders. In: Stevenson DK, ed. *Fetal and neonatal brain injury: mechanisms, management and the risks of practice.* 3rd ed. West Nyack, NY: Cambridge University Press; 2003:745; **B** from Scher MS. Pathological myoclonus of the newborn: electrographic and clinical correlations. *Pediatr Neurol.* 1985;1:342-348.)

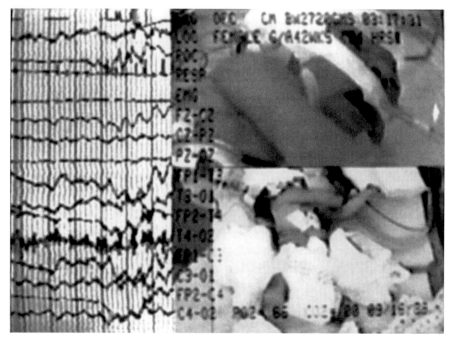

Figure 8-6 Segment of a video-electroencephalogram (EEG) of a 42-week gestation, <growth-restricted female, obtained before 24 hours of age, demonstrating stereotypic posturing and eye opening with no coincident electrographic seizure. The child presented with nonimmune hydrops fetalis with significant neocortical injury from a fetal period. The EEG background is markedly slow and suppressed, representing a severe interictal electrographic abnormality. (From Scher MS. Seizures in the newborn infant. *Clin Perinatol.* 1997;24:74.)

coincident video/EEG/polygraphic recordings help avoid misdiagnosis as seizures and inappropriate treatment.

Electrographic Seizure Criteria

Over the last few decades, electrographic/polysomnographic studies have become invaluable tools for the assessment of suspected seizures.[7,16,24,31,41-43] Technical and interpretative skills of normal and abnormal neonatal EEG sleep patterns must be mastered before one can develop a confident visual analysis style for seizure recognition.[11,12,44-46]

Collaboration with the EEG technologist is always an essential part of the diagnostic process, because physiologic and nonphysiologic artifacts can masquerade as EEG seizures. The physician must also anticipate expected behaviors for a specific gestational maturity, medication use, and state of arousal in the context of potential artifacts. Synchronized video/EEG documentation permits careful off-line analysis for more accurate documentation. Specific newborns may express both electrographic seizures and nonepileptic events, based on the particular brain regions affected that subserve these phenomena.

As in the epileptic older child and adult, it is generally accepted that the epileptic seizure in an infant is a clinical paroxysm of altered brain function with the simultaneous presence of an electrographic event on a surface EEG recording. Therefore, when one is assessing the suspected clinical event in the neonate, coincident EEG or preferably synchronized video/EEG/polygraph monitoring is a useful tool to distinguish an epileptic from a nonepileptic event. One study concluded that two thirds of clinical manifestations are either unrecognized or misinterpreted by experienced neonatal staff.[47] This conclusion reaffirms earlier findings that more than 50% of neonatal seizures are only electrographic[48]; in one study, 58% of infants who initially expressed electroclinical seizures demonstrated uncoupling of clinical and EEG patterns after phenobarbital and phenytoin administration.[49]

Uncoupling of the clinical and electrographic expressions of neonatal seizures after administration of AEDs also contributes to an underestimation of the true seizure duration, including status epilepticus (Fig. 8-7). One study estimated that 58% of neonates expressed persistent electrographic seizures despite resolution of their clinical seizure behaviors after receiving either of two AEDs,[49] termed *electroclinical uncoupling*. Other pathophysiologic mechanisms beside medication effect also might explain uncoupling.[9]

Some authorities advocate the use of single- or dual-channel computerized devices for continuous prolonged monitoring,[50] given the multiple logistical challenges to the use of conventional multichannel recording devices at the cribside of a critically ill newborn. This specific device may fail to detect focal or regional seizures if the single-channel recording is not near the brain region involved with seizure expression, is sufficiently short in duration, or is low in amplitude.[4] For example, a study reported that fewer than 3 out of 10 neonates with suspected seizure findings on a single-channel device could be verified as having seizures by conventional EEG. Others have suggested that modified four-, five-, or nine-channel EEG can efficiently detect seizures when verified by continuous video/EEG telemetry.[4,51] In one study, one centrally placed channel detected 78% of electrographic seizures,[52] whereas in another, a frontally placed channel detected only 46% of seizures.[53]

Epilepsy monitoring services for older children and adults regularly utilize intracerebral or surface electrocorticography to detect seizures in patients who are considered possible candidates for epilepsy surgery, after surface-recorded synchronized video/EEG recordings with multiple electrodes have been utilized. Such recording strategies, however, are not ethically appropriate or practical for the

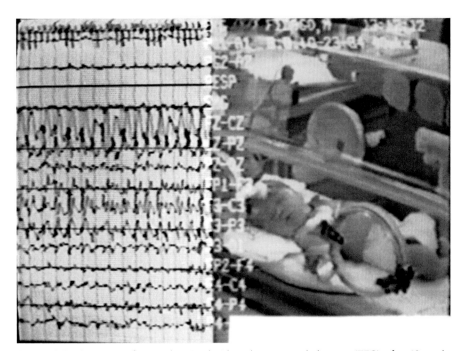

Figure 8-7 Segment of a synchronized video-electroencephalogram (EEG) of a 40-week-gestation, 1-day-old male with electrographic status epilepticus in the left central midline regions after administration of antiepileptic medication. Focal right shoulder clonic activity was only intermittently shown, whereas continuous electrographic seizures were documented mostly without clinical expression. This phenomenon of uncoupling of electrical and clinical seizure activities is associated with use of antiepileptic drugs (see text). (From Scher MS, Painter MJ. Controversies concerning neonatal seizures. *Pediatr Clin North Am.* 1989;36:290.)

neonatal patient on the basis of current technologies. Subcortical foci are consequentially difficult to definitively eliminate from consideration, as discussed later.

Ictal EEG Patterns: A More Reliable Marker for Surface-Recorded Seizure Onset, Duration, and Severity

Neonatal EEG seizure patterns commonly consist of a repetitive sequence of waveforms that evolve in frequency, amplitude, electrical field, and/or morphology. Four types of ictal patterns have been described: focal ictal patterns with normal background, focal ictal patterns with abnormal background, multifocal ictal patterns,[44] and focal monorhythmic periodic patterns of various frequencies. It is generally suggested that a minimal duration of 10 seconds for the evolution of discharges is required to distinguish electrographic seizures from repetitive but nonictal epileptiform discharges (see Figs. 8-1A, 8-2A and B).[16,54,55] Although most seizures occur spontaneously, there may be environmental triggers that evoke neonatal seizures in encephalopathic infants, such as painful or tactile stimuli.[56,57] Such instances may be useful in either the consideration of diagnostic possibilities or the planning of clinical paths. Clinical neurophysiologists separately classify brief or prolonged repetitive discharges that lack an electrographic evolution as nonictal abnormal epileptiform patterns but not confirmatory of seizures.[58] The unique features of neonatal electrographic seizure duration and topography that should be recognized by the neurophysiologist are discussed here.

Seizure Duration and Topography

Few studies have quantified minimal or maximal seizure durations in neonates.[7,16,55] Most notably, the definition of the most severe expression of seizures, status epilepticus, which potentially promotes brain injury, can be problematic. For the older patient, status epilepticus is defined as at least 30 minutes of continuous seizures or two consecutive seizures with an interictal period during which the patient fails to return to full consciousness. This definition is not easily applied to the neonate, for whom the level of arousal may be difficult to assess because of immaturity, disease, or medications. One study arbitrarily defined neonatal status epilepticus as continuous seizure activity for at least 30 minutes, or 50% of the recording time[55]; 33% or 11 of 34 full-term infants in the study had status epilepticus with a mean duration of 29.6 minutes prior to AED use, and 9% or 3 out of the 34 preterm infants also had status epilepticus with an average duration of 5.2 minutes per seizure (i.e., 50% of the recording time). The mean seizure duration was longer in the full-term infants (5 minutes) than in the preterm infants (2.7 minutes). Given that more than 20% of this study group fit the criteria for status epilepticus on the basis of EEG documentation, this study raises concerns regarding the underdiagnosis of the more severe form of seizures that potentially contribute to brain injury if only clinical criteria are applied.

Most neonatal electrographic seizures arise focally from one brain region. Generalized synchronous and symmetric repetitive discharges can also occur. In one study, 56% of seizures were seen in a single location at onset; specific sites were temporal-occipital (15%), temporal-central (15%), central (10%), frontotemporal central (6%), frontotemporal (5%), and vertex (5%). Multiple locations at the onset of the electrographic seizures were noted in 44%.[16] Electrographic discharges may be expressed as specific EEG frequency ranges from fast to slow, including beta, alpha, theta, or delta activities. Multiple electrographic seizures can also be expressed independently in anatomically unrelated brain regions.

Subcortical Seizures versus Nonictal Functional Decortication

Experimental animal models offer seemingly contradictory neuronal mechanisms to explain clinical events that do not have coincident EEG confirmation. Most clinical neurophysiologists require documentation of an ictal pattern by surface EEG electrodes. However, subcortical seizures with only intermittent propagation to the surface may occur. At the other end of the spectrum, nonictal brainstem release phenomena must be considered, particularly if EEG seizures are never expressed.[24] A more integrated electroclinical approach has been suggested to classify clinical events as seizures or nonepileptic movement disorders on the basis of documentation by synchronized video/EEG monitoring.[7]

Brainstem Release Phenomena

As recommended by Mizrahi and Kellaway,[15] synchronized video/EEG/polygraph monitoring provides the physician with documentation of a suspicious event with a concurrent electrographic pattern on surface recordings. The temporal relationship between clinical and electrographic phenomena based on synchronized video/EEG/ polygraph monitoring has been described. After analysis of 415 clinical seizures in 71 babies, these authors found clonic seizure activity to have the best correlation with coincident electrographic seizures. Subtle clinical events, on the other hand, had a more inconsistent relationship with coincident EEG seizure activity, suggesting a nonepileptic brainstem release phenomenon for at least a proportion of such events. Functional decortication resulting from neocortical damage without coincident EEG seizures has therefore been suggested,[24] such as with tonic posturing, as illustrated in Figure 8-3A. Newborns with nonseizure brainstem release activity may express a different functional pattern of metabolic dysfunction, detected as altered glucose uptake on single-photon emission computed tomography (SPECT) studies, from that seen in neonates with seizures.[59] Documentation of increased prolactin levels with clinical seizures has also been suggested,[60] but such levels have not yet been correlated with electrographic seizures in newborns.

Electroclinical Dissociation Suggesting Subcortical Seizures

Experimental studies of immature animals also support the possibility that subcortical structures may initiate seizures, which subsequently, although intermittently, propagate to the cortical surface.[61-63] Although EEG depth recordings in adults and adolescents help document subcortical seizures both with and without clinical expression, this technology is not applicable or appropriate to the neonate. Only one anecdotal report of a human infant documented seizures possibly emanating from deep gray matter structures.[64]

Electroclinical dissociation (ECD) is one proposed mechanism by which subcortical seizures may only intermittently appear on surface-recorded EEG studies.[8] ECD has been defined as a reproducible clinical event that occurs both with and without coincidental electrographic seizures. In one group of 51 infants with electroclinical seizures, 33 infants simultaneously expressed both electrical and clinical seizure phenomena. Extremity movements were more significantly associated with synchronized electroclinical seizures. However, a subset of 18 neonates (34%) also expressed ECD on EEG recordings. For neonates who expressed ECD, the clinical seizure component always preceded the electrographic seizure expression, suggesting that a subcortical focus may have initiated the seizure state. Some of these children also expressed synchronized electroclinical seizures, even on the same EEG record. It may be useful to classify clinical events without either simultaneous or disassociated electrographic patterns as nonepileptic movement disorders mediated by alternative neuronal pathways, which thus require different treatments.

Controversy remains whether subcortical seizures or nonictal functional decortication best categorizes suspicious clinical behaviors without coincident EEG seizure documentation. This dilemma should encourage the clinician to use the EEG as a neurophysiologic yardstick by which more exact seizure start and end points can be assigned before offering pharmacologic treatment with AEDs.[31] Neonates certainly exhibit electrographic seizures that go undetected unless EEG is utilized.[16,48,65-69] Two examples are neonates who are pharmacologically paralyzed for ventilatory assistance (Fig. 8-8A) and those who have clinical seizures that are suppressed by the use of AEDs (see Fig. 8-8B).[16,49,65,67,68] In one cohort of 92 infants, 60% of whom were pretreated with AEDs, 50% of neonates had electrographic seizures with no clinical accompaniment.[49] Both clinical and electrographic seizure criteria were

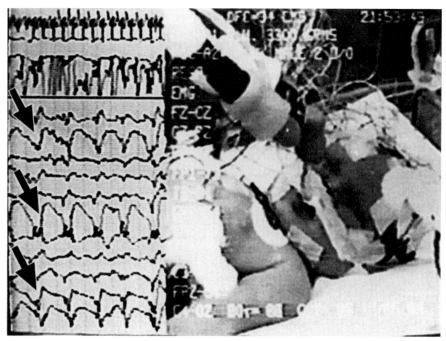

A

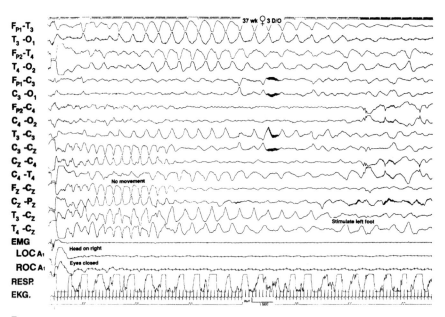

B

Figure 8-8 A, Segment of a synchronized video-electroencephalogram (EEG) record of a 38-week-gestation, 2-day-old male who is pharmacologically paralyzed for ventilatory care. A seizure is seen in the right posterior quadrant and midline *(arrows)*. **B,** EEG segment for a 37-week-gestation, 3-day-old female after antiepileptic drug use with multifocal electrical seizures in the delta frequency range in the temporal and midline regions. Note the marked suppression of normal EEG background. (From Scher MS, Painter MJ. Controversies concerning neonatal seizures. *Pediatr Clin North Am.* 1989;36:287.)

noted for 45% of 62 preterm and 53% of 33 full-term infants. Seventeen infants were pharmacologically paralyzed when the EEG seizures were first documented. In a later cohort of 60 infants, none of whom was pretreated with AEDs, 7% of infants had only electrographic seizures prior to AED administration[49] and 25% expressed electroclinical uncoupling after AED use.

The underestimation of seizures in the newborn period may also result from inadequate monitoring for specific neurologic signs. Autonomic changes in respirations, blood pressure, oxygenation, heart rate, pupillary size, skin color, and salivation are examples of subtle ictal signs (Fig. 8-9). In one study, autonomic seizures accompanied electrographic seizures in 37% of 19 preterm neonates.[48] Newer classifications of neonatal seizures emphasize documentation of autonomic findings on EEG recordings.[7]

Variation in the Incidence of Neonatal Seizures Based on Clinical versus EEG Criteria

Overestimation and underestimation of neonatal seizures are consequentially reported whether clinical or electrical criteria are used. With use of clinical criteria, seizure incidences ranged from 0.5% in term infants to 22.2% in preterm neonates.[70-73] Discrepancies in incidence reflect not only varying postconceptional ages of the

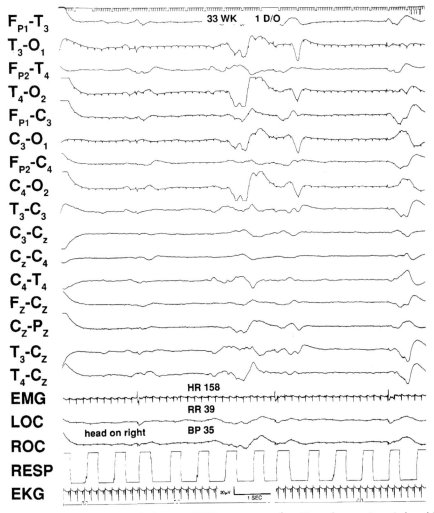

Figure 8-9   A, Electroencephalogram (EEG) segments of a 33-week-gestation, 1-day-old male before seizures associated with drops in heart rate and blood pressure measurements.
Continued

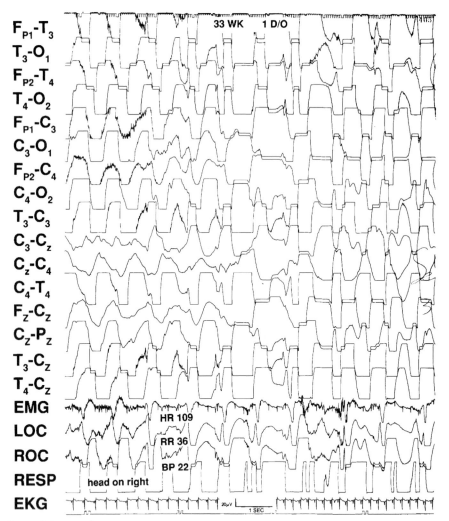

Figure 8-9, cont'd   **B,** EEG segment of neonate in **A** after seizure onset with accompanying drops in heart rate and blood pressure.

study populations chosen but also poor interobserver reliability[74] and the hospital setting in which the diagnosis was made. Hospital-based studies,[48] which include infants from high-risk deliveries, generally report a higher seizure incidence. Population studies,[75] which include less medically ill infants from general nurseries, report lower percentages. Incidence figures based only on clinical criteria without EEG confirmation include neonates with false-positive results who demonstrate either normal or nonepileptic pathologic neonatal behaviors. Conversely, the group without scalp-generated EEG seizure findings may include a subset of neonates with false-negative findings who express seizures only from subcortical brain regions and not on the cortical surface. Closer consensus between clinical and EEG criteria is still needed.

Seizures in the Clinical Context of Maternal-Fetal-Placental-Neonatal Disease: Developing a Diagnostic Algorithm

When initiating a diagnostic plan for the neonate with seizures, one must assume that the presence of seizures reflects a complex phenotype related to etiology, anatomic localization, and time course. Once seizures are confirmed by EEG with or without accompanying clinical events, the clinician must place these events into the context of clinical, historical, and laboratory findings to determine the pathogenesis, brain region, and timing of seizures.

Clinical Findings

It is diagnostically relevant to establish on physical examination whether the newborn is encephalopathic, as expressed by decreased level of arousal and altered muscle tone in the context of seizure occurrence. Focal neurologic deficits such as a hemiparesis may be helpful in the context of focal or regional diseases, such as arterial or venous stroke and hemorrhage. Neonates with sustained hypertonicity include subsets of children who either have acute injury to deep brain regions or have experienced intracranial trauma and/or hemorrhage. Alternatively, the hypertonic neonate with or without contractures can suggest a more chronic insult to motor pathways, including in the brainstem.[26,27] Growth restriction, microcephaly, and body stigmata may also suggest chronic and possibly congenital disorders. Other physical findings may be helpful, such as neurocutaneous lesions on skin inspection, hepatosplenomegaly, or ophthalmologic examination. Careful inspection of clouding of the lens or altered anatomy of the fundus or retina in the eye by the pediatric ophthalmologist, for example, may document evidence of genetic or acquired disease, such as corneal clouding, cataracts, chorioretinitis, optic atrophy, and coloboma.

Etiology

Asphyxia is the most common etiology associated with neonatal seizures, representing one type of neonatal encephalopathy. Diagnostic criteria for determining whether hypoxic-ischemic insults may have occurred during the intrapartum period have been suggested by an interdisciplinary consortium.[76] Maternal, fetal, placental, and neonatal disease entities must be considered to facilitate a diagnosis and potential treatment plan.[77-80] Seizures in neonates after asphyxia may support acute intrapartum and/or antepartum disease conditions in addition to ongoing postnatal evolution of the disease process. If intrapartum asphyxia is a possibility, does the child with seizures also express clinical and laboratory signs of evolving cerebral edema? Cerebral edema emerges to a maximum expression on neuroimaging over a 72-hour period after the onset of asphyxia. The presence of a bulging fontanel with neuroimaging evidence of asphyxia-related brain injuries and cerebral edema (i.e., obliterated ventricular outline and abnormal diffusion-weighted magnetic resonance images) may support a more recent asphyxial disease process, during or around the intrapartum period.

Although asphyxia may have occurred during parturition or close to delivery, the etiologies may be more complex, limiting the clinician's ability to predict the emergence of a neonatal encephalopathy reflective of a specific time course or etiology. For example, investigators from one institution were unable to predict perinatal brain injury on the basis of specific clinical characteristics, except for postnatal clinical signs of evolving intrapartum hypoxic-ischemic encephalopathy.[81] This retrospective review documented a high percentage of maternal/placental diseases not related to conventional causes of intrapartum asphyxia, including chorioamnionitis/funisitis and fetal thrombotic vasculopathy, that resulted in signs of neonatal encephalopathy that mimic and/or overlap with signs of classic asphyxia. The fetal inflammatory response syndrome, which may occur with or without sepsis and can affect both full-term as well as preterm neonates through the adverse effects of chorioamnionitis/funisitis, has been described.[82,83] Vascular lesions of the placenta, such as fetal thrombotic vasculopathy, can be the result of diverse conditions, including maternal/fetal thrombophilia and preeclampsia.[78] Systemic diseases reflected by imaging findings or by biochemical studies of the heart, kidney, or alimentary tract may suggest genetic or acquired diseases that also manifest as neonatal seizures.

Alternatively, failure to document evolving clinical signs of decreased arousal, altered muscle tone with seizures, or the presentation of encephalomalacia or cystic brain lesions on neuroimaging shortly after birth (with or without encephalopathy) supports the occurrence of a more chronic disease process with remote antepartum brain injury. Liquefaction necrosis does not produce a cystic cavity until more than 2 weeks after the presumed in utero asphyxial event,[84] so a cavity visible on neuroimaging immediately after birth suggests antepartum maternal, placental, or fetal disease. Isolated seizures in an otherwise asymptomatic neonate without accompanying encephalopathic signs suggests a disease process that began either remotely before labor or during the postnatal period as a result of craniocerebral trauma, intracranial infection or hemorrhage, worsening cardiovascular disease, drug toxicity, or an inherited metabolic disease. Fetal injury alternatively may occur after ischemic-hypoperfusion events from circulatory disturbances, such as maternal shock from trauma or illness, chorioamnionitis, or placental fetal vasculopathy, and a small percentage of infants with such injury may present with neonatal seizures.[85,86]

Diagnostic Considerations

Evaluation includes a careful review of the medical history, determination of serum glucose, electrolyte, magnesium, calcium, and phosphorus levels, and, when indicated, determination of serum ammonia, lactate, and pyruvate levels, which may identify correctable metabolic conditions not requiring antiepileptic medications. Spinal fluid analyses, including cell count, protein, glucose, lactate, pyruvate, amino acid measurements, and culture studies to consider central nervous system infection, intracranial hemorrhage, and metabolic disease, may be indicated from the history and clinical examination. Absence of multiorgan dysfunction may alert the clinician to other etiologies for seizures beside intrapartum asphyxia. Signs of chronic in utero stress, such as growth restriction, early hypertonicity after neonatal depression, and joint contractures, are selected clues that suggest longstanding antepartum stress to the fetus. Careful review of placental and cord specimens can also be extremely useful. Neuroimaging, preferably using magnetic resonance imaging, can help localize and grade the severity and possibly time a brain insult.[87] Altered signals on diffusion-weighted images suggest a more recent time course, whereas the absence of characteristic lesions associated with asphyxia (e.g., basal ganglia, periatrial) redirect the clinician to consider alternative explanations. Identification of genetic or syndromic conditions can contribute to the expression of neonatal encephalopathies independent of asphyxial injury,[88] and several may even mimic the brain lesions seen after asphyxia (i.e., sulfite oxidase and related defects).[88] Ancillary studies may also be considered including long-chain fatty acids and chromosomal/DNA analyses, as deemed necessary by family history and clinical examination findings. Serum studies to determine folinic acid levels and biotinidase activity and spinal fluid studies that consider glucose cotransporter deficiency are the evaluations to detect reversible neonatal encephalopathies that may respond to supplements or dietary modification.[88] Finally, serum and urine organic acid and amino acid determinations may be needed to delineate a specific biochemical disorder for the child with a persistent metabolic acidosis. Lysosomal enzyme studies are also occasionally considered to diagnose specific enzymatic deficiencies in children with neonatal seizures who have storage disease.

Principles of Therapy

The goal for treating neonatal seizures remains the prevention of long-term brain damage in the context of the medical management of the underlying etiology for a brain disorder. However, the therapeutic treatment algorithm is as complex as seizure recognition and etiologic determination. The three-tiered objective of medical management for neonatal seizures is the initial treatment of etiologic factors that may be responsible for seizure generation followed by the cessation of seizures of epileptic origin with either traditional anticonvulsant medications or etiology-specific therapeutic agents. These goals may not be achievable because many etiologic factors are not determined for all neonates and the potential causes for seizures are as yet unknown. As discussed in previous sections, certain clinical seizures with no electrographic expression on surface recordings may in fact be nonepileptic in physiologic origin and therefore may not require treatment or respond to traditional anticonvulsant medications. Alternative treatment choices that stop or lessen nonepileptic movement disorders need to be developed and tested. Even with recognition of seizures requiring treatment, commercially available anticonvulsant medications may be ineffective despite high doses of one or multiple anticonvulsant medications. Finally, there is a double-edged sword to therapeutic interventions to prevent seizures. Antiepileptic medications used to control seizures may have short-term negative consequences such as causing cerebral perfusion secondary to systemic hypotension, contributing to adverse consequences on brain growth and development. Long-term effects of brain growth and maturation are also concerns, on the basis of experimental evidence.

There are three stages in the current acute management of neonates with seizures: (1) initial medical management; (2) etiology-specific therapy; and (3) anticonvulsant medication treatment. These stages should be patient-specific for the clinical profile of the individual neonate. A hypothesized fourth level of treatment is discussed, which refers to the current level of understanding about seizure generation in the immature brain related to specific etiologies, brain region, and timing of injury as reflected in pathophysiologic mechanisms.

General principles of medical management should always include maintaining the newborn's airway, providing adequate ventilation, and preserving cardiovascular circulation. In neonates with seizures, particularly those with recurrent or prolonged seizures, elevations in respiration, heart rate, and blood pressure may occur. Measures must therefore be taken to ensure adequate ventilatory support and circulatory perfusion of neonates with seizures during the initial stage of evaluation and therapy. This approach potentially avoids the harmful side effects that may occur as a result of recurrent seizures that can compromise multiorgan system function, leading to secondary brain damage. Experimental evidence of brain injury after rapid introduction of hyperoxemia, hypercapnia, or hypocapnia[89] highlights the importance of medical management of acid-base balance and ventilation. Vulnerable brain regions within the brainstem, diencephalon, and cortex must be considered in the management of metabolic acidosis and alkalosis both during resuscitation and over the early postresuscitative period. A 2011 report on a rodent model documented an increased risk for brain injury expressed as seizures with the overly rapid introduction of brain alkalosis, suggesting the need to validate these findings in human clinical studies.[90]

If a specific reason for seizures has been identified as potentially treatable, specific therapy needs to be initiated. Examples are hypoglycemia, hypocalcemia, and hypomagnesemia. Although uncommon, other inherited metabolic conditions are potentially reversible neonatal encephalopathies with seizures; for example, pyridoxine deficiency may respond to a specific nutritional supplementation, such as pyridoxine 50 to 500 mg with coincident EEG monitoring. Specific cases may respond more effectively to the active metabolite pyridoxal phosphate, although the myoclonic and tonic clinical events may have an inconsistent association with synchronized video-EEG documentation.[91] Other reversible epileptic encephalopathies associated with metabolic disturbances are folinic acid deficiency, biotinidase deficiency, and glucose cotransporter deficiency. Supplemental treatments with folinic acid and biotin and initiation of the ketogenic diet, respectively, are definitive treatments for these conditions. Some metabolic disorders of metabolism can mimic clinical and neuroimaging findings of postasphyxial encephalopathy, such as sulfite oxidase/ molybdenum deficiencies, but lack therapeutic agents to effectively reverse the encephalopathy and seizures of these conditions.[88]

Emergency Anticonvulsant Drug Treatment

It remains controversial which first-line anticonvulsant agents should be used for neonatal seizure management. There have traditionally been three drug categories: barbiturates, phenytoin, and benzodiazepines. Table 8-4 lists loading doses. Subsequent doses may be required for persistent seizure activity that did not respond to the initial loading doses. Adverse events must be anticipated with the administration

Table 8-4 ANTICONVULSANT DRUGS FOR NEONATAL SEIZURES

Drug	Loading Dose	Maintenance Dose	Withdrawal	Side Effects	Monitoring
Phenobarbital	20 mg/kg IV max. 40 mg/kg	3-5 mg/kg per 24 hr IV or PO	Irritability, altered sleep, tremors	Drowsiness	Blood pressure
Midazolam	>35 wks GA: 0.05 mg/kg IV (in 10 min)	0.15 mg/kg/hr	If seizure-free for 24 hr	Temporary reduction of blood pressure and cerebral blood flow	Blood pressure
Lidocaine	2 mg/kg IV	6 mg/kg/hr IV	After 24 hr of treatment: 4 mg/kg/hr After 36 hr: 2 mg/kg/hr After 48 hr: stop	Arrhythmia, seizures, hypotension	ECG, EEG, blood pressure
Clonazepam	0.15 mg/kg IV repeat 1× or 2×	0.1 mg/kg per 24 hr	If seizure-free for 24 hr		
Phenytoin	20 mg/kg IV (infusion rate 1 mg/kg/min)	3-4 mg/kg per 24 hr IV	At removal of IV lines	Dysrhythmia	EEG
Pyridoxine	50-100 mg	50-100 mg	If no effect: stop		EEG
Thiopental	10 mg/kg IV	Increase dose until EEG shows burst suppression.	After 24 hr	Hypotension	EEG, blood pressure

From van de Bor M. The recognition and management of neonatal seizures. *Curr Paediatr.* 2002;12:382-387.
ECG, Electrocardiogram; *EEG*, electroencephalogram; *GA*, gestational age; *IV*, intravenous; *PO*, by mouth.

of these anticonvulsant medications, including alteration in levels of arousal, systemic hypotension, bradycardia, respiratory depression, and cardiac arrhythmias.

A relative consensus still exists regarding the choice of phenobarbital as a first-line AED, with benzodiazepines and phenytoin remaining the second and third.[92] This practice has been historically because of convention but is not supported given the dearth of evidence-based studies.[93,94] Nonetheless, studies with phenobarbital continue to be disseminated in the peer-reviewed literature for the general use as an anticonvulsant after asphyxia,[95] as well in combination with therapeutic hypothermia, although the pharmacokinetics may be altered.[96,97] Additional AEDs in the benzodiazepine family of drugs continue to be suggested. Controversy remains regarding these choices, given the few evidence-based studies that question the efficacy of these specific AEDs to control seizures.[98]

If the decision to treat neonates with anticonvulsant medications is reached, important questions must be addressed with respect to who should be treated, when to begin treatment, which drug to use, and for how long neonates should be treated. Some authorities suggest that only neonates with clinical seizures should receive medications and that brief electrographic seizures need not be treated. Others suggest more aggressive treatment of EEG seizures, because uncontrolled seizures potentially have an adverse effect on immature brain development. An alternative observation suggests that early administration of an anticonvulsant, such as phenobarbital, may have adverse effects on outcome in term infants.

Phenobarbital and phenytoin, nonetheless, remain the most widely used anticonvulsant medications; benzodiazepines, levetiracetam, primidone, and valproic acid have been reported over the last several decades. The half-life of phenobarbital ranges from 45 to 173 hours in the neonate[99-101]; the initial loading dose is recommended at 20 mg/kg, with a maintenance dose of 3 to 4 mg/kg/day. Therapeutic levels are generally suggested to be between 16 and 40 μg/mL; however, there is no consensus with the respect to drug maintenance.

The preferred loading dose of phenytoin is 15 to 20 mg/kg.[100,101] Serum levels of phenytoin are difficult to maintain because this drug is rapidly redistributed to body tissues. Blood drug levels cannot be well maintained with an oral preparation.

Benzodiazepines may also be used to control neonatal seizures. The drug most widely used is diazepam. One study suggests a half-life of 54 hours in preterm infants to 18 hours in full-term infants.[102] Intravenous administration is recommended because the drug is slowly absorbed after an intramuscular injection. Diazepam is highly protein-bound; alteration of bilirubin binding is low. Recommended intravenous doses for acute management should begin at 0.5 mg/kg. Midazolam has been suggested as an alternative benzodiazepine. It has been recommended to give a bolus of 0.2 mg/kg followed by 20 to 400 μg/kg/hr titrated to blood pressure as tolerated until seizures are controlled, with weaning from the drug 12 to 24 hours after the bolus.[103] Deposition into muscle precludes the use of either phenytoin or diazepam as a maintenance anticonvulsant medication, because profound hypotonia and respiratory depression may result, particularly if barbiturates have also been administered. Lidocaine rather than benzodiazepine infusion has more recently been used.[104] A bolus of 2 mg/kg is recommended over 10 minutes, to be followed by decreasing infusion rates every 12 hours of 6, 4, and 2 mg/kg/hr, with the serum lidocaine level kept below 9 mg/L. This medication needs to be discontinued within 48 hours to avoid cardiotoxicity.

The medication levetiracetam (Keppra) has been reported to reduce or stop neonatal seizures on the basis of anecdotal evidence.[105] Because the medication has an intravenous preparation, it can be readily given to the sick neonate with intravenous access. It has no know drug interactions and is excreted by the kidney, although the pharmacokinetics and safety profile are unknown; the half-life in neonates is longer than that in adults, approximately 18 hours. A starting loading dose is 20 mg/kg but a loading dose high as 60 mg/kg has been reported before seizures are lessened or controlled. Long-term effects on brain maturation are unknown.

Efficacy of Treatment

Conflicting studies report varying efficacy with phenobarbital and phenytoin. Most studies only apply a clinical end point to seizure cessation. One study[99] found that only 36% of neonates with clinical seizures showed response to phenobarbital,[99] and another study noted cessation of clinical seizures with phenobarbital in only 32% of neonates.[100] With doses as high as 40 mg/kg,[106] the rate of seizure control was reported to be 85%. A later study reported that the earlier administration of high-dose phenobarbital in a group of asphyxiated infants was associated with a 27% reduction in clinical seizures and better outcome than that of a group who did not receive high dosages.[107] However, coincident EEG studies are now suggested to verify the resolution of electrographic seizures, given the uncoupling that abolishes only the clinical expression of seizures. Another report suggests that 30% of neonates have persistent electrographic seizures after suppression of clinical seizure behaviors following drug administration.[49] With EEG as an end point to judge cessation of seizures, another study found neither phenobarbital nor phenytoin to be effective to control seizure activity.[109] At this time evidence is extremely limited, with only two randomized controlled trials supporting the use of specific types of antiepileptic medications in the newborn period, with long-term prediction of efficacy.[93,94]

The use of measurements of free or drug-bound fractions of anticonvulsants has been suggested to better assess both efficacy and potential toxicity of anticonvulsants in pediatric populations.[109] Drug binding in neonates with seizures has only recently been reported and can be altered in a sick neonate with organ dysfunction. Toxic side effects may result from elevated free fractions of a drug that adversely affect cardiovascular and respiratory function. To guard against untoward effects, evaluation of treatment and efficacy must take into account both total and free anticonvulsants fractions in the context of the progression or resolution of systemic illness.

Once an anticonvulsant drug is chosen, the clinician must closely monitor to ensure that seizures are not worsened by the administration of the drug choice. AEDs may cause worsening of seizures by either aggravating previous seizures or triggering new seizure types, as described in four neonates after midazolam was administered.[110]

Discontinuation of Drug Use

Whether to maintain or discontinue anticonvulsant drug use is also uncertain.[111,112] Discontinuation of drugs before discharge from the neonatal unit is generally recommended, because clinical assessments of arousal, tone, and behavior will no longer be hampered by medication effect. However, in newborns with neuroimaging evidence of congenital or destructive brain lesions and those with persistently abnormal neurologic findings at the time of discharge a slower tapering of medication over several weeks or months may be required. Conventional wisdom suggests that most children with neonatal seizures uncommonly experience recurrence during the first 2 years of life. Therefore, prophylactic anticonvulsant administration need not be maintained past 3 months of age unless the child is considered at high risk. This approach is supported by a study suggesting a low risk of seizure recurrence after early withdrawal of anticonvulsant therapy in the neonatal period.[113] Also, older infants who present with specific epileptic syndromes, such as infantile spasms, will not show response to the conventional anticonvulsants that were initially begun during the neonatal period. This honeymoon period without seizures commonly persists for many years in most children before isolated or recurrent seizures appear.

The potential damage to the developing central nervous system by anticonvulsants also emphasizes the need to consider early discontinuation of these agents in the newborn period. Adverse effects on the morphology and metabolism of neuronal cells have been extensively reported from collective research performed over the last few decades.[114]

Novel Drug Approaches

A 2008 National Institutes of Health workshop concluded that no one therapeutic choice will fit the needs of all neonates with seizures.[2] Selective therapies are needed that are specific to the disease mechanism affecting the immature brain in the context of changes over time in a brain region–specific manner. Mechanisms of seizure generation, propagation, and termination are different during early brain development from those in older children. These age-related mechanisms have been partially elucidated.[115] Given that traditional anticonvulsant medications have unacceptable efficacy to stop neonatal seizures for specific subsets of newborns, alternative medication options must be developed.

Novel approaches to treat neonatal seizures are now being proposed and studied. These strategies have different rationales, as follows: (1) single or combination therapies focused on the signaling pathways for a specific etiology of brain disorder (e.g., stroke, asphyxia etc); (2) alteration of receptor actions within neural networks important for neurotransmission to reduce the likelihood of depolarization and seizure generation; and (3) selective alteration of the action of a specific receptor associated with a specific genetic form of neonatal seizures. This section gives examples of each of these approaches:

Single or Synergistic Treatments for General Neonatal Disease States

One class of medications is the N-methyl-D-aspartate antagonists, such as topiramate,[116] which may be useful in the treatment of asphyxia and stroke because it reduces the excitatory and harmful effects of extracellular glutamate. Combination therapies such as therapeutic hypothermia with topiramate further lessened the severity of brain injury after stroke in a rodent model.[117] Such an approach suggests that treatment of the underlying cause with single or synergistic drugs may indirectly reduce the risk of seizures by reducing brain injury and therefore treating the underlying cause of neonatal seizures.

A variety of experimental models of asphyxia-induced seizure activity in immature animal brains have indicated a certain degree of efficacy with these drugs.

Such models provide data regarding pharmacologic and physiologic characteristics of neuronal responses after an asphyxial stress, which causes excessive release of excitotoxic neurotransmitters,[118] such as glutamate. Specific cell membrane receptors, termed *metabotropic glutamate receptors (MGluRs)*, are sensitive to extracellular glutamate release and may play a role in epileptogenesis and seizure-induced brain damage.[119] One class of membrane receptor, for example, has been studied in rat pups after hypoxia-induced seizures, suggesting that downregulation of MGluRs can be associated with epileptogenesis in the absence of cell loss.[115] Molecular subclasses of MGluRs will lead to investigations of novel drugs to block these membrane receptors as the mode of treatment for neonatal seizures[120] due to injury after ischemia and postasphyxia inflammation-induced brain damage, with up regulation of MGluR4.[120] One such experimental drug is talampanel,[121] a noncompetitive AMPAR (alpha-amino-3-hydroxy-5-methyl-4-isoxazole-propionic acid receptor) antagonist with actions that are beneficial over both the short and long term. The administration of this drug to neonatal rats that sustained global hypoxic injury both acutely suppressed seizures in a dose-dependent manner and prevented later apoptosis in the adult animals. Such an experimental drug represents the more comprehensive neuroprotective treatment by addressing both antiepileptogenic and anticonvulsant actions in the immature brain that sustained injury.

Treatments That Alter Neurotransmission

Another therapeutic approach considers drugs that alter neurotransmission in the immature neuron to reduce seizure risk. Experimental studies demonstrate enhanced seizure susceptibility in the developing brain because γ-aminobutyric acid (GABA) exerts a depolarizing excitatory rather than repolarizing inhibitory action in immature subjects.[122] This paradoxic action of GABA early in development may be due in part to age-related differences in chloride homeostasis.[123] Chloride transport is a function of two membrane pumps with different time courses of expression. Early in development (e.g., in the rat, 3 to 15 days after birth), the Na^+-K^+-2Cl^- cotransporter (NKCC1) imports large amounts of chloride into the neuron (along with sodium and potassium to maintain electroneutrality). This pump sets the chloride equilibrium potential positive to the resting potential so that when the $GABA_A$ receptor is activated, chloride flows out of the neuron, depolarizing it. Over time, NKCC1 expression diminishes, and another chloride transporter, KCC2, is expressed. KCC2 has the opposite effect, extruding chloride out of the neuron. This makes the equilibrium potential more negative than the resting potential, so that $GABA_A$ receptor activation allows extracellular chloride to flow into the neuron, hyperpolarizing it and endowing GABA with inhibitory action.

Researchers have termed this process the *developmental switch* in chloride homeostasis. This maturational aspect to the chloride ion may influence seizure susceptibility in the neonatal brain. The additional depolarization that is due to $GABA_A$ receptor activation augments excitation that may be initiated by the glutamate neurotransmission. As a result there is a shift in the excitation-inhibition balance toward excessive excitation and thus toward seizure activity. These conclusions have been suggested by Dzhala and colleagues,[124] who described the developmental profile of NKCC1 in the human neonate. In the early postnatal period, levels of NKCC1 rise to a peak and then decline to adult levels. This rearrangement of membrane receptors occurs over the first few months of life. In the same period, KCC2 expression gradually rises to adult levels.

Blocking NKCC1 function in the immature neuron with a commonly used diuretic, bumetanide, prevents the accumulation of intercellular chloride, which therefore counteracts the depolarizing action of $GABA_A$ receptor activation. Bumetanide reduces kainic-induced seizures in neonatal, but not adult, rats and burst firing in hippocampus slices. As further evidence for genetically engineered mice that lack NKCC1, bumetanide is not effective in ameliorating seizures, supporting its role as a specific inhibitor of NKCC1. Therefore, bumetanide is now considered one promising anticonvulsant with a developmental target, namely the immature chloride cotransporter NKCC1. Some investigators claim that this particular diuretic can be safely used for the neonate, although its long-term safety profile needs to be better studied. It has also been suggested that pharmacologic agents that can diminish bursting behavior in neonatal neurons can add a level of seizure control. In another study, Dzhala and colleagues[124] demonstrated that bumetanide rapidly suppresses synchronous bursts of network activity in hippocampus slices harvested between 4 and 8 days after birth in a rat model. This finding supports the use of this agent as a potential antiepileptic medication in this age group. These investigators have further illustrated that the combined use of bumetanide with phenobarbital may be synergistic by blocking chloride ion efflux from the cell, thus enhancing a more negative GABA equilibrium potential with the use of phenobarbital.[125] Clinical trials need to demonstrate that bumetanide or other similar diuretics can inhibit seizure activity in humans,[126] although a case report anecdotally supports this anticonvulsant effect.[127] A research protocol is now underway in one U.S. children's hospital to study a randomized control trial of bumetanide alone and with add-on phenobarbital is being studied to confirm the findings in the animal studies. Research is also needed to establish that these agents can reach the brain in appropriate concentrations and lack short- as well as long-term adverse effects.

There are still crucial issues regarding the theory that GABA-mediated excitation may have an important action contributing to human neonatal seizures amenable to the treatment, as discussed earlier. It is yet unknown why some GABAergic agents, such as phenobarbital and benzodiazepine, fail to have adequate efficacy for human neonatal seizure control. Although seizures can be halted in a percentage of newborns, additional understanding of epileptogenesis in the immature brain must consider the etiology-specific aspects of GABA-mediated mechanisms of seizures as they relate to asphyxia, infection, and trauma. A specific etiology may alter seizure threshold by epigenetic modification, changing the specific genetic variability within individuals. On the basis of upregulation or downregulation of genetic expression, individuals who suffer asphyxia, infection, or trauma may have variable vulnerability or resistance to GABA-mediated mechanisms for seizures. This generalization is further complicated by the timing and the specific brain region of damage, which may have occurred remotely during the antepartum as opposed to the intrapartum or neonatal period and have selectively affected deep gray matter as well as neocortical structures. Finally, the occurrence of status epilepticus can alter the action of brain-derived neurotrophic factor (BDNF) and the downstream pathways that enhance epileptogenesis through upregulation of specific subunits of the GABA receptor that promote further seizures.[128]

Selective Alteration of a Specific Receptor

A third example of an approach to the treatment for neonatal seizures involves the receptor affected by a specific genetic defect. Loss-of-function mutations in the KCNQ potassium channels have been identified with benign familial neonatal seizures. Selective neuronal KCNQ channel openers, such as flupirtine, are effective in diminishing the severity of clinical and electrographic expression of neonatal seizures in an animal model.[129]

Summary

One must consider the question whether neonatal seizures cause brain injury or are surrogates of injury resulting from etiologies varied in either brain location or periods beginning during fetal life.[130] This issue is further complicated by alterations in the genetic expression of neuronal networks after prolonged seizures that further lower the threshold for seizures. The neurologist must place events leading to seizures in the context of clinical, historical, and laboratory findings to determine both the pathogenesis and timing of neonatal seizures specific to an accompanying encephalopathy or in the absence of a clinically apparent brain disorder. A new classification of neonatal seizures must integrate electrographic expression, brain region, etiology, and timing to facilitate the choice of anticonvulsant medication during the neonatal period. This classification scheme will also be relevant in the choice of anticonvulsants during childhood if epilepsy is later expressed.[131]

Recognition and classification of seizures remain problematic, because neonatal seizures represent a complex phenotype. The clinician should rely on synchronized video/EEG/polygraph recordings to correlate suspicious behaviors with electrographic seizures, because clinical phenomena without coincident electrographic seizure events represent other types of neuronal network dysfunction, requiring different diagnostic, prognostic, and therapeutic strategies. This monitoring technique will limit misdiagnosis and overtreatment of nonepileptic abnormal behaviors and will define an exact end point with anticonvulsants for cortically propagated seizures. This practice must be integrated with an appreciation of pathophysiologic mechanisms responsible for brain injury in a variety of anatomic sites during antepartum periods from maternal-fetal-placental disease as well as during the intrapartum or neonatal period.[131]

Gaps in Knowledge

1. How long should a neonate who experiences seizures in the neonatal intensive care unit be treated?
2. Are electrical or clinical seizures more detrimental to normal brain structure and function?
3. Is there a need to incorporate two-tiered recording paradigms in future studies to combine results from screening devices with more traditional comprehensive neurophysiologic protocols?
4. Should targeted antiseizure medications be developed?

References

1. Scher MS. *Seizures in the neonate: diagnostic and therapeutic considerations.* In: *Intensive care of the fetus and neonate.* Elsevier-Mosby; 2005.
2. Silverstein FS, Jensen FE, Inder T, et al. Improving the treatment of neonatal seizures: National Institute of Neurological Disorders and Stroke workshop report. *J Pediatr.* 2008;153:12-15.
3. Scher MS. *Neonatal seizures: an expression of fetal or neonatal brain disorders.* Cambridge, UK: Cambridge University Press; 2002.
4. Clancy RR. Prolonged electroencephalogram monitoring for seizures and their treatment. *Clin Perinatol.* 2006;33:649-665, vi.
5. Ray S. Question 1. Is cerebral function monitoring as accurate as conventional EEG in the detection of neonatal seizures? *Arch Dis Child.* 2011;96:314-316.
6. Proposal for revised clinical and electroencephalographic classification of epileptic seizures. From the Commission on Classification and Terminology of the International League Against Epilepsy. *Epilepsia.* 1981;22:489-501.
7. Mizrahi EM, Kellaway P. *Diagnosis and management of neonatal seizures.* Philadelphia: Lippincott-Raven; 1998.
8. Weiner SP, Painter MJ, Geva D, et al. Neonatal seizures: electroclinical dissociation. *Pediatr Neurol.* 1991;7:363-368.
9. Biagioni E, Ferrari F, Boldrini A, et al. Electroclinical correlation in neonatal seizures. *Eur J Paediatr Neurol.* 1998;2:117-125.
10. Volpe JJ. *Neonatal seizures.* Philadelphia: W.B. Saunders; 2001.
11. Scher MS. Normal electrographic-polysomnographic patterns in preterm and fullterm infants. *Semin Pediatr Neurol.* 1996;3:2-12.
12. Scher MS. *Electroencephalography of the newborn: normal and abnormal features.* Philadelphia: Lippincott Williams and Wilkins; 2005.
13. Fenichel GM, Olson BJ, Fitzpatrick JE. Heart rate changes in convulsive and nonconvulsive neonatal apnea. *Ann Neurol.* 1980;7:577-582.
14. da Silva O, Collado Guzman GM, Young GB. The value of standard electroencephalograms in the evaluation of the newborn with recurrent apneas. *J Perinatol.* 1998;18:377-380.
15. Mizrahi EM, Kellaway P. Characterization and classification of neonatal seizures. *Neurology.* 1987;37:1837-1844.
16. Bye AM, Flanagan D. Spatial and temporal characteristics of neonatal seizures. *Epilepsia.* 1995;36:1009-1016.

8

17. Boylan GB, Pressler RM, Rennie JM, et al. Outcome of electroclinical, electrographic, and clinical seizures in the newborn infant. *Dev Med Child Neurol.* 1999;41(12):819-825.

18. Clancy R, Malin S, Laraque D, et al. Focal motor seizures heralding stroke in full-term neonates. *Am J Dis Child.* 1985;139:601-606.

19. Levy SR, Abroms IF, Marshall PC, Rosquete EE. Seizures and cerebral infarction in the full-term newborn. *Ann Neurol.* 1985;17:366-370.

20. Scher MS, Klesh KW, Murphy TF, Guthrie RD. Seizures and infarction in neonates with persistent pulmonary hypertension. *Pediatr Neurol.* 1986;2:332-339.

21. Holmes GL. *Diagnosis and management of seizures in children.* Philadelphia: WB Saunders; 1987.

22. Karayiannis NB, Srinivasan S, Bhattacharya R, et al. Extraction of motion strength and motor activity signals from video recordings of neonatal seizures. *IEEE Trans Med Imaging.* 2001;20:965-980.

23. Rose AL, Lombroso CT. A study of clinical, pathological, and electroencephalographic features in 137 full-term babies with a long-term follow-up. *Pediatrics.* 1970;45:404-425.

24. Kellaway P, Hrachovy R. *Status epilepticus in newborns: a perspective on neonatal seizures.* New York: Raven Press; 1983.

25. Sarnat HB. *Anatomic and physiologic correlates of neurologic developments in prematurity.* Orlando, FL: Grune & Stratton; 1984.

26. Scher MS. Neonatal hypertonia: I. Classification and structural-functional correlates. *Pediatr Neurol.* 2008;39:301-306.

27. Scher MS. Neonatal hypertonia: II. Differential diagnosis and proposed neuroprotection. *Pediatr Neurol.* 2008;39:373-380.

28. Scher MS. Pathologic myoclonus of the newborn: electrographic and clinical correlations. *Pediatr Neurol.* 1985;1:342-348.

29. Coulter DL, Allen RJ. Benign neonatal sleep myoclonus. *Arch Neurol.* 1982;39:191-192.

30. Resnick TJ, Moshé SL, Perotta L, Chambers HJ. Benign neonatal sleep myoclonus. Relationship to sleep states. *Arch Neurol.* 1986;43:266-268.

31. Clancy RR. The contribution of EEG to the understanding of neonatal seizures. *Epilepsia.* 1996; 37(Suppl 1):S52-S59.

32. Shuper A, Zalzberg J, Weitz R, Mimouni M. Jitteriness beyond the neonatal period: a benign pattern of movement in infancy. *J Child Neurol.* 1991;6:243-245.

33. Parker S, Zuckerman B, Bauchner H, et al. Jitteriness in full-term neonates: prevalence and correlates. *Pediatrics.* 1990;85:17-23.

34. Hakamada S, Watanabe K, Hara K, Miyazaki S. Development of the motor behavior during sleep in newborn infants. *Brain Dev.* 1981;3:345-350.

35. Sexson WR, Thigpen J, Stajich GV. Stereotypic movements after lorazepam administration in premature neonates: a series and review of the literature. *J Perinatol.* 1995;15:146-149; quiz 150-141.

36. Scher MS, Belfar H, Martin J, Painter MJ. Destructive brain lesions of presumed fetal onset: antepartum causes of cerebral palsy. *Pediatrics.* 1991;88:898-906.

37. Brown P, Rothwell JC, Thompson PD, et al. The hyperekplexias and their relationship to the normal startle reflex. *Brain.* 1991;114:1903-1928.

38. Andermann F, Andermann E. Startle disorders of man: hyperekplexia, jumping and startle epilepsy. *Brain Dev.* 1988;10:213-222.

39. Barth PJ. Inherited progressive disorders of the fetal brain: a field in need of recognition. In: Fukuyama Y, Suzuki Y, Kamoshita S, et al, eds. *Fetal and perinatal neurology.* Basel: Karger; 1992.

40. Lyon G, Adams RD, Kolodny EH. Hypoglycemia. In: *Neurology of hereditary metabolic disease in children.* New York, NY: McGraw-Hill; 1996.

41. Watanabe K, Kuroyanagi M, Hara K, Miyazaki S. Neonatal seizures and subsequent epilepsy. *Brain Dev.* 1982;4:341-346.

42. Scher MS. Seizures in the newborn infant. Diagnosis, treatment, and outcome. *Clin Perinatol.* 1997;24:735-772.

43. Oliveira AJ, Nunes ML, da Costa JC. Polysomnography in neonatal seizures. *Clin Neurophysiol.* 2000;111(Suppl 2):S74-S80.

44. Lombroso CT. Neonatal polygraphy in full-term and premature infants: a review of normal and abnormal findings. *J Clin Neurophysiol.* 1985;2:105-155.

45. Hrachovy R, Mizrahi EM, Kellaway P. *Electroencephalography of the newborn.* In: Daly D, Pedley TA, eds. *Current practice of clinical electroencephalography.* 2nd ed. New York: Raven Press; 1990;201-242.

46. Stockard-Pope JE, Werner SS, Bickford RG. *Atlas of neonatal electroencephalography.* New York: Raven Press; 1992.

47. Murray DM, Boylan GB, Ali I, et al. Defining the gap between electrographic seizure burden, clinical expression and staff recognition of neonatal seizures. *Arch Dis Child Fetal Neonatal Ed.* 2008;93: F187-F191.

48. Scher MS, Aso K, Beggarly ME, et al. Electrographic seizures in preterm and full-term neonates: clinical correlates, associated brain lesions, and risk for neurologic sequelae. *Pediatrics.* 1993;91: 128-134.

49. Scher MS, Alvin J, Gaus L, et al. Uncoupling of EEG-clinical neonatal seizures after antiepileptic drug use. *Pediatr Neurol.* 2003;28:277-280.

50. Hellstrom-Westas L. Comparison between tape-recorded and amplitude-integrated EEG monitoring in sick newborn infants. *Acta Paediatr.* 1992;81:812-819.

51. Alfonso I, Jayakar P, Yelin K, et al. Continuous-display four-channel electroencephalographic monitoring in the evaluation of neonates with paroxysmal motor events. *J Child Neurol.* 2001;16: 625-628.

52. Shellhaas RA, Clancy RR. Characterization of neonatal seizures by conventional EEG and single-channel EEG. *Clin Neurophysiol.* 2007;118:2156-2161.
53. Wusthoff CJ, Shellhaas RA, Clancy RR. Limitations of single-channel EEG on the forehead for neonatal seizure detection. *J Perinatol.* 2009;29:237-242.
54. Clancy RR, Legido A. The exact ictal and interictal duration of electroencephalographic neonatal seizures. *Epilepsia.* 1987;28:537-541.
55. Scher MS, Hamid MY, Steppe DA, et al. Ictal and interictal electrographic seizure durations in preterm and term neonates. *Epilepsia.* 1993;34:284-288.
56. Scher MS. Stimulus-evoked electrographic patterns in neonates: an abnormal form of reactivity. *Electroencephalogr Clin Neurophysiol.* 1997;103:679-691.
57. Takenouchi T, Yap VL, Engel M, Perlman JM. Stimulus-induced seizure in sick neonates—novel observations with potential clinical implications. *Epilepsia.* 2010;51:308-311.
58. Sheth RD. Electroencephalogram confirmatory rate in neonatal seizures. *Pediatr Neurol.* 1999;20:27-30.
59. Alfonso I, Papazian O, Litt R, et al. Single photon emission computed tomographic evaluation of brainstem release phenomenon and seizure in neonates. *J Child Neurol.* 2000;15:56-58.
60. Kiliç S, Tarim O, Eralp O. Serum prolactin in neonatal seizures. *Pediatr Int.* 1999;41:61-64.
61. Caveness WF, Kato M, et al. Propagation of focal motor seizures in the pubescent monkey. *Ann Neurol.* 1980;7:213-221, 232-235.
62. Hosokawa S, Iguchi T, Caveness WF, et al. Effects of manipulation of the sensorimotor system on focal motor seizures in the monkey. *Ann Neurol.* 1980;7:222-229, 236-237.
63. Browning RA. Role of the brain-stem reticular formation in tonic-clonic seizures: lesion and pharmacological studies. *Fed Proc.* 1985;44:2425-2431.
64. Danner R, Shewmon DA, Sherman MP. Seizures in an atelencephalic infant. Is the cortex essential for neonatal seizures? *Arch Neurol.* 1985;42:1014-1016.
65. Staudt F, Roth JG, Engel RC. The usefulness of electroencephalography in curarized newborns. *Electroencephalogr Clin Neurophysiol.* 1981;51:205-208.
66. Coen RW, McCutchen CB, Wermer D, et al. Continuous monitoring of the electroencephalogram following perinatal asphyxia. *J Pediatr.* 1982;100:628-630.
67. Goldberg RN, Goldman SL, Ramsay RE, Feller R. Detection of seizure activity in the paralyzed neonate using continuous monitoring. *Pediatrics.* 1982;69:583-586.
68. Eyre JA, Oozeer RC, Wilkinson AR. Continuous electroencephalographic recording to detect seizures in paralysed newborn babies. *Br Med J (Clin Res Ed).* 1983;286:1017-1018.
69. O'Meara MW, Bye AM, Flanagan D. Clinical features of neonatal seizures. *J Paediatr Child Health.* 1995;31:237-240.
70. Seay AR, Bray PF. Significance of seizures in infants weighing less than 2,500 grams. *Arch Neurol.* 1977;34:381-382.
71. Eriksson M, Zetterstrom R. Neonatal convulsions. Incidence and causes in the Stockholm area. *Acta Paediatr Scand.* 1979;68:807-811.
72. Ronen GM, Penney S, Andrews W. The epidemiology of clinical neonatal seizures in Newfoundland: a population-based study. *J Pediatr.* 1999;134:71-75.
73. Saliba RM, Annegers FJ, Waller DK, et al. Risk factors for neonatal seizures: a population-based study, Harris County, Texas, 1992-1994. *Am J Epidemiol.* 2001;154:14-20.
74. Lanska MJ, Lanska DJ, Baumann RJ, et al. Interobserver variability in the classification of neonatal seizures based on medical record data. *Pediatr Neurol.* 1996;15:120-123.
75. Lanska MJ, Lanska DJ, Baumann RJ, Kryscio RJ. A population-based study of neonatal seizures in Fayette County, Kentucky. *Neurology.* 1995;45:724-732.
76. ACOG. *Neonatal encephalopathy and cerebral palsy: Defining the pathogenesis and pathophysiology. American College of Obstetrics and Gynecology.* Washington, DC: American College of Obstetricians and Gynecologists; 2003.
77. Scher MS. Fetal and neonatal neurologic case histories: assessment of brain disorders in the context of fetal-maternal-placental disease. Part 2: Neonatal neurologic consultations in the context of adverse antepartum and intrapartum events. *J Child Neurol.* 2003;18:155-164.
78. Redline RW. Disorders of placental circulation and the fetal brain. *Clin Perinatol.* 2009;36:549-559.
79. Locatelli A, Incerti M, Paterlini G, et al. Antepartum and intrapartum risk factors for neonatal encephalopathy at term. *Am J Perinatol.* 2010;27:649-654.
80. Wintermark P, Boyd T, Gregas MC, et al. Placental pathology in asphyxiated newborns meeting the criteria for therapeutic hypothermia. *Am J Obstet Gynecol.* 2010;203:579 e571-579.
81. Takenouchi T, Kasdorf E, Engel M, et al. Changing pattern of perinatal term brain injury—implications for diagnosis and preventative strategies. *Pediatrics.* [in press].
82. Shalak LF, Laptook AR, Jafri HS, et al. Clinical chorioamnionitis, elevated cytokines, and brain injury in term infants. *Pediatrics.* 2002;110:673-680.
83. Romero R, Gotsch F, Pineles B, Kusanovic JP. Inflammation in pregnancy: its roles in reproductive physiology, obstetrical complications, and fetal injury. *Nutr Rev.* 2007;65:S194-S202.
84. Friede RL. *Porencephaly, hydranencephaly, multilocular cystic encephalopathy. Reaction of immature nervous tissue to necrosis.* In: RL Friede, ed. *Developmental neuropathology.* New York: Springer Verlag; 1975:102-122.
85. Miller V. Neonatal cerebral infarction. *Semin Pediatr Neurol.* 2000;7:278-288.
86. de Vries LS, Groenendaal F, Eken P, et al. Infarcts in the vascular distribution of the middle cerebral artery in preterm and fullterm infants. *Neuropediatrics.* 1997;28:88-96.

87. Leth H, Toft PB, Herning M, et al. Neonatal seizures associated with cerebral lesions shown by magnetic resonance imaging. *Arch Dis Child Fetal Neonatal Ed.* 1997;77:F105-F110.

88. Enns GM. Inborn errors of metabolism masquerading as hypoxic-ischemic encephalopathy. *NeoReviews.* 2005;6:e549-e558.

89. Zhou W, Liu W. Hypercapnia and hypocapnia in neonates. *World J Pediatr.* 2008;4:192-196.

90. Helmy MM, Tolner EA, Vanhatalo S, et al. Brain alkalosis causes birth asphyxia seizures, suggesting therapeutic strategy. *Ann Neurol.* 2011;69:493-500.

91. Schmitt B, Baumgartner M, Mills PB, et al. Seizures and paroxysmal events: symptoms pointing to the diagnosis of pyridoxine-dependent epilepsy and pyridoxine phosphate oxidase deficiency. *Dev Med Child Neurol.* 2010;52:e133-e142.

92. Carmo KB, Barr P. Drug treatment of neonatal seizures by neonatologists and paediatric neurologists. *J Paediatr Child Health.* 2005;41:313-316.

93. Booth D, Evans DJ. Anticonvulsants for neonates. *Cochrane Database Syst Rev.* 2004; (4):CD004218.

94. Evans DJ, Levene MI, Tsakmakis M. Anticonvulsants for preventing mortality and morbidity in full term newborns with perinatal asphyxia. *Cochrane Database Syst Rev.* 2007;(3):CD001240.

95. Singh D, Kumar P, Narang A. A randomized controlled trial of phenobarbital in neonates with hypoxic ischemic encephalopathy. *J Matern Fetal Neonatal Med.* 2005;18:391-395.

96. Meyn Jr DF, Ness J, Ambalavanan N, Carlo WA. Prophylactic phenobarbital and whole-body cooling for neonatal hypoxic-ischemic encephalopathy. *J Pediatr.* 2010;157:334-336.

97. Filippi L, la Marca G, Cavallaro G, et al. Phenobarbital for neonatal seizures in hypoxic ischemic encephalopathy: a pharmacokinetic study during whole body hypothermia. *Epilepsia.* 2011;52: 794-801.

98. Sankar R, Painter MJ. Neonatal seizures: after all these years we still love what doesn't work. *Neurology.* 2005;64:776-777.

99. Painter MJ, Pippenger C, MacDonald H, Pitlick W. Phenobarbital and diphenylhydantoin levels in neonates with seizures. *J Pediatr.* 1978;92:315-319.

100. Lockman LA, Kriel R, Zaske D, et al. Phenobarbital dosage for control of neonatal seizures. *Neurology.* 1979;29:1445-1449.

101. Painter MJ, Pippenger C, Wasterlain C, et al. Phenobarbital and phenytoin in neonatal seizures: metabolism and tissue distribution. *Neurology.* 1981;31:1107-1112.

102. Smith BT, Masotti RE. Intravenous diazepam in the treatment of prolonged seizure activity in neonates and infants. *Dev Med Child Neurol.* 1971;13:630-634.

103. Castro Conde JR, Hernández Borges AA, Doménech Martínez E, et al. Midazolam in neonatal seizures with no response to phenobarbital. *Neurology.* 2005;64:876-879.

104. Malingré MM, Van Rooij LG, Rademaker CM, et al. Development of an optimal lidocaine infusion strategy for neonatal seizures. *Eur J Pediatr.* 2006;165:598-604.

105. Shoemaker MT, Rotenberg JS. Levetiracetam for the treatment of neonatal seizures. *J Child Neurol.* 2007;22:95-98.

106. Gal P, Toback J, Boer HR, et al. Efficacy of phenobarbital monotherapy in treatment of neonatal seizures—relationship to blood levels. *Neurology.* 1982;32:1401-1404.

107. Hall RT, Hall FK, Daily DK. High-dose phenobarbital therapy in term newborn infants with severe perinatal asphyxia: a randomized, prospective study with three-year follow-up. *J Pediatr.* 1998;132: 345-348.

108. Painter MJ, Scher MS, Stein AD, et al. Phenobarbital compared with phenytoin for the treatment of neonatal seizures. *N Engl J Med.* 1999;341:485-489.

109. Painter MJ, Minnigh MB, Gaus L, et al. Binding profiles of anticonvulsants in neonates with seizures. *Ann Neurol.* 1987;22:413.

110. Montenegro MA, Guerreiro MM, Caldas JP, et al. Epileptic manifestations induced by midazolam in the neonatal period. *Arq Neuropsiquiatr.* 2001;59:242-243.

111. Camfield PR, Camfield CS. Neonatal seizures: a commentary on selected aspects. *J Child Neurol.* 1987;2:244-251.

112. Scher MS, Painter MJ. Controversies concerning neonatal seizures. *Pediatr Clin North Am.* 1989;36:281-310.

113. Hellström-Westas L, Blennow G, Lindroth M, et al. Low risk of seizure recurrence after early withdrawal of antiepileptic treatment in the neonatal period. *Arch Dis Child Fetal Neonatal Ed.* 1995; 72:F97-F101.

114. Mizrahi EM. Acute and chronic effects of seizures in the developing brain: lessons from clinical experience. *Epilepsia.* 1999;40(Suppl 1):S42-S50.

115. Sanchez RM, Jensen FE. Maturational aspects of epilepsy mechanisms and consequences for the immature brain. *Epilepsia.* 2001;42:577-585.

116. Koh S, Jensen FE. Topiramate blocks perinatal hypoxia-induced seizures in rat pups. *Ann Neurol.* 2001;50:366-372.

117. Liu Y, Barks JD, Xu G, Silverstein FS. Topiramate extends the therapeutic window for hypothermia-mediated neuroprotection after stroke in neonatal rats. *Stroke.* 2004;35:1460-1465.

118. Jensen FE, Wang C. Hypoxia-induced hyperexcitability in vivo and in vitro in the immature hippocampus. *Epilepsy Res.* 1996;26:131-140.

119. Aronica EM, Gorter JA, Paupard MC, et al. Status epilepticus-induced alterations in metabotropic glutamate receptor expression in young and adult rats. *J Neurosci.* 1997;17:8588-8595.

120. Lie AA, Becker A, Behle K, et al. Up-regulation of the metabotropic glutamate receptor mGluR4 in hippocampal neurons with reduced seizure vulnerability. *Ann Neurol.* 2000;47:26-35.

121. Aujla PK, Fetell MR, Jensen FE. Talampanel suppresses the acute and chronic effects of seizures in a rodent neonatal seizure model. *Epilepsia.* 2009;50:694-701.
122. Brooks-Kayal AR. Rearranging receptors. *Epilepsia.* 2005;46(Suppl 7):29-38.
123. Staley KJ. Wrong-way chloride transport: is it a treatable cause of some intractable seizures? *Epilepsy Curr.* 2006;6:124-127.
124. Dzhala VI, Talos DM, Sdrulla DA, et al. NKCC1 transporter facilitates seizures in the developing brain. *Nat Med.* 2005;11:1205-1213.
125. Dzhala VI, Brumback AC, Staley KJ. Bumetanide enhances phenobarbital efficacy in a neonatal seizure model. *Ann Neurol.* 2008;63:222-235.
126. Haglund MM, Hochman DW. Furosemide and mannitol suppression of epileptic activity in the human brain. *J Neurophysiol.* 2005;94:907-918.
127. Kahle KT, Barnett SM, Sassower KC, Staley KJ. Decreased seizure activity in a human neonate treated with bumetanide, an inhibitor of the Na(+)-K(+)-2Cl(-) cotransporter NKCC1. *J Child Neurol.* 2009; 24:572-576.
128. Brooks-Kayal AR, Raol YH, et al. Alteration of epileptogenesis genes. *Neurotherapeutics.* 2009;6: 312-318.
129. Raol YH, Lapides DA, Keating JG, et al. A KCNQ channel opener for experimental neonatal seizures and status epilepticus. *Ann Neurol.* 2009;65:326-336.
130. Scher MS. Neonatal seizures and brain damage. *Pediatr Neurol.* 2003;29:381-390.
131. Scher MS. Neonatal seizure classification: a fetal perspective concerning childhood epilepsy. *Epilepsy Res.* 2006;70(Suppl 1):S41-S57.

8

CHAPTER 9

Glucose and Perinatal Brain Injury: Questions and Controversies

Jerome Y. Yager, MD

Hypoglycemia remains a common though controversial problem of the newborn infant.[1-3] Such controversy persists around issues related, in the first place, to definition and subsequent diagnosis,[4] the relevance of "asymptomatic" versus "symptomatic" hypoglycemia, incidence rates, underlying pathophysiology, treatment, and, of course, neurodevelopmental outcome. Importantly, contributing to the persistence of neonatal hypoglycemia as a cause of morbidity in the newborn is the increasing prevalence of both type 1 and type 2 diabetes both worldwide and being diagnosed in younger women of childbearing age.[5,6] Confounding these issues are improvements in obstetric and neonatal intensive care, which have allowed for the survival of low-birth-weight infants, with their attendant complications of prematurity, respiratory distress, altered metabolism, and higher risks of disorders such as hypoxia-ischemia, seizures, and sepsis.

The adult is completely independent with respect to nutritional requirements. The fetus, on the other hand is fully dependent on the placental transfer of glucose and other nutritional requirements. The newborn is in a transition phase between these two states of complete dependence and independence. For normal cerebral development and consequent function to proceed, an adequate amount of metabolizable substrate must be supplied to the brain during the perinatal period. Glucose is the primary energy substrate for both the adult and newborn brain under physiologic conditions. However, other organic substrates are capable of supplementing glucose during conditions whereby the normal balance of supply and demand for energy production are superceded.[7-9]

At birth, the previously consistent supply of maternal glucose is abruptly terminated. Immediately after birth, hepatic glycogen stores are broken down to maintain reasonable amounts of nutritional support. Glucose-6-phosphatase, the rate-limiting enzyme for this to occur, is expressed at low levels in the newborn, increasing to adult values within the first few days of life.[10] To rapidly adapt, an endocrine stress response involving insulin and glucagon drives hepatic glycogenolysis, lipolysis, and fatty acid oxidation, which generate lactate and ketone bodies as alternative fuels important in maintaining cerebral energy metabolism. Estimated rates of glucose metabolism in the 1-day-old newborn are threefold greater than those in older newborns and infants.[11] Moreover, measured rates of glucose oxidation suggest that only about 70% of the energy needs of the brain are met through the metabolism of glucose. Hence, the newborn is adapted for utilizing ketone bodies, which can be 5- to 40-fold greater than in the adult, and lactate, which contributes significantly in the first few hours of life.

Despite the obvious importance of glucose for cerebral energy utilization, particularly during the complex transition from fetal to newborn life, questions remain regarding the role of hypoglycemia, per se, to brain damage and neurodevelopmental outcome. It is, therefore, the intent of this chapter to provide the reader with a general review of glucose metabolism and its alternative substrates in the newborn brain, to describe the recognized derangements associated with hypoglycemia, and finally to review the clinical aspects of hypoglycemia. Furthermore, a case history is presented that exemplifies aspects of neonatal hypoglycemia, highlighting questions and controversies around this complex issue.

Glucose Metabolism in the Fetus and Newborn

In most species studied, including humans, glucose serves as the primary organic fuel for energy production under physiologic circumstances.[9,12] In the fetus, a linear relationship has been observed between the glucose level in the mother and that in the fetus.[13-16] At birth, blood glucose concentration in the newborn is about 80% to 90% that in the mother.[17] This linear relationship has been seen during all states of maternal euglycemia, hyperglycemia, and hypoglycemia, and is important in that it implies at least a one-to-one relationship between maternal and fetal glucose needs.

At the time of birth, glucose concentrations in the term healthy newborn fall within the first hour of life, recovering and becoming more stable by 3 hours of age, and gradually increasing for at least the first 96 hours, when infants receive exogenous nutrition.[17-21] In preparation for birth, a doubling of the glycogen stores occurs at 36 weeks of gestation. At birth, plasma insulin levels fall, together with a marked surge in glucagon levels, leading to a mobilization of glycogen stores, which are rapidly depleted within the first 12 to 24 hours of life.[22,23] Glucagon levels remain high through the first week of life. Subsequent glucose concentrations, in the normal newborn, depend on feeding practices. Although some studies have suggested feeding intervals to be a major determinant of blood glucose concentrations,[24] others have not found this to be the case.[21] Nevertheless, "low" blood glucose concentrations in appropriately fed term infants are very rare.

Preterm Infants

It is a generally held belief that blood glucose concentrations in the preterm infant are lower than those in the term infant. Although studies now suggest that this is not likely the case, given current policies of early feeding and intravenous glucose supplementation,[24] the theoretical risks certainly apply. In this regard, the preterm infant has not as yet had the opportunity afforded the term infant to build up glycogen stores, typically in the last 4 weeks of gestation. Moreover, the rate-limiting enzyme for glyconeogenesis is significantly lower in the preterm than in the term infant,[10] so the preterm's ability to break down even these stores is limited. The capability of the preterm to mount a response with alternative substrates may also be impaired. Hawdon and colleagues[24] compared 156 term infants with 62 preterms and found that although blood glucose concentrations were not statistically different, preterms were unable to mount a significant ketone body response at the lower end of the blood glucose values. Other investigators have found preterms to variably mount an inadequate glycemic response to glucagon, suggesting features of insulin resistance.[25]

Table 9-1 INCIDENCE OF HYPOGLYCEMIA CLASSIFIED BY BIRTH WEIGHT AND GESTATIONAL AGE

	Blood Glucose Concentrations	
Birth Weight	<1.6 mmol/L (30 mg/dL) (%)	<1.1 mmol/L (20 mg/dL) (%)
Small for Gestational Age* Preterm	67	40
Term	25	21
Post-term	18	9
Appropriate for Gestational Age* Preterm	15	3
Term	10	2
Post-term	5	0
Large for Gestational Age* Preterm	38	13
Term	4	2
Post-term	7	0
Number of Episodes†:	>0.6 to <1.6 mmol/L (>11 to <30 mg/dL)	>1.6 to <2.6 mmol/L (>30 to <45 mg/dL)
2-5	30	58
>6	2	21

*Modified from the data of Lubchenco LO, Bard H. Incidence of hypoglycemia in newborn infants classified by birth weight and gestational age. *Pediatrics.* 1971;47:831-838.
†Modified from the data of Duvanel CB, Fawer CL, Cotting J, et al. Long-term effects of neonatal hypoglycemia on brain growth and psychomotor development in small-for-gestational-age preterm infants. *J Pediatr.* 1999;134:492-498.

Intrauterine Growth Restriction

Clearly, intrauterine growth restriction (IUGR), which exposes the fetus to an environment in which nutrition is restricted due to either placental insufficiency or maternal lack of nutrition, predisposes the newborn to hypoglycemia. Previous reports (Table 9-1) have certainly indicated a higher prevalence of hypoglycemia in small babies than in those within the normal weight range.[26,27] Other reports are more controversial, with some reporting similar glucose concentrations in small-for-gestational age (SGA) and appropriate-for-gestational age (AGA) babies,[17,28] again likely the result of more aggressive nutritional management. Still others continue to show differences between the two weight groups, with SGA babies displaying lower glucose concentrations than AGA babies.[29] In either case, IUGR babies display altered metabolic profiles that include reduced glycogen stores, limited oxidation of free fatty acids, and functional hyperinsulinism.[22] When this problem is combined with a relatively larger brain size, one can see the predisposition of these babies to neurologic injury from a hypoglycemic insult.

Cerebral Metabolism of Glucose

The ontogeny of regional changes in cerebral glucose utilization has important implications regarding the sensitivity of the immature brain to hypoglycemia. With use of the 2-deoxyglucose technique (2-DG) technique, regional cerebral glucose utilization (rCGU) in the perinatal animal has been shown to be high in brainstem gray matter structures, declining in a caudal-to-rostral fashion toward the cerebral cortex.[30] Using positron emission tomography (PET) with ^{18}F-2-deoxyglucose as the isotope, Chugani and associates[31-34] and other groups[35,36] measured regional CGU

9

in humans from birth through adulthood. In infants 5 weeks of age, regional CGU was highest in the sensorimotor cortex, thalamus, midbrain-brainstem, and cerebellar vermis. By 3 months of age, maximal glucose utilization had shifted to the parietal, temporal, and occipital cortices and to the basal ganglia, with subsequent increases in frontal and various association regions of the cerebral cortex occurring by 8 months of age. Little further change in regional CGU was observed between 8 and 18 months, with adult values being reached by 2 years.

Alternative Substrates to Glucose

The perinatal brain is capable of incorporating and metabolizing alternate substrates, most notably lactic acid and the ketone bodies β-hydroxybutyrate and acetoacetate. In vitro studies of regional energy status and the availability of alternate substrates in rats has shown newborn brain lactate concentrations to be elevated by six times those of adult brain concentrations, and β-hydroxybutyrate levels to be double those in of the adult, mature brain.[37]

With respect to the latter, both animal and human studies of the newborn have shown an enhanced capacity for the cerebral extraction of ketone bodies from blood, in comparison with older infants and adults. The investigation of ketone body utilization in the suckling rat suggest they may account for between 20% and 35% of cerebral energy metabolism in this age group.[7,8,38] Ketone body utilization peaks at postnatal day (PD) 14, and subsequently diminishes by PD 21, at a time during which CGU is increasing and glucose becomes the major substrate for energy metabolism. These findings coincide with the capacity of the immature blood-brain barrier to transport ketone bodies at a threefold greater rate than glucose.[39] Furthermore, those enzymes linked to ketone body metabolism in the brain display a rapid increase in activity after birth and a subsequent decline after weaning, in contrast to the pattern displayed by the key enzymes of glycolysis, whose activity increases with advancing age in an inverse relation to those of ketogenesis.[40]

Although ketone bodies appear to play a role in normal energy metabolism of the immature brain, whether they do under pathophysiologic circumstances of glucose deprivation seems unlikely. Data from human infants suggest that the capacity for hepatic ketone synthesis in the neonate is restricted. The findings demonstrate (1) low blood ketone levels, (2) a failure of ketone bodies to rise with fasting, and (3) a failure of ketone bodies to rise with hypoglycemia.[41,42] In contrast, lactic acid has been shown to be an important source of energy during hypoglycemia. Elegant studies in the newborn dog during normoglycemia show that 95% of cerebral energy requirements are met by glucose with ketone bodies and lactate, which contribute 1% and 4%, respectively.[43] With insulin-induced hypoglycemia, and a concomitant reduction in CGU, lactate was able to support 58% of cerebral oxidative metabolism. Subsequent experiments showed that under these conditions there was no significant decline in brain high-energy phosphate levels.[44] Other investigators have also shown a preferential utilization of lactate over either glucose or ketone bodies in the newborn rat and dog, and a sparing effect on glucose utilization during hypoglycemia.[45-49]

Glucose Transporters

The mechanism by which glucose is transported from blood into brain across cell membranes occurs by an Na^+-glucose co-transporter protein that is energy independent. These facilitative glucose transporter proteins are a family of structurally related proteins. Twelve glucose transporters have been identified and labeled as GLUT 1 through 12.[50] Within the brain, GLUT 1 and 3 are predominant. GLUT 1, the most prevalent of the glucose transporters, is highly expressed in all blood-tissue barriers, including the blood-brain barrier. GLUT 3 is the predominant isoform in neurons. GLUT 5 has been detected in the microglia of both humans and rats.

The expression of glucose transporter proteins, not surprisingly, reflects the energy demands of the brain. Hence, analysis of cerebral cortical microvessels and membranes in the newborn rat demonstrates that all GLUT proteins are low during the first week of life. During the second and third postnatal weeks, GLUT proteins increase, particularly in the deep gray matter structures of the thalamus and hypothalamus, coincident with enhanced utilization of glucose as a fuel. Similarly, and in an almost linear fashion, GLUT proteins in the cortex and hippocampus increase from 20% to 100% of adult values between 7 and 30 postnatal days during a recognized period of rapid neuronal maturation and synaptogenesis.[51-53]

Definitions

Ambiguity surrounding a precise definition of neonatal hypoglycemia continues[54] and has been emphasized by a number of reviews.[4,55] Koh and associates,[56] as far back as 1988, surveyed 36 pediatric textbooks and 178 pediatric consultants in a search for agreement on the definition of neonatal hypoglycemia. Perhaps not surprisingly, there was none, with definitions ranging from less than 1 mmol/L to less than 4 mmol/L. In 1937, Hartmann and Jaudon[12] published a series of 286 neonates and infants with significant hypoglycemia as determined by recurrent or persistent low "true" blood glucose values. Only those infants with clinical manifestations were considered. These authors defined hypoglycemia as being mild (2.2-2.78 mmol/L) (39.6-50 mg/dL), moderate (1.11-2.22 mmol/L) (19-38 mg/dL), or extreme (less than 1.11 mmol/L) (19 mg/dL). Their approach incorporated the important concept that the definition of hypoglycemia must represent a continuum of values that deviate from the biologic norm. This latter concept is particularly relevant today, as definitions of treatable hypoglycemia take into account gestational age, multisystem organ complications, and neurophysiologic and/or clinical symptomatology.

Difficulty in arriving at an absolute value for hypoglycemia in the newborn stems from the obvious factors that encompass a dynamic and vulnerable biologic process. *Hypoglycemia* simply refers to an abnormally low blood glucose concentration. In this context, the definition of abnormal becomes relevant, given that hypoglycemia, or euglycemia for that matter, is an evolving, dynamic process, itself dependent on a large number of variables.

Absolute glucose concentrations below which the term *hypoglycemia* can be applied have been defined on the basis of statistical measures (within 2 standard deviations of the mean). Hence, serial plasma glucose determinations in term healthy newborn infants revealed an initial drop to 55 to 60 mg/dL (3.05 mmol/L) within the first 2 hours of life, followed by a rise to 70 mg/dL (3.88 mmol/L) from 3 to 72 hours, and levels in excess of 80 mg/dL (4.44 mmol/L) beyond the 3rd day.[20] Values below the 5th percentile were therefore considered by the investigators as representing statistical hypoglycemia (see Table 9-1).

Lubchenco and Bard[27] studied the incidence of hypoglycemia as determined by gestational age and birth weight. Their work showed that preterm infants who were AGA displayed a mean glucose concentration of 48 mg/dL (2.6 mmol/L), compared with 54 mg/dL (3.0 mmol/L) in term AGA infants. In SGA infants born at term, there was a further shift, with mean glucose concentrations being 44 mg/dL (2.4 mmol/L).

Of later studies that have looked at glucose concentrations in healthy, term infants, Hoseth and colleagues[18] evaluated 223 term breast-fed newborns serially over the first 96 hours, and found lowest blood glucose values to occur within the first hours of life, with an overall range of 1.4 to 5.3 mmol/L (median 3.1) (25-95 mg/dL) (median 55.8 mg/dL). Similar results were reported by a study of more 200 term healthy newborns,[21] in which a mean glucose concentration of 2.8 mmol/L (50.8 mg/dL) was found. In both of the preceding studies, 12% to 14% of the children had blood glucose values lower than 2.6 mmol/L (46.8 mg/dL), mostly during the first day of life.

A meta-analysis[57] reviewing 10 studies, inclusive of 723 healthy term AGA infants, suggested parameters that are less than the 5th percentile of norm be considered for the definition of neonatal hypoglycemia.[57] In this regard, thresholds for hypoglycemia would be on a sliding scale based on time after birth and include values of less than 1.6, 2.2, and 2.67 mmol/L (28.8, 39.6, 48 mg/dL) at 1 to 2, 3 to 47, and 48 to 72 hours of age, respectively.

9

On the basis of these findings, it is reasonable to state that normal glucose concentrations in term healthy infants have a wide range, with the lowest concentrations occurring during the first few hours of life. Within this range, the risk of neurologic sequelae is remote, and routine measurement of blood glucose has been suggested to be unnecessary.[54]

Controversy and Question

The preceding data do not, however, direct themselves to the more controversial and clinically relevant questions that remain somewhat unanswered. Hence, the definition of neonatal hypoglycemia remains nonspecific and is dependent on gestational age, appropriateness of fetal growth, the age of the newborn at the time of sampling, and whether or not the infant has fed. Given these parameters, current data suggest that hypoglycemia is not clinically evident, nor perhaps relevant, until the blood glucose level is less than 1.1 mmol/L (19.8 mg/dL). We therefore need to ask whether there are other parameters or markers of hypoglycemia that suggest an association with resultant encephalopathy.

Symptomatic Versus Asymptomatic Hypoglycemia

Most common among the features of hypoglycemic encephalopathy is an alteration in the level of consciousness, described as lethargy or somnolescence. Irritability, high-pitched cry, or exaggerated primitive reflexes may also be found. Newborns are often described as being jittery, and this state may progress to seizures, apnea, hypotonia, and coma.[58]

In this regard, a number of investigators have shown that perhaps the more relevant way to define hypoglycemia is to do so on the basis of whether or not the infant is symptomatic. Koivisto and associates[59] reported on 151 children, divided into the following groups: (1) symptomatic-convulsive group (n = 8), (2) symptomatic-nonconvulsive group (n = 77), and (3) asymptomatic group (n = 66). In this group of patients, feeding was not initiated for the first 24 hours of life. Symptoms were characterized by the presence of tremor, cyanosis, pallor, limpness, irritability, apathy, or tachypnea, which disappeared with glucose therapy. Hypoglycemia was defined as a glucose concentration less than 20 mg/dL (1.1 mmol/L). The findings indicated that 50% of the symptomatic-convulsive group and 12% of the symptomatic-nonconvulsive group had neurologic abnormalities on follow-up compared with only 6% of both the asymptomatic and control groups. In a study by Singh and coworkers,[60] 107 babies with severe hypoglycemia (less than 25 mg/dL) were evaluated over 15 months. Symptoms were present in 40%. Neurodevelopment in asymptomatic babies was normal.

Moore and Perlman[61] described three cases of profound hypoglycemia in term breast-fed newborns, in whom seizures developed following discharge from hospital. All were symptomatic, with pallor, jitteriness, and poor feeding, but had nevertheless been home on early discharge. All of the patients showed glucose concentrations lower than 1.1 mmol/L. Late follow-up suggested that two of the three infants were normal, and one showed significant developmental delay.

Alkalay and coworkers[62] reviewed reports of hypoglycemia over the last 4 decades. Their criterion for inclusion, albeit retrospective, was the presence of neurologic sequelae believed to be directly or primarily the result of hypoglycemia. The study was inclusive of both AGA and SGA babies as well as preterms. Their findings indicated that, of the study patients reported, more than 95% had plasma glucose concentrations lower than 25 mg/dL (1.4 mmol/L). The incidence in this group with neurologic abnormality was 21%.

In order to correlate a critical threshold of blood glucose concentration with neurologic dysfunction, several studies have evaluated neurophysiologic parameters in association with hypoglycemia. Koh and associates[63] reported abnormalities in sensory evoked potentials in children when blood glucose concentrations fell below 2.6 mmol/L (46.8 mg/dL). Unfortunately, only 5 of 17 children investigated were younger than 1 month of age. Cowett and colleagues,[64] studying term and preterm infants, found no such correlation, and Pryds and coworkers[65] also found no correlation between hypoglycemic glucose concentrations and brain auditory evoked response (BAER) and electroencephalography (EEG) patterns.

In a 2011 study, Caksen and associates[66] examined 110 infants with hypoglycemia using magnetic resonance imaging (MRI). There seemed to be no difference in glucose concentrations between the symptomatic and asymptomatic patients, all of whom had mean values less than 1.0 mmol/L (18 mg/dL). However, the symptomatic infants were more likely than the asymptomatic infants to have abnormal MRI findings.

Duration of Hypoglycemia

Alkalay and colleagues[62] found that the minimal age that hypoglycemia was detected was 10 hours, suggesting that a prolonged period of hypoglycemia was required before neurologic sequelae or symptomatology becomes evident.[62] Others have similarly suggested prolonged hypoglycemia as a prerequisite for damage. Lucas and coworkers[67] determined the neurologic outcome of 661 preterm infants. Moderate hypoglycemia, defined in their study as less than 2.6 mmol/L (46.8 mg/dL), occurred in 433 infants, of which 104 displayed recurrent events on three or more separate days. A strong correlation existed between the number of separate days on which hypoglycemia was recorded and reduced mental and motor development scores at 18 months corrected age. When hypoglycemia was present on five or more days, the incidence of cerebral palsy or developmental delay was increased by a factor of 3.5.

A later study conducted by Duvanel and coworkers[26] illustrated similar results. Eighty-five SGA preterm newborns were tested for hypoglycemia (defined as <2.6 mmol/L) (46.8 mg/dL). In their cohort, 73% met the criteria for hypoglycemia, and recurrent episodes were once again strongly correlated with persistent neurodevelopmental and physical growth deficits to 5 years of age.

A primate study determining the effect of prolonged insulin-induced hypoglycemia on outcome also showed that the longer the duration of hypoglycemia, the greater the degree of abnormal behavioral outcome.[68] However, even in those in which hypoglycemia was produced for 10 hours, the effects were transient and were reversible when training was done for the behavioral task. Blood glucose concentrations were lower than 25 mg/dL. Unfortunately, no neuropathologic examination was reported for this group of animals.

In our own laboratory, my colleagues and I have completed a study in newborn rat pups undergoing insulin-induced hypoglycemia to various degrees and for variable durations. Neuropathologic assessment was determined following a series of behavioral tests. In this experiment, the mortality rate was significantly increased among rat pups that had profound levels of hypoglycemia, less than 1.0 mmol/L (18 mg/dL). In survivors of prolonged hypoglycemia (>12 hours), behavioral assessments were no different from those in controls. However, brain pathology indicated a significant increase in cell death among those with severe hypoglycemia in specific nuclei of the thalamus. Moreover, these pathologic alterations were accompanied by alterations in excitatory amino acid release and free radical production (unpublished data).

In a more mature model of recurrent hypoglycemia, moderate hypoglycemia, rat pups received 5 U/kg of insulin twice daily from postnatal days 10 to 19. Although glucose levels were not recorded, those pups receiving insulin displayed heightened levels of anxiety during juvenile age equivalent and diminished social play behavior as adolescents. Although the model used was not a model of neonatal hypoglycemia, the study confirms the need for a prolonged period of hypoglycemia in order to obtain an abnormal phenotype.[69]

To provide basic guidelines by which to define hypoglycemia, Cornblath and associates[70] issued a consensus statement regarding operational thresholds for blood glucose concentrations. They defined *operational threshold* as that concentration of plasma or blood glucose at which clinicians should consider intervention. In that regard, they believed that healthy, asymptomatic full-term infants need not have routine blood glucose monitoring. On the other hand, any infant with clinical manifestations compatible with hypoglycemia should be tested, and intervention taken for those with values lower than 45 mg/dL (2.5 mmol/L). For infants at risk for hypoglycemia because of alterations in maternal metabolism, intrinsic neonatal problems, or endocrine or metabolic disturbances, glucose monitoring should begin as soon after birth as possible. For those with glucose values less than 36 mg/dL (2.0 mmol/L), close surveillance should be maintained, and intervention recommended if concentrations remain low, regardless of the presence or absence of symptoms. In those infants in whom very low concentrations are detected (less than 20-25 mg/dL; 1.1-1.4 mmol/L), therapeutic intervention should be initiated immediately. Newborn infants being fed by continuous parenteral nutrition will have persistently high insulin levels. As a result, their ability to manifest significant ketogenesis and the means by which to utilize alternative substrates will be impaired. Under these circumstances, prudence suggests maintaining glucose concentrations in the higher therapeutic ranges (>45 mg/dL; 2.5 mmol/L).

Although this consensus statement certainly addresses many of the concerns regarding under what circumstances clinicians should be vigilant in their approach to the diagnosis and treatment of hypoglycemia, it does not answer several other important questions about the newborn in particular. Before one attempts to answer these questions, further understanding of the epidemiology and pathophysiology of hypoglycemia would be in order.

Causes of Hypoglycemia

Although it is not the intent of this chapter to discuss the underlying causes of hypoglycemia, a list of etiologies is given in Box 9-1.

Incidence

The reported incidence of hypoglycemia depends on those variables also specific to its definition. Sexson and associates[23] found that 8.1% of 232 infants had glucose values less than 30 mg/dL (1.6 mmol/L) in the first hours of life, with 20.6% having glucose concentrations less than 40 mg/dL (2.2 mmol/L). Using less than 30 mg/dL as a definition of hypoglycemia, Lubchenco and colleagues[27] studied the incidence of hypoglycemia according to gestational age and weight and found the overall incidence to be 32% for SGA infants, 10% for AGA infants, and 11.5% for large-for-gestational age (LGA) infants. With a definition of less than 20 mg/dL, the incidence obviously decreases. Of the 73% of SGA infants studied by Duvanel and

---

Box 9-1   DIFFERENTIAL DIAGNOSIS OF SEVERE RECURRENT HYPOGLYCEMIA

Hyperinsulinism:
- Betacell hyperplasia
- Nesidioblastosis
- Macrosomia
- Beckwith-Wiedemann syndrome

Endocrine abnormalities:
- Panhypopituitarism
- Hypothyroidism
- Growth hormone deficiency
- Cortisol deficiency

Hereditary metabolic disorders:
- Abnormalities of carbohydrate metabolism
- Amino acid disorders (maple syrup urine disease)
- Organic acid disorders
- Fatty acid oxidation defects

Glucose transporter defects

coworkers[26] who had hypoglycemia, 30% would have had six or more episodes with glucose values between 1.6 and 2.6 mmol/L (28.8 and 46.8 mg/dL) (see Table 9-1).

Pathophysiology of Hypoglycemia

Cerebral Blood Flow, Glucose Utilization, and Cerebral Energy Metabolism

Because glucose is the major metabolic fuel for cerebral energy production, there is an inextricable link between the demands for energy production and the supply and extraction of substrate. In that regard, studies in newborn dogs displayed an inverse linear relationship between blood glucose concentrations and cerebral blood flow (CBF).[71] Therefore, increases in CBF ranging from 150% to 450% of normal occurred as blood glucose concentrations decreased from 40 mg/dL to less than 5 mg/dL (2.2 to <0.3 mmol/L). Increases followed ontogeny and were more predominant in brainstem structures than in other major regions of the brain. The same phenomenon is seen in human infants. Pryds and colleagues[65] found that CBF increased to 200% above normal at levels of blood glucose below 30 mg/dL (1.6 mmol/L).

Vannucci's group of collaborators found similar results and, importantly, looked at the alterations in white matter glucose utilization during hypoglycemia.[72] In this study blood glucose concentrations were reduced to about 1.0 mmol/L (18 mg/dL). Hypoglycemia was associated with increases in regional CBF ranging from 170% (white matter) to 250% (thalamus). In both of the former studies, there was a direct relation between CBF and mean arterial pressure. Regional CGU was unchanged in 11 of the 16 structures measured but significantly was reduced by 30% to 45% in the occipital white matter structures and cerebellum. Calculations of the extent to which glucose transport into the brain during hypoglycemia was enhanced by the increases in CBF suggested that glucose delivery contributed minimally (<10%) to the maintenance of CGU. Earlier studies had also shown that with hypoglycemia to glucose levels as low as less than 1.0 mmol/L (18 mg/dL), the cerebral metabolic rate for oxygen ($CMRO_2$) decreased to 50% of normal. At this same level, cerebral metabolic rates for lactate increased tenfold, and lactate became the dominant fuel for oxidative metabolism in the newborn dog brain.[43] Later experiments using a similar experimental paradigm of hypoglycemia showed that high-energy phosphate reserves (phosphocreatine, adenosine triphosphate [ATP]) remained within normal concentrations.[44] From this group of studies, the investigators concluded that CBF autoregulation is lost during hypoglycemia in the newborn, and that, rather than glucose delivery, low-energy demands serve to maintain glucose homeostasis and preclude tissue glucose deficiencies. They further hypothesized that alternative cerebral energy fuels, predominantly in the form of lactate, substitute for glucose when the blood glucose level is less than 1 mmol/L.

Cerebral Biochemical Alterations During Hypoglycemia

Little work has actually been done on the biochemical pertubations that arise as a result of hypoglycemia in the immature brain. Much of what is known in this regard is derived from experiments done in the adult animal exposed to insulin-induced hypoglycemia. However, given the information discussed in the previous section, important comparisons between the adult and newborn brain can be made, and perhaps some tentative conclusions drawn.

As in the newborn, CBF increases during hypoglycemia. In the adult, this is where the similarities end. Hence in adult models of hypoglycemia, cerebral levels of high-energy phosphates (ATP, phosphocreatine) plummet to levels less than 20% of normal as blood glucose concentrations fall below 1 mmol/L (<18 mg/dL). In concert with this depletion of high-energy reserves, neurophysiologic monitoring reveals an isoelectric electroencephalogram, a marked increase in intracellular calcium, and tenfold and fourfold rises in extracellular concentrations of the excitatory amino acids (EAAs) aspartate and glutamate, respectively.[73-75] Hence, at least in the adult, it now appears that the mechanism of neuronal death due to

Table 9-2 COMPARISON OF PATHOPHYSIOLOGIC MECHANISMS RESPONSIBLE FOR BRAIN DAMAGE IN ADULT VS NEWBORN ANIMALS

Mechanism	Adult	Newborn
Cerebral blood flow	Increased	Increased
Cerebral uptake of glucose	Increased	Increased
Cerebral energy reserves	Decreased	Neutral
Utilization of alternate substrates	Neutral	Increased
Glucose utilization	Increased	Decreased

hypoglycemia is similar to that of hypoxia-ischemia (energy depletion → excitatory amino acid release → Ca^{2+} influx → free radical production → cell death).

As indicated earlier, the preservation of cerebral energy status in the newborn, even at very low concentrations of glucose, is accompanied by a preservation of neurophysiologic function as demonstrated by electroencephalography. A possible underlying cause of cellular injury in the newborn may, however, be related to the release of excitatory amino acids. Silverstein and coworkers[76] induced hypoglycemia by insulin injection in 7-day-old immature rats. Blood glucose concentrations gradually diminished over time to 30 to 40 mg/dL in the first hour after injection, 20 mg/dL in the second hour, and to less than 5 mg/dL by 3 to 4 hours after injection. These results indicated a direct correlation between decreasing glucose levels and increasing concentrations of extracellular glutamate. In hypoglycemic newborn human infants, Aral and colleagues[77] also reported their finding of increased concentrations of glutamate and aspartate in cerebrospinal fluid.

Beyond the preceding experimental data, there is very little information regarding the underlying mechanisms of hypoglycemic brain injury in the newborn. In comparing the newborn response to hypoglycemia with that of the adult response (Table 9-2), several important differences become evident, particularly as related to the controversy surrounding hypoglycemic brain injury. In this regard, then, the newborn appears to respond to hypoglycemia with physiologic alterations that appear to protect the brain from damage. Hence, CBF increases, glucose utilization drops, alternate substrates are able to substitute for demands of energy production, and as a result, cerebral energy reserves are preserved, at least in experimental animals. These metabolic adaptations beg the question as to whether or not hypoglycemia per se does cause brain damage, certainly an area of ongoing controversy.

Hypoglycemia and Brain Damage

Evidence of pathologic injury to the brain due to neonatal hypoglycemia has been particularly difficult to obtain. In this regard, in vitro cell culture studies as well as animal models of pure hypoglycemia have been helpful in documenting the effects of significantly low blood glucose levels on brain pathology.

In vitro nuclear magnetic resonance (NMR) studies on energy metabolism of neurons and astroglia under various pathologic conditions have shown that hypoglycemia per se does not significantly alter the high-energy reserves of either neurons or glia, even at levels as low as 0.1 mmol/L.[78] In our own laboratory, immature astrocytes in culture were exposed to a substrate-free medium (absence of glucose and amino acids). Under these circumstances, which do not allow for the utilization of any alternative substrate, the immature cells were able to survive for almost twice as long as the mature astrocytes. Although not strictly an indication of the effects of hypoglycemia, this finding clearly points out the resistance of immature cells to substrate deprivation.[79]

Brierly and colleagues[80] investigated the effects of insulin-induced hypoglycemia in a group of adolescent primates. Physiologic parameters were controlled. Six of the 10 animals in which blood glucose was lowered to less than 20 mg/dL

(1.1 mmol/L) for 2 hours or more displayed selective neuronal necrosis throughout the cerebral cortices, with particular vulnerability in the parieto-occipital region, as well as the hippocampus, caudate, and putamen. Similar findings were present in primates exposed to severe (<20 mg/dL) and prolonged hypoglycemia (>6 hours). In these animals neuropathologic alterations occurred primarily in the basal ganglia, cerebral cortex, and hippocampus.[81]

Using the adult rat, Auerand colleagues[82-87] have done extensive work defining the neuropathologic consequences of severe hypoglycemia. In a series of papers, this group defined the timing, evolution, and distribution of hypoglycemic brain damage in the rat. These investigators defined severe hypoglycemia as that level of blood glucose that caused electrocerebral silence.[88] Their previous studies had shown that glucose concentrations under these circumstances were between 0.12 and 1.36 mmol/L. Over the course of these investigations, they described several important features of hypoglycemic brain damage that distinguishes it from ischemic injury, as follows: (1) infarction of brain tissue does not occur with hypoglycemia; (2) a superficial to deep gradient in the density of neuronal necrosis is seen in the cerebral cortex; (3) the caudate putamen is involved more heavily near the white matter and near the angle of the lateral ventricle; and (4) the hippocampus shows dense neuronal necrosis at the crest of the dentate gyrus (which is always spared in ischemia), and a gradient of increasing damage in the medial aspect of CA1.[83,84,89] Interestingly, white matter injury was not particularly dealt with in these studies.

For the human neonate, there is clearly a paucity of neuropathologic papers allowing some insight into the distribution of injury in the newborn brain as a result of hypoglycemia. Anderson and colleagues[90] described six neonates who had been diagnosed with hypoglycemia and died within the first year of life of other, non-CNS–related causes. Blood glucose concentrations were less than 20 mg/dL in all cases. In four of the neonates, the duration of hypoglycemia was more than 36 hours. All infants were symptomatic. Histopathologically, these investigators observed widespread necrosis of neuronal and glial cells in the cerebral cortex, hippocampus, and basal ganglia. They commented on a greater degree of involvement in the occipital region than the frontal region. They also noted no predilection for the boundary zones between major blood vessels, which often distinguishes ischemic lesions. Larroche and associates[91] emphasized the white matter–damaging potential of hypoglycemia and demonstrated prominent periventricular leukomalacia in their series of newborns dying of hypoglycemia.

Neuroimaging Abnormalities

The recognition of specific patterns of abnormality on computed tomography (CT) and MRI of infants with diagnosed hypoglycemia has been a relatively recent finding in the literature. Spar and colleagues[92] described a newborn who had had well-documented hypoglycemia for at least 15 hours. MRI performed at 19 days of age demonstrated a predominance of bilateral tissue loss in the parenchyma of the occipital lobes. Barkovich and coworkers[93] described five patients who suffered from hypoglycemia in the newborn period and emphasized the findings of white matter damage in the parietal and occipital lobes. Globus pallidus injury was present in only one of the infants described. Kinnala and associates[94] published their findings in 18 full-term infants with blood glucose values less than 45 mg/dL (2.5 mmol/L). All were symptomatic. Only 3 of the infants reported had hypoglycemia for more than 24 hours, with the longest duration being 33 hours. The mean blood glucose value was 25 mg/dL (1.4 mmol/L), with only 2 of the infants displaying values below 5 mg/dL (0.3 mmol/L). Four of the infants showed hyperintensity lesions on T1-weighted images either in the occipital periventricular regions or in the thalamus. Ninety-four percent of the infants were developmentally normal at follow-up. Murakami and colleagues[95] confirmed these latter results in a retrospective review of brain MRI in 8 term infants, all of whom were symptomatic and had blood glucose concentrations below 20 mg/dL (1.1 mmol/L). Once again, abnormalities were consistently found in the parieto-occipital white matter in all but one of the children.

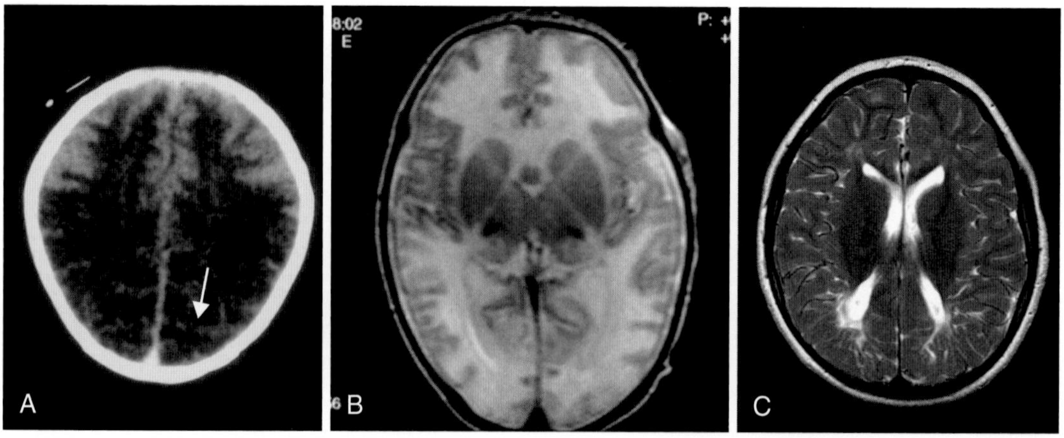

9

Figure 9-1 Series of images from term infant, normal Apgar scores, and hypoglycemia at 20 hours of age. **A,** Computed tomography scan on day 3 of life. Note the areas of attenuation bilaterally in the occipital regions. **B,** T2-weighted magnetic resonance (MR) image on day 10 of life. Loss of cortex in the occipital region and hyperintense putamen are noted. **C,** T2-weighted MR image scan at 7 years of age displaying chronic alterations with focal white matter and cortical injury in the occipital regions.

Within the last decade, a pattern of predominantly parieto-occipital white matter abnormalities, often in association with abnormal signal in the deep gray matter structures of the thalamus and/or basal ganglia, has been identified on follow-up of children who had experienced symptomatic hypoglycemia as neonates. Although the number of studies and patients is few overall, the abnormalities appear to be relatively distinct for the syndrome of neonatal hypoglycemia. Alkalay and coworkers[96] reported a single case of term hypoglycemia and reviewed the literature of associated imaging findings. Blood glucose values were always less than 25 mg/dL (1.4 mmol/L), they were generally low for a prolonged period, and patients were symptomatic. When neuroimaging was done in this group, findings were abnormal, with more than 80% showing consistent abnormalities of the occipital lobes, similar to those displayed in Figure 9-1.

A later study correlated brain MRI findings and neurodevelopmental outcome with symptomatic hypoglycemia. Burns and associates[97] examined 35 term infants who had symptomatic hypoglycemia (mean glucose concentration of <1.0 mmol/L [18 mg/dL]) without evidence of other complicating features such as hypoxia-ischemia. White matter injury was present in 94% of the patients, although in only 29% was a predominantly posterior localization noted. Cortical abnormalities were seen in 51%, of whom 40% had deep gray matter thalamic and basal ganglia lesions. Of the total, 65% displayed neurodevelopmental abnormalities at 18 months of age, correlating in large part to the severity of the white matter lesions.

In this study, the majority of blood glucose values recorded (86%) were less than 1.5 mmol/L (27 mg/dL). Interestingly, however, two thirds were reported as being only transient in nature, resolving readily with treatment, with the other third prolonged or recurrent.

These neuroimaging findings are metabolically consistent with studies by Mujsce and associates[72] that showed a reduction in CGU in the occipital white matter of newborn dogs during insulin-induced hypoglycemia. These findings occurred in spite of the preservation of glucose utilization in other regions of the brain and an increase in brainstem structures. These data suggest an uncoupling of supply and demand requirements for glucose in this region of the newborn brain and an outstripping of the available substrate supply for energy production, resulting in the enhanced sensitivity of the occipital regions.

Given the preceding findings, several aspects of hypoglycemia and its effect on the newborn brain can be summarized as follows:

1. The definition of hypoglycemia within statistical boundaries has been reasonably consistent as being abnormal if less than 2.5 mmol/L (45 mg/dL), and severely so if less than 1.1 mmol (20 mg/dL).
2. The definition of and risk for hypoglycemia are not static, but depend on the gestational age of the infant at birth, weight of the infant, and timing of the evaluation of glucose as it relates to the age of the infant from birth and whether or not feeding has been implemented.
3. A consistent association of hypoglycemia and neurologic injury has occurred only when the infant, in addition to evidence of low blood glucose concentrations, been symptomatic and generally continued to have hypoglycemia for a prolonged period.

Controversy and Question

These parameters provide important information regarding the approach to hypoglycemia in the otherwise healthy infant, but because glucose is a metabolically active substance in constant flux, confounding factors may influence whether or not hypoglycemia contributes to brain injury and at what level. Hence, disorders that the newborn faces alter the metabolic requirements of the brain, tipping the balance of supply and demand toward injury. Common problems in the newborn whereby the demand for glucose may outstrip its supply include hypoxia-ischemia and seizures, the latter being a complication of both hypoxia-ischemia and hypoglycemia itself. In these circumstances,[98] we ask the following question:

Does hypoglycemia contribute to the brain damage caused by hypoxia-ischemia or seizures in the newborn infant?

Hypoglycemia and Hypoxia-Ischemia, Seizures

Hypoglycemia is deleterious when superimposed on hypoxia-ischemia. Vannucci and Vannucci[99] subjected newborn rat pups to anoxia in 100% nitrogen. The experimental group was rendered hypoglycemic to a blood glucose value of 0.75 mmol/L (14 mg/dL) by intraperitoneal insulin injection. Normoglycemic animals survived 10 times as long as animals that were hypoglycemic. In newborn dogs made hypoglycemic in combination with asphyxia, brain ATP concentrations fell by 61%, but in puppies with hypoglycemia alone, ATP was preserved.

In determining the combined effects of substrate utilization and hypoxia-ischemia in the neonate,[9] Yager and colleagues[100] subjected 7-day-old rat pups to hypoglycemia by either fasting for 12 hours or subcutaneously injecting insulin. Both control and experimental rat pups underwent hypoxia-ischemia by exposure to 8% oxygen combined with unilateral common carotid artery ligation. Although hypoglycemia was only mild in nature—5.4, 4.3, and 3.4 mmol/L (97, 77, and 61 mg/dL) for control, insulin, and fasted groups respectively—brain damage was significantly greater in the insulin-treated animals than in either of the other two groups. Fasted animals had the least damage, presumably owing to the enhanced ketogenesis and alternative substrate utilization displayed by this group.

Seizures are associated with an increase in energy demands, and hence a several-fold increase in glucose utilization. The increased demand produces a decrease in brain glucose stores, placing the brain in a vulnerable position. Hence it is not surprising that during hypoglycemia, supplies of glucose are further depleted and a deficit in energy reserves might be expected. Thus in the newborn puppy, significant depletion of cerebral high-energy phosphate stores, as measured by nuclear magnetic resonance spectroscopy using ^{31}P, occurred when seizures and hypoglycemia were combined, in comparison with seizures alone.[101] In a model of neonatal hypoxia-ischemia and subsequent seizures, Wirrell and colleagues[102] showed that rat pups experiencing seizures and hypoxia-ischemia had significantly greater brain damage, particularly in the hippocampus, than animals who were only exposed to hypoxia-ischemia. In a follow-up study, these investigators found that the former group of rat pups displayed a prolonged and irrecoverable period of brain energy depletion, accompanied also by diminished brain glucose concentrations during the postischemic seizures. The investigators concluded that it was this relative

9

decrease in the concentration of brain glucose, compared with controls, during the postischemic seizures, that was responsible for the increase in brain damage seen in this model.[103] These data serve to highlight the importance of controlling seizures, particularly in the presence of hypoglycemia.

In the human newborn, several studies have reviewed the effects of compounding hypoglycemia and perinatal asphyxia. Salhab and associates[104] retrospectively reviewed 185 term infants with perinatal asphyxia defined by a cord pH of less than 7.00. Fifteen percent (27) of the infants had an initial blood glucose level less than 40 mg/dL (2.2 mmol/L). These researchers found a significant contribution of hypoglycemia to abnormal outcome, compared with infants with blood glucose values higher than 40 mg/dL. They did not comment in this study about the duration of hypoglycemia. Additional complicating features were also present.

Reviews on the subject of hypoglycemic brain injury in the newborn have consistently come to similar conclusions.[105] In one, 4021 patients admitted to a neonatal intensive care unit between 1990 and 2006 were reviewed.[106] Sixty newborns were identified as having met study criteria for hypoglycemia, in whom there was an equal distribution of males and females. The patients were divided into two groups, one of which had abnormal developmental outcome (developmental delay, cerebral palsy, or epilepsy), and the other had normal outcome. The two groups had equal incidences of SGA births. Those individuals who had abnormal outcomes were significantly more likely to have severe hypoglycemia, glucose level less than 15 mg/dL, for a prolonged duration (14 hours or more) than those with normal outcomes. In addition, however, those newborns in the abnormal outcome group were more likely to have other perinatal risk factors, such as hypoxia and neonatal seizures, which were believed to contribute to the hypoglycemic brain injury syndrome.

CASE HISTORY

Not infrequently, medicolegal questions arise surrounding the contribution of perinatal asphyxia to children who have developmental disability.[98] Among the confounding factors is often hypoglycemia; the following case history illustrates this situation.

A male infant was born at 42 weeks of gestation following a normal pregnancy. Delivery was forceps assisted. Birth weight was 3.27 kg. Thick meconium was present, and the infant was suctioned for significant amounts. Apgar scores were 2 and 4 at 1 and 5 minutes, respectively. Approximately 3.5 hours after birth, during which the infant still displayed evidence of a neonatal encephalopathy, clinical seizures developed. Blood glucose was determined to be 54 mg/dL (3.0 mmol/L). Seizures persisted intermittently that day. Blood glucose concentrations measured at 14 and 24 hours after delivery were 20 and 59 mg/dL (1.1 and 3.3 mmol/L), respectively. Electroencephalography revealed multifocal areas of electrographic seizures. Computed tomography demonstrated bilateral occipital infarcts. Now in his teens, this young man has bilateral cortical blindness and mild developmental delay.

Clearly this infant illustrates a number of complexities. First, there is some evidence of perinatal asphyxia (although a cord pH value was not available), with respect to modestly depressed Apgar scores. Although he has cortical blindness, there is minimal developmental delay, suggesting that the majority of injury was in fact, in the occipital cortical regions. The question is to what extent, if any, did hypoglycemia contribute to the injury?

Although he did not have severe hypoglycemia at birth, depressed glucose levels certainly persisted for at least 24 hours. They were concurrent with repetitive seizures, a circumstance of increased metabolic demand on a background of a diffuse brain insult. Clinically this child did express a neonatal encephalopathy with both altered neurologic status and seizures. The outcome suggests that the injury, however, was relatively restricted to the occipital cortices. Hence, in the current scenario, hypoglycemia on the background of perinatal asphyxia not only contributed to the brain damage incurred but also may have had the greatest effect, despite only one value that would have been categorized as indicating severe hypoglycemia.

The findings are consistent with the available data suggesting that the otherwise normal neonatal brain is relatively tolerant of hypoglycemia but that, when superimposed on a brain that has been compromised by hypoxia-ischemia and/or seizures, hypoglycemia may exact damage, even when the blood glucose values are only borderline for the diagnosis of hypoglycemia.[102]

Outcome

Given the complexities surrounding the definition and diagnosis of hypoglycemia in the newborn period, it is not surprising that there are difficulties in determining the neurologic morbidity surrounding this clinical entity. Several important papers on definition (discussed previously) and those looking at clinical prognosis allow us to make important observations regarding the thresholds to be assumed for the hypoglycemic neonate. Hence, Lucas and colleagues[67] detailed the neurologic outcome of a multicenter study of 661 preterm infants weighing less than 1850 g. Developmental outcome was determined at 18 months of age. The researchers excluded variables independent of glucose concentrations and found that reduced mental and motor developmental scores were inversely related to the number of days that glucose concentrations were less than 2.6 mmol/L (47 mg/dL), whereas with values above this level, no relationship was found. The relative risk of neurodevelopmental impairment in infants with hypoglycemia in comparison with those with no hypoglycemia was 3.5 times as great for those with blood glucose values less than 2.6 mmol/L for more than 5 days.

A study by Stenninger and associates[107] reviewed the long-term neurologic morbidity in 13 children with neonatal hypoglycemia defined as blood glucose concentrations less than 1.5 mmol/L (27 mg/dL), and compared them with 15 children who had not had neonatal hypoglycemia. Neurodevelopmental assessments were done at approximately 7.75 years of age. These investigators found that children with neonatal hypoglycemia had significantly more difficulties in a screening test for minimal brain dysfunction and were more likely to be hyperactive, impulsive, and inattentive. These children also had lower developmental scores than controls.

Brand and coworkers[108] evaluated 75 healthy term LGA babies of nondiabetic mothers. The value of glucose considered to be significant for hypoglycemia was less than 2.2 mmol/L (<40 mg/dL). Treatment with intravenous glucose was started if a baby was symptomatic. The researchers concluded that transient neonatal hypoglycemia was not harmful to psychomotor development when evaluated at 4 years of age.

A systematic review[109] of neurodevelopment following neonatal hypoglycemia in the first week of life evaluated 18 studies.[109] Sixteen of the studies were judged to be of poor quality and two of high quality, although they could not be pooled for data analysis. Unfortunately, the review concluded that "none of the studies provided a valid estimate of the effect of hypoglycemia on neurodevelopment,"[109] a further indication that this topic requires significantly more research into the overall outcome of infants experiencing hypoglycemia at birth in the various scenarios that may occur.[55]

Treatment

Despite the issues surrounding neonatal hypoglycemia, a review of the literature as has been outlined in this chapter clearly allows for the appropriate recognition of those infants at risk for significant hypoglycemia and the institution of a plan for monitoring and therapeutic intervention. Given the information available to us today, it appears that term infants born without complication and without symptomatology are highly unlikely to be at risk of neurodevelopmental abnormalities unless one of the following conditions applies:

1. Blood glucose concentrations are less than 1.1 mmol/L (<20 mg/dL).
2. The newborn is symptomatic.
3. Hypoglycemia is prolonged (hours).

In evaluating a newborn whose perinatal course has been complicated by SGA status, perinatal asphyxia, seizures, sepsis, or other disorders that suggest an imbalance between substrate supply and demand for cerebral energy production, a broader definition of hypoglycemia should be used. Hence, under these circumstances, infants displaying blood glucose concentrations below 40 mg/dL (<2.2 mmol/L), particularly on more than one occasion, should be aggressively treated and followed up. Newer techniques of continuous blood glucose monitoring of the newborn will provide a much greater and more accurate determination of glucose concentrations following birth and will allow for early identification of those at risk.[110]

Clearly there are infants who will require specific forms of therapy for underlying metabolic and endocrinologic abnormalities. In the vast majority of infants, glucose administration alone will be the predominant therapeutic intervention. Although in the past relatively large boluses of high concentration glucose have been advised, it is probably best to avoid hyperglycemia and its attendant risks of rebound hypoglycemia. Lilien and associates[111] have shown that a minibolus of 200 mg/kg (2 mL of 10% glucose over 1 minute) immediately followed by a continuous infusion of 8 mg/kg/min results in the rapid correction of blood glucose concentrations and stable values of between 70 and 80 mg/dL (3.8 and 4.4 mmol/L). Continuous monitoring is required, of course, and after glucose concentrations appear to have stabilized for 12 to 24 hours, the infusion can be decreased by 2 mg/kg/min every 6 to 12 hours. In rare circumstance in which hypoglycemia does not respond to this regimen or to infusions of up to 12 mg/kg/min, or it recurs with tapering of the dosage, hydrocortisone can be administered at a dose of 5 mg/kg every 12 hours.

Conclusions

Despite the fact that hypoglycemia remains a common disorder of the newborn, consensus has been difficult to reach regarding definition, diagnosis, outcome, and treatment. The following important points, however, can be made:

- The definition of hypoglycemia is not absolute and is highly dependent on the age, weight, timing of evaluation, whether the baby was fed, and extenuating and complicating factors. Hence, it should be assessed on a per-patient basis.
- Healthy term infants of appropriate weight who are fed early are not at risk for hypoglycemic injury.
- Significant hypoglycemia, with the potential to result in abnormal neurodevelopmental outcome, occurs in those newborns in whom (1) blood glucose levels are less than 1.1 mmol/L (<20 mg/dL), (2) hypoglycemia is prolonged, and (3) neurologic symptoms are present.
- A high level of sensitivity for hypoglycemia needs to be applied to all newborns who are compromised by SGA status, perinatal asphyxia, seizures, sepsis, or other pathologies that increase metabolic requirements. In these circumstances, a broader definition should be applied, and glucose concentrations of 40 mg/dL or higher should be maintained.

With improved neuroradiologic techniques such as MRI and positron emission tomography becoming increasingly available, studies to determine the correlation between hypoglycemia and outcome will further help to clarify issues surrounding the effects of hypoglycemia on brain pathology and neurobehavioral outcome.

Long-term epidemiologic studies correlating the severity and duration of hypoglycemia with neurologic consequences are required, and they can be complemented by appropriate parallel investigations in animal models of neonatal hypoglycemia.

Currently, increasing attention to the rising incidence of gestational diabetes will ultimately help provide the opportunity for prevention of neonatal hypoglycemia. Several guidelines are currently available for the close monitoring of maternal diabetes and the placement of appropriate protocols for blood glucose monitoring of the newborn after delivery.[112]

References

1. Aynsley-Green A, Hawdon JM. Hypoglycemia in the neonate: current controversies. *Acta Paediatr Jpn*. 1997;39:S12-S16.
2. Kalhan S, Peter-Wohl S. Hypoglycemia: what is it for the neonate? *Am J Perinatol*. 2000;17: 11-18.
3. Hawdon JM. Best practice guidelines: neonatal hypoglycaemia. *Early Hum Dev*. 2010;86:261.
4. Rozance PJ, Hay Jr WW. Describing hypoglycemia—definition or operational threshold? *Early Hum Dev*. 2010;86:275-280.
5. Hotu S, Carter B, Watson PD, et al. Increasing prevalence of type 2 diabetes in adolescents. *J Paediatr Child Health*. 2004;40:201-204.
6. Jensen DM, Damm P, Moelsted-Pedersen L, et al. Outcomes in type 1 diabetic pregnancies: a nationwide, population-based study. *Diabetes Care*. 2004;27:2819-2823.
7. Nehlig A. Respective roles of glucose and ketone bodies as substrates for cerebral energy metabolism in the suckling rat. *Dev Neurosci*. 1996;18:426-433.
8. Nehlig A, Pereira de Vasconcelos A. Glucose and ketone body utilization by the brain of neonatal rats. *Prog Neurobiol*. 1993;40:163-221.
9. Vannucci RC, Yager JY. Glucose, lactic acid, and perinatal hypoxic-ischemic brain damage. *Pediatr Neurol*. 1992;8:3-12.
10. Burchell A, Gibb L, Waddell ID, et al. The ontogeny of human hepatic microsomal glucose-6-phosphatase proteins. *Clin Chem*. 1990;36:1633-1637.
11. Bier DM, Leake RD, Haymond MW, et al. Measurement of "true" glucose production rates in infancy and childhood with 6,6-dideuteroglucose. *Diabetes*. 1977;26:1016-1023.
12. Hartmann A, Jaudon JC. Hypoglycemia. *J Pediatr*. 1937:1-36.
13. Aynsley-Green A. Metabolic and endocrine interrelations in the human fetus and neonate. *Am J Clin Nutr*. 1985;41:399-417.
14. Aynsley-Green A, Soltesz G, Jenkins PA, Mackenzie IZ. The metabolic and endocrine milieu of the human fetus at 18-21 weeks of gestation. II. Blood glucose, lactate, pyruvate and ketone body concentrations. *Biol Neonate*. 1985;47:19-25.
15. Soltesz G, Harris D, Mackenzie IZ, Aynsley-Green A. The metabolic and endocrine milieu of the human fetus and mother at 18-21 weeks of gestation. I. Plasma amino acid concentrations. *Pediatr Res*. 1985;19:91-93.
16. Bozzetti P, Ferrari MM, Marconi AM, et al. The relationship of maternal and fetal glucose concentrations in the human from midgestation until term. *Metabolism*. 1988;37:358-363.
17. Heck LJ, Erenberg A. Serum glucose levels in term neonates during the first 48 hours of life. *J Pediatr*. 1987;110:119-122.
18. Hoseth E, Joergensen A, Ebbesen F, Moeller M. Blood glucose levels in a population of healthy, breast fed, term infants of appropriate size for gestational age. *Arch Dis Child Fetal Neonatal Ed*. 2000;83:F117-F119.
19. Tanzer F, Yazar N, Yazar H, Icagasioglu D. Blood glucose levels and hypoglycaemia in full term neonates during the first 48 hours of life. *J Trop Pediatr*. 1997;43:58-60.
20. Srinivasan G, Pildes RS, Cattamanchi G, et al. Plasma glucose values in normal neonates: a new look. *J Pediatr*. 1986;109:114-117.
21. Diwakar KK, Sasidhar MV. Plasma glucose levels in term infants who are appropriate size for gestation and exclusively breast fed. *Arch Dis Child Fetal Neonatal Ed*. 2002;87:F46-F48.
22. Ward Platt M, Deshpande S. Metabolic adaptation at birth. *Semin Fetal Neonatal Med*. 2005;10: 341-350.
23. Sexson WR. Incidence of neonatal hypoglycemia: a matter of definition. *J Pediatr*. 1984;105:149-150.
24. Hawdon JM, Ward Platt MP, Aynsley-Green A. Patterns of metabolic adaptation for preterm and term infants in the first neonatal week. *Arch Dis Child*. 1992;67:357-365.
25. Jackson L, Burchell A, McGeechan A, Hume R. An inadequate glycaemic response to glucagon is linked to insulin resistance in preterm infants? *Arch Dis Child Fetal Neonatal Ed*. 2003;88: F62-F66.
26. Duvanel CB, Fawer CL, Cotting J, et al. Long-term effects of neonatal hypoglycemia on brain growth and psychomotor development in small-for-gestational-age preterm infants. *J Pediatr*. 1999;134: 492-498.
27. Lubchenco LO, Bard H. Incidence of hypoglycemia in newborn infants classified by birth weight and gestational age. *Pediatrics*. 1971;47:831-838.
28. Hawdon JM, Weddell A, Aynsley-Green A, Ward Platt MP. Hormonal and metabolic response to hypoglycaemia in small for gestational age infants. *Arch Dis Child*. 1993;68:269-273.
29. Bazaes RA, Salazar TE, Pittaluga E, et al. Glucose and lipid metabolism in small for gestational age infants at 48 hours of age. *Pediatrics*. 2003;111:804-809.
30. Duckrow RB, LaManna JS, Rosenthal M. Disparate recovery of resting and stimulated oxidative metabolism following transient ischemia. *Stroke*. 1981;12:677-686.

31. Chugani HT, Phelps ME, Mazziotta JC. Positron emission tomography study of human brain functional development. *Ann Neurol.* 1987;22:487-497.
32. Chugani HT, Phelps ME. Maturational changes in cerebral function in infants determined by 18FDG positron emission tomography. *Science.* 1986;231:840-843.
33. Chugani HT, Hovda DA, Villablanca JR, et al. Metabolic maturation of the brain: a study of local cerebral glucose utilization in the developing cat. *J Cereb Blood Flow Metab.* 1991;11:35-47.
34. Chance B, Leigh Jr JS, Nioka S, et al. An approach to the problem of metabolic heterogeneity in brain: ischemia and reflow after ischemia. *Ann N Y Acad Sci.* 1987;508:309-320.
35. Kinnala A, Nuutila P, Ruotsalainen U, et al. Cerebral metabolic rate for glucose after neonatal hypoglycaemia. *Early Hum Dev.* 1997;49:63-72.
36. Kinnala A, Suhonen-Polvi H, Aarimaa T, et al. Cerebral metabolic rate for glucose during the first six months of life: an FDG positron emission tomography study. *Arch Dis Child Fetal Neonatal Ed.* 1996;74:F153-F157.
37. Lust WD, Pundik S, Zechel J, et al. Changing metabolic and energy profiles in fetal, neonatal, and adult rat brain. *Metab Brain Dis.* 2003;18:195-206.
38. Cremer JE. Substrate utilization and brain development. *J Cereb Blood Flow Metab.* 1982;2: 394-407.
39. DeVivo DC, Leckie MP, Agrawal HC. The differential incorporation of beta-hydroxybutyrate and glucose into brain glutamate in the newborn rat. *Brain Res.* 1973;55:485-490.
40. Booth RF, Patel TB, Clark JB. The development of enzymes of energy metabolism in the brain of a precocial (guinea pig) and non-precocial (rat) species. *J Neurochem.* 1980;34:17-25.
41. Anday EK, Stanley CA, Baker L, Delivoria-Papadopoulos M. Plasma ketones in newborn infants: absence of suckling ketosis. *J Pediatr.* 1981;98:628-630.
42. Stanley CA, Anday EK, Baker L, Delivoria-Papadopolous M. Metabolic fuel and hormone responses to fasting in newborn infants. *Pediatrics.* 1979;64:613-619.
43. Hernandez MJ, Vannucci RC, Salcedo A, Brennan RW. Cerebral blood flow and metabolism during hypoglycemia in newborn dogs. *J Neurochem.* 1980;35:622-628.
44. Vannucci RC, Nardis EE, Vannucci SJ, Campbell PA. Cerebral carbohydrate and energy metabolism during hypoglycemia in newborn dogs. *Am J Physiol.* 1981;240:R192-R199.
45. Young RS, Petroff OA, Chen B, et al. Preferential utilization of lactate in neonatal dog brain: in vivo and in vitro proton NMR study. *Biol Neonate.* 1991;59:46-53.
46. Vicario C, Medina JM. Metabolism of lactate in the rat brain during the early neonatal period. *J Neurochem.* 1992;59:32-40.
47. Miller AL, Kiney CA, Staton DM. Effects of lactate on glucose metabolism of developing rat brain. *Brain Res.* 1984;316:33-40.
48. Maran A, Cranston I, Lomas J, et al. Protection by lactate of cerebral function during hypoglycaemia. *Lancet.* 1994;343:16-20.
49. Dombrowski Jr GJ, Swiatek KR, Chao KL. Lactate, 3-hydroxybutyrate, and glucose as substrates for the early postnatal rat brain. *Neurochem Res.* 1989;14:667-675.
50. Simpson IA, Carruthers A, Vannucci SJ. Supply and demand in cerebral energy metabolism: the role of nutrient transporters. *J Cerebr Blood Flow Metab.* 2007;27:1766-1791.
51. Powers WJ, Rosenbaum JL, Dence CS, et al. Cerebral glucose transport and metabolism in preterm human infants. *J Cereb Blood Flow Metab.* 1998;18:632-638.
52. Vannucci SJ, Maher F, Simpson IA. Glucose transporter proteins in brain: delivery of glucose to neurons and glia. *Glia.* 1997;21:2-21.
53. Vannucci SJ. Developmental expression of GLUT1 and GLUT3 glucose transporters in rat brain. *J Neurochem.* 1994;62:240-246.
54. Nicholl R. What is the normal range of blood glucose concentrations in healthy term newborns? *Arch Dis Child.* 2003;88:238-239.
55. Hay Jr WW, Raju TN, Higgins RD, et al. Knowledge gaps and research needs for understanding and treating neonatal hypoglycemia: workshop report from Eunice Kennedy Shriver National Institute of Child Health and Human Development. *J Pediatr.* 2009;155:612-617.
56. Koh TH, Eyre JA, Aynsley-Green A. Neonatal hypoglycaemia—the controversy regarding definition. *Arch Dis Child.* 1988;63:1386-1388.
57. Alkalay AL, Sarnat HB, Flores-Sarnat L, et al. Population meta-analysis of low plasma glucose thresholds in full-term normal newborns. *Am J Perinatol.* 2006;23:115-119.
58. Volpe JJ. *Neurology of the newborn,* 4th ed. Philadelphia: WB Saunders; 2001.
59. Koivisto M, Blanco-Sequeiros M, Krause U. Neonatal symptomatic and asymptomatic hypoglycaemia: a follow-up study of 151 children. *Dev Med Child Neurol.* 1972;14:603-614.
60. Singh M, Singhal PK, Paul VK, et al. Neurodevelopmental outcome of asymptomatic & symptomatic babies with neonatal hypoglycaemia. *Ind J Med Res.* 1991;94:6-10.
61. Moore AM, Perlman M. Symptomatic hypoglycemia in otherwise healthy, breastfed term newborns. *Pediatrics.* 1999;103:837-839.
62. Alkalay AL, Flores-Sarnat L, Sarnat HB, et al. Plasma glucose concentrations in profound neonatal hypoglycemia. *Clin Pediatr (Phila).* 2006;45:550-558.
63. Koh TH, Aynsley-Green A, Tarbit M, Eyre JA. Neural dysfunction during hypoglycaemia. *Arch Dis Child.* 1988;63:1353-1358.
64. Cowett RM, Howard GM, Johnson J, Vohr B. Brain stem auditory-evoked response in relation to neonatal glucose metabolism. *Biol Neonate.* 1997;71:31-36.
65. Pryds O, Greisen G, Friis-Hansen B. Compensatory increase of CBF in preterm infants during hypoglycaemia. *Acta Paediatr Scand.* 1988;77:632-637.

66. Caksen H, Guven AS, Yilmaz C, et al. Clinical outcome and magnetic resonance imaging findings in infants with hypoglycemia. *J Child Neurol*. 2011;26:25-30.
67. Lucas A, Morley R, Cole TJ. Adverse neurodevelopmental outcome of moderate neonatal hypoglycaemia. *BMJ*. 1988;297:1304-1308.
68. Schrier A, Wilhelm PB, Church RM, et al. Neonatal hypoglycemia in the rhesus monkey: Effect on development and behavior. *Infant Behav Dev*. 1990;13:189-207.
69. Moore H, Craft TK, Grimaldi LM, et al. Moderate recurrent hypoglycemia during early development leads to persistent changes in affective behavior in the rat. *Brain Behav Immun*. 2010;24:839-849.
70. Cornblath M, Hawdon JM, Williams AF, et al. Controversies regarding definition of neonatal hypoglycemia: suggested operational thresholds. *Pediatrics*. 2000;105:1141-1145.
71. Anwar M, Vannucci RC. Autoradiographic determination of regional cerebral blood flow during hypoglycemia in newborn dogs. *Pediatr Res*. 1988;24:41-45.
72. Mujsce DJ, Christensen MA, Vannucci RC. Regional cerebral blood flow and glucose utilization during hypoglycemia in newborn dogs. *Am J Physiol*. 1989;256:H1659-H1666.
73. Butcher SP, Sandberg M, Hagberg H, Hamberger A. Cellular origins of endogenous amino acids released into the extracellular fluid of the rat striatum during severe insulin-induced hypoglycemia. *J Neurochem*. 1987;48:722-728.
74. Sandberg M, Butcher SP, Hagberg H. Extracellular overflow of neuroactive amino acids during severe insulin-induced hypoglycemia: in vivo dialysis of the rat hippocampus. *J Neurochem*. 1986;47:178-184.
75. Uematsu D, Greenberg JH, Reivich M, Karp A. Cytosolic free calcium and NAD/NADH redox state in the cat cortex during in vivo activation of NMDA receptors. *Brain Res*. 1989;482:129-135.
76. Silverstein FS, Simpson J, Gordon KE. Hypoglycemia alters striatal amino acid efflux in perinatal rats: an in vivo microdialysis study. *Ann Neurol*. 1990;28:516-521.
77. Aral YZ, Gucuyener K, Atalay Y, et al. Role of excitatory amino acids in neonatal hypoglycemia. *Acta Paediatr Jpn*. 1998;40:303-306.
78. Alves PM, Fonseca LL, Peixoto CC, et al. NMR studies on energy metabolism of immobilized primary neurons and astrocytes during hypoxia, ischemia and hypoglycemia. *NMR Biomed*. 2000;13:438-448.
79. Hertz L, Yager JY, Juurlink BH. Astrocyte survival in the absence of exogenous substrate: comparison of immature and mature cells. *Int J Dev Neurosci*. 1995;13:523-527.
80. Brierly JB, Brown AW, Meldrum BS. The neuropathology of insulin induced hypoglycemia in primate. In: Brierly JB, Meldrum BS, eds. Philadelphia: JB Lippincott; 1971.
81. Myers RE, Kahn KJ. Insulin induced hypoglycemia in the non-human primate. II: Long term neuropathological consequences. In: Brierly JB, Meldrum BS, ed. Philadelphia: JB Lippincott; 1971.
82. Auer R, Kalimo H, Olsson Y, Wieloch T. The dentate gyrus in hypoglycemia: pathology implicating excitotoxin-mediated neuronal necrosis. *Acta Neuropathol (Berl)*. 1985;67:279-288.
83. Auer RN, Kalimo H, Olsson Y, Siesjo BK. The temporal evolution of hypoglycemic brain damage. I. Light- and electron-microscopic findings in the rat cerebral cortex. *Acta Neuropathol (Berl)*. 1985;67:13-24.
84. Auer RN, Kalimo H, Olsson Y, Siesjo BK. The temporal evolution of hypoglycemic brain damage. II. Light- and electron-microscopic findings in the hippocampal gyrus and subiculum of the rat. *Acta Neuropathol (Berl)*. 1985;67:25-36.
85. Auer RN, Siesjo BK. Biological differences between ischemia, hypoglycemia, and epilepsy. *Ann Neurol*. 1988;24:699-707.
86. Auer RN, Siesjo BK. Hypoglycaemia: brain neurochemistry and neuropathology. *Baillieres Clin Endocrinol Metab*. 1993;7:611-625.
87. Auer RN, Wieloch T, Olsson Y, Siesjo BK. The distribution of hypoglycemic brain damage. *Acta Neuropathol (Berl)*. 1984;64:177-191.
88. Auer RN, Olsson Y, Siesjo BK. Hypoglycemic brain injury in the rat. Correlation of density of brain damage with the EEG isoelectric time: a quantitative study. *Diabetes*. 1984;33:1090-1098.
89. Kalimo H, Auer RN, Siesjo BK. The temporal evolution of hypoglycemic brain damage. III. Light and electron microscopic findings in the rat caudoputamen. *Acta Neuropathol (Berl)*. 1985;67:37-50.
90. Anderson JM, Milner RD, Strich SJ. Effects of neonatal hypoglycaemia on the nervous system: a pathological study. *J Neurol Neurosurg Psychiatry*. 1967;30:295-310.
91. Larroche JC. Developmental pathology of the neonate. In: Larroche JC, ed. New York: Excerpta Medica; 1977.
92. Spar JA, Lewine JD, Orrison Jr WW. Neonatal hypoglycemia: CT and MR findings. *AJNR Am J Neuroradiol*. 1994;15:1477-1478.
93. Barkovich AJ, Ali FA, Rowley HA, Bass N. Imaging patterns of neonatal hypoglycemia. *AJNR Am J Neuroradiol*. 1998;19:523-528.
94. Kinnala A, Rikalainen H, Lapinleimu H, et al. Cerebral magnetic resonance imaging and ultrasonography findings after neonatal hypoglycemia. *Pediatrics*. 1999;103:724-729.
95. Murakami Y, Yamashita Y, Matsuishi T, et al. Cranial MRI of neurologically impaired children suffering from neonatal hypoglycaemia. *Pediatr Radiol*. 1999;29:23-27.
96. Alkalay AL, Flores-Sarnat L, Sarnat HB, et al. Brain imaging findings in neonatal hypoglycemia: case report and review of 23 cases. *Clin Pediatr (Phila)*. 2005;44:783-790.
97. Burns CM, Rutherford MA, Boardman JP, Cowan FM. Patterns of cerebral injury and neurodevelopmental outcomes after symptomatic neonatal hypoglycemia. *Pediatrics*. 2008;122:65-74.
98. Williams AF. Neonatal hypoglycaemia: clinical and legal aspects. *Semin Fetal Neonatal Med*. 2005;10:363-368.

9

99. Vannucci RC, Vannucci SJ. Cerebral carbohydrate metabolism during hypoglycemia and anoxia in newborn rats. *Ann Neurol.* 1978;4:73-79.
100. Yager JY, Heitjan DF, Towfighi J, Vannucci RC. Effect of insulin-induced and fasting hypoglycemia on perinatal hypoxic-ischemic brain damage. *Pediatr Res.* 1992;31:138-142.
101. Young RS, Cowan BE, Petroff OA, et al. In vivo 31P and in vitro 1H nuclear magnetic resonance study of hypoglycemia during neonatal seizure. *Ann Neurol.* 1987;22:622-628.
102. Wirrell EC, Armstrong EA, Osman LD, Yager JY. Prolonged seizures exacerbate perinatal hypoxic-ischemic brain damage. *Pediatr Res.* 2001;50:445-454.
103. Yager JY, Armstrong EA, Miyashita H, Wirrell EC. Prolonged neonatal seizures exacerbate hypoxic-ischemic brain damage: correlation with cerebral energy metabolism and excitatory amino acid release. *Dev Neurosci.* 2002;24:367-381.
104. Salhab WA, Wyckoff MH, Laptook AR, Perlman JM. Initial hypoglycemia and neonatal brain injury in term infants with severe fetal acidemia. *Pediatrics.* 2004;114:361-366.
105. Rozance PJ, Hay WW. Hypoglycemia in newborn infants: features associated with adverse outcomes. *Biol Neonate.* 2006;90:74-86.
106. Montassir H, Maegaki Y, Ogura K, et al. Associated factors in neonatal hypoglycemic brain injury. *Brain Dev.* 2009;31:649-656.
107. Stenninger E, Flink R, Eriksson B, Sahlen C. Long-term neurological dysfunction and neonatal hypoglycaemia after diabetic pregnancy. *Arch Dis Child Fetal Neonatal Ed.* 1998;79:F174-F179.
108. Brand PL, Molenaar NL, Kaaijk C, Wierenga WS. Neurodevelopmental outcome of hypoglycaemia in healthy, large for gestational age, term newborns. *Arch Dis Child.* 2005;90:78-81.
109. Boluyt N, van Kempen A, Offringa M. Neurodevelopment after neonatal hypoglycemia: a systematic review and design of an optimal future study. *Pediatrics.* 2006;117:2231-2243.
110. Beardsall K. Measurement of glucose levels in the newborn. *Early Hum Dev.* 2010;86:263-267.
111. Lilien LD, Pildes RS, Srinivasan G, et al. Treatment of neonatal hypoglycemia with minibolus and intravenous glucose infusion. *J Pediatr.* 1980;97:295-298.
112. Williams A, Modder J. Management of pregnancy complicated by diabetes—maternal glycaemic control during pregnancy and neonatal management. *Early Hum Dev.* 2010;86:269-273.

CHAPTER 10

Hyperbilirubinemia and the Risk for Brain Injury

Steven M. Shapiro, MD, MSHA

10

CASE HISTORY

BB is a white male, born at term gestation weighing 2980 g in August 2005 to a 25-year-old G1P0 mother, blood type B$^+$, via spontaneous vaginal delivery. Apgar scores were 8 and 9 at 1 and 5 minutes, respectively. He was blood type A$^+$, had a large cephalohematoma, and appeared jaundiced at 24 hours of life. He passed an automated auditory brainstem response (ABR) screening and was discharged at 58 hours with a transcutaneous bilirubin level of 13.2 mg/dL and a serum bilirubin level of 14 mg/dL. One day later at follow-up, the pediatrician said he looked fine. He returned at 6 days of age with a history of lethargy but had regained his birth weight. The pediatrician estimated that the bilirubin level was about 5 mg/dL. On day 7 BB was more lethargic and feeding was more difficult. On day 8 he was noted to have a high-pitched cry, downward deviation of the eyes, and episodic and then continual extension of arms, legs, neck, and trunk. He was evaluated in an emergency room, where a spinal tap and analysis was normal except for yellow cerebrospinal fluid. Total bilirubin level at 211 hours (8.8 days) of age was 45.6 mg/dL. He was placed under phototherapy lights with blanket underneath, was intubated because of low O$_2$ saturation, and received a double-volume exchange transfusion at 214 hours of age. Pre- and post-exchange total bilirubin values were 35.8 and 20.9 mg/dL, respectively. BB was intubated and sedated. Five days later, emerging from sedation, he was hypotonic with setting sun sign, and with episodic O$_2$ desaturation. He was treated with phenobarbital for seizures. Electroencephalography (EEG) findings were normal except for some sharp waves over the left temporal region. The episodes improved with treatment for reflux. He was discharged after a 10-day hospitalization. He has subsequently demonstrated feeding issues, incoordination of suck and swallow, hypertonia and dystonia, and delayed motor development. ABRs at 2.5 weeks and 2 months of age were absent, a finding consistent with auditory neuropathy/dyssynchrony, despite normal distortion product otoacoustic emissions (OAEs). Magnetic resonance imaging (MRI) done at 11 days of age showed increased signal intensity in the globus pallidus bilaterally on both T1- and T2-weighted images and a resolving cephalohematoma. Because of reflux and failure to thrive, a gastrostomy tube was placed with Nissen fundoplication. Treatment with diazepam was instituted to treat increased tone. Phenobarbital dosage was tapered and then discontinued. Clonic activity has been noted several times, but video EEG has repeatedly demonstrated that these episodes are not seizures. At 1.5 years of age, BB has not developed speech or language, has not responded to sound amplification, and cannot sit or crawl. A cochlear implant is planned.

This case highlights the risk of visual assessment of jaundice. The serum bilirubin level at discharge, 14 mg/dL, is at the 95th percentile of the hour-specific nomogram developed by Bhutani and colleagues.[1] The bilirubin at the 95th percentile, the significant cephalohematoma, and an A/B blood group abnormality were predictive of a high subsequent bilirubin level. The child had symptoms of acute bilirubin encephalopathy (ABE) that were not recognized until it was too late to prevent the extreme hyperbilirubinemia, and now the child has all the clinical signs, symptoms, and laboratory findings of kernicterus.

The classic form of brain injury due to hyperbilirubinemia is called *kernicterus*. Kernicterus was originally a pathologic term referring to the yellow staining (*icterus*) of the deep nuclei of the brain (*kern*, relating to the basal ganglia). The terms *acute bilirubin encephalopathy* and *chronic bilirubin encephalopathy* are used to describe the clinical symptoms associated with the neuropathology. In modern times, the use of the term kernicterus has expanded to include clinical bilirubin encephalopathy, and modern testing, such MRI and brainstem auditory evoked potentials (BAEPs)—also known as brainstem auditory evoked responses (BAERs) and auditory brainstem responses (ABRs)—has shown objective evidence of both neuropathologic lesions (MRI) and abnormal neurologic function (BAEPs).

Classic kernicterus is a well-described clinical syndrome that involves (1) a dystonic or athetoid movement disorder, (2) an auditory processing disturbance with or without hearing loss, (3) ocular motor impairment, especially impairment of upward gaze, (4) dysplasia of the enamel of deciduous (baby) teeth, and, perhaps less well known, (5) hypotonia and ataxia due to cerebellar involvement. More subtle forms of brain injury due to excess of hyperbilirubinemia have also been described in different terms—for example, subtle kernicterus, chronic bilirubin encephalopathy of the subtle type, and bilirubin-induced neurologic disorders (BINDs). These describe more subtle neurodevelopmental disorders in children with less than all of the clinical features of classic kernicterus, or with mild or subtle manifestations of the classic abnormalities. Finally, the newest term *kernicterus spectrum disorder* (KSD) encompasses a range of sequelae of bilirubin neurotoxicity from classic kernicterus to subtle BIND.

Classic kernicterus is a rare disorder. Its incidence in Denmark has been estimated to be 1 per 110,000 live births, whereas the incidence of extreme hyperbilirubinemia, defined as at or above criteria for performing exchange transfusion (median 28.8 mg/dL, range 22.5-40.3 mg/dL), was 25 per 100,000.[2,3] A population-based survey in northern California found that 150 per 100,000 had total serum bilirubin (TSB) levels of 25 mg/dL or higher, and 10 per 100,000 of 30 mg/dL or higher.[4,5] A review by Bhutani and Johnson[6] estimated that risk of kernicterus in infants with TSB levels above 25 mg/DL to be about 1 in 17.6 in Canada and 1 in 16.2 in Denmark, with the risk rising to about 1 in 7 for TSB levels exceeding 30 mg/dL.

The incidence of extreme hyperbilirubinemia and kernicterus depends on the care infants receive in the first few weeks of life, the vigilance of screening, and the ability to treat excessive hyperbilirubinemia should it occur. Incidence and prevalence studies are complicated by the lack of specific objective definitions of kernicterus or BIND and the inconsistency of reporting kernicterus or excessive hyperbilirubinemia in most countries.

Further, the incidence and prevalence of subtler neurodevelopmental disorders, such as auditory processing disorders and visual motor disabilities due to hyperbilirubinemia, are a subject of speculation without adequate data or documentation.

Precisely how to determine the risk of brain injury in a hyperbilirubinemic newborn is important not only for choosing the level of care but also for optimally allocating health care resources. The precise determination of risk of brain injury will allow not only better guidelines for treatment to prevent brain damage but also the reduction or elimination of unnecessary treatments. This chapter discusses new concepts of pathogenesis, approaches or strategies for diagnosis and treatment, gaps in knowledge, and recommendations for treatment.

10

Pathogenesis

Bilirubin neurotoxicity is highly selective, targeting specific neurons in the central nervous system (CNS). The clinical expression and neuropathology of kernicterus are likewise highly selective. The movement disorders dystonia and athetosis correspond to lesions in the basal ganglia (globus pallidus and subthalamic nucleus), cerebellum, and brainstem nuclei having to do with auditory, vestibular, and oculomotor function and truncal tone. Any explanation of pathogenesis must account for the selective neurotoxicity of bilirubin.

It may be useful to compartmentalize the concept of bilirubin neurotoxicity into (1) what causes the cell to be exposed to excess bilirubin, (2) what causes the cell to be able to handle or not handle this excess bilirubin, and (3) the molecular mechanisms of cell damage and cell protection. Bilirubin exposure is a combination of bilirubin production, binding, and excretion. Bilirubin is excreted out of the cell, the CNS, and the circulation. The ability of cells to handle excess bilirubin may vary. Risk factors may be compartmentalized, too, and, of course, may affect one or more compartments. For example, acidosis decreases binding and increases unbound free bilirubin (Bf), thus exposing the cell to more bilirubin. However, pH might also affect cell enzymes, energy production, and transport. Other risk factors, such as prematurity, inflammation, and isoimmunization, may act in one or more specific compartments. It is important that clinicians start thinking about what is going on at the cellular level in the CNS of a child with bilirubin toxicity.

It appears that bilirubin damages cells by both apoptotic and necrotic mechanisms and affects mitochondrial energy metabolism. Studies in cultured cells by the Brites group[7-10] has begun to define the role of apoptosis, mitochondria, and other molecular mechanisms of bilirubin neurotoxicity. Purified bilirubin can induce apoptosis in cultured rat brain neurons[8,9] by triggering the release of cytochrome c from mitochondria with caspase-3 activation and cleavage of poly(ADP-ribose) polymerase, confirming the role of one of the pathways that underlies induction of apoptosis.[11] Studies have shown that bilirubin facilitates transmitter release in cochlear nucleus neurons via presynaptic protein kinase A activation, which might provide insight into the cellular mechanism underlying bilirubin-induced hearing dysfunction.[12] Apoptotic changes are found in the cerebellum[11,13] and brainstem of jaundiced Gunn rats[13] and in the basal ganglia of kernicteric human infants, accounting for prominent signs of bilirubin neurotoxicity in each. Furthermore, Falcao and colleagues[14] have also raised the possibility that neuroinflammation may be a significant contributor to bilirubin neurotoxicity. Comprehensive reviews have been published about the molecular mechanism of bilirubin neurotoxicity.[10,15,16]

The blood-brain barrier (BBB) excludes large molecules including albumin and albumin-bound bilirubin from most of the CNS and transports substances into and out of the CNS.[10] The endothelial cells of the blood-brain barrier restrict diffusion of many toxic compounds to adjacent neurons and astrocytes but do not restrict the free diffusion of unconjugated bilirubin, which is permeable with single-pass uptake estimated to be as high as 28% in rats.[17] Bilirubin rapidly diffuses through lipid membranes[18] and through phosphatidylcholine vesicle membranes as the uncharged diacid.[19] The concentration gradient for TSB from plasma to cerebrospinal fluid in humans[20,21] and jaundiced Gunn rats[22,23] is thus probably due to the lower concentrations of binding proteins in the cerebrospinal fluid.

Specific transporters for bilirubin, such as multidrug resistance protein 1 (MRP1),[10] member of the multidrug resistance–associated protein subfamily of adenosine triphosphate (ATP)–binding cassette transporters, may protect the CNS from exposure to excessive levels of bilirubin. The Tiribelli group has provided evidence that bilirubin is removed from cells via MRP1.[10,15,24,25] MRP1 transports bilirubin with an affinity that is 10 times greater than that of other substrates[25] and may represent a mechanism by which bilirubin is transported out of the CNS and excreted into the circulation. These researchers hypothesize that when this transport system is overwhelmed, toxic bilirubin can accumulate in the cell.

Braun and Schulman[26] have proposed that bilirubin interferes with intracellular calcium homeostasis and have demonstrated decreased activity of calcium and calmodulin-dependent protein kinase II (CaMKII) in the Gunn rat model of kernicterus. Bilirubin inhibits CaMKII in vitro,[27] and its developmental expression is impaired in jaundiced (jj) Gunn rats.[28] Further, there is selective decrease in expression of calcium-binding proteins (CBPs) in specific brainstem areas susceptible to bilirubin neurotoxicity in the CNS of kernicteric Gunn rats.[29,30] CaMKII regulates neurotransmitter release, calcium-regulated ion conductance, and neuroskeletal dynamics[31] and can trigger programmed cell death (apoptosis).

It has also been proposed that bilirubin and increased calcium cause damage through an excitotoxic, N-methyl-D-aspartame (NMDA)–dependent mechanism,[32-34] although there is also evidence against this hypothesis.[35] My colleagues and I[36] have found that MK-801, an NMDA channel blocker, does not protect against bilirubin neurotoxicity in vitro in hippocampal neurons, nor does it protect against auditory dysfunction in vivo in the Gunn rat model of ABE.

Another study used the Gunn rat to investigate bilirubin-induced auditory deficits.[37] In vivo ABRs revealed severe auditory deficits within 18 hours of exposure to high bilirubin levels. Extracellular multielectrode array recordings following hyperbilirubinemia in an in vitro preparation of the auditory brainstem demonstrated transmission failure indicative of damage at a presynaptic site in the medial nucleus of the trapezoid body, and multi-photon imaging demonstrated that giant synapses in this nucleus were destroyed. These neurons express high levels of nitric oxide synthase (NOS); nitric oxide has been implicated in mechanisms of bilirubin toxicity elsewhere in the brain,[38] and antagonism of neuronal NOS by 7-nitroindazole was found to protect hearing during bilirubin exposure.[37]

Neurons are susceptible to apoptotic death from oxidative stress. Work from the Snyder laboratory has begun to define the role of bilirubin and its precursor, biliverdin, in normal cells.[39-43] Bilirubin and heme oxygenase 2, the enzyme that catalyzes its formation, have neuroprotective antioxidant properties. Depleting cultured HeLA cells and cortical neurons of biliverdin reductase by RNA interference leads to increased oxidative activity and renders cells more susceptible to caspase-dependent death from hyperoxia and hydrogen peroxide toxicity.[41] The antioxidant activity is comparable to that of glutathione, long assumed to be the principal cellular antioxidant.[41] Hippocampal cultures from heme oxygenase 2 (but not 1) knockout mice are more susceptible to hydrogen peroxide toxicity,[39] and heme oxygenase 2 knockout mice are more susceptible to focal cerebral ischemia and excitotoxic injury.[44] Bilirubin, despite its extremely low concentration in the cell, is recycled to greatly increase its effect.[41] Bararano and colleagues[41] have proposed that the potent physiologic antioxidant action of bilirubin is amplified when the detoxification of reactive oxygen species oxidizes bilirubin back to biliverdin, which is then reduced again by biliverdin reductase to form bilirubin. As this redox-amplification cycle is repeated, the antioxidant effect of bilirubin is multiplied. Although this redox-amplification cycle has been proposed to constitute the principal physiologic function of bilirubin, it should be noted that a protective action of modest levels of bilirubin does not alter the well-established dangers of kernicterus associated with major elevations of serum bilirubin.[43]

Windows of developmental susceptibility of the CNS to bilirubin toxicity may exist. Cerebellar neurons undergoing early differentiation at the time of bilirubin exposure are highly susceptible to bilirubin neurotoxicity, whereas slightly more or slightly less mature neurons may show only transient changes.[45] Bilirubin-induced cell death, glutamate release, cytokine production, and activation of transcription factors involved in inflammation are enhanced in undifferentiated astrocytes and neurons in comparison with more mature cells.[14,46] Falcao and associates[47] have shown that both messenger RNA and protein levels of MRP1 increase with cell differentiation, and suggest that the development expression of MRP1 may explain the susceptibility of premature babies to bilirubin neurotoxicity.

It is likely that prolonged exposure of neurons to bilirubin causes cell death and that the developmental stage of the neuron determines whether the cell can handle the bilirubin load. The hyperbilirubinemia must be sufficient to permit Bf to enter the neuron and exceed the neuron's capacity to handle it. Neuronal exposure to extremely high bilirubin levels for relatively short amounts of time probably affects the cell differently from exposure to relatively lower but still excessive levels for a longer time. The developmental stage of the neuron, for unknown reasons, probably determines in part whether or not the cell can handle the bilirubin load.

Bilirubin is on the one hand a powerful antioxidant that has protective properties and modulates cell growth; however, in excess, has deleterious properties that cause cell death and apoptosis in part due to oxidative stress. Cells exposed to bilirubin increase expression of a multifunctional neuroprotective protein DJ-1, an adaptive response that maintains cellular oxidative stress homeostasis.[48]

Dogan and coworkers[49] have demonstrated a relationship between serum total bilirubin and antioxidants and oxidative stress by studying oxidant and antioxidant status in 36 neonates with hyperbilirubinemia requiring phototherapy limits per the 2004 American Academy of Pediatrics (AAP) guidelines, 33 with kernicterus (ABE on examination and absence of ABRs), and 25 age-matched healthy controls. Plasma total antioxidant capacity and serum total oxidant status were significantly higher in the hyperbilirubinemia and kernicterus groups than in controls, and total free sulfhydryl values were significantly elevated in the hyperbilirubinemia group. The investigators found a relationship between serum total bilirubin, antioxidants, and oxidative stress that could be expressed by a quadratic correlation curve. They suggested that that after a certain point, kernicterus occurs with a direct toxic effect on the cell. Certainly, more studies on the role of oxidant and antioxidant status in hyperbilirubinemic and kernicteric infants will be of great interest.

Approaches: Strategies for Diagnosis and Treatment

Strategies for diagnosis and treatment of hyperbilirubinemia are well known. The AAP guidelines for the treatment of hyperbilirubinemia[50] are a significant improvement over previous guidelines. Following these guidelines has undoubtedly prevented many cases of kernicterus, although a study using data derived from diagnosis coding showing no change in reported cases of kernicterus cast some doubt on the effect of guidelines on the incidence of kernicterus.[51] How many cases of kernicterus actually occur and the types and number of cases of subtle bilirubin encephalopathy or bilirubin-induced neurologic disorders (BINDs) that occur is unknown. The amount of excessive treatment and its associated cost to the health care system is also unknown. In part, objective methods of determining kernicterus and BINDs are needed in any study that purports to determine the incidence of kernicterus; accepting diagnosis codes as the dependent measure in incidence studies fails to account for a bias of cases not being recognized or reported.

However, some concerns with current guidelines should be mentioned. First is the failure to highly recommend a predischarge bilirubin measurement as an indispensable part of risk assessment (rather than saying that this is one of two recommended options, the other being risk factor summation). Second is the lack of clear guideline for bilirubin/jaundice assessment at the first and subsequent follow-up visits. As shown by the pilot kernicterus registry[52] and my personal experience, infants who have severe hyperbilirubinemia and kernicterus are often those whose jaundice at a follow-up visit is not considered severe or extensive enough to warrant a serum bilirubin measurement. This failure can be the result of forgetting that before an infant becomes pumpkin orange, full-body jaundice usually is associated with a clearly deeper yellow in the face and belly than in the legs and feet (Johnson, personal communication, 2007). The observer may therefore assume that full-body jaundice is not yet present and that the bilirubin level is below rather than at or above 15 mg/dL. Third, a child with a bilirubin level of 11 to 12 mg/dL (jaundice below the umbilicus but not yet to the thighs) also needs to be followed closely and the measurement confirmed by a TSB measurement or transcutaneous bilirubin evaluation. Such follow-up represents a problem, of course, because not all doctors' offices have transcutaneous bilirubin meters. Finally, the guidelines fail to take into account new methods of measuring unbound (free) bilirubin and binding, which in the future are likely to lead to better, more effective preventive treatment strategies.[53,55,56] Basing screening and treatment decisions on TSB value alone is not likely to improve the sensitivity and specificity of detecting and preventing kernicterus. Using new strategies to assess individual binding—perhaps a two-step method using TSB and clinical criteria to determine risk category, and then using Bf to determine binding and more precisely TSB action levels for a particular infant—might improve sensitivity and specificity.

Acute Bilirubin Encephalopathy (Acute Kernicterus)

In newborns with ABE, symptoms progress from lethargy and decreased feeding to variable or fluctuating tone (hypotonia and hypertonia), high-pitched cry, retrocollis and opisthotonus, impairment of upward gaze (setting sun sign), fever, seizures, and death. BAEPs are absent or abnormal,[57-59] and these findings are reversible with double-volume exchange transfusion.[60,61] MRI reveals abnormal signal bilaterally in specific subdivisions of the basal ganglia, globus pallidus, and subthalamic nucleus.[62-66] Abnormalities are found within days after the peak total serum bilirubin level[67] and are initially hyperintense on T1-weighted images, and later become normal or hypointense on T1- and hyperintense on T2-weighted images.[67,68] The subthalamic nucleus is smaller and so is not easily seen on some MR images, so abnormalities of this structure may be subtle and easily overlooked.[67] In some patients, abnormalities may normalize.

The diagnosis of acute encephalopathy can usually be made in term or near-term newborns through clinical examination (mental status, tone, posture, cry, setting sun sign, and late signs of opisthotonus, seizures, and fever) and laboratory values (measurements of TSB, unconjugated and conjugated bilirubin, pH, and albumin). Some clinicians believe that hyperbilirubinemia from Rh disease (or hemolysis) is more likely to be damaging than that from other causes (perhaps because of a more rapid rate of rise or rapid rate of bilirubin production). Current illnesses such as sepsis may increase risk. New diagnostic methodology is currently based on BAEP and MRI, both of which give specific diagnostic information in newborns and can usually distinguish encephalopathy due to bilirubin from encephalopathy due to other causes.

Because the auditory system is sensitive to bilirubin neurotoxicity, the BAEP test is a sensitive, objective measure of early CNS dysfunction due to bilirubin. Early changes, such as increased latency and decreased amplitude of waves III and V, herald the onset of bilirubin neurotoxicity, probably at a reversible stage. Wave III arises from the cochlear nuclei in the pons, and wave V arises from the lateral lemniscus in the midbrain, a pathway terminating in the inferior colliculus. The use of interwave intervals, such as I-III, III-V, and I-V, reflects conduction time. The earliest BAEP indicators of bilirubin neurotoxicity are I-III and the somewhat more reliably measured I-V. As bilirubin neurotoxicity progresses, BAEP abnormalities progress to absence of waves III and V and, finally, to complete absence of all waves, including I. Clinically, BAEP wave amplitudes are usually too variable to serve as criteria for BAEP normality, although they are useful when serial studies can be compared with a baseline, and the use of amplitude ratios III:I and V:I helps decrease variability.

The automated ABR (AABR) device has been used to assess auditory function in hyperbilirubinemic newborns in the neonatal intensive care unit (NICU). The AABR matches the BAEP (also known as ABR) response to a predesigned template and is reported as either present (pass) or absent (refer). Absence of AABRs in the presence of hyperbilirubinemia, especially in a neonate who has become hyperbilirubinemic and whose AABR result has changed from pass to refer, is evidence of abnormal auditory function and may reflect significant bilirubin neurotoxicity. Unfortunately, the AABR as opposed to the BAEP does not distinguish CNS from middle or inner ear dysfunction (neither due to bilirubin), and current devices are not able to detect the early changes of bilirubin neurotoxicity. However, the ease of use and availability of AABR at all times in the NICU make it a clinically useful device to consider as part of an evaluation of when to treat sick neonates.

A prospective observational study in late preterm and term neonates with severe jaundice concluded that auditory neuropathy spectrum disorder (ANSD) is a common manifestation of acute bilirubin neurotoxicity.[69] In infants with hyperbilirubinemia at a level at which AAP guidelines would suggest exchange transfusion, a comprehensive auditory evaluation was performed before discharge. Six of 13 neonates (46%) had audiologic findings of acute ANSD. There were no detectable differences in clinical variables, including hemolysis, peak total bilirubin and peak bilirubin-to-albumin molar ratio, between the 6 neonates who had ANSD and the 7 who had normal audiologic findings, and only 2 of the 6 with ANSD had clinical signs and symptoms of ABE. Thus, ANSD is a common manifestation of acute bilirubin neurotoxicity in late preterm and term infants and may occur without clinical signs and symptoms of ABE.

Difficulties in obtaining MRI in sick neonates in most centers preclude its use for making clinical decisions such as when to intervene—in other words, when to perform an exchange transfusion. However, MRI is useful to establish kernicterus, and in many cases findings are abnormal almost immediately after the fact. If rescue treatments are shown to be neuroprotective after severe hyperbilirubinemia, then MRI and ABR testing may be critically important to identify patients and determine response to treatment.

Findings of other neuroimaging techniques, such as head computed tomography and ultrasound scans, are generally normal in kernicterus, though hyperechogenicity is occasionally seen and was reported in one of eight preterm and term infants with abnormal MRI findings in one study.[67] Cerebrospinal fluid measurements of bilirubin and binding, as well as other substances, such as indicators of neuroinflammation, may become useful in the future. Magnetic resonance spectroscopy has currently unrealized potential to reveal abnormalities of brain energy metabolism.

New strategies for the diagnosis of ABE have been proposed. The first is a BIND score, similar to an Apgar score, to be used in infants with significant hyperbilirubinemia. This score, proposed by an ad hoc BIND study group,[70] rates neurologic symptoms such as muscle tone, posture, cry, and mental status on the basis of Volpe's description of ABE,[71] on a scale of 0 to 9 in infants with high TSB values (Table 10-1) and can be used much like an Apgar score. It has not yet been validated in any study. Although it seems simple to use, crying, a major component, is difficult to assess objectively and cannot be assessed when the infant is intubated.

The BIND score can be used retrospectively to track the clinical progression of ABE from nonspecific, subtle encephalopathy (score 1-3) through progressive toxicity (score 4-6) to advanced toxicity (score 7-9). However, ABE in premature infants may occur with different or no clinical signs.

Table 10-1   BILIRUBIN-INDUCED NEUROLOGIC DYSFUNCTION (BIND) SCORE FROM 0 (BEST) TO 9 (WORST)

Mental status (0-3)	0 = Normal 1 = Sleepy, poor feeding 2 = Lethargic, irritable 3 = Semicoma, coma, seizures
Muscle tone (0-3)	0 = Normal 1 = Neck stiffness, mild hypertonia or hypotonia 2 = Arching neck and/or trunk 3 = Opisthotonus
Cry (0-3)	0 = Normal 1 = High-pitched 2 = Shrill 3 = Inconsolable

Diagnosis of Chronic Bilirubin Encephalopathy (Chronic Kernicterus)

Examination in older children and adults often involves determining whether cerebral palsy or neurodevelopmental problems are due to neonatal hyperbilirubinemia. Beyond the newborn period, kernicterus is diagnosed through a combination of history, physical examination, and laboratory tests, especially MRI and BAEP testing (Table 10-2).

In all cases, there should be a history of jaundice and, hopefully, laboratory confirmation of an increased serum bilirubin level; the higher the bilirubin, the more significantly it is modified by its duration and risk factors. Important is whether the child is neurologically symptomatic at the time of the hyperbilirubinemia. History of neonatal neurologic signs or symptoms, such as abnormal tone, cry, posturing, abnormal eye movements, and positions (including setting sun sign), at the time of or following hyperbilirubinemia should be sought. The history should include an estimate of the amount and duration of hyperbilirubinemia, other risk factors, such as gestational age, sepsis, academia, and hypoalbuminemia, and a search for etiology such as Rh or ABO isoimmunization, glucose-6-phosphate dehydrogenase (G6PD) deficiency, Gilbert's syndrome, Crigler-Najjar syndrome, spherocytosis, and third spacing of blood (e.g., a large intraventricular hemorrhage, cephalohematoma, caput, or other bruising). A history of muscle cramps, delayed gross or fine motor development, delayed speech, hearing loss, and dental enamel dysplasia is sought. A history of past or present sucking and swallowing dysfunction, gastroesophageal reflux, constipation, and failure to thrive can often be obtained. Inconsistency of hearing or sound localization in a young child raises the suspicion of a subtle auditory neuropathy/dyssynchrony, also known as ANSD.

History of BAEPs and AABRs obtained early in life should be sought. One should note that hearing screening with OAEs detects peripheral auditory problems of the inner ear. OAE screening is unaffected by bilirubin toxicity, and babies with severe ANSD with deafness have normal OAEs. BAEPs improve in a minority of children with time, in our experience; improvement in BAEPs does not mean that the auditory system has returned to normal. An MRI of the brain showing an abnormal globus pallidus with or without an abnormal subthalamic nucleus is nearly pathognomonic of kernicterus. Initially, these abnormalities are hyperintense on T1-weighted images. Later, they are more hyperintense onT2-weighted images but normalize or become hypointense on T1-weighted images. Metabolic disorders such as glutaric academia and mitochondrial encephalopathies can be excluded by history and specific laboratory tests if necessary.

On physical examination of the older child, one specifically looks for athetosis (slow writhing movements), dystonia (abnormal tone, fixed postures, cocontraction

Table 10-2 DIAGNOSIS OF KERNICTERUS OR BILIRUBIN-INDUCED NEUROLOGIC DYSFUNCTION (BIND) IN OLDER CHILDREN

Neonatal history	Magnitude and duration of hyperbilirubinemia; other risk factors (sepsis, acidosis, Rh isoimmunization); neonatal neurologic signs or symptoms during or following peak hyperbilirubinemia (abnormal tone, cry, posturing/opisthotonus, eye movements/setting sun sign)
Subsequent history	Auditory neuropathy spectrum disorder (ANSD); hearing loss; delayed speech; dental enamel dysplasia (or capped teeth); abnormal muscle tone—especially dystonia and/or variable hypotonia/hypertonia; muscle cramps; swallowing problems, gastroesophageal reflux
Examination	Athetosis, dystonia, dystonia and variable hypo-/hypertonia (± true velocity-dependent hypertonia, i.e., spasticity), ataxia, impaired upward gaze (may resolve); staining or flaking of baby teeth (enamel hypoplasia) unless capped; hearing impairment
Laboratory/imaging	Magnetic resonance imaging: abnormal signal in globus pallidus ± subthalamic nucleus, but findings may be normal, and initially abnormal findings may recover Auditory: brain auditory evoked potentials (BAEPs) abnormal consistent with ANSD—increased waves I-III and I-V, absent III and V, or all waves absent with normal cochlear microphonic responses and normal otoacoustic emissions (OAEs) (although initially normal OAEs may become abnormal, but abnormal BAEPs and ANSD may recover, in which case central auditory processing disorders may later be found)

10

of agonist and antagonist muscles), variable hypotonia/hypertonia, spasticity, ataxia, incoordination, impaired upgaze, staining or flaking of deciduous teeth (enamel hypoplasia), dysarthria, hearing impairment, and difficulty localizing sound. Improvement of impaired upward gaze has been described, but it is difficult to examine upward gaze in older infants and young children, who have learned to turn their heads to compensate for gaze pareses. Spasticity suggest a nonbilirubin, nonkernicteric etiology, and in fact, a retrospective study used spasticity as a criterion to exclude nonkernicteric causes of athetoid/dystonic cerebral palsy.[54] However, some children clearly have both kernicterus and other etiologies for their cerebral palsy and neurodevelopmental disabilities.

Laboratory evaluation consists of MRI and BAEP (ABR) testing. Other testing may show the presence or absence of other conditions, such as seizures, metabolic disorders, Gilbert's or Crigler-Najjar syndrome, liver disease if the older child remains jaundiced, G6PD deficiency or partial deficiency, and spherocytosis. The MRI may show abnormal signal in the globus pallidus and/or subthalamic nucleus, but normal MRI findings do not exclude the diagnosis. MRI abnormalities may or may not improve with time. Few other etiologies cause discrete bilateral lesions in the globus pallidus and/or subthalamic nucleus, and most of these are metabolic conditions with a different history and onset, such as glutaric aciduria with a sudden onset of encephalopathy or abnormal movements during an acute febrile illness or episode of vomiting. In addition, the MRI usually shows more extensive areas of damage in these other conditions. MRI findings consistent with kernicterus may occur with additional lesions in the putamen and cortex, or with periventricular leukomalacia, in children with conditions in addition to kernicterus. I suggest the term *kernicterus plus syndrome* for these children—that is, kernicterus plus other neonatal encephalopathies, such as hypoxia-ischemia, stroke, encephalitis, and intraventricular hemorrhage.

10

The BAEP may be absent or abnormal with an increase of conduction time between waves I and III and I and V. The cochlear microphonic (CM) response, which can be obtained at the time of BAEP testing, should be present even in the absence of BAEP neural waves (I through V). Occasionally, giant CM responses may occur and are often mistaken for BAEP waves by inexperienced readers. Cochlear microphonics can be distinguished from BAEP waves by the fact that the former do not change their latencies with intensity (whereas BAEP waves do), and phase-reverse with phase reversal of the click stimulus (whereas BAEP waves do not). BAEPs may or may not improve with time. OAEs, initially normal, may disappear with time for unknown reasons, possibly related to overstimulation of the cochlea. A full audiology evaluation is usually advisable. As with MRI, an abnormal BAEP result in the presence of ANSD is consistent with bilirubin neurotoxicity, but a normal BAEP result does not rule out kernicterus.

Recommendations for Treatment

The concentrations of unconjugated bilirubin (UCB) or TSB, unbound or free bilirubin (Bf), and hydrogen ion (pH) are all important determinants of neuronal injury by bilirubin. Because Bf measurement is not readily available clinically, estimates of binding have been used, such as the bilirubin-to-albumin molar ratio. Wennberg and colleagues[55] concluded that clinical evidence indicates that Bf is better than UCB in discriminating risk for neurotoxicity in patients with severe hyperbilirubinemia.[55] Ahlfors[55a] argues that the issue is not whether Bf is a better measure than UCB (or TcB) but that measuring both UCB and Bf permits a better understanding of the miscible (diffusible) pool of bilirubin, bilirubin binding, the risk of neurotoxicity, and when to treat a particular baby.[74a] Ahlfors makes an analogy to blood gases, in which both pH and CO_2 are measured because knowing both values, even though they are related, makes for better treatment decisions. He argues that it is not possible to identify a single total bilirubin level at which to intervene for all babies of the same gestation because binding varies from baby to baby. Measuring both Bf and TSB can identify the unique binding in the individual baby and thus identify the unique TSB at which to intervene for that child. Ahlfors argues that arbitrary TSB cutoffs determined primarily by consensus do not necessarily protect patients, and that measuring Bf in addition to TSB would better determine the total bilirubin level one is trying to avoid in a particular baby. Asking questions such as "What bilirubin level is too high?" is like asking "At what pO_2 do we intubate?" It just is not that simple! We need more information.

Neonatal hyperbilirubinemia with signs of acute encephalopathy should be considered a neurologic emergency and treated immediately to reduce the duration of exposure to excessive bilirubin and to try to move some bilirubin out of the CNS. Anecdotal evidence suggests that exchange transfusion may in part reverse neurotoxicity. During the wait for blood for exchange transfusion, intense phototherapy (e.g., a double bank of phototherapy lamps overhead as close to the infant as possible, plus intense light from below) and, if the infant is not encephalopathic, gavage feedings with preferably elemental formula[72-74] to promote fecal excretion of bilirubin are recommended.

Some treatments could be easily implemented with current technology and in the current health care delivery system. The first recommendation is to improve the emergency treatment of infants with extremely high bilirubin levels with a bilirubin crash cart. Both the intensity of treatment and speed in initiating therapy can be improved. There is often delay from the time the child is first identified until a treatment occurs. A protocol for emergency rooms for dealing with children with extreme hyperbilirubinemia should be implemented. The idea of such a bilirubin crash cart has been proposed: an incubator outfitted with high-intensity phototherapy lights above and underneath, all the necessary tubes for blood collection, and a protocol for the emergency treatment of all infants admitted with severe jaundice.[74a,74b] There is no reason to wait for laboratory results before the yellow- or orange-colored infant is started on high-intensity phototherapy. The first set of laboratory tests should include all that is necessary to order blood for an exchange transfusion. Nasogastric tubes should be available to administer elemental formula to help with gut elimination of bilirubin in nonencephalopathic babies who can tolerate nasogastric feeding.[75] There is no need to withhold treatment while blood samples are being sent, while abnormal laboratory values are being confirmed, and while other procedures such as spinal taps are being done to rule out other conditions such as meningitis. The patient should be rushed to the NICU without administrative delay for further treatment and line placement. In infants with isoimmune hemolytic disease and a rising TSB value in spite of intensive phototherapy or within 2 to 3 mg/dL of exchange level, intravenous immunoglobulin (IVIG) should be administered.[50,73,76] If infants need to be transferred to another center for an exchange transfusion, then treatment including high-intensity phototherapy should be administered during the transport, and preparations for exchange should be made while the infant is being transported.

My reviews of medical records of infants with subsequent kernicterus reveal that treatment mistakes occur both in the emergency room and in the NICU. Mistakes sometimes encountered in the emergency room are as follows:

1. The dose of phototherapy is not considered—it is not recognized that the proximity of phototherapy lights from the infant is important.
2. Infants are put on NPO status (nothing by mouth) because it is not recognized that oral or nasogastric feeding with elemental formula helps promote bilirubin excretion in healthy, nonencephalopathic infants.[74]
3. Unnecessary delay in treatment occurs because treating physicians believe that the initial level "can't be that high."
4. Initiation of phototherapy or preparation for exchange transfusions is delayed until after other investigations (e.g., sepsis workups or lumbar punctures) are done.
5. Infants with very high total and high conjugated bilirubin levels are not treated in fear of "bronze baby syndrome."
6. Infants are not treated because the bilirubin level is so high and the infant so encephalopathic that it is believed to be "too late to treat." (My colleagues and I believe that it is never too late to treat acute, symptomatic bilirubin encephalopathy, because the duration of excessive hyperbilirubinemia is related to outcome.[77,78])
7. Treatment is neglected or forgotten during emergency treatment of critical, life-threatening neonatal illness. (We call this critical illness kernicterus—for example, surgical treatment of another urgent, life-threatening illness such as cyanotic congenital heart disease or necrotizing endocarditis with perforation leads to discontinuation of phototherapy in the operating and recovery rooms and subsequent development of kernicterus.)

A second recommendation that could be implemented with current technology is universal bilirubin screening. Current AAP guidelines do not recommend a predischarge bilirubin measurement as an indispensable part of risk assessment but, rather, say that it is one of two recommended options, the other being risk factor summation. A comparison of two recommended approaches for identifying newborns at risk of significant hyperbilirubinemia concluded that use of a predischarge bilirubin measurement expressed as a risk zone on an hour-specific bilirubin nomogram is more accurate and generates wider risk stratification than a clinical risk factor score.[79] Systems that are not universal or that rely on subjective assessment of jaundice by health care providers with different levels of training allow some preventable cases of kernicterus to slip through the system. Other recommendations that can be accomplished with existing resources are standardizing laboratory bilirubin measurements and introducing a system of reporting elevated bilirubin levels (e.g., ≥25 mg/dL) to enable a better appreciation of the true epidemiology of this problem.

There is also a lack of clear guidelines for bilirubin and jaundice assessments at follow-up visits. As previously discussed, infants who later have kernicterus are often put at risk because their jaundice was not considered severe or extensive enough to warrant a transcutaneous or serum bilirubin measurement. Some clinicians and health care workers forget that before an infant becomes pumpkin orange, full-body jaundice is often associated with a clearly deeper yellow in the face and belly than in the legs and feet. This situation leads the observer to assume that full-body jaundice is not yet present and that the bilirubin level is below, rather than above, 15 mg/dL. In addition, levels of 11 to 12 mg/dL need to be closely followed and confirmed either by transcutaneous bilirubin evaluation or serum bilirubin measurement.

A TSB level below which the risk of neurotoxicity is minimal has yet to be established (and may never be established for TSB alone; e.g., in infants with bilirubin displacers—substances that displace bilirubin from albumin—such as sulfonamide[80] or benzyl alcohol,[81] may have kernicterus at extremely low bilirubin levels). Until better information is obtained, the use of the level at which phototherapy is recommended for a particular child can be used as a rough guideline below which hyperbilirubinemia is probably not significant if other clinical factors, including other illness, acidosis, and the presence of bilirubin displacers, are excluded. The use of BAEPs, especially serial BAEPs that are improving, could be a good guide to the lack of ongoing bilirubin neurotoxicity.

Once the child is stable, consideration should be given to obtaining an MRI of the head. Contrast is not necessary. Currently I recommend an MRI of the head with special attention to the globus pallidus (i.e., T1-weighted, T2-weighted, FLAIR sequences through the basal ganglia), and a BAEP test with special attention to interwave intervals and cochlear microphonics to determine the presence or absence of ANSD. The addition of thin sections with contiguous cuts and coronal sections through the basal ganglia may be helpful but are generally not necessary. It is not often appreciated that OAEs, also known as distortion product otoacoustic emissions (DPOAEs), do not detect the auditory abnormality due to hyperbilirubinemia. Children completely deaf with severe ANSD have normal OAEs as neonates and in infancy. Therefore, one must obtain a BAEP (ABR) test for diagnostic information. Because the number of children who have abnormalities that then improve is unknown, early testing is important, with serial testing if results are abnormal. A good neurologic examination with special attention to muscle tone and eye movements is important. Serial neurologic evaluations during the first few months of life can be helpful in determining whether brain injury has occurred. Early identification and treatment with physical therapy, occupational therapy, and speech therapy can be helpful. Some children with classic kernicterus have failure to thrive because of swallowing difficulties, gastroesophageal reflux, and excessive metabolic demands from their movement disorders. These children often benefit from placement of nasogastric or gastrostomy tubes, although they continue to be fed orally. If severe ANSD is present or the child is deaf or severely hearing impaired, cochlear implantation has proved beneficial. I agree with current recommendations for this procedure to be done as soon as possible. The parents of a large majority of patients with kernicterus who have undergone cochlear implantation have reported benefit. In severe cases, medications to treat dystonia and hypertonia are important. Benzodiazepines and baclofen have been useful. Anecdotal reports have suggested no benefit of bilateral deep brain stimulators in teenagers with severe dystonic kernicterus; we follow a 7-year-old with severe motor-predominant dystonic kernicterus who showed modest clinical improvements 6 to 12 months after implantation of bilateral deep brain stimulators in the globus pallidus interna.

Gaps in Knowledge

Although there has been significant progress in the understanding of how bilirubin causes brain damage, significant gaps in knowledge remain. An important gap in basic science knowledge relates to specific cellular and regional selectivity of CNS bilirubin toxicity. The current methods of assessing risk for kernicterus and BIND— that is, TSB measurement—do not measure the amount of bilirubin in brain tissue. Thus, some infants with relatively low TSB values may have BIND, and undoubtedly many with relatively high TSB levels may be treated unnecessarily to prevent kernicterus in a few infants. Research is needed to investigate the sensitivity and reliability of new methods to better detect BIND, including clinical examination of newborn infants, additional biochemical measures of bilirubin toxicity such as Bf, and neurophysiology such as BAEPs.

Through the decades from the 1950s to the 1980s, clinical practice evolved to essentially eliminate classic kernicterus; however, a reemergence of kernicterus occurred in the 1990s and continues to the present, in association with changes in medical practice and health care delivery. Clearly, universal screening of infants combined with close follow-up, monitoring, and aggressive phototherapy treatment at relatively low bilirubin levels could eliminate most of the new cases of kernicterus, but the prevention of a devastating but very rare disorder must be balanced against the costs and possible risks, although minimal with current treatment, of overtreating very large numbers of babies. More precise determination of who is at risk for brain injury is needed to ensure that no baby unnecessarily gets kernicterus yet the number of babies overtreated is minimized. The concentration of bilirubin when toxicity is increased is a difficult issue for physicians in practice, who must balance the gain in value of an early visit against the worry about whether increased surveillance will result in greater use of resources (phototherapy), more parental anxiety, and reduced breast-feeding. However, the benefits of an early visit may not only be to screen for and prevent significant hyperbilirubinemia but also to reduce parental anxiety and, through education, increase breast-feeding.

A more precise definition of kernicterus is needed. The definition of classic kernicterus is well established in the literature, but new clinical cases have led to the concept of a spectrum of kernicterus and BIND. Cases of auditory-predominant or motor-predominant kernicterus have been described, in which some of the classic features of kernicterus (auditory dysfunction or movement disorders) are prominent, with other features absent or much less pronounced. I have seen a small number of cases of auditory-predominant kernicterus occurring in 30- to 32-week-gestation infants with TSB levels in the range of 20 to 25 mg/dL.[82,83]

Precisely which hyperbilirubinemic infants to treat and when they should be treated have not been precisely determined. The role of bilirubin in common neurodevelopmental disorders, such as auditory processing disorders, cognitive disorders, sensory motor disorders, autism, and attention-deficit/hyperactivity disorder (ADHD), has yet to be established. The genetic influences and susceptibilities are not completely known—for example, why males are more susceptible than females. Identification of precisely when and how bilirubin becomes neurotoxic both on a cellular (molecular) basis and in the whole organism will necessarily improve understanding how and when to treat hyperbilirubinemic newborns. Better basic science can thus be expected to lead to a better treatment paradigm for jaundiced newborns.

Whether total or unconjugated bilirubin levels determine risk when the conjugated bilirubin value is elevated is not completely resolved. Classic kernicterus was reported in an Rh-sensitized infant with TSB of 45.2 mg/dL, of which 31.6 mg/dL was direct,[84] and in a term infant with bronze baby syndrome in which the maximum TSB was 18 mg/dL and direct was 4.1 mg/dL.[85] Ebbesen[86] found that infants with elevated direct bilirubin (6.4 to 9.9 mg/dL) and bronze baby syndrome had a decrease in reserve albumin-binding capacity and suggested that conjugated bilirubin may compete with unconjugated bilirubin for the bilirubin binding site for albumin. The AAP recommends that when guidelines for phototherapy and exchange transfusion are used, the conjugated bilirubin level should not be subtracted from the total.[50] The guidelines go on to state, "In unusual situations in which the direct bilirubin level is 50% or more of the total bilirubin, there are no good data to provide guidance for therapy, and consultation with an expert in the field is recommended."[50] The recommendation to use TSB to determine treatment seems prudent for now.

Following the 2004 AAP guidelines undoubtedly will prevent most kernicterus, although how much potentially preventable BIND occurs because the guidelines are followed is unknown. The amount of unnecessary treatment and its associated cost to the health care system is also unknown. Although the emotional cost to children and their families of a lifetime of disability from kernicterus is immeasurable, the financial cost to society of caring for a child with kernicterus over a lifetime is huge, and preventing one case of kernicterus will pay for much preventive screening. I support universal screening for hyperbilirubinemia; a systematic screening program will obviously prevent some additional cases of kernicterus, although how many more is currently unknown.

A significant gap in knowledge is determining when bilirubin neurotoxicity occurs in the premature infant. Guidelines that exist for administration of phototherapy and exchange transfusion are not evidence based. Whether bilirubin encephalopathy contributes to neurodevelopmental disabilities or learning disorders in this population is unknown. I suspect that, if present, bilirubin is likely to cause problems similar to those seen with classic kernicterus, for example, auditory process disorders. However, the damage or developmental consequences of excessive bilirubin on the very immature CNS may be fundamentally different from the effects on a more mature system.

The New Frontier—Bilirubin-Induced Neurologic Disorders in Preterm Infants: Part of a Kernicterus Spectrum Disorder

Kernicterus and BINDs in preterm infants present difficult but important challenges for the future. Because almost all prematurely born infants have hyperbilirubinemia, it is problematic to determine whether hyperbilirubinemia is the cause of subsequent neurodevelopmental disabilities. Nonetheless, the relative rarity of ANSD in the general population and in the population of children with hearing loss (0.23%) contrasts greatly with its accounting for 24% of at-risk infants from a regional perinatal center NICU.[87] Our retrospective analysis of children with kernicterus indicating an association of auditory-predominant kernicterus with earlier gestational age at the time of peak TSB[88,89] suggests that the developing central auditory nervous system may be selectively sensitive to bilirubin neurotoxicity in premature neonates.

Kernicterus in preterm infants may occur without the typical neurologic signs of ABE[54] or with neurologic signs different from those in term infants[90] yet may have sequelae similar to those in infants born at term, either classic kernicterus or isolated kernicterus, with or without MRI abnormalities that appear to normalize after 1 year corrected age. A retrospective study from Japan of eight preterm infants with a diagnosis of athetoid cerebral palsy made by consensus between pediatric neurologists and physical therapists[54] concluded that premature infants (<34 weeks of gestation, several of whom were born at less than 26 weeks of gestation and/or with 1000-g birth weight) with athetoid cerebral palsy had features similar to those in term infants with kernicterus. Peak mean bilirubin level was 12.2 ± 3.9 mg/dL (range 7.1-17.4), measured at an average 23 ± 17.5 days of age. Infants met guidelines for and received phototherapy as recommended in Japan. One infant's bilirubin level exceeded that recommended for exchange transfusion based on birth weight, but the infant did not receive transfusion because of body weight at the time. None showed classic ABE during the neonatal period. Abnormal muscle tone and dystonic posture were recognized within 6 months corrected age in all. In infancy, MRI in all seven showed abnormalities of high intensity in the globus pallidus bilaterally, but MRI after 1 year corrected age showed no abnormal findings. BAEPs, measured after discharge, were abnormal bilaterally in all seven infants evaluated. The researchers noted that a lack of acute neurologic symptoms of preterm infants was characteristic in infants whom developed kernicterus and concluded that the absence of characteristic neurologic symptoms does not exclude the possibility of kernicterus in preterm infants.

The issue of MRI abnormalities that disappear with time presents difficulties for diagnosis and recognition that sequelae are due to bilirubin neurotoxicity. MRI and single-photon emission computed tomography (SPECT) from three of the patients from the study just described found high-intensity areas in the globus pallidus in the neonatal period, but on later MRI, only one had abnormalities, which were subtle.[91] However, SPECT performed at the time of the later MRI showed decreased perfusion in all three patients.

Govaert and associates[90] performed serial MRI and head ultrasonography (HUS) of the globus pallidus in five preterm and three term infants with kernicterus and described the clinical context in very low-birth-weight preterm infants.[90] As newborns, the infants were rigid and had severe apnea before demonstrating hypertonic quadriplegia in infancy. The investigators documented a shift from acute mainly T1 hyperintensity to permanent T2 hyperintensity in the globus pallidus in the late neonatal period and found that subthalamic, not thalamic, involvement differentiated kernicterus from ischemic or metabolic disorders. They concluded that acidotic very low-birth-weight preterm infants with low serum albumin levels, and bilirubin/albumin ratios above exchange transfusion thresholds recommended by Ahlfors,[55] experience pallidal injury and hearing loss following accepted TSB levels (i.e., below exchange levels of bilirubin <13 mg/dL for low risk, <10 mg/dL for high risk infants <1250 g birth weight[92a]).

Wennberg and colleagues[92] pointed out that 150,000 to 200,000 premature infants undergo phototherapy each year in the United States to avoid TSB levels thought to require exchange transfusion. Two measurable plasma variables that might explain the variation and the response to TSB are the unbound, unconjugated bilirubin concentration (free bilirubin) and the plasma concentration of photoisomers, although the question of whether photic isomers are toxic has not been convincingly resolved. These issues and questions are likely more important in the prevention of kernicterus and BIND in prematurely born infants.

Gkoltsiou and associates[93] studied serial brain MRI and head ultrasound (HUS) findings in 11 infants with unconjugated bilirubin levels higher than 400 μmol/L (23.4 mg/dL) and/or neonatal or later neurologic signs suggestive of kernicterus. All infants were symptomatic at the time of peak TSB. Two infants were born at 26 and 27 weeks of gestational age (GA), 4 at 35 or 36 weeks GA, and 5 at 37 to 40 weeks. Term or near-term infants had classic signs, whereas preterm infants had mainly apnea and desaturation, similar to those described by Govaert and associates.[90] MRI showed abnormal signal in the globus pallidus in all except 1, the 27-week GA child. Head ultrasound showed mild increase in echogenicity in the globus pallidus or basal ganglia in 4 of 10 infants, with (GA of 26, 35, 35, and 37 weeks). These investigators concluded that severe cerebral palsy occurred with relatively low TSB levels in preterm infants but only with high levels in full-term infants and that the occurrence of neurologic damage at relatively low TSB levels in preterm infants highlights the need for further study to identify infants at risk for neurotoxicity. They believed that head ultrasound and MRI at preterm and term age were not reliable in excluding significant damage to the globus pallidus and suggested that when kernicterus is suspected, MRI should be performed by at least 5 months post-term age.

Amin and coworkers[94] found an association of apnea with ABE in premature infants with transient bilirubin encephalopathy. They studied 100 infants of 28 to 32 weeks' GA and identified 34 with bilirubin encephalopathy, as defined by abnormal ABR progression in temporal relation to hyperbilirubinemia. Abnormal ABR progression was defined as deterioration in ABR type or prolongation of the latency of wave V compared with previous ABRs and was associated with elevated bilirubin values, specifically of unbound bilirubin. A blinded retrospective chart review revealed that infants with abnormal ABR progression had significantly more apneic and bradycardic events, required more prolonged treatment with continuous positive airway pressure (CPAP) and methylxanthines, and had higher bilirubin values, specifically of unbound bilirubin, than those with normal ABR progression. The researchers concluded that premature infants with transient bilirubin encephalopathy, as defined by abnormal ABR progression in relation to hyperbilirubinemia, have more concurrent apneic events and require more prolonged respiratory support and medications.

Acknowledgments

The author appreciates suggestions and comments from Drs. Charles E. Ahlfors, Vinod K. Bhutani, Thor W. Hansen, Lois H. Johnson, M. Jeffrey Maisels, Michael J. Painter, Ann C. Rice, Richard P. Wennberg, Ann R. Stark, and Jon F Watchko.

10

References

1. Bhutani VK, Johnson L, Sivieri EM. Predictive ability of a predischarge hour-specific serum bilirubin for subsequent significant hyperbilirubinemia in healthy term and near-term newborns. *Pediatrics.* 1999;103:6-14.
2. Bjerre JV, Ebbesen F. [Incidence of kernicterus in newborn infants in Denmark.] *Ugeskr Laeger.* 2006;168:686-691.
3. Ebbesen F. Recurrence of kernicterus in term and near-term infants in Denmark. *Acta Paediatr.* 2000;89:1213-1217.
4. Newman TB, Escobar GJ, Gonzales VM. Frequency of neonatal bilirubin testing and hyperbilirubinemia in a large health maintenance organization. *Pediatrics.* 1999;104:1198-1203.
5. 5 Newman TB, Liljestrand P, Escobar GJ. Infants with bilirubin levels of 30 mg/dL or more in a large managed care organization. *Pediatrics.* 2003;111:1303-1311.
6. Bhutani VK, Johnson L. Kernicterus in the 21st century: frequently asked questions. *J Perinatol.* 2009;29(Suppl 1):S20-S24.
7. Rodrigues CM, Sola S, Silva R, Brites D. Bilirubin and amyloid-beta peptide induce cytochrome c release through mitochondrial membrane permeabilization. *Mol Med.* 2000;6:936-946.
8. Silva RF, Rodrigues CM, Brites D. Bilirubin-induced apoptosis in cultured rat neural cells is aggravated by chenodeoxycholic acid but prevented by ursodeoxycholic acid. *J Hepatol.* 2001;34:402-408.
9. Rodrigues CMP, Sola S, Brites D. Bilirubin induces apoptosis via the mitochondrial pathway in developing rat brain neurons. *Hepatology.* 2002;35:1186-1195.
10. Ostrow JD, Pascolo L, Brites D, Tiribelli C. Molecular basis of bilirubin-induced neurotoxicity. *Trends Mol Med.* 2004;10:65-70.
11. 11 Hanko E, Hansen TW, Almaas R, et al.. Bilirubin induces apoptosis and necrosis in human NT2-N neurons. *Pediatr Res.* 2005;57:179-184.
12. Li CY, Shi HB, et al. Protein kinase A and C signaling induces bilirubin potentiation of GABA/glycinergic synaptic transmission in rat ventral cochlear nucleus neurons. *Brain Res.* 2010;1348:30-41.
13. Conlee JW, Shapiro SM. Morphological changes in the cochlear nucleus and nucleus of the trapezoid body in Gunn rat pups. *Hear Res.* 1991;57:23-30.
14. Falcao AS, Fernandes A, Brito MA, et al. Bilirubin-induced immunostimulant effects and toxicity vary with neural cell type and maturation state. *Acta Neuropathol (Berl)..* 2006;112:95-105.
15. Ostrow JD, Pascolo L, Shapiro SM, Tiribelli C. New concepts of bilirubin encephalopathy. *Eur J Clin Invest.* 2003;33:988-997.
16. Watchko JF. Kernicterus and the molecular mechanisms of bilirubin-induced CNS injury in newborns. *Neuromolec Med.* 2006;8:513-530.
17. Ives NK, Gardiner RM. Blood-brain barrier permeability to bilirubin in the rat studied using intracarotid bolus injection and in situ brain perfusion techniques. *Pediatr Res.* 1990;27:436-441.
18. Hayward D, Schiff D, Fedunec S, et al. Bilirubin diffusion through lipid membranes. *Biochim Biophys Acta.* 1986;860:149-153.
19. Zucker SD, Goessling W, Hoppin AG. Unconjugated bilirubin exhibits spontaneous diffusion through model lipid bilayers and native hepatocyte membranes. *J Biol Chem.* 1999;274(16):10852-10862.
20. Amatuzio DS, Weber LJ, Nesbitt S. Bilirubin and protein in the cerebrospinal fluid of jaundiced patients with severe liver disease with and without hepatic coma. *J Lab Clin Med.* 1953;41:615-618.
21. Berman LB, Lapham LW, Pastore E. Jaundice and xanthochromia of the spinal fluid. *J Lab Clin Med.* 1954;44:273-279.
22. Sawasaki Y, Yamada N, Nakajima H. Developmental features of cerebellar hypoplasia and brain bilirubin levels in a mutant (Gunn) rat with hereditary hyperbilirubinemia. *J Neurochem.* 1976;27:577-583.
23. Rodriguez Garay EA, Scremin OU. Transfer of bilirubin-14 C between blood, cerebrospinal fluid, and brain tissue. *Am J Physiol.* 1971;221:1264-1270.
24. Gennuso F, Fernetti C, Tirolo C, et al. Bilirubin protects astrocytes from its own toxicity by inducing up-regulation and translocation of multidrug resistance-associated protein 1 (Mrp1). *Proc Natl Acad Sci U S A.* 2004;101:2470-2475.
25. Rigato I, Pascolo L, Fernetti C, et al. The human multidrug-resistance-associated protein MRP1 mediates ATP-dependent transport of unconjugated bilirubin. *Biochem J.* 2004;383(Pt 2):335-341.
26. Braun AP, Schulman H. The multifunctional calcium/calmodulin-dependent protein kinase: from form to function. *Annu Rev Physiol.* 1995;57:417-445.
27. Churn SB. Multifunctional calcium and calmodulin-dependent kinase II in neuronal function and disease. *Adv Neuroimmunol.* 1995;5:3.
28. Conlee JW, Shapiro SM, Churn SB. Expression of the alpha and beta subunits of Ca^{2+}/calmodulin kinase II in the cerebellum of jaundiced Gunn rats during development: a quantitative light microscopic analysis. *Acta Neuropathol (Berl).* 2000;99:393-401.
29. Shaia WT, Shapiro SM, Heller AJ, et al. Immunohistochemical localization of calcium-binding proteins in the brainstem vestibular nuclei of the jaundiced Gunn rat. *Hear Res.* 2002;173:82-90.
30. Spencer RF, Shaia WT, Gleason AT, et al. Changes in calcium-binding protein expression in the auditory brainstem nuclei of the jaundiced Gunn rat. *Hear Res.* 2002;171:129-141.
31. Greengard P. Neuronal phosphoproteins. Mediators of signal transduction. *Mol Neurobiol.* 1987;1:51-119.

32. Hoffman DJ, Zanelli SA, Kubin J, et al. The in vivo effect of bilirubin on the N-methyl-D-aspartate receptor/ion channel complex in the brains of newborn piglets. *Pediatr Res*. 1996;40:804-808.
33. McDonald JW, Shapiro SM, Silverstein FS, Johnston MV. Role of glutamate receptor-mediated excitotoxicity in bilirubin-induced brain injury in the Gunn rat model. *Exp Neurol*. 1998;150:21-29.
34. Grojean S, Koziel V, Vert P, Daval JL. Bilirubin induces apoptosis via activation of NMDA receptors in developing rat brain neurons. *Exp Neurol*. 2000;166:334-341.
35. Warr O, Mort D, Attwell D. Bilirubin does not modulate ionotropic glutamate receptors or glutamate transporters. *Brain Res*. 2000;879:13-16.
36. Shapiro SM, Sombati S, Geiger AS, Rice AC. NMDA channel antagonist MK-801 does not protect against bilirubin neurotoxicity. *Neonatology*. 2007;92:248-257.
37. Haustein MD, Read DJ, Steinert JR, et al. Acute hyperbilirubinaemia induces presynaptic neurodegeneration at a central glutamatergic synapse. *J Physiol*. 2010;588:4683-4693.
38. Brito MA, Vaz AR, Silva SL, et al. N-methyl–aspartate receptor and neuronal nitric oxide synthase activation mediate bilirubin-induced neurotoxicity. *Mol Med*. 2010;16:372-380.
39. Dore S, Takahashi M, Ferris CD, et al. Bilirubin, formed by activation of heme oxygenase-2, protects neurons against oxidative stress injury. *Proc Natl Acad Sci U S A*. 1999;96:2445-2450.
40. Dore S, Goto S, Sampei K, et al. Heme oxygenase-2 acts to prevent neuronal death in brain cultures and following transient cerebral ischemia. *Neuroscience*. 2000;99:587-592.
41. Baranano DE, Rao M, Ferris CD, Snyder SH. Biliverdin reductase: a major physiologic cytoprotectant. *Proc Natl Acad Sci U S A*. 2002;99:16093-16098.
42. Greenberg DA. The jaundice of the cell. *Proc Natl Acad Sci U S A*. 2002;99:15837-15839.
43. Sedlak TW, Snyder SH. Bilirubin benefits: cellular protection by a biliverdin reductase antioxidant cycle. *Pediatrics*. 2004;113:1776-1782.
44. Dore S, Sampei K, Goto S, et al. Heme oxygenase-2 is neuroprotective in cerebral ischemia. *Mol Med*. 1999;5:656-663.
45. Conlee JW, Shapiro SM. Development of cerebellar hypoplasia in jaundiced Gunn rats treated with sulfadimethoxine: a quantitative light microscopic analysis. *Acta Neuropathol*. 1997;93:450-460.
46. Falcao AS, Fernandes A, Brito MA, et al. Bilirubin-induced inflammatory response, glutamate release, and cell death in rat cortical astrocytes are enhanced in younger cells. *Neurobiol Dis*. 2005; 20:199-206.
47. Falcao AS, Bellarosa C, Fernandes A, et al. Role of multidrug resistance-associated protein 1 expression in the in vitro susceptibility of rat nerve cell to unconjugated bilirubin. *Neuroscience*. 2007;144: 878-888.
48. Deganuto M, Cesaratto L, Bellarosa C, et al. A proteomic approach to the bilirubin-induced toxicity in neuronal cells reveals a protective function of DJ-1 protein. *Proteomics*. 2010;10:1645-1657.
49. Dogan M, Peker E, Kirimi E, et al. Evaluation of oxidant and antioxidant status in infants with hyperbilirubinemia and kernicterus. *Hum Exp Toxicol*. 2011;30:1751-1760.
50. American Academy of Pediatrics Subcommittee on Hyperbilirubinemia. Management of hyperbilirubinemia in the newborn infant 35 or more weeks of gestation. *Pediatrics*. 2004;114:297-316.
51. Brooks JC, Fisher-Owens SA, Wu YW, et al. Evidence suggests there was not a "resurgence" of kernicterus in the 1990s. *Pediatrics*. 2011;127:672-679.
52. Johnson L, Brown AK. A pilot registry for acute and chronic kernicterus in term and near-term infants. *Pediatrics*. 1999;104:736.
53. Ahlfors CE, Wennberg RP. Bilirubin-albumin binding and neonatal jaundice. *Semin Perinatol*. 2004; 28:334-339.
54. Okumura A, Kidokoro H, Shoji H, et al. Kernicterus in preterm infants. *Pediatrics*. 2009;123: e1052-e1058.
55. Wennberg RP, Ahlfors CE, Bhutani VK, et al. Toward understanding kernicterus: a challenge to improve the management of jaundiced newborns. *Pediatrics*. 2006;117:474-485.
55a. Ahlfors CE, Ligand LW, Vashon WA. *The potential role of unbound bilirubin measurements for the management of jaundiced newborns*. Presented at the 22nd Annual Audrey K. Brown Kernicterus Symposium, Pediatric Academic Societies' 2006 Annual Meeting, San Francisco, May 1, 2006.
56. Ahlfors CE. Bilirubin-albumin binding and free bilirubin. *J Perinatol* 2001;21(Suppl 1):S40-S42, discussion S59-S62.
57. Wennberg RP, Ahlfors CE, Bickers R, et al. Abnormal auditory brainstem response in a newborn infant with hyperbilirubinemia: improvement with exchange transfusion. *J Pediatr*. 1982;100:624-626.
58. Amin SB, Ahlfors C, Orlando MS, et al. Bilirubin and serial auditory brainstem responses in premature infants. *Pediatrics*. 2001;107:664-670.
59. Funato M, Tamai H, Shimada S, Nakamura H. Vigintiphobia, unbound bilirubin, and auditory brainstem responses. *Pediatrics*. 1994;93:50-53.
60. Nwaesei CG, Van Aerde J, Boyden M, Perlman M. Changes in auditory brainstem responses in hyperbilirubinemic infants before and after exchange transfusion. *Pediatrics*. 1984;74:800-803.
61. Wennberg R. Bilirubin transport and toxicity. *Mead Johnson Symp Perinat Dev Med*. 1982;19:25-31.
62. Sugama S, Soeda A, Eto Y: Magnetic resonance imaging in three children with kernicterus. *Pediatr Neurol*. 2001;25:328-331.
63. Martich-Kriss V, Kollias SS, Ball WS Jr. MR findings in kernicterus. *AJNR Am J Neuroradiol*. 1995;16:819-821.
64. Yilmaz Y, Alper G, Kilicoglu G, et al. Magnetic resonance imaging findings in patients with severe neonatal indirect hyperbilirubinemia. *J Child Neurol*. 2001;16:452-455.
65. Penn AA, Enzmann DR, Hahn JS, Stevenson DK. Kernicterus in a full term infant. *Pediatrics*. 1994;93:1003-1006.

66. Johnston MV, Hoon AH Jr. Possible mechanisms in infants for selective basal ganglia damage from asphyxia, kernicterus, or mitochondrial encephalopathies. *J Child Neurol*. 2000;15:588-591.
67. Govaert P, Lequin M, Swarte R, et al. Changes in globus pallidus with (pre)term kernicterus. *Pediatrics*. 2003;112:1256-1263.
68. Harris MC, Bernbaum JC, Polin JR, et al. Developmental follow-up of breastfed term and near-term infants with marked hyperbilirubinemia. *Pediatrics*. 2001;107:1075-1080.
69. Saluja S, Agarwal A, Kler N, Amin S. Auditory neuropathy spectrum disorder in late preterm and term infants with severe jaundice. *Int J Pediatr Otorhinolaryngol*. 2010;74:1292-1297.
70. Johnson L, Brown AK, Bhutani VK. BIND: a clinical score for bilirubin induced neurologic dysfunction in newborns. *Pediatrics*. 1999;104:746-747.
71. Volpe JJ. Bilirubin and brain injury. In: Volpe JJ, ed. *Neurology of the newborn*. Philadelphia: WB Saunders; 2001:490-514.
72. Hansen TW. Acute management of extreme neonatal jaundice: the potential benefits of intensified phototherapy and interruption of enterohepatic bilirubin circulation. *Acta Paediatr*. 1997;86:843-846.
73. Smitherman H, Stark AR, Bhutan VK. Early recognition of neonatal hyperbilirubinemia and its emergent management. *Semin Fetal Neonatal Med*. 2006;11:214-224.
74. Gourley GR, Kreamer B, Cohnen M, Kosorok MR. Neonatal jaundice and diet. *Arch Pediatr Adolesc Med*. 1999;153:1002-1003.
74a. Johnson L, Bhutani VK, Karp K, et al. Clinical report from the pilot USA kernicterus registry (1992 to 2004). *J Perinatol*. 2009;29(Suppl 1):S25-S45.
74b. Hansen TW. The role of phototherapy in the crash-cart apporach to extreme neonatal jaundice. *Sem Perinatol*. 2011;35:171-174.
75. Gourley GR, Arend RA. Beta-glucuronidase and hyperbilirubinaemia in breast-fed and formula-fed babies. *Lancet*. 1986;1(8482):644-646.
76. Gottstein R, Cooke RW. Systematic review of intravenous immunoglobulin in haemolytic disease of the newborn. *Arch Dis Child Fetal Neonatal Ed*. 2003;88:F6-F10.
77. Johnson L, Boggs TR. Bilirubin-dependent brain damage: incidence and indications for treatment. In: Odell GB, Schaffer R, Sionpoulous AP, eds: *Phototherapy in the newborn: an overview*. Washington, DC: National Academy of Sciences; 1974:122-149.
78. de Vries LS, Lary S, Dubowitz LMS. Relationship of serum bilirubin levels to ototoxicity and deafness in high-risk, low birth-weight infants. *Pediatrics*. 1985;76:351-354.
79. Keren R, Bhutani VK, Luan X, et al. Identifying newborns at risk of significant hyperbilirubinaemia: a comparison of two recommended approaches. *Arch Dis Child*. 2005;90:415-421.
80. Silverman WA, Andersen DH, Blanc WA, Crozier DN. A difference in mortality rate and incidence of kernicterus among premature infants allotted to two prophylactic antibacterial regimens. *Pediatrics*. 1956;18:614-625.
81. Jardine DS, Rogers K. Relationship of benzyl alcohol to kernicterus, intraventricular hemorrhage, and mortality in preterm infants. *Pediatrics*. 1989;83:153-160.
82. Shapiro SM, Bhutani VK, Johnson L. Hyperbilirubinemia and kernicterus. *Clin Perinatol*. 2006;33:387-410.
83. Shapiro SM. Definition of the clinical spectrum of kernicterus and bilirubin-induced neurologic dysfunction (BIND). *J Perinatol*. 2005;25:54-59.
84. Grobler JM, Mercer MJ. Kernicterus associated with elevated predominantly direct-reacting bilirubin. *S Afr Med J*. 1997;87:1146.
85. Clark CF, Torii S, Hamamoto Y, Kaito H. The "bronze baby" syndrome: postmortem data. *J Pediatr*. 1976;88:461-464.
86. Ebbesen F. Low reserve albumin for binding of bilirubin in neonates with deficiency of bilirubin excretion and bronze baby syndrome. *Acta Paediatr Scand*. 1982;71:415-420.
87. Berg AL, Spitzer JB. Newborn hearing screening in the NICU: profile of failed auditory brainstem response/passed otoacoustic emission. *Pediatrics*. 2005;116:933-938.
88. Powers KM, Miller S, et al. Exposure to excessive hyperbilirubinemia earlier in neurodevelopment is associated with auditory-predominant kernicterus subtype. 37th Annual Meeting of the Child Neurology Society, Santa Clara, CA. *Ann Neurol*. 2008;64(Suppl 12):S105.
89. Shapiro SM, Power KM. Kernicterus subtypes and their association with signs of neonatal encephalopathy. *Ann Neurol*. 2010;68(Suppl 14):S117-S118.
90. Govaert P, Lequin M, Swarte R, et al. Changes in globus pallidus with (pre)term kernicterus. *Pediatrics*. 2003;112:1256-1263.
91. Okumura A, Hayakawa F, Maruyama K, et al. Single photon emission computed tomography and serial MRI in preterm infants with kernicterus. *Brain Dev*. 2006;28:348-352.
92. Wennberg RP, Ahlfors CE, Aravkin AY. Intervention guidelines for neonatal hyperbilirubinemia: an evidence based quagmire. *Curr Pharm Des*. 2009;15:2939-2945.
92a. Pearlman MA, Gartner LM, Lee K, et al. Absence of kernicterus in low-birth-weight infants from 1971 through 1976: comparison with findings in 1966 and 1967. *Pediatrics*. 1978;62:460-466.
93. Gkoltsiou K, Tzoufi M, Counsell S, et al. Serial brain MRI and ultrasound findings: relation to gestational age, bilirubin level, neonatal neurologic status and neurodevelopmental outcome in infants at risk of kernicterus. *Early Hum Dev*. 2008;84:829-838.
94. Amin SB, Charafeddine L, Guillet R. Transient bilirubin encephalopathy and apnea of prematurity in 28 to 32 weeks gestational age infants. *J Perinatol*. 2005;25:386-390.
95. Morris BH, Oh W, Tyson JE, et al. Aggressive vs. conservative phototherapy for infants with extremely low birth weight. *N Engl J Med*. 2008;359:1885-1896.

CHAPTER 11

Neonatal Meningitis: Current Treatment Options

David Kaufman, MD, Santina Zanelli, MD, Joseph B. Cantey, MD, and Pablo J. Sánchez, MD

Bacterial meningitis occurs in approximately 0.4 neonates per 1000 live births. It is defined as inflammation of the meninges that is manifested by an elevated number of white blood cells in the cerebrospinal fluid (CSF). It often is associated with elevated protein content and a low glucose concentration in CSF. Meningitis generally occurs as a consequence of hematogenous dissemination of bacteria via the choroid plexus and into the central nervous system (CNS) during a sepsis episode. Invasion of the meninges occurs in about 10% to 20% of infants with bacteremia. Rarely, meningitis develops secondary to extension from infected skin through the soft tissues and skull, as may occur with an infected cephalohematoma or direct spread from skin surfaces as in infants with myelomeningocele or other congenital malformations of the neural tube. In addition, a ventriculoperitoneal shunt or ventricular reservoir may be the primary site of infection. A potential but infrequent complication of meningitis is brain abscess that results from hematogenous spread of bacteria into tissue that has suffered anoxic injury or severe vasculitis with hemorrhage or infarction.

Virtually all organisms that cause neonatal infection or sepsis can result in CNS disease with severe consequences to the developing brain.[1-4] A list of these pathogens

Table 11-1   CAUSATIVE AGENTS OF NEONATAL MENINGITIS*

1. Bacteria	Aerobic: Gram-positive: group B streptococcus, group A streptococcus, *Enterococcus* spp., viridans streptococci, *Staphylococcus aureus*, coagulase-negative staphylococci, *Listeria monocytogenes*, others[†] Gram-negative: *Escherichia coli*, *Klebsiella* spp., *Enterobacter* spp., *Serratia* spp., *Proteus* spp., *Citrobacter* spp., *Salmonella* spp., *Pseudomonas aeruginosa*, *Haemophilus influenzae*, *Neisseria gonorrhoeae*, others[†]
	Anaerobic: Gram-positive: *Clostridium* spp., *Peptostreptococcus* spp. Gram-negative: *Bacteroides fragilis*
	Genital mycoplasmas: *Ureaplasma urealyticum*, *Mycoplasma hominis*
	Spirochetes: *Treponema pallidum*, *Borrelia burgdorferi*
	Mycobacteria: *Mycobacterium tuberculosis*
2. Viruses	Herpes simplex virus, cytomegalovirus, enteroviruses, human immunodeficiency virus, varicella-zoster virus, rubella virus, human parvovirus B19, lymphocytic choriomeningitis virus
3. Fungi	*Candida* spp., *Malassezia* spp., *Aspergillus* spp., *Trichosporon beigelii*, *Cryptococcus*, *Coccidioides immitis*
4. Protozoa	*Toxoplasma gondii*

*For a more complete listing, see Palazzi DL, Klein JO, Baker CJ. Bacterial sepsis and meningitis. In: Remington JS, Klein JO, Wilson CB, Baker CJ, eds. *Infectious diseases of the fetus and newborn infant.* 6th ed. Philadelphia: WB Saunders; 2006: 247-295.
†For others, see Giacoia GP. Uncommon pathogens in newborn infants. *J Perinatol.* 1994;14:134-144.

is shown in Table 11-1. It is imperative that a correct and timely diagnosis with a specific organism be made because treatment decisions vary with causative agent.

The case of a preterm infant is presented and discussed to illustrate and highlight the multifaceted nature of this disease. It is the objective of this chapter to review the current management of neonatal bacterial meningitis, in the hope of ameliorating the destructive nature of many of these organisms and ultimately improving the outcome of these high-risk infants.

Question 1: What Risk Factors Predispose this Infant to Early-Onset Bacterial Meningitis?

Because meningitis is a complication of bacteremia, the risk factors are similar to those for neonatal sepsis, namely prematurity, prolonged rupture of fetal membranes (18 to 24 hours or longer), and maternal intrapartum fever or chorioamnionitis.[5]

CASE HISTORY

A preterm infant weighing 1004 g was born at 28 weeks of gestation to a 24-year-old mother by cesarean section. The pregnancy was complicated by premature rupture of membranes 2 weeks before delivery, and the mother demonstrated intrapartum fever and was diagnosed with chorioamnionitis. She received antenatal steroids and antimicrobial therapy consisting of ampicillin and gentamicin. At delivery, the infant was floppy with poor respiratory effort, and required intubation and admission to the neonatal intensive care unit (NICU). Apgar scores were 3 at 1 minute and 7 at 5 minutes. The infant's vital signs were stable, and antimicrobial therapy with ampicillin and gentamicin was initiated after a blood culture specimen was obtained. Hyaline membrane disease was diagnosed, and the infant received exogenous surfactant therapy.

Likewise, clinical signs suggestive of bacterial meningitis are similar to those of neonatal sepsis. In the full-term infant, fever, lethargy, hypotonia, irritability, apnea, poor feeding, high-pitched cry, emesis, seizures, and bulging fontanel are prominent clinical signs, whereas in preterm infants, respiratory decompensation consisting of an increased number of apneic episodes predominates. *Neonates with meningitis are not asymptomatic.*[6]

Maternal antepartum antibiotic use has been associated with early-onset meningitis caused by gram-negative bacilli.[7] The widespread and routine use of intrapartum antimicrobial chemoprophylaxis since 1996 has significantly reduced the rate of early-onset group B streptococcal (GBS) infection by more than 70%.[4,5,8] At the same time, there has not been an increase in early-onset bacterial infections caused by gram-negative organisms among all newborns in the United States.[9,10] However, among very low-birth-weight (VLBW) infants, those with birth weights of 1500 g or less, a shift toward more gram-negative infections has occurred.[4,11] Among the NICUs of the National Institute of Child Health and Human Development (NICHD) Neonatal Research Network centers, intrapartum antimicrobial chemoprophylaxis resulted in a significant decrease in early-onset GBS infection while the rate of infections due to *Escherichia coli* increased significantly from about 3 to 7 cases per 1000 live births.[4,11,12] The majority of *E. coli* isolates were resistant to ampicillin, an antibiotic that is often used for intrapartum GBS chemoprophylaxis.

Question 2: Do Infants with Meningitis Have Positive Blood Culture Results?

As many as 40% of infants with meningitis whose gestational age is 34 weeks or less do not have a positive blood culture result at the time of diagnosis.[13] Similarly, among VLBW infants, almost half of cases of meningitis occur with sterile blood cultures.[14,15] Therefore, it is imperative that if sepsis or meningitis is suspected, a lumbar puncture be performed.[16,17] Evaluation of CSF indices and Gram stain not only will establish a diagnosis but also will help guide therapy.[18] Normal CSF indices are provided in Table 11-2.[19-26]

Meningitis in preterm infants admitted to the NICU with respiratory distress syndrome is very uncommon.[27-30] Therefore, performance of a lumbar puncture in these infants in whom sepsis is not suspected is not mandatory. Similar data are available for full-term infants.[6,31] However, if the blood culture yields a pathogenic organism, then evaluation of CSF should be done.[17,32] Delay in performance of a lumbar puncture because of cardiorespiratory instability, extreme prematurity, or concern for increase in blood pressure due to pain with a lumbar puncture and the risk of intraventricular hemorrhage in extremely preterm infants only delays the diagnosis and leads to prolonged and possibly inappropriate antibiotic use.[14]

CONTINUATION OF CASE HISTORY

The infant was extubated and started on continuous positive airway pressure (CPAP) therapy on the first day of age. Trophic feedings were initiated on the second day of age, and a percutaneous intravenous central venous catheter (PICC) was placed for parenteral nutrition. The infant achieved full enteral feedings on the 20th day. Over the subsequent 2 days, the infant demonstrated lethargy, hyperglycemia, and increased episodes of apnea that resulted in re-initiation of mechanical ventilation. Two blood culture specimens were obtained, and antimicrobial therapy with oxacillin and gentamicin was initiated.

11

Table 11-2 CEREBROSPINAL FLUID INDICES IN NEONATES

Birth Weight (g)	Age (Days)	No. of Samples	Red Blood Cells (/mm³), Mean ± SD (Range)	White Blood Cells (/mm³), Mean ± SD (Range)	Polymorphonuclear Leukocytes (%), Mean ± SD (Range)	Glucose (mg/dL), Mean ± SD (Range)	Protein (mg/dL), Mean ± SD (Range)
Preterm Neonate*							
≤1000	0-7	6	335 ± 709 (0-1780)	3 ± 3 (1-8)	11 ± 20 (0-50)	70 ± 17 (41-89)	162 ± 37 (115-222)
	8-28	17	1465 ± 4062 (0-19 050)	4 ± 4 (0-14)	8 ± 17 (0-66)	68 ± 48 (41-89)	159 ± 77 (95-370)
	29-84	15	808 ± 1843 (0-6850)	4 ± 3 (0-11)	2 ± 9 (0-36)	49 ± 22 (41-89)	137 ± 61 (76-260)
1001-1500	0-7	8	407 ± 853 (0-2450)	4 ± 4 (1-10)	4 ± 10 (0-28)	74 ± 19 (41-89)	136 ± 35 (85-176)
	8-28	14	1101 ± 2643 (0-9750)	7 ± 11 (0-44)	10 ± 19 (0-60)	59 ± 23 (41-89)	137 ± 46 (54-227)
	29-84	11	661 ± 1198 (0-3800)	8 ± 8 (0-23)	11 ± 19 (0-48)	47 ± 13 (41-89)	122 ± 47 (45-187)
Full-Term Neonate†							
	0-30	108	≤1000	7.3 ± 13.9 (0-130), median 4	0.8 ± 6.2 (0-65), median 0	51.2 ± 12.9 (62% of serum glucose)	64.2 ± 24.2

*Data from Rodriguez AF, Kaplan SL, Mason EO Jr. Cerebrospinal fluid values in the very low birth weight infant. *J Pediatr.* 1990;116:971-974.
†Data from Ahmed A, Hickey SM, Ehrett S, et al. Cerebrospinal fluid values in the term neonate. *Pediatr Infect Dis J.* 1996;15:298-303.

Question 3: What is the Optimal Evaluation for Possible Late-Onset Sepsis in Preterm Infants in the NICU?

Infants in the NICU in whom late-onset sepsis is suspected should undergo a complete evaluation consisting of a complete blood cell count, a urinalysis and culture, and CSF evaluation. Unfortunately, there is no laboratory or clinical finding that has a sensitivity of 100% for the diagnosis of neonatal sepsis.[33,34] Such laboratory tools as complete blood cell (CBC) count and measurements of C-reactive protein (CRP), interleukin-6 (IL-6), IL-8, IL-10, and procalcitonin have suboptimal sensitivity and specificity to replace the blood culture as the gold standard, but these tests may be useful to support a diagnosis of infection when their results are abnormal and accompanied by clinical signs of infection.[35-37] Polymerase chain reaction (PCR) analysis for detection of bacterial and fungal DNA ultimately may be the answer.

Performance of a CBC count with platelets is important for reasons other than diagnosis. Neonatal sepsis may result in neutropenia, which is associated with a high mortality rate. The finding of an absolute neutrophil count of 500/mm^3 or less may prompt the administration of intravenous immunoglobulin (IVIG, 500-1000 mg/kg); the use of IGIV has been associated with improvement in the peripheral neutrophil count presumably secondary to neutrophil egression from the bone marrow.[38,39] Granulocyte transfusions also have been found to be beneficial, but the lack of timely availability and donor screening has limited their routine use.[40] Recombinant granulocyte colony-stimulating factor (G-CSF) or granulocyte-macrophage CSF have been used with some success and can be considered if IVIG is unsuccessful in improving the neutrophil count.[40,41] Because elevated concentrations of G-CSF are often detected in urine of infected infants, a lack of response may be due to dysfunction rather than quantity of endogenous G-CSF.[39] Another reason for performance of a CBC count is evaluation of platelet count because disseminated intravascular coagulation may result in severe thrombocytopenia. In addition, thrombocytopenia may be an early marker of disseminated candidiasis or even bacterial sepsis.[42,43]

Debate continues as to whether multiple blood cultures should be performed. Certainly, with bacterial organisms that are frequent blood culture contaminants, such as coagulase-negative staphylococci (CoNS), the diagnosis of sepsis is best confirmed by the finding of two or more positive blood culture results in specimens from multiple sites.[44,45] Controversy exists about whether one of the blood cultures should be obtained from a PICC or other central venous catheter if either is present,[46] because the specimen collection may cause the catheter to become infected or even clotted. Moreover, a positive culture result for blood obtained only from the catheter may represent hub colonization rather than true infection. Certainly, if blood culture specimens are obtained from indwelling venous or arterial catheters, guidelines should be in place to minimize contamination as well as how long the blood remains stagnant in the catheter. It is clear, however, that the isolation of CoNS from only one blood culture specimen when only one is obtained is problematic and of uncertain significance. Because many of these positive culture results represent contamination with skin microflora, the practice of obtaining only one blood culture specimen often leads to prolonged and unnecessary antibiotic therapy. In addition, performance of two blood cultures may increase the likelihood of isolating a causative agent. This practice leads to more prudent antibiotic use—a major goal in the NICU, where antimicrobial resistance is an emerging but preventable problem.

Urine culture is an important part of the evaluation because urinary tract infection is relatively common in neonates older than 72 hours.[47,48] Urine should be obtained by suprapubic bladder aspiration whenever possible, and the finding of any growth is significant. Alternatively, a catheterized urine specimen may be obtained, with the recognition that urethral or perineal bacterial or fungal contamination in these small infants may complicate the assessment of results. In general, growth of a single isolate with a colony count of 10^4 or greater is considered indicative of a true pathogen, whereas lesser colony counts are more indicative of contamination. Bag specimens should never be obtained for the evaluation of possible urinary tract infection.

Chest radiographs should be obtained if respiratory decompensation is present. A lumbar puncture should always be performed in the infants evaluated for possible late-onset sepsis for reasons stated in the answer to Question 2. Risk factors for meningitis in preterm infants include low gestational age and prior bloodstream infection.[14] In VLBW infants, the average age of late-onset meningitis is 26 days (median 19 days; range 4-102 days).[14] Therapeutic decisions with regard to antibiotic choices can be made only if one knows whether the CNS is involved.

Question 4: What is the Empiric Antimicrobial Choice for Possible Late-Onset Sepsis in the NICU?

In general, antimicrobial therapy for neonatal sepsis depends on the agents commonly seen in that particular nursery and their susceptibility pattern. For early-onset sepsis, ampicillin combined with an aminoglycoside, usually gentamicin, has been the empiric therapy of choice because GBS, other streptococcal species, *Listeria monocytogenes*, and gram-negative bacilli predominate in this disorder.

For late-onset sepsis, a penicillinase-resistant, semisynthetic penicillin such as oxacillin or nafcillin in combination with an aminoglycoside is the preferred choice.[45,49,50] For CNS infections, nafcillin is preferred because of its better penetration. Approximately 50% of all bloodstream infections are due to CoNS, so some experts recommend vancomycin instead of semisynthetic penicillin, to which CoNS are almost uniformly resistant. This practice has led to widespread use of vancomycin in NICUs with its attendant risk for emergence of vancomycin-resistant organisms.

The use of a penicillinase-resistant penicillin antibiotic such as oxacillin to treat for possible staphylococcal infection in the infant is based on the goal of reducing vancomycin use in NICUs. Clinical experience suggests that such a practice is safe.[49-53] Bloodstream infections due to CoNS are rarely fulminant or fatal, and they are not associated with a higher case-fatality rate than that seen among uninfected VLBW infants.[54,55] The short-term clinical outcomes of CoNS bacteremia is similar whether the initial antibiotic therapy is vancomycin or another agent that does not reliably treat CoNS infections.[52,53] In addition, only one of five evaluations for sepsis yields a causative organism.[54] The fact that results of more than 80% of blood cultures that yield CoNS are positive by 24 hours of incubation makes it possible for the clinician to change antibiotic therapy in a timely fashion if needed.[56] An additional concern about vancomycin therapy has been the association of prior vancomycin use with subsequent development of gram-negative bacteremia among hospitalized pediatric patients.[57] The emergence of community-associated methicillin-resistant *Staphylococcus aureus* (CA-MRSA) in NICUs may limit the use of such a policy in NICUs where the prevalence of CA-MRSA is high.[58,59] However, routine screening for MRSA and appropriate isolation precautions for colonized infants can control if not eradicate MRSA in NICUs.[60]

Aminoglycosides have been the time-honored choice for empiric treatment of infections due to gram-negative bacilli.[61] Once-daily or extended dosing of gentamicin is used frequently in both full-term and preterm infants on the basis of sound pharmacodynamic and pharmacokinetic considerations.[62] Such a dosing schedule may maximize the bactericidal activity of the aminoglycoside while minimizing its potential toxicity. A retrospective review by Jackson and colleagues[63] reported the occurrence of hypocalcemia in 3.5% of term and near-term newborns who received gentamicin once daily for 4 days or longer after a change in dosing regimen from every 12 hours to every 24 hours. Although aminoglycosides are known to enhance urinary calcium excretion, it is not known whether this is potentiated by higher doses of gentamicin.

Aminoglycosides have the distinct advantage of exerting less selective pressure for development of resistance in closed units such as an NICU, thus minimizing the risk of emergence of resistant bacteria.[64] This situation is in contrast to the rapid emergence of cephalosporin resistance when these agents are provided routinely for possible late-onset sepsis.[65,66] When used for empiric therapy of early-onset infection, cefotaxime has been associated with neonatal death.[67] However, CSF penetration of aminoglycosides is poor, so their use in meningitis is problematic. If a lumbar puncture is not performed as part of the initial evaluation for possible sepsis, and only an aminoglycoside is used, effective therapy for gram-negative meningitis is not provided. Delay in the determination of whether a neonate has meningitis will delay optimal therapy for this condition.

CONTINUATION OF CASE HISTORY

> Within 24 hours of specimen collection, the blood cultures yielded gram-negative rods. Cefotaxime was added to the antibiotic regimen. *E. coli* was subsequently identified from the blood cultures. A lumbar puncture was then performed that demonstrated 4160 white blood cells/mm^3 (90% polymorphonuclear cells, 10% mononuclear cells), 8320 red blood cells/mm^3, a protein value of 433 mg/dL, and a glucose value of 84 mg/dL (serum glucose 180 mg/dL). Culture of CSF yielded *E. coli*.

Question 5: What is the Treatment of Meningitis in Neonates, and in Particular that due to Gram-Negative Bacilli?

Table 11-3 provides the recommended antimicrobial treatment for neonatal meningitis based on causative organism.[68] The recommended antimicrobial dosages are provided in Table 11-4. The treatment of gram-negative meningitis initially includes the addition of a third- or fourth-generation cephalosporin, such as cefotaxime or cefepime,[69,70] or a carbapenem antibiotic, such as meropenem.[61,71-73] Piperacillin/tazobactam, a combination antibiotic that combines the extended-spectrum penicillin antibiotic piperacillin and the β-lactamase inhibitor tazobactam, is being used increasingly in NICUs as a second agent for gram-negative infections. Although this antibiotic also has broad coverage against many gram-positive and anaerobic bacteria, the tazobactam component does not reliably cross the blood-brain barrier, and therefore it should not be used for the treatment of meningitis.

Meningitis caused by gram-negative enteric bacilli is challenging because eradication of the organism from CSF is often delayed. Moreover, many of these pathogens are now resistant to ampicillin, and aminoglycoside concentrations are typically low in CSF. Cefotaxime, which has superior in vitro and CSF bactericidal activity, is the agent of choice. It is combined with an aminoglycoside, at least until sterilization of CSF has been achieved. There is little experience with and no human studies of once-daily dosing of aminoglycosides for neonatal meningitis, although from a pharmacodynamic standpoint, such a dosing schedule may be preferred because it should achieve higher CSF concentrations.[61,74] Continued treatment of gram-negative bacillary meningitis is based on in vitro susceptibility test results. Ampicillin may be used in the infrequent cases in which the organism is susceptible.

Of concern is the production by gram-negative bacteria of both chromosomally determined β-lactamases and plasmid-determined extended-spectrum β-lactamases (ESBLs), both of which can result in resistance to the third-generation cephalosporin antibiotics, even during therapy.[75-77] Chromosomally determined β-lactamases are seen in *Enterobacter* spp., *Serratia* spp., *Pseudomonas aeruginosa*, *Citrobacter* spp., and indole-positive *Proteus*, whereas ESBLs are present in the Enterobacteriaceae, especially *Klebsiella pneumoniae* and *E. coli*. Treatment of infections due to gram-negative bacteria that produce ESBLs with a third-generation cephalosporin such

Table 11-3 RECOMMENDED THERAPY FOR NEONATAL MENINGITIS

Meningitis	Therapy	Comment
Initial therapy, cerebrospinal fluid abnormal but organism unknown	Ampicillin IV *AND* gentamicin IV, IM *AND* cefotaxime IV	Cefotaxime is added if meningitis suspected or cannot be excluded Alternatives to ampicillin in nursery-acquired infections: vancomycin or nafcillin
Bacteroides fragilis spp. *fragilis**	Metronidazole IV	Alternative: meropenem
Coliform bacteria[†]	Cefotaxime IV, IM *AND* gentamicin	Discontinue gentamicin when clinical and microbiologic responses documented Alternative: ampicillin if organism susceptible; meropenem or cefepime for multiresistant organisms Lumbar intrathecal or intraventricular gentamicin usually not beneficial
Chryseobacterium (*Flavobacterium*) *meningosepticum*	Vancomycin IV *AND* rifampin IV, PO	Alternatives: clindamycin, ciprofloxacin
Group A streptococcus[†]	Penicillin G or ampicillin IV	
Group B streptococcus*	Ampicillin or penicillin G IV *AND* gentamicin IV, IM	Discontinue gentamicin when clinical and microbiologic responses documented
Enterococcal spp.[‡]	Ampicillin IV, IM *AND* gentamicin IV, IM; for ampicillin-resistant organisms: vancomycin *AND* gentamicin	Gentamicin only if synergy documented
Other streptococcal species[†]	Penicillin or ampicillin IV, IM	
Gonococcal[§]	Ceftriaxone IV, IM *OR* cefotaxime IV, IM	Duration of therapy uncertain (5-10 days?)
Haemophilus influenzae[‡]	Cefotaxime IV, IM	Ampicillin if β-lactamase negative
Listeria monocytogenes[‡]	Ampicillin IV, IM *AND* gentamicin IV, IM	Gentamicin is synergistic in vitro with ampicillin but can be discontinued when sterilization achieved
Staphylococcus epidermidis (or any coagulase-negative staphylococci)[§]	Vancomycin IV	Add rifampin if culture results persistently positive Alternative: linezolid
Staphylococcus aureus[†]	Methicillin-susceptible *S. aureus*: nafcillin IV Methicillin-resistant *S. aureus*: vancomycin IV	Gentamicin may provide synergy; rifampin if culture results persistently positive
Pseudomonas aeruginosa[†]	Ceftazidime IV, IM *AND* aminoglycoside IV, IM	Meropenem OR cefepime AND aminoglycoside are suitable alternatives

Table 11-3 RECOMMENDED THERAPY FOR NEONATAL MENINGITIS—cont'd

Meningitis	Therapy	Comment
Candida spp.[¶]	Amphotericin B deoxycholate (AmB-D) × 3-6 wk	Alternatives: AmB–lipid complex, AmB-liposomal, fluconazole (for susceptible strains [*Candida krusei* usually resistant]) Addition of fluconazole to amphotericin if culture results persistently positive
Ureaplasma urealyticum[†]	Doxycycline IV OR azithromycin IV	Alternatives: chloramphenicol; ciprofloxacin
Mycoplasma hominis[†]	Clindamycin OR doxycycline IV	Alternatives: chloramphenicol; ciprofloxacin

Adapted from Bradley JS, Nelson JD. *2006-2007 Nelson's pocket book of pediatric antimicrobial therapy.* 16th ed. Buenos Aires: Alliance for World Wide Editing; 2006.
*Minimum duration of therapy: 14 days.
[†]Minimum duration of therapy: 21 days; for gram-negative meningitis, at least 14 days after cerebrospinal fluid is sterilized, whichever is longer.
[‡]Minimum duration of therapy: 10 days.
[§]Minimum duration of therapy: 7 to 10 days.
[¶]Minimum duration of therapy: 4 weeks (or 30 mg/kg total dose of amphotericin deoxycholate).

Table 11-4 ANTIMICROBIAL DOSAGES FOR NEONATES WITH MENINGITIS

		Dosage (mg/kg/day) and Intervals of Administration				
		Chronologic Age < 28 Days				
		Body Weight ≤ 2000 g		Body Weight > 2000 g		Chronologic Age > 28 Days
Antibiotic	Route	0-7 Days Old	8-28 Days Old	0-7 Days Old	8-28 Days Old	
Amphotericin B: Deoxycholate	IV	1 q24h	1 q24h	1 q24h	1 q24h	1 q24h
Lipid complex	IV	5 q24h	5 q24h	5 q24h	5 q24h	5 q24h
Liposomal	IV	5 q24h	5 q24h	5 q24h	5 q24h	5 q24h
Ampicillin	IV, IM	100 div q12h	150 div q8h	150 div q8h	200 div q6h	200 div q6h
Azithromycin	IV	10 q24h	10 q24h	10 q24h	10 q24h	10 q24h
Cefepime*	IV, IM	90 div q8h	90-150 div q8h*	90 div q8h	90-150 div q8h*	150 div q8h
Cefotaxime	IV, IM	100-200 div q12h	150-300 div q8h	100-200 div q12h	150-300 div q8h	150-300 div q6-8h
Ceftazidime	IV, IM	100-200 div q12h	150-300 div q8h	100-200 div q12h	150-300 div q8h	150-300 div q8h
Ceftriaxone	IV, IM	50 q24h	80-100 q24h	50 q24h	80-100 q24h	100 q24h
Clindamycin	IV, IM	15 div q12h	20-30 div q8h	20-30 div q8h	20-30 div q8h	30 div q6h
Fluconazole	IV	12 q72h	12 q48h	12 q24h	12 q24h	12 q24h
Linezolid	IV	20 div q12h	30 div q8h	30 div q8h	30 div q8h	30 div q8h

11

Table 11-4   ANTIMICROBIAL DOSAGES FOR NEONATES WITH MENINGITIS—cont'd

		Dosage (mg/kg/day) and Intervals of Administration				
		Chronologic Age < 28 Days				Chronologic Age > 28 Days
		Body Weight ≤ 2000 g		Body Weight > 2000 g		
Antibiotic	Route	0-7 Days Old	8-28 Days Old	0-7 Days Old	8-28 Days Old	
Meropenem	IV	80 div q12h	120 div q8h	80 div q12h	120 div q8h	120 div q8h
Metronidazole	IV, PO	7.5 div q24h	15 div q12h	15 div q12h	30 div q12h	30 div q6h
Nafcillin, oxacillin	IV	100 div q12h	150-200 div q8h	150 div q8h	150-200 div q6h	150-200 div q6h
Penicillin G, crystalline	IV	200,000 U div q12h	300,000 U div q8h	300,000 U div q8h	400,000 U div q6h	400,000 U div q6h
Piperacillin	IV	200 div q12h	300 div q8h	200 div q12h	300 div q8h	400 div q6h
Rifampin	IV, PO	10-20 q24h	10-20 q24h	10-20 q24h	10-20 q24h	10-20 q24h
Ticarcillin	IV	200 div q12h	300 div q8h	300 div q8h	300 div q6h	300 div q6h
Voriconazole	IV, PO	8-20 div q12h	8-20 div q12	8-20 div q12 h	8-20 div q12 h	8-20 div q12 h
Acyclovir	IV	20 q12h	20 q12h	20 q8h	20 q8h	
Amikacin[†]	IV, IM	7.5 q24h	10 q24	15 q24h	15 q24h	
Ganciclovir	IV	6 q24h	6 q18h	6 q12h	6 q12h	
Gentamicin[‡]	IV, IM	2.5 q24h	3 q18h	4 q24h	4 q24h	
Tobramycin[‡]	IV, IM	2.5 q24h	3 q18h	4 q24h	4 q24h	
Vancomycin[§]	IV	15 q24h	15 q18h[‖]	15 q12h[‖]	15 q8h[‖]	

Adapted from Bradley JS, Nelson JD. 2006-2007 Nelson's pocket book of pediatric antimicrobial therapy. 16th ed. Buenos Aires: Alliance for World Wide Editing; 2006.

div, Divided; *IM,* intramuscular; *IV,* intravenous; *PO,* by mouth.

*Cefepime for severe infections (e.g., meningitis or pseudomonas infections) should be given at 90 mg/kg/day div q8h for the first 2 weeks of age, after which the dosing increases to 150 mg/kg/day q8h.

[†]Desired serum concentrations: 20-30 µg/mL (peak), < 10 µg/mL (trough).

[‡]Desired serum concentrations: 5-12 µg/mL (peak), < 2.0 µg/mL (trough).

[§]Desired serum concentrations: 20-40 µg/mL (peak), < 10-15 µg/mL (trough).

[‖]At 28 days of age (4 weeks), vancomycin is dosed at 20 mg/kg/dose. The interval remains the same.

as cefotaxime has been associated with significantly higher mortality in adults.[75] It is therefore recommended that such infections should be treated with a carbapenem antibiotic (meropenem or imipenem), possibly in combination with an aminoglycoside.[76] Studies on the impact of these organisms in NICUs and the appropriate antimicrobial therapy of neonatal infections with these organisms are needed.

The treatment of GBS meningitis is ampicillin or penicillin G. No GBS resistance to penicillin G in the United States has been documented despite its extensive use in mothers and neonates. However, a report from Japan suggests that the organism may be capable of developing penicillin resistance.[78] Despite the in vitro resistance of GBS to aminoglycosides, the addition of gentamicin to a penicillin agent provides synergy. In general, gentamicin can be discontinued once CSF sterilization is documented by a second lumbar puncture performed 24 to 48 hours after initiation of therapy. For more severe cases of meningitis, some experts continue gentamicin for about 1 week; the benefit of such an approach is unproven.

Similar considerations are applicable in the preterm infant in whom meningitis develops in the NICU. Potential pathogens include *S. aureus*, coagulase-negative staphylococci, enterococci, and multiple drug–resistant organisms such as MRSA and gentamicin- or cephalosporin-resistant gram-negative enteric bacilli. Empiric therapy may include a combination of ampicillin, nafcillin, or vancomycin and an aminoglycoside, cefotaxime, or even meropenem, depending on the predominant pathogens seen in that NICU. Ceftazidime or meropenem in combination with an aminoglycoside should be used for *P. aeruginosa* meningitis. *Chryseobacterium* (formerly *Flavobacterium*) *meningosepticum*, a multiple drug–resistant gram-negative bacillus, is a rare cause of meningitis that requires treatment with vancomycin and rifampin, or even ciprofloxacin.

Meningitis due to anaerobic bacteria is uncommon, and is usually caused by *Bacteroides fragilis* and *Clostridium* spp., mostly *Clostridium perfringens*.[79] The mortality rate is high. Penicillin, ampicillin, cephalosporins, and vancomycin are active against many gram-positive anaerobes. They have little if any activity against most anaerobic gram-negative bacilli; metronidazole is the agent of choice for meningitis secondary to these organisms. Carbapenem antibiotics such as meropenem and imipenem have excellent anaerobic activity against both gram-positive and negative organisms and also can be used.

The treatment of neonatal infections caused by *Ureaplasma* spp. and *Mycoplasma hominis* is complicated by the susceptibility patterns of these organisms because they usually are resistant to most antibiotics commonly used in neonates.[80] For infections due to *Ureaplasma* spp., doxycycline is recommended, with azithromycin as an alternative. For *M. hominis*, doxycycline or clindamycin is preferred, with ciprofloxacin as an alternative. Although the exact duration of therapy is not known, a 10- to 14-day course seems reasonable when there is associated clinical improvement and microbiologic eradication during that period.

Neonatal fungal infection of the CNS is usually caused by *Candida* spp.[81] Amphotericin deoxycholate remains the treatment of choice,[82] and it has been used successfully as monotherapy.[83] Amphotericin B lipid formulations may be used if renal toxicity occurs while the infant is receiving the deoxycholate preparation. Fluconazole has excellent CNS penetration and is frequently added to amphotericin therapy in cases of persistent fungemia or poor clinical response.[84-87] There is limited experience in neonates with the use of newer azoles such as voriconazole that are active against more resistant fungi such as *C. krusei* and *C. glabrata*.[88,89] Concern exists for CNS penetration of echinocandins such as caspofungin and micofungin although higher doses of the latter in animal models have been successful.[42,90-96]

CONTINUATION OF CASE HISTORY

A second lumbar puncture was performed 24 hours after diagnosis of meningitis, and the CSF showed 6900 white blood cells/mm^3 (90% polymorphonuclear cells, 10% mononuclear cells), 2400 red blood cells/mm^3, a protein value of 550 mg/dL, and a glucose value of 21 mg/dL. Culture of CSF again yielded *E. coli* that was resistant to ampicillin but susceptible to cefotaxime, ceftazidime, and gentamicin with minimum inhibitory concentrations (MICs) of 2 μg/mL.

Question 6: Should Other Therapies Be Considered?

Meningitis secondary to gram-negative bacilli is associated with persistently positive CSF culture results despite appropriate therapy. The median duration of positive CSF culture results is 3 days, and the duration of positivity has been correlated with worse long-term prognosis and higher mortality.[97] In addition, the duration of a positive CSF culture result will affect the total length of therapy. For these reasons, it is recommended that daily or every-other-day lumbar punctures be performed in order to determine both occurrence and timing of CSF sterilization.

Both lumbar intrathecal and intraventricular gentamicin have been used for treatment of gram-negative meningitis.[98-100] Ventriculitis occurs in at least 70% of cases, and the ventricular fluid is poorly accessible to systemically administered antibiotics. However, among infants who received parenteral gentamicin alone or parenteral plus intrathecal therapy (1 mg/day for at least 3 days), no differences in either case-fatality rate or neurologic residua were observed by the Neonatal Meningitis Cooperative Study Group.[98] These investigators subsequently studied the use of intraventricular gentamicin (2.5 mg); there was higher mortality among infants who received intraventricular gentamicin (43%) in combination with ampicillin and gentamicin than in those who received systemic antibiotics alone (13%).[99] Subsequent evaluation of ventricular fluid from infants who received intraventricular gentamicin showed significantly greater concentrations of tumor necrosis factor and interleukin-1β in their CSF, indicating that greater inflammatory injury may result from this form of therapy.[100] In general, intraventricular therapy is not recommended, although it remains an option in those infants in whom a ventricular drain is already in place and CSF culture results are persistently positive.

CONTINUATION OF CASE HISTORY

Cranial ultrasound scans performed on days 2 and 7 after presentation did not demonstrate abscess formation or new intracranial hemorrhage but did show mild ventricular dilation, and echogenic debris and septations were visualized within the ventricular system (Fig. 11-1). The infant continued to receive cefotaxime and was nearing 21 days of therapy.

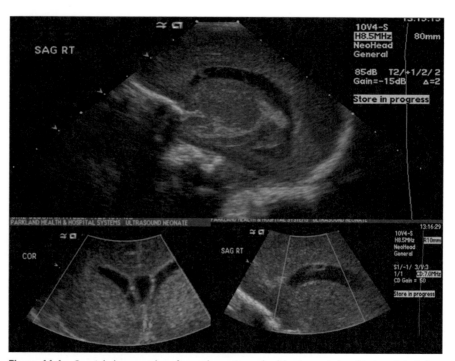

Figure 11-1 Cranial ultrasound performed on a 2-week-old extremely low-birth-weight infant with meningitis caused by *Escherichia coli*. Echogenic debris and septation consistent with purulent material can be seen within the dilated lateral ventricle.

Question 7: What is the Duration of Treatment for Meningitis in Neonates?

Unfortunately, there are no randomized studies of duration of antibiotic therapy for neonatal meningitis. In general, duration of therapy depends on the causative organism, site(s) of infection, clinical severity, and course. It is usually 7 days for uncomplicated bacteremia, 7 to 10 days for sepsis and pneumonia, and 14 to 21 days for meningitis, depending on the causative agent. Normalization of levels of C-reactive protein or other inflammatory markers such as IL-8 and IL-10 has been utilized to discontinue antibiotic therapy.[101,102] Although this approach seems reasonable, more studies involving high-risk neonates with serious infections such as meningitis are needed before such a strategy can be recommended routinely.

For meningitis due to gram-negative bacilli, the duration of antimicrobial therapy is a minimum of 21 days or 2 weeks after the first sterile CSF culture result, whichever is longer. Earlier discontinuation of antimicrobial therapy may result in infection relapse. Performance of another lumbar puncture after 21 days of treatment in infants with gram-negative enteric meningitis and before discontinuation of antibiotic therapy is useful to determine the adequacy of therapy. Markedly abnormal CSF findings, such as glucose concentration lower than 25 mg/dL, protein content higher than 300 mg/dL, or more than 50% polymorphonuclear cells, without other explanation warrant continued antimicrobial therapy in order to prevent relapse.

For meningitis due to GBS, a minimum of 14 days of antimicrobial therapy is recommended. The decision of whether to perform an end of therapy lumbar puncture in the neonate with this disorder can be based on the clinical course. If the infant has experienced a complication such as seizures, significant hypotension, or prolonged positive CSF culture results, or if neuroimaging findings are abnormal, the lumbar puncture is probably prudent.

The optimal duration of therapy for meningitis due to other microorganisms is not known. Meningitis secondary to *S. aureus* should be treated with at least 3 weeks of antibiotic therapy. In general, cerebral abscess requires more prolonged therapy, 4 to 6 weeks, depending on whether the abscess is surgically drained or there is persistence of abnormalities on neuroimaging.

Question 8: When Should Neuroimaging Be Considered, and What Type of Examination is Recommended?

The timing and the reason for performing neuroimaging studies are important considerations in the decision about which type of study should be performed. Cranial ultrasonography is safe, convenient, and readily available; it can be done at the bedside and does not require sedation. It provides rapid and reliable information on ventricular size and presence or absence of hydrocephalus.[103] It is therefore useful to perform an ultrasound scan early in the course, when the infant's condition is too critical for transport to the radiology department. Cranial ultrasonography also provides information on periventricular white matter injury; initially, ischemia may be manifested by increased periventricular echogenicity, which may progress to cystic periventricular leukomalacia in later studies (Fig. 11-2).[104,105] Ultrasonography, however, does not allow for optimal evaluation of parenchymal abnormalities such as infarct and abscess nor of the presence of subdural empyema, all known complications of neonatal meningitis.

Computed tomography (CT) provides information on whether the course of meningitis has been complicated by a cerebral abscess, hydrocephalus, or subdural collections. In general, however, this modality should be avoided unless neuroimaging is required on an emergency basis because its use has been associated with subsequent neurodevelopmental impairment and increased risk for cancer.[106,107]

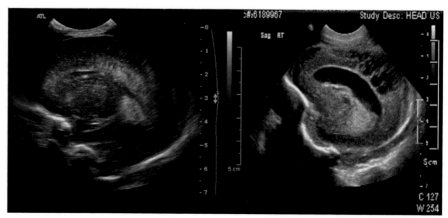

Figure 11-2   Cranial ultrasound scan performed on an extremely low-birth-weight infant with meningitis. Echogenic periventricular white matter *(left)* with subsequent progression to cystic periventricular leukomalacia *(right)* is shown.

Magnetic resonance imaging (MRI) is the best currently available modality for evaluation of the neonatal brain.[108] It provides excellent information on the status of the white matter, cortex, subdural and epidural spaces, and even the posterior fossa in cases of tuberculous meningitis (Fig. 11-3). In addition, it has been used in preterm infants to predict neurodevelopmental outcome.[109] For these reasons, infants in whom cerebral injury is suspected, because of abnormalities on ultrasonography, seizures, persistent CSF abnormalities, or meningitis due to organisms such as *Citrobacter koseri* (formerly *C. diversus*) or fungi that are associated with abscess formation, should undergo brain MRI.[110] Cerebral abscess complicates the course of about 70% of cases of *C. koseri* meningitis, whereas it occurs in less than 10% of cases of meningitis due to other gram-negative enteric bacilli (Fig. 11-4).[111,112] Microabscesses also are not infrequent with neonatal fungal meningitis. For these reasons, many experts recommend that at least one brain MRI be performed in every case of neonatal meningitis. The timing of the MRI is important, in that MRI performed near the end of therapy will more likely detect the extent of the CNS injury. On the other hand, if the head ultrasound scan or clinical course raises concern about obstructive hydrocephalus or intracranial abscess, earlier MRI is warranted. In addition, all infants with meningitis require hearing evaluation.

Question 9: Should Other Adjunctive Therapies Be Provided to an Infant with Meningitis?

Dexamethasone has been shown in some studies to decrease neurologic morbidity in older infants and children with meningitis.[113-115] No studies are available in neonates, and its use is not recommended. In a rabbit model of *E. coli* meningitis, the addition of dexamethasone to standard antibiotic therapy was associated with an increase in hippocampal neuronal apoptosis.[113] IVIG has not been shown to improve outcome in neonatal sepsis and meningitis and should not be used routinely.[114,115]

The prolonged use of broad-spectrum antimicrobial agents, especially third-generation cephalosporins and carbapenems, has been associated with the development of systemic candidiasis in preterm infants with a birth weight less than 1500 g.[116] Prophylactic fluconazole has been shown to decrease the incidence of candidiasis in these infants,[117-119] and it use should be considered in preterm infants with meningitis who require prolonged broad-spectrum antimicrobial therapy.[120] No data from randomized controlled clinical trials are available in infants with a birth weight higher than 1500 g.

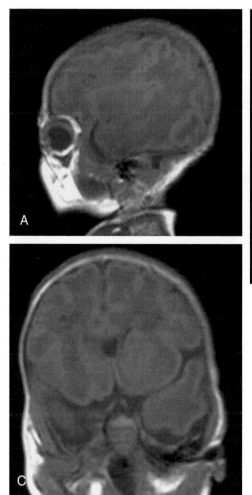

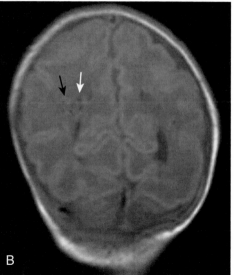

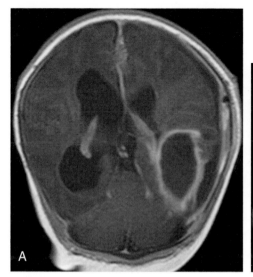

Figure 11-3 Magnetic resonance imaging of the brain of an infant who 4 weeks earlier had *Pseudomonas aeruginosa* sepsis and meningitis. **A,** On the T2-weighted image, small foci of high signal can be seen in the periventricular white matter in the frontoparietal and occipital regions. These represent areas of cystic encephalomalacia, consistent with periventricular leukomalacia. **B,** Small foci of hemosiderin deposition *(black arrow)* can be seen in the posterior right temporo-occipital region along with cystic encephalomalacia changes *(white arrow)*. **C,** Coronal image of periventricular white matter.

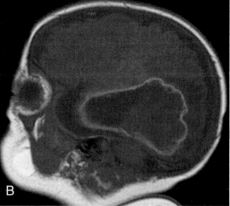

Figure 11-4 A, Magnetic resonance image of the brain of a 3-week-old full-term infant with meningitis and cerebral abscess caused by *Serratia marcescens*. **B,** Following gadolinium administration, a large ring-enhancing lesion is shown that extends from the posterior aspect of the temporal lobe into the adjacent parietal and occipital white matter.

Question 10: What If the Infant's CSF Is Abnormal but Routine Bacterial Cultures of CSF and Blood Are Sterile?

The most frequent reason for a sterile CSF culture despite CSF changes indicative of meningitis is previous antimicrobial therapy. However, intraventricular hemorrhage can result in inflammatory changes such as pleocytosis with predominance of polymorphonuclear cells, elevated protein concentration, and hypoglycorrhachia in the absence of an infectious process, making the performance of a lumbar puncture before initiation of antimicrobial therapy important.

When an infant in whom sepsis and meningitis is suspected has abnormal CSF indices but routine bacterial cultures are sterile, a second lumbar puncture should be performed. Pathogens that can produce aseptic meningitis should be excluded (see Table 11-1), especially because specific therapy is available for some of them. CSF specimens should be sent for anaerobic, *Mycoplasma*, fungal, and viral cultures, as well as testing for herpes and polymerase chain reaction (PCR) analysis for enteroviruses.

CONTINUATION OF CASE HISTORY

The infant's CSF indices were markedly improved after 21 days of cefotaxime, and MRI revealed only mild ventriculomegaly. At discharge to home at 3 months of age, the infant passed an automated auditory brainstem response test. At 22 months of corrected gestational age, the infant had mild impairment in both mental and psychomotor development indices of the Bayley Scales of Infant Development.

Question 11: What is the Outcome of Meningitis in Neonates?

Despite improvements in neonatal care and antibiotic therapy for meningitis, significant morbidity and mortality persist.[121] Among preterm infants with a birth weight of 1000 g or less, those with meningitis are more likely to have low (<70) Bayley mental and psychomotor indices, cerebral palsy, vision impairment, and head circumference lower than the 10th percentile than uninfected infants of similar birth weight and gestation.[125]

Among infants with gram-negative enteric meningitis, the case-fatality rate and morbidity remain high. Approximately 20% to 30% of affected infants die, and neurologic sequelae are found in 35% to 50% of survivors.[98,99,126] These include hydrocephalus (30%), seizure disorder (30%), developmental delay (30%), cerebral palsy (25%), and hearing loss (15%). Ten percent have severe sequelae, defined as failure to develop beyond the age at which the disease occurred or requirement for custodial care. It is hoped that prediction of late morbidity will be aided by the use of brain MRI performed toward the end of therapy.

Among infants with GBS meningitis, the mortality is about 25%, and among survivors, another 25% to 30% of children have major neurologic sequelae, such as spastic quadriplegia, profound mental retardation, hemiparesis, deafness, and cortical blindness; 15% to 20% have mild to moderate sequelae; and 50% to 60% are normal when compared with sibling controls.[127,128] The occurrence of seizures during the acute illness has been associated with a poor prognosis; infants who had seizures were more likely to die or sustain major sequelae than those who did not. On the other hand, children not identified early as having major sequelae performed intellectually, socially, and academically in a manner similar to other family members.[127,128]

Conclusions

Meningitis is a serious life-threatening infection for which early therapy is mandatory to improve both short- and long-term outcomes. Early therapy is possible only with the timely recognition of its occurrence, thus making performance of a lumbar puncture for CSF analysis and culture the key to rapid institution of effective antimicrobial therapy. Ultimately, however, the prevention of neonatal meningitis will be achieved when neonatal sepsis is controlled, an elusive but not impossible goal in neonatal medicine today.

References

1. Kaufman D, Fairchild KD. Clinical microbiology of bacterial and fungal sepsis in very-low-birth-weight infants. *Clin Microbiol Rev.* 2004;17:638-680, table of contents.
2. Palazzi DLKJO, Baker CJ. Bacterial sepsis and meningitis. In: Jack S, Remington JOK, Christopher BW, Carol JB, eds. *Infectious diseases of the fetus and newborn infant.* 6th ed. Philadelphia: Elsevier Saunders; 2006:1328.
3. Giacoia GP. Uncommon pathogens in newborn infants. *J Perinatol.* 1994;14:134-144.
4. Stoll BJ, Hansen NI, Sanchez PJ, et al. Early onset neonatal sepsis: the burden of group B streptococcal and *E. coli* disease continues. *Pediatrics.* 2011;127:817-826.
5. Verani JR, McGee L, Schrag SJ. Prevention of perinatal group B streptococcal disease—revised guidelines from CDC, 2010. *MMWR Recomm Rep.* 2010;59(RR-10):1-36.
6. Johnson CE, Whitwell JK, Pethe K, et al. Term newborns who are at risk for sepsis: are lumbar punctures necessary? *Pediatrics.* 1997;99:E10.
7. Smith PB, Cotten CM, Garges HP, et al. A comparison of neonatal Gram-negative rod and Gram-positive cocci meningitis. *J Perinatol.* 2006;26:111-114.
8. Schrag SJ, Zywicki S, Farley MM, et al. Group B streptococcal disease in the era of intrapartum antibiotic prophylaxis. *N Engl J Med.* 2000;342:15-20.
9. Schrag SJ, Hadler JL, Arnold KE, et al. Risk factors for invasive, early-onset Escherichia coli infections in the era of widespread intrapartum antibiotic use. *Pediatrics.* 2006;118:570-576.
10. Baltimore RS, Huie SM, Meek JI, et al. Early-onset neonatal sepsis in the era of group B streptococcal prevention. *Pediatrics.* 2001;108:1094-1098.
11. Stoll BJ, Hansen N, Fanaroff AA, et al. Changes in pathogens causing early-onset sepsis in very-low-birth-weight infants. *N Engl J Med.* 2002;347:240-247.
12. Stoll BJ, Hansen NI, Higgins RD, et al. Very low birth weight preterm infants with early onset neonatal sepsis: the predominance of gram-negative infections continues in the National Institute of Child Health and Human Development Neonatal Research Network, 2002-2003. *Pediatr Infect Dis J.* 2005;24:635-639.
13. Garges HP, Moody MA, Cotten CM, et al. Neonatal meningitis: what is the correlation among cerebrospinal fluid cultures, blood cultures, and cerebrospinal fluid parameters? *Pediatrics.* 2006;117:1094-1100.
14. Stoll BJ, Hansen N, Fanaroff AA, et al. To tap or not to tap: high likelihood of meningitis without sepsis among very low birth weight infants. *Pediatrics.* 2004;113:1181-1186.
15. Cohen-Wolkowiez M, Smith PB, Mangum B, et al. Neonatal *Candida* meningitis: significance of cerebrospinal fluid parameters and blood cultures. *J Perinatol.* 2007;27:97-100.
16. Wiswell TE, Baumgart S, Gannon CM, Spitzer AR. No lumbar puncture in the evaluation for early neonatal sepsis: will meningitis be missed? *Pediatrics.* 1995;95:803-806.
17. Malbon K, Mohan R, Nicholl R. Should a neonate with possible late onset infection always have a lumbar puncture? *Arch Dis Child.* 2006;91:75-76.
18. Greenberg RG, Smith PB, Cotten CM, et al. Traumatic lumbar punctures in neonates: test performance of the cerebrospinal fluid white blood cell count. *Pediatr Infect Dis J.* 2008;27:1047-1051.
19. Ahmed A, Hickey SM, Ehrett S, et al. Cerebrospinal fluid values in the term neonate. *Pediatr Infect Dis J.* 1996;15:298-303.
20. Bonadio WA. The cerebrospinal fluid: physiologic aspects and alterations associated with bacterial meningitis. *Pediatr Infect Dis J.* 1992;11:423-431.
21. Pappu LD, Purohit DM, Levkoff AH, Kaplan B. CSF cytology in the neonate. *Am J Dis Child.* 1982;136:297-298.
22. Portnoy JM, Olson LC. Normal cerebrospinal fluid values in children: another look. *Pediatrics.* 1985;75:484-487.
23. Rodriguez AF, Kaplan SL, Mason EO Jr. Cerebrospinal fluid values in the very low birth weight infant. *J Pediatr.* 1990;116:971-974.
24. Sarff LD, Platt LH, McCracken GH Jr. Cerebrospinal fluid evaluation in neonates: comparison of high-risk infants with and without meningitis. *J Pediatr.* 1976;88:473-477.
25. Naidoo BT. The cerebrospinal fluid in the healthy newborn infant. *S Afr Med J.* 1968;42(35):933-935.
26. O'Shea TM, Klinepeter KL, Meis PJ, Dillard RG. Intrauterine infection and the risk of cerebral palsy in very low-birthweight infants. *Paediatr Perinat Epidemiol.* 1998;12:72-83.
27. Eldadah M, Frenkel LD, Hiatt IM, Hegyi T. Evaluation of routine lumbar punctures in newborn infants with respiratory distress syndrome. *Pediatr Infect Dis J.* 1987;6:243-246.

11

28. Hendricks-Munoz KD, Shapiro DL. The role of the lumbar puncture in the admission sepsis evaluation of the premature infant. *J Perinatol.* 1990;10:60-64.

29. MacMahon P, Jewes L, de Louvois J. Routine lumbar punctures in the newborn—are they justified? *Eur J Pediatr.* 1990;149:797-799.

30. Weiss MG, Ionides SP, Anderson CL. Meningitis in premature infants with respiratory distress: role of admission lumbar puncture. *J Pediatr.* 1991;119:973-975.

31. Isaacs D, Dobson S. When to do a lumbar puncture in a neonate. *Arch Dis Child.* 1989;64:1513-1514.

32. Ansong AK, Smith PB, Benjamin DK, et al. Group B streptococcal meningitis: cerebrospinal fluid parameters in the era of intrapartum antibiotic prophylaxis. *Early Hum Dev.* 2009;85(10 Suppl):S5-S7.

33. Laborada G, Rego M, Jain A, et al. Diagnostic value of cytokines and C-reactive protein in the first 24 hours of neonatal sepsis. *Am J Perinatol.* 2003;20:491-501.

34. Verboon-Maciolek MA, Thijsen SF, Hemels MA, et al. Inflammatory mediators for the diagnosis and treatment of sepsis in early infancy. *Pediatr Res.* 2006;59:457-461.

35. Manroe BL, Weinberg AG, Rosenfeld CR, Browne R. The neonatal blood count in health and disease. I. Reference values for neutrophilic cells. *J Pediatr.* 1979;95:89-98.

36. Mouzinho A, Rosenfeld CR, Sanchez PJ, Risser R. Revised reference ranges for circulating neutrophils in very-low-birth-weight neonates. *Pediatrics.* 1994;94:76-82.

37. Engle WD, Rosenfeld CR, Mouzinho A, et al. Circulating neutrophils in septic preterm neonates: comparison of two reference ranges. *Pediatrics.* 1997;99:E10.

38. Christensen RD, Brown MS, Hall DC, et al. Effect on neutrophil kinetics and serum opsonic capacity of intravenous administration of immune globulin to neonates with clinical signs of early-onset sepsis. *J Pediatr.* 1991;118:606-614.

39. Christensen RD, Calhoun DA, Rimsza LM. A practical approach to evaluating and treating neutropenia in the neonatal intensive care unit. *Clin Perinatol.* 2000;27:577-601.

40. Cairo MS, Worcester CC, Rucker RW, et al. Randomized trial of granulocyte transfusions versus intravenous immune globulin therapy for neonatal neutropenia and sepsis. *J Pediatr.* 1992;120:281-285.

41. Shaw CK, Thapalial A, Shaw P, Malla K. Intravenous immunoglobulins and haematopoietic growth factors in the prevention and treatment of neonatal sepsis: ground reality or glorified myths? *Int J Clin Pract.* 2007;61:482-487.

42. Benjamin DK Jr, DeLong ER, Steinbach WJ, et al. Empirical therapy for neonatal candidemia in very low birth weight infants. *Pediatrics.* 2003;112:543-547.

43. Manzoni P, Mostert M, Galletto P, et al. Is thrombocytopenia suggestive of organism-specific response in neonatal sepsis? *Pediatr Int.* 2009;51:206-210.

44. Struthers S, Underhill H, Albersheim S, et al. A comparison of two versus one blood culture in the diagnosis and treatment of coagulase-negative staphylococcus in the neonatal intensive care unit. *J Perinatol.* 2002;22:547-549.

45. Rubin LG, Sanchez PJ, Siegel J, et al. Evaluation and treatment of neonates with suspected late-onset sepsis: a survey of neonatologists' practices. *Pediatrics.* 2002;110:e42.

46. Schulman J, Stricof R, Stevens TP, et al. Statewide NICU central-line-associated bloodstream infection rates decline after bundles and checklists. *Pediatrics.* 2011;127:436-444.

47. Bauer S, Eliakim A, Pomeranz A, et al. Urinary tract infection in very low birth weight preterm infants. *Pediatr Infect Dis J.* 2003;22:426-430.

48. Subcommittee on Urinary Tract Infection, Steering Committee on Quality Improvement and Management. Urinary tract infection: clinical practice guideline for the diagnosis and management of the initial UTI in febrile infants and children 2 to 24 months. *Pediatrics.* 2011;128:595-610.

49. Sanchez PJ. Bacterial and fungal infections in the neonate: current diagnosis and therapy. *Adv Exp Med Biol.* 2004;549:97-103.

50. Chiu CH, Michelow IC, Cronin J, et al. Effectiveness of a guideline to reduce vancomycin use in the neonatal intensive care unit. *Pediatr Infect Dis J.* 2011;30:273-278.

51. Karlowicz MG, Buescher ES, Surka AE. Fulminant late-onset sepsis in a neonatal intensive care unit, 1988-1997, and the impact of avoiding empiric vancomycin therapy. *Pediatrics.* 2000;106:1387-1390.

52. Krediet TG, Jones ME, Gerards LJ, Fleer A. Clinical outcome of cephalothin versus vancomycin therapy in the treatment of coagulase-negative staphylococcal septicemia in neonates: relation to methicillin resistance and mec A gene carriage of blood isolates. *Pediatrics.* 1999;103:E29.

53. Lawrence SL, Roth V, Slinger R, et al. Cloxacillin versus vancomycin for presumed late-onset sepsis in the neonatal intensive care unit and the impact upon outcome of coagulase negative staphylococcal bacteremia: a retrospective cohort study. *BMC Pediatr.* 2005;5:49.

54. Stoll BJ, Hansen N, Fanaroff AA, et al. Late-onset sepsis in very low birth weight neonates: the experience of the NICHD Neonatal Research Network. *Pediatrics.* 2002;110:285-291.

55. Jean-Baptiste N, Benjamin DK Jr, Cohen-Wolkowiez M, et al. Coagulase-negative staphylococcal infections in the neonatal intensive care unit. *Infect Control Hosp Epidemiol.* 2011;32:679-686.

56. Garcia-Prats JA, Cooper TR, Schneider VF, et al. Rapid detection of microorganisms in blood cultures of newborn infants utilizing an automated blood culture system. *Pediatrics.* 2000;105:523-527.

57. Van Houten MA, Uiterwaal CS, Heesen GJ, et al. Does the empiric use of vancomycin in pediatrics increase the risk for gram-negative bacteremia? *Pediatr Infect Dis J.* 2001;20:171-177.

58. Healy CM, Hulten KG, Palazzi DL, et al. Emergence of new strains of methicillin-resistant *Staphylococcus aureus* in a neonatal intensive care unit. *Clin Infect Dis.* 2004;39:1460-1466.

59. Chuang YY, Huang YC, Lee CY, et al. Methicillin-resistant *Staphylococcus aureus* bacteraemia in neonatal intensive care units: an analysis of 90 episodes. *Acta Paediatr*. 2004;93:786-790.
60. Haley RW, Cushion NB, Tenover FC, et al. Eradication of endemic methicillin-resistant Staphylococcus aureus infections from a neonatal intensive care unit. *J Infect Dis*. 1995;171:614-624.
61. de Hoog M, Mouton JW, van den Anker JN. New dosing strategies for antibacterial agents in the neonate. *Semin Fetal Neonatal Med*. 2005;10:185-194.
62. Nestaas E, Bangstad HJ, Sandvik L, Wathne KO. Aminoglycoside extended interval dosing in neonates is safe and effective: a meta-analysis. *Arch Dis Child Fetal Neonatal Ed*. 2005;90:F294-F300.
63. Jackson GL, Sendelbach DM, Stehel EK, et al. Association of hypocalcemia with a change in gentamicin administration in neonates. *Pediatr Nephrol*. 2003;18:653-656.
64. de Man P, Verhoeven BA, Verbrugh HA, et al. An antibiotic policy to prevent emergence of resistant bacilli. *Lancet*. 2000;355:973-978.
65. Acolet D, Ahmet Z, Houang E, et al. *Enterobacter cloacae* in a neonatal intensive care unit: account of an outbreak and its relationship to use of third generation cephalosporins. *J Hosp Infect*. 1994;28:273-286.
66. Bryan CS, John JF Jr, Pai MS, Austin TL. Gentamicin vs cefotaxime for therapy of neonatal sepsis. Relationship to drug resistance. *Am J Dis Child*. 1985;139:1086-1089.
67. Clark RH, Bloom BT, Spitzer AR, Gerstmann DR. Empiric use of ampicillin and cefotaxime, compared with ampicillin and gentamicin, for neonates at risk for sepsis is associated with an increased risk of neonatal death. *Pediatrics*. 2006;117:67-74.
68. Bradley JNJ. *Nelson's pocket book of pediatric antimicrobial therapy*. 16th ed. Buenos Aires: AWWE; 2006-2007.
69. Ellis JM, Rivera L, Reyes G, et al. Cefepime cerebrospinal fluid concentrations in neonatal bacterial meningitis. *Ann Pharmacother*. 2007;41:900-901.
70. Capparelli E, Hochwald C, Rasmussen M, et al. Population pharmacokinetics of cefepime in the neonate. *Antimicrob Agents Chemother*. 2005;49:2760-2766.
71. Shah D, Narang, M. Drug therapy: Meropenem. *Indian Pediatr*. 2004;42:443-450.
72. Odio CM, Puig JR, Feris JM, et al. Prospective, randomized, investigator-blinded study of the efficacy and safety of meropenem vs. cefotaxime therapy in bacterial meningitis in children. Meropenem Meningitis Study Group. *Pediatr Infect Dis J*. 1999;18:581-590.
73. van den Anker JN, Pokorna P, Kinzig-Schippers M, et al. Meropenem pharmacokinetics in the newborn. *Antimicrob Agents Chemother*. 2009;53:3871-3879.
74. Ahmed A, Paris MM, Trujillo M, et al. Once-daily gentamicin therapy for experimental *Escherichia coli* meningitis. *Antimicrob Agents Chemother*. 1997;41:49-53.
75. Wong-Beringer A, Hindler J, Loeloff M, et al. Molecular correlation for the treatment outcomes in bloodstream infections caused by *Escherichia coli* and *Klebsiella pneumoniae* with reduced susceptibility to ceftazidime. *Clin Infect Dis*. 2002;34:135-146.
76. Patterson JE. Extended spectrum beta-lactamases: a therapeutic dilemma. *Pediatr Infect Dis J*. 2002;21:957-959.
77. Sinha AK, Kempley ST, Price E, et al. Early onset *Morganella morganii* sepsis in a newborn infant with emergence of cephalosporin resistance caused by depression of AMPC beta-lactamase production. *Pediatr Infect Dis J*. 2006;25:376-377.
78. Kimura KWJKH, Suzuki S, et al. Emergence of penicillin-resistant group B streptococci. Presented at 46th Annual Interscience Conference on Antimicrobial Agents and Chemotherapy (ICAAC). San Francisco; 2006.
79. Brook I. Anaerobic infections in the neonate. *Adv Pediatr*. 1994;41:369-383.
80. Cassell GH, Waites KB, Watson HL, et al. *Ureaplasma urealyticum* intrauterine infection: role in prematurity and disease in newborns. *Clin Microbiol Rev*. 1993;6:69-87.
81. Fernandez M, Moylett EH, Noyola DE, Baker CJ. Candidal meningitis in neonates: a 10-year review. *Clin Infect Dis*. 2000;31:458-463.
82. Frattarelli DA, Reed MD, Giacoia GP, Aranda JV. Antifungals in systemic neonatal candidiasis. *Drugs*. 2004;64:949-968.
83. Butler KM, Rench MA, Baker CJ. Amphotericin B as a single agent in the treatment of systemic candidiasis in neonates. *Pediatr Infect Dis J*. 1990;9:51-56.
84. Gurses N, Kalayci AG. Fluconazole monotherapy for candidal meningitis in a premature infant. *Clin Infect Dis*. 1996;23:645-646.
85. Black KE, Baden LR. Fungal infections of the CNS: treatment strategies for the immunocompromised patient. *CNS Drugs*. 2007;21:293-318.
86. Wade KC, Benjamin DK Jr, Kaufman DA, et al. Fluconazole dosing for the prevention or treatment of invasive candidiasis in young infants. *Pediatr Infect Dis J*. 2009;28:717-723.
87. Watt K, Benjamin DK Jr, Cohen-Wolkowiez M. Pharmacokinetics of antifungal agents in children. *Early Hum Dev*. 2011;87(Suppl 1):S61-S65.
88. Steinbach WJ, Benjamin DK Jr. New antifungal agents under development in children and neonates. *Curr Opin Infect Dis*. 2005;18:484-489.
89. Santos RP, Sanchez PJ, Mejias A, et al. Successful medical treatment of cutaneous aspergillosis in a premature infant using liposomal amphotericin B, voriconazole and micafungin. *Pediatr Infect Dis J*. 2007;26:364-366.
90. Odio CM, Araya R, Pinto LE, et al. Caspofungin therapy of neonates with invasive candidiasis. *Pediatr Infect Dis J*. 2004;23:1093-1097.
91. Heresi GP, Gerstmann DR, Reed MD, et al. The pharmacokinetics and safety of micafungin, a novel echinocandin, in premature infants. *Pediatr Infect Dis J*. 2006;25:1110-1115.

92. Hope WW, Smith PB, Arrieta A, et al. Population pharmacokinetics of micafungin in neonates and young infants. *Antimicrob Agents Chemother*. 2010;54:2633-2637.

93. Ascher S, Smith PB, Benjamin DK Jr. Safety of micafungin in infants: insights into optimal dosing. *Expert Opin Drug Safe*. 2011;10:281-286.

94. Manzoni P, Rizzollo S, Franco C, et al. Role of echinocandins in the management of fungal infections in neonates. *J Matern Fetal Neonatal Med*. 2010;23(Suppl 3):49-52.

95. Cohen-Wolkowiez M, Benjamin DK Jr, Piper L, et al. Safety and pharmacokinetics of multiple-dose anidulafungin in infants and neonates. *Clin Pharmacol Ther*. 2011;89:702-707.

96. Benjamin DK Jr, Smith PB, Arrieta A, et al. Safety and pharmacokinetics of repeat-dose micafungin in young infants. *Clin Pharmacol Ther*. 2010;87:93-99.

97. Greenberg RG, Benjamin DK Jr, Cohen-Wolkowiez M, et al. Repeat lumbar punctures in infants with meningitis in the neonatal intensive care unit. *J Perinatol*. 2011;31:425-429.

98. McCracken GH Jr, Mize SG. A controlled study of intrathecal antibiotic therapy in gram-negative enteric meningitis of infancy. Report of the Neonatal Meningitis Cooperative Study Group. *J Pediatr*. 1976;89:66-72.

99. McCracken GH Jr, Mize SG, Threlkeld N. Intraventricular gentamicin therapy in gram-negative bacillary meningitis of infancy. Report of the Second Neonatal Meningitis Cooperative Study Group. *Lancet*. 1980;1(8172):787-791.

100. McCracken GH Jr, Mustafa MM, Ramilo O, et al. Cerebrospinal fluid interleukin 1-beta and tumor necrosis factor concentrations and outcome from neonatal gram-negative enteric bacillary meningitis. *Pediatr Infect Dis J*. 1989;8:155-159.

101. Franz AR, Steinbach G, Kron M, Pohlandt F. Reduction of unnecessary antibiotic therapy in newborn infants using interleukin-8 and C-reactive protein as markers of bacterial infections. *Pediatrics*. 1999;104:447-453.

102. Franz AR, Bauer K, Schalk A, et al. Measurement of interleukin 8 in combination with C-reactive protein reduced unnecessary antibiotic therapy in newborn infants: a multicenter, randomized, controlled trial. *Pediatrics*. 2004;114:1-8.

103. Perlman JM, Rollins N, Sanchez PJ. Late-onset meningitis in sick, very-low-birth-weight infants. Clinical and sonographic observations. *Am J Dis Child*. 1992;146:1297-1301.

104. Faix RG, Donn SM. Association of septic shock caused by early-onset group B streptococcal sepsis and periventricular leukomalacia in the preterm infant. *Pediatrics*. 1985;76:415-419.

105. Perlman JM. White matter injury in the preterm infant: an important determination of abnormal neurodevelopment outcome. *Early Hum Dev*. 1998;53:99-120.

106. Brenner DJ. Estimating cancer risks from pediatric CT: going from the qualitative to the quantitative. *Pediatr Radiol*. 2002;32:228-233; discussion 42-44.

107. Frush DP, Donnelly LF, Rosen NS. Computed tomography and radiation risks: what pediatric health care providers should know. *Pediatrics*. 2003;112:951-957.

108. Counsell SJ, Tranter SL, Rutherford MA. Magnetic resonance imaging of brain injury in the high-risk term infant. *Seminars in perinatology*. 2010;34:67-78.

109. Woodward LJ, Anderson PJ, Austin NC, et al. Neonatal MRI to predict neurodevelopmental outcomes in preterm infants. *N Engl J Med*. 2006;355:685-694.

110. Shah DK, Daley AJ, Hunt RW, et al. Cerebral white matter injury in the newborn following *Escherichia coli* meningitis. *Eur J Paediatr Neurol*. 2005;9:13-17.

111. Graham DR, Band JD. Citrobacter diversus brain abscess and meningitis in neonates. *JAMA*. 1981;245(19):1923-1925.

112. Doran TI. The role of *Citrobacter* in clinical disease of children: review. *Clin Infect Dis*. 1999;28:384-394.

113. Lebel MH, Freij BJ, Syrogiannopoulos GA, et al. Dexamethasone therapy for bacterial meningitis. Results of two double-blind, placebo-controlled trials. *N Engl J Med*. 1988;319:964-971.

114. Schaad UB, Kaplan SL, McCracken GH Jr. Steroid therapy for bacterial meningitis. *Clin Infect Dis*. 1995;20:685-690.

115. Wald ER, Kaplan SL, Mason EO Jr, et al. Dexamethasone therapy for children with bacterial meningitis. Meningitis Study Group. *Pediatrics*. 1995;95:21-28.

116. Spreer A, Gerber J, Hanssen M, et al. Dexamethasone increases hippocampal neuronal apoptosis in a rabbit model of *Escherichia coli* meningitis. *Pediatr Res*. 2006;60:210-215.

117. Wynn JL, Seed PC, Cotten CM. Does IVIg administration yield improved immune function in very premature neonates? *J Perinatol*. 2010;30:635-642.

118. Ohlsson A, Lacy J. Intravenous immunoglobulin for suspected or subsequently proven infection in neonates. *Cochrane Database System Rev*. 2010;(3):CD001239.

119. Cotten CM, McDonald S, Stoll B, et al. The association of third-generation cephalosporin use and invasive candidiasis in extremely low birth-weight infants. *Pediatrics*. 2006;118:717-722.

120. Kaufman D, Boyle R, Hazen KC, et al. Fluconazole prophylaxis against fungal colonization and infection in preterm infants. *N Engl J Med*. 2001;345:1660-1666.

121. Kaufman D, Boyle R, Hazen KC, et al. Twice weekly fluconazole prophylaxis for prevention of invasive *Candida* infection in high-risk infants of <1000 grams birth weight. *J Pediatr*. 2005;147:172-179.

122. Manzoni P, Stolfi I, Pugni L, et al. A multicenter, randomized trial of prophylactic fluconazole in preterm neonates. *N Engl J Med*. 2007;356(24):2483-2495.

123. Uko S, Soghier LM, Vega M, et al. Targeted short-term fluconazole prophylaxis among very low birth weight and extremely low birth weight infants. *Pediatrics*. 2006;117:1243-1252.

124. de Louvois J, Halket S, Harvey D. Neonatal meningitis in England and Wales: sequelae at 5 years of age. *Eur J Pediatr.* 2005;164:730-734.
125. Stoll BJ, Hansen NI, Adams-Chapman I, et al. Neurodevelopmental and growth impairment among extremely low-birth-weight infants with neonatal infection. *JAMA.* 2004;292:2357-2365.
126. Unhanand M, Mustafa MM, McCracken GH Jr, et al. Gram-negative enteric bacillary meningitis: a twenty-one-year experience. *J Pediatr.* 1993;122:15-21.
127. Edwards MS, Rench MA, Haffar AA, et al. Long-term sequelae of group B streptococcal meningitis in infants. *J Pediatr.* 1985;106:717-722.
128. Wald ER, Bergman I, Taylor HG, et al. Long-term outcome of group B streptococcal meningitis. *Pediatrics.* 1986;77:217-221.

11

CHAPTER 12

Neonatal Herpes Simplex Virus and Congenital Cytomegalovirus Infections

David W. Kimberlin, MD

- ● Question 1: When Does Infection Occur?
- ● Question 2: What Are the Risk Factors for Neonatal Infection?
- ● Question 3: What Are the Clinical Manifestations of Neonatal Infection and Disease?
- ● Question 4: What Are the Treatments and Outcomes for HSV and CMV Brain Infections in Neonates?
- ● Question 5: Do All Babies with HSV and CMV Infections Have to Be Treated?
- ● Question 6: What Is the Appropriate Diagnostic Approach to a Baby Suspected of Having HSV or CMV Infection?
- ● Question 7: How Should the Response to Treatment Be Monitored?
- ● Question 8: What Are the Biggest Gaps in our Current Understanding of the Natural History, Diagnosis, and Management of These Infections?
- ● Conclusions

Among the numerous viral pathogens that cause central nervous system (CNS) infections in the neonatal period, herpes simplex virus (HSV) and cytomegalovirus (CMV) are unique in their therapeutic management. Both have commercially available antiviral drugs that treat the virus, as well as evidence-based data documenting the benefit of antiviral therapy. Neonatal HSV infection is primarily acquired in the peripartum period, whereas congenital CMV infection is the most common viral infection acquired in utero. Utilization of antiviral therapy to improve disease outcomes is influenced by these differences, with antiviral therapy of neonatal HSV disease aimed primarily at improving mortality and antiviral therapy of congenital CMV infections targeting improvement in longer term audiologic outcomes. Additionally, the extent of data and clinical experience differs for the two viruses, with antiviral treatment of neonatal HSV disease being required in all cases but antiviral management of congenital CMV infection being an option rather than a requirement.

The studies conducted by the National Institute of Allergy and Infectious Diseases (NIAID) Collaborative Antiviral Study Group (CASG) over the past 30 years have defined the benefits and toxicities of antiviral treatment of these two diseases. In conducting controlled investigations of these rare infections, the CASG also has characterized the natural history of infection with these viruses in neonates. Although tremendous advances have been achieved over the past decades, questions and controversies remain for both neonatal HSV disease and congenital CMV infection.

CASE HISTORY

In the summer of July, an 8 day-old white male infant was brought to your office by his mother because he felt warm to her and was more fussy than usual. A rectal temperature in your office was 38.3° C. Physical findings were normal. Notably, the baby was well grown and there was no hepatospleno-megaly or cutaneous rash. The baby was admitted to the hospital for a rule-outsepsis evaluation. Cerebrospinal fluid (CSF) contained 38 white blood cells/mm^3 with 92% mononuclear cells on differential, 236 red blood cells/mm^3, a protein level of 110 mg/dL, and a glucose level of 38 mg/dL. In order to check electrolytes, you ordered a complete metabolic profile. Electrolyte values are normal, but the alanine aminotransferase (ALT) (an incidental laboratory value also on the panel) was elevated, at 430 U/L. As a consequence, you considered perinatal viral infections in the differential diagnosis of his febrile illness. Results of CSF and blood polymerase chain reaction (PCR) assays for HSV DNA were both positive.

Question 1: When Does Infection Occur?

Neonatal HSV Disease

Herpes simplex virus disease of the newborn is acquired at one of three distinct times: intrauterine (in utero), peripartum (perinatal), and postpartum (postnatal). Among infected infants, the time of transmission for the overwhelming majority (≈85%) of neonates is in the peripartum period.[1] An additional 10% of infected neonates acquire the virus postnatally, and the final 5% are infected with HSV in utero.[1]

Congenital CMV Infection

Cytomegalovirus infection can occur at any of these three distinct times as well (intrauterine, peripartum, and postpartum). Congenital infection, however, is synonymous with in utero acquisition and is clearly associated with long-term morbidity. In contrast, peripartum transmission can produce acute illness but rarely has long-term sequelae. Infection of women both immediately prior to and during pregnancy puts the fetus at risk for congenital CMV infection.[2,3] In utero transmission occurs following primary maternal infection, as is the case with toxoplasmosis and rubella, and also in recurrent infections, including reinfection with a different strain of the virus[4] or reactivation of latent virus.[5]

Question 2: What Are the Risk Factors for Neonatal Infection?

Neonatal HSV Infection

The five factors known to influence transmission of HSV from mother to neonate are as follows:
1. Type of maternal infection (primary vs. recurrent)[6-10]
2. Maternal antibody status[10-13]
3. Duration of rupture of membranes[9]
4. Integrity of mucocutaneous barriers (e.g., use of fetal scalp electrodes)[10,14,15]
5. Mode of delivery (cesarean section vs. vaginal)[10]

A woman with no pre-existing antibody to HSV-1 or HSV-2 who then acquires either virus has first episode primary infection. A woman with antibody to one serotype of HSV who then acquires the virus of the other serotype (e.g., has HSV-1 antibody and acquires HSV-2) has first episode nonprimary infection. A woman with reactivation of latent virus has recurrent infection. Infants born to mothers who have a first episode of genital HSV infection near term are at much greater risk for development of neonatal herpes than infants whose mothers have recurrent genital herpes.[6-10] This increased risk is due both to lower concentrations of transplacentally passaged HSV-specific antibodies (which also are less reactive to expressed

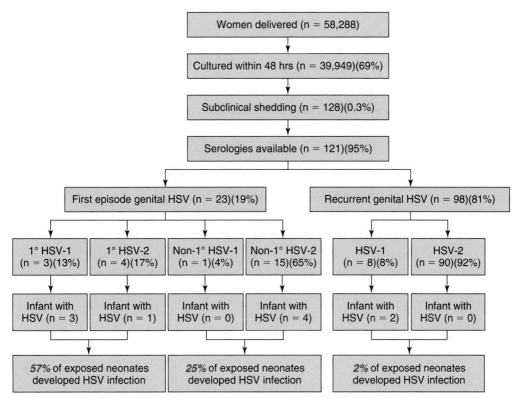

Figure 12-1 Risk of neonatal herpes simplex virus (HSV) infection as function of type of maternal infection. 1°, Primary infection. (Data from Brown ZA, Wald A, Morrow RA, et al. Effect of serologic status and cesarean delivery on transmission rates of herpes simplex virus from mother to infant. *JAMA.* 2003;289:203-209.)

polypeptides) in women with primary infection[12] and to the higher quantities of HSV that are shed for a longer period in the maternal genital tract in comparison with women with recurrent genital HSV infection.[16]

The largest assessment of the influence of type of maternal infection on likelihood of neonatal transmission is a landmark study involving almost 60,000 women in labor who did not have clinical evidence of genital HSV infection, approximately 40,000 of whom underwent vaginal culture for HSV within 48 hours of delivery (Fig. 12-1). Of these, 121 women were identified who were asymptomatically shedding HSV and for whom sera were available for serologic analysis. In this large trial, 57% of babies delivered to women with first-episode primary infection had neonatal HSV infection, compared with 25% of babies delivered to women with first episode nonprimary infection and 2% of babies delivered to women with recurrent HSV infection (see Fig. 12-1).[10]

The duration of rupture of membranes and mode of delivery also appear to affect the risk for acquisition of neonatal infection. A small study published in 1971 demonstrated that cesarean delivery in a woman with active genital lesions can reduce the infant's risk of acquiring HSV if performed within 4 hours of rupture of membranes.[9] On the basis of this observation, it has been recommended for more than 3 decades that women with active genital lesions at the time of onset of labor be delivered by cesarean section.[17] It was not until 2003, however, that cesarean delivery was definitively proven to be effective in the prevention of HSV transmission to the neonate from a mother actively shedding virus from the genital tract.[10] Importantly, neonatal infection has occurred in spite of cesarean delivery performed prior to the rupture of membranes.[18,19]

Congenital CMV Infection

Intrauterine CMV infection usually is the result of acquisition of infection by a susceptible woman from a child in the family or day care environment early during her gestation.[20-22] Multiple studies in Sweden and the United States have shown that the rate of CMV infection is much higher in children who attend day care than those who do not.[21,23-25] Many initially seronegative children become infected with CMV from their day care peers. CMV infection then is transmitted horizontally from child to child, most likely through the spread of saliva on hands and toys.[26,27] Infected children excrete large amounts of CMV for extended periods, exposing parents and other caregivers who may become pregnant.

In perinatal transmission, the amount of maternal shedding of virus directly correlates with the risk of perinatal infection. Infected breast milk and exposure to CMV in the genital tract lead to high rates of peripartum and postnatal CMV transmission.[28] Infants who breast-feed from CMV-seropositive women have an estimated rate of infection between 39% and 59%. The risk is greater when the maternal viral load is higher than 7×10^3 genome equivalents/mL. Excretion of the virus in breast milk is greatest between 2 weeks and 2 months postpartum. Infected infants usually begin to excrete CMV in saliva and urine between 3 weeks and 3 months after birth. Many of these infants excrete CMV chronically (for years), providing an opportunity to infect caretakers or others in contact with them.

Question 3: What Are the Clinical Manifestations of Neonatal Infection and Disease?

Neonatal HSV Disease

Herpes simplex virus infections acquired either peripartum or postpartum can be classified as (1) disseminated disease involving multiple visceral organs, including lung, liver, adrenal glands, skin, eye, and the brain (disseminated disease); (2) central nervous system disease, with or without skin lesions (CNS disease); or (3) disease limited to the skin, eyes, and/or mouth (SEM disease). This classification system is predictive of both morbidity and mortality.[29-33]

Neonatal HSV disseminated disease is manifest by hepatitis that is often severe, disseminated intravascular coagulopathy, and pneumonitis. The mean age at presentation (±SE) is 11.4 ± 0.8 days (see Case History).[30] Central nervous system involvement is a common component of this category of infection, occurring in about 60% to 75% of infants with disseminated disease.[34] Although the presence of a vesicular rash can greatly facilitate the diagnosis of HSV infection, more than 20% of neonates with disseminated HSV disease do not have cutaneous vesicles during the course of their illness.[18,30,35,36] Events associated with disseminated neonatal HSV infection that can result in death relate primarily to the severe coagulopathy, liver dysfunction, and pulmonary involvement of the disease.

Clinical manifestations of neonatal HSV CNS disease include seizures (both focal and generalized), lethargy, irritability, tremors, poor feeding, temperature instability, and bulging fontanelle. The mean age at presentation (±SE) is 19.7 ± 1.6 days.[30] Between 60% and 70% of babies classified as having CNS disease have associated skin vesicles at any point in the disease course.[30,35] With CNS neonatal HSV disease, mortality is usually the product of devastating brain destruction, with resulting acute neurologic and autonomic dysfunction.

SEM disease is the most favorable of the presenting categories of neonatal HSV infection. By definition, infection in babies with SEM disease has not progressed to multiorgan, visceral involvement and does not involve the CNS. Presenting signs and symptoms can include skin vesicles in approximately 80% of patients, fever, lethargy, and/or conjunctivitis.[30] The mean age at presentation (±SE) is 12.0 ± 2.2 days.[30] There is a high degree of likelihood that, in the absence of antiviral therapy, SEM disease will progress to one of the more severe categories of neonatal HSV infection.[18]

Congenital CMV Infection

Congenital CMV infection is the most frequent known viral cause of mental retardation[37] and the leading nongenetic cause of neurosensory hearing loss in many countries, including the United States.[38-40] It also is the most common congenital infection in humans, with approximately 1% of all live births in the United States being infected with CMV ($\approx$40,000 babies per year).[41] CMV can be acquired in utero during any trimester of pregnancy. Of those fetuses infected, approximately 10% are symptomatic at birth, about 20% of whom will die in the neonatal period; of the survivors, 90% will have significant neurologic sequelae.[42-47] The majority of these infants will have sensorineural hearing loss (SNHL), mental retardation, micro-cephaly, seizures, and/or paresis/paralysis.[39,48-51] These impairments frequently result in spastic quadriplegia requiring lifelong dependence on a wheelchair, along with cognitive and speech impairments that dramatically limit their ability to interact with and function in the world. Between 25% and 40% of all childhood SNHL is caused by intrauterine CMV infection.[52] Fetuses can be infected with CMV at any point throughout gestation. However, infections occurring earlier in gestation (first or early second trimesters) are more likely to result in severe forms of encephaloclastic injury. Most infants ($\approx$90%) with congenital CMV infection have no detectable clinical abnormalities at birth (asymptomatic infection), and about 10% of these children experience SNHL. Because most infants with congenital CMV have asymptomatic infection, approximately 70% of CMV-associated cases of SNHL occur in this group (Table 12-1).

CMV-associated SNHL is extremely variable with respect to the age of onset, laterality, degree of deficit, and continued deterioration of loss (progression) during early childhood.[38,49,51] About half of all children with CMV-associated SNHL have normal hearing at birth (delayed-onset SNHL) and therefore are not identified by newborn hearing screening.[38] Delayed-onset SNHL, threshold fluctuations, and/or progressive loss of hearing are observed in both symptomatic and asymptomatic infection. The age of onset of delayed-onset SNHL can range from 6 to 197 months. However, the median age is 33 and 44 months for symptomatic and asymptomatic children, respectively.[38,49] Therefore, neither routine physical examination in the nursery nor newborn hearing screening will identify the majority of children with CMV-associated SNHL at birth.

The natural history of congenitally acquired CMV infection is well described.[38,42,49,53-56] In contrast, outcomes of perinatally and postnatally acquired CMV infections are less well characterized. It is generally agreed that postnatal acquisition of CMV in term infants does not lead to symptomatology or disease.[57] In preterm infants, initial case reports suggested that perinatally and postnatally acquired CMV infections could produce severe disease.[58-63] Results of later, larger series and case-controlled trials suggest that symptomatic disease in preterm babies is less common than asymptomatic infection and that long-term sequelae are

Table 12-1 UNITED STATES PUBLIC HEALTH IMPACT OF CONGENITAL CYTOMEGALOVIRUS INFECTION

	Estimated Number
No. of live births per year	4,000,000
Rate of congenital CMV infection	1%
No. of infected infants	40,000
No. of infants symptomatic at birth (5-7%):	2,800
No. with fatal disease ($\pm$12%)	336
No. with sequelae (90% of survivors)	2,160
No. of infants asymptomatic at birth (93-95%)	37,200
No. with late sequelae (15%)	5,580
Total no. with sequelae or fatal outcome	8,076

From Centers for Disease Control and Prevention: U.S. public health impact of congenital cytomegalovirus infection. *MMWR CDC Surveill Summ.* 1992;41:35-39.

Table 12-2   MORTALITY AND MORBIDITY OUTCOMES AMONG 295 INFANTS WITH NEONATAL HERPES SIMPLEX VIRUS INFECTION, EVALUATED BY THE NATIONAL INSTITUTES OF ALLERGY AND INFECTIOUS DISEASES COLLABORATIVE ANTIVIRAL STUDY GROUP BETWEEN 1974 AND 1997

Extent of Disease	Treatment			
	Placebo[33]	Vidarabine[31]	Acyclovir[31] 30 mg/kg/day	Acyclovir[29] 60 mg/kg/day
Disseminated Disease	n = 13	n = 28	n = 18	n = 34
Dead	11 (85%)	14 (50%)	11 (61%)	10 (29%)
Alive	2 (15%)	14 (50%)	7 (39%)	24 (71%)
Normal	1 (50%)	7 (50%)	3 (43%)	15 (63%)
Abnormal	1 (50%)	5 (36%)	2 (29%)	3 (13%)
Unknown	0 (0%)	2 (14%)	2 (29%)	6 (25%)
Central Nervous System Infection	n = 6	n = 36	n = 35	n = 23
Dead	3 (50%)	5 (14%)	5 (14%)	1 (4%)
Alive	3 (50%)	31 (86%)	30 (86%)	22 (96%)
Normal	1 (33%	13 (42%)	8 (27%)	4 (18%)
Abnormal	2 (67%)	17 (55%)	20 (67%)	9 (41%)
Unknown	0 (0%)	1 (3%)	2 (7%)	9 (41%)
Skin, Eye, or Mouth Infection	n = 8	n = 31	n = 54	n = 9
Dead	0 (0%)	0 (0%)	0 (0%)	0 (0%)
Alive	8 (100%)	31 (100%)	54 (100%)	9 (100%)
Normal	5 (62%)	22 (71%)	45 (83%)	2 (22%)
Abnormal	3 (38%)	3 (10%)	1 (2%)	0 (0%)
Unknown	0 (0%)	6 (19%)	8 (15%)	7 (78%)

Adapted from Kimberlin DW: Advances in the treatment of neonatal herpes simplex infections. *Rev Med Virol.* 2001;11: 157-163.

rare.[64-68] Nevertheless, severe disseminated CMV disease can occur in premature infants, including life-threatening pneumonitis, hepatitis, and thrombocytopenia.[69]

Question 4: What Are the Treatments and Outcomes for HSV and CMV Brain Infections in Neonates?

Neonatal HSV Disease

In the pre-antiviral era, 85% of patients with disseminated neonatal HSV disease died by 1 year of age, as did 50% of patients with CNS neonatal HSV disease (Table 12-2).[33] Evaluations of two different doses of vidarabine and of a lower dose of acyclovir (30 mg/kg/day for 10 days) documented that both of these antiviral drugs reduce mortality to comparable degrees,[31,33,70] with mortality rates at 1 year from disseminated disease decreasing to 54% and from CNS disease decreasing to 14% (see Table 12-2).[31] Despite its lack of therapeutic superiority, the lower dose of acyclovir quickly supplanted vidarabine as the treatment of choice for neonatal HSV disease because of its favorable safety profile and ease of administration. Unlike acyclovir, vidarabine had to be administered over prolonged infusion times and in large volumes of fluid.

    With utilization of a higher dose of acyclovir (60 mg/kg/day administered in 3 divided daily doses for 21 days), 12-month mortality is further reduced to 29%

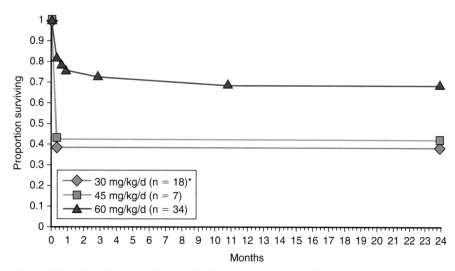

Figure 12-2 Mortality in patients with disseminated neonatal herpes simplex virus (HSV) disease given different dosages of acyclovir. *, Historical controls. (From Kimberlin DW, Lin CY, Jacobs RF, et al. Safety and efficacy of high-dose intravenous acyclovir in the management of neonatal herpes simplex virus infections. *Pediatrics.* 2001;108:230-238.)

for disseminated neonatal HSV disease and to 4% for CNS HSV disease (Figs. 12-2 and 12-3).[29] Differences in mortality at 24 months between patients treated with the higher dose of acyclovir and the lower dose of acyclovir are statistically significant after stratification for disease category (CNS vs. disseminated) ($P = 0.0035$; odds ratio [OR] 3.3; 95% confidence [CI] 1.5-7.3).[29] Lethargy and severe hepatitis are associated with death among patients with disseminated disease, as are prematurity and seizures in patients with CNS disease.[30]

For neonates with disseminated or CNS neonatal HSV disease, improvements in morbidity rates with antiviral therapies have not been as dramatic as those of mortality. In the pre-antiviral era, 50% of survivors of disseminated neonatal HSV infections were developing normally at 12 months of age (see Table 12-2).[33] With utilization of the higher dose of acyclovir for 21 days, this percentage has increased

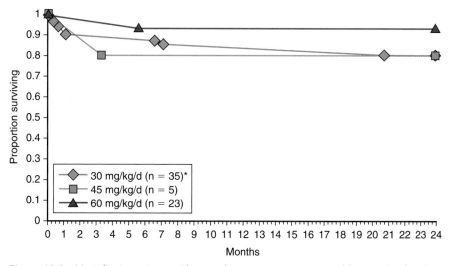

Figure 12-3 Mortality in patients with central nervous system neonatal herpes simplex virus disease given different dosages of acyclovir. *, Historical controls. (From Kimberlin DW, Lin CY, Jacobs RF, et al. Safety and efficacy of high-dose intravenous acyclovir in the management of neonatal herpes simplex virus infections. *Pediatrics.* 2001;108:230-238.)

12

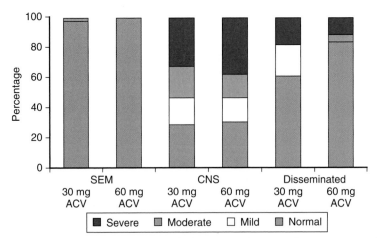

Figure 12-4 Morbidity among patients with disseminated or central nervous system herpes simplex virus and known outcomes after 12 months of life. *ACV*, Acyclovir. (From Kimberlin DW, Lin CY, Jacobs RF, et al. Safety and efficacy of high-dose intravenous acyclovir in the management of neonatal herpes simplex virus infections. *Pediatrics.* 2001;108:230-238.)

to 83% (Fig. 12-4).[29] In the case of CNS neonatal HSV disease, 33% of patients in the pre-antiviral era were developing normally at 12 months of age (see Table 12-2), whereas 31% of higher dose acyclovir recipients develop normally at 12 months today (see Fig. 12-4).[29,33] Although these differences are not dramatic, it is important to note that as more neonates survive neonatal HSV disease, on the basis of the mortality data presented previously, the total numbers of patients who subsequently develop normally is higher today even though the percentages of survivors with normal development are not dramatically different. Seizures at or before the time of initiation of antiviral therapy are associated with increased risk of morbidity both in patients with CNS disease and in patients with disseminated infection.[30]

Unlike disseminated or CNS neonatal HSV disease, morbidity following SEM disease has dramatically improved during the antiviral era. Prior to utilization of antiviral therapies, 38% of patients with SEM disease experienced developmental difficulties at 12 months of age (see Table 12-2).[33] With vidarabine and lower dose acyclovir, these percentages were reduced to 12% and 2%, respectively.[31] In the high-dose acyclovir study, no patients with SEM disease demonstrated neurologic sequelae at 12 months of life (see Fig. 12-4).[29]

Babies with neonatal HSV disease should be treated with intravenous acyclovir at a dose of 60 mg/kg/day delivered intravenously in three doses.[29,71] The dosing interval of intravenous acyclovir may need to be increased in premature infants, according to their creatinine clearance.[72] Duration of therapy is 21 days for patients with disseminated or CNS neonatal HSV disease, and 14 days for patients with SEM HSV infection.[71] All patients with CNS HSV involvement should undergo a second lumbar puncture at the end of intravenous acyclovir therapy to determine that results of PCR assay of the CSF specimen performed by a reliable laboratory are negative and to document the end of therapy CSF indices.[30] Those patients whose CSF PCR results remain positive should continue to receive intravenous antiviral therapy until PCR results are negative.[30,73]

The primary apparent toxicity associated with the use of intravenous acyclovir administered at 60 mg/kg/day is neutropenia, with approximately one fifth of patients demonstrating an absolute neutrophil count (ANC) of 1000/μL or lower.[29] Although the neutropenia resolves either during continuation of intravenous acyclovir or following its cessation, it is prudent to monitor neutrophil counts at least twice weekly throughout the course of intravenous acyclovir therapy, with consideration being given to decreasing the dose of acyclovir or administering granulocyte colony-stimulating factor (GCSF) if the absolute neutrophil count remains below 500/μL for a prolonged time.[29]

Congenital CMV Infection

Administration of parenteral ganciclovir for 6 weeks beginning within the first month of life improves audiologic outcomes among patients with symptomatic congenital CMV disease involving the CNS.[74] From 1991 through 1999, 100 patients with symptomatic congenital CMV disease involving the CNS were enrolled in a pivotal CASG study. Patients were randomly allocated to ganciclovir treatment [6 mg/kg/dose administered intravenously (IV) every 12 hours for 6 weeks] or to no treatment. Infants in the no-treatment arm were managed in an identical fashion to those receiving active drug. The primary study end point was improvement in brainstem evoked response (BSER) audiometry results by one gradation between baseline and the 6-month follow-up (or, for those patients with normal hearing at baseline, normal brainstem evoked response audiometry results at both times). Audiologic analyses were performed on best evaluable ear ("functional" assessment) and on total evaluable ears ("biologic" assessment). The best ear assessment correlates with functional hearing impairment in daily living (e.g., a person with mild hearing impairment in one ear and severe hearing-impairment in the other ear will function essentially as a mildly hearing-impaired person).[75,76] Total ear assessment further assesses the biologic effects of ganciclovir therapy.

Of these 100 subjects, 42 patients met all study entry criteria, had undergone both baseline and 6-month follow-up brainstem evoked response audiometric examinations, and thus were evaluable for the primary end point. Twenty-one (84%) of 25 ganciclovir recipients either had improvement in hearing in their best ear between baseline and 6 months or had normal hearing at both times, compared with 10 (59%) of 17 patients in the no-treatment group (adjusted P value = 0.06; OR 5.03; 95% CI 0.84-45.94). Inclusion in the better ear analysis of two additional patients who did not meet all entry criteria yielded an adjusted P value of 0.03. None (0%) of 25 ganciclovir recipients had worsening in hearing in their better ear between baseline and 6 months, compared with 7 (41%) of 17 patients in the no-treatment group (adjusted P value < 0.001; OR 21.11; 95% CI 2.84-∞). Five (21%) of 24 ganciclovir recipients had worsening in hearing in their better ear between baseline and 1 year or more, compared with 13 (68%) of 19 patients in the no-treatment group (adjusted P value = 0.002; OR 10.26; 95% CI 1.79-81.92). Ganciclovir-treated patients had a more rapid median time to normalization of alanine aminotransferase value (19 days) than patients in the no-treatment group (66 days) (P = 0.03). Ganciclovir-treated patients had better weight gain (P = 0.02) and growth in head circumference (P < 0.01) at 6 weeks after study enrollment than did patients who did not receive antiviral therapy.

Denver developmental assessments were performed during the conduct of the parenteral ganciclovir study. Post hoc blinded analysis of the results demonstrated that patients receiving 6 weeks of intravenous ganciclovir experienced fewer developmental delays at 6 months and 12 months of age,[77] suggesting that there may be a neurodevelopmental benefit to antiviral therapy as well.

Twenty-nine (63%) of 46 ganciclovir-treated patients demonstrated grade 3 or 4 neutropenia during the 6 weeks of study drug administration, compared with 9 (21%) of 43 patients in the no-treatment group over the same period (P < 0.01). Fourteen (48%) of the 29 required dosage adjustments, although in only 4 patients was the drug permanently discontinued. The mean time (±SD) of onset of grade 3 or 4 neutropenia was 14.2 (±12.3) days for patients receiving ganciclovir, and 14.3 (±13.1) days for the no-treatment group. Neutropenia resolved in 12.8 (±13.6) days in ganciclovir-treated patients, and 14.2 (±13.5) days in the no-treatment group. In all affected patients, neutropenia resolved without treatment.

The CASG has completed a phase I/II pharmacokinetic/pharmacodynamic investigation of oral valganciclovir in babies with symptomatic congenital CMV disease.[78] This study identified the oral dose of valganciclovir of 16 mg/kg administered twice daily as the dose that reliably achieves the same ganciclovir blood concentrations as the previously studied intravenous ganciclovir dose of 6 mg/kg/dose administered every 12 hours. Valganciclovir is commercially available in the

12

United States in liquid formulation, so this is now a viable treatment option in lieu of parenteral therapy in neonates who can tolerate oral medication.

Question 5: Do All Babies with HSV and CMV Infections Have to Be Treated?

Neonatal HSV Disease

Yes. Neonatal HSV disease has significant mortality and morbidity, and all affected babies require parenteral acyclovir therapy.

Congenital CMV Infection

No. Antiviral therapy administered for 6 weeks improves audiologic outcomes, and may improve developmental outcomes, for babies with symptomatic congenital CMV disease involving the CNS (e.g., microcephaly, chorioretinitis, periventricular calcifications, sensorineural hearing loss, abnormal CSF indices, or CMV DNA detected in CSF by PCR assay). However, the toxicities from the therapy are not inconsequential, and if parenteral ganciclovir is utilized it usually necessitates insertion of permanent or semipermanent intravenous access as well as prolonged hospitalization. Therefore, antiviral therapy is not recommended routinely in neonates and young infants because of possible toxicities but may be considered on a case by case basis.[79]

Question 6: What Is the Appropriate Diagnostic Approach to a Baby in Whom HSV or CMV Infection is Suspected?

Neonatal HSV Disease

For diagnosis of neonatal HSV infection, the following specimens should be obtained: (1) swabs of the mouth, nasopharynx, conjunctivae, and rectum ("surface cultures") for HSV culture; (2) specimens of skin vesicles and CSF for HSV culture and PCR; (3) whole blood for HSV PCR; and (4) whole blood for alanine aminotransferase.[71] Positive cultures obtained from any of the surface sites more than 12 to 24 hours after birth indicate viral replication and, therefore, are suggestive of infant infection rather than merely contamination after intrapartum exposure. As with any PCR assay, false-negative and false-positive results can occur. Red blood cells in spinal fluid historically has been associated with HSV CNS infections. The data suggesting this association are older and reflect a time when the hemorrhagic encephalitis produced by HSV was more advanced at the time of diagnosis. As a consequence of enhanced appreciation for HSV CNS infections and of rapid diagnostic testing such as PCR, most CNS HSV infections today do not have a significant amount of blood in the CSF. Whole-blood PCR may be of benefit in the diagnosis of neonatal HSV disease, but its use should not supplant the standard workup of such patients (which includes surface cultures and CSF PCR); no data exist to support use of serial blood PCR assay to monitor response to therapy. Rapid diagnostic techniques also are available, such as direct fluorescent antibody (DFA) staining of vesicle scrapings or enzyme immunoassay detection of HSV antigens. These techniques are as specific but slightly less sensitive than culture. Typing HSV strains differentiates between HSV-1 and HSV-2 isolates. Radiographs and clinical manifestations can suggest HSV pneumonitis, and elevated transaminase values can suggest HSV hepatitis; both are seen commonly in neonatal HSV disseminated disease. Histologic examination of lesions for the presence of multinucleated giant cells and eosinophilic intranuclear inclusions typical of HSV (e.g., with the Tzanck test) has low sensitivity and should not be performed.

Serologic diagnosis of neonatal HSV infection is not of great clinical value. The presence of transplacentally acquired maternal IgG confounds the assessment of the neonatal antibody status during acute infection, especially given the large proportions of the adult American population who are HSV-1– and HSV-2–seropositive. Serial antibody assessment may be useful in the very specific circumstance of a mother who has a primary infection late in gestation and transfers very little or no antibody to the fetus. In general, however, serologic studies play no role in the diagnosis of neonatal HSV disease.

Congenital CMV Infection

Proof of congenital infection requires isolation of CMV from urine, stool, respiratory tract secretions, or CSF obtained within 2 to 4 weeks of birth.[79] The sensitivity of CMV DNA detection by PCR of dried blood spots is low,[80] limiting use of this type of specimen for widespread screening for congenital CMV. A positive PCR result from a neonatal dried blood spot confirms congenital infection, but a negative result does not rule out congenital infection. Differentiation between intrauterine and perinatal infection is difficult later than 2 to 4 weeks of age unless clinical manifestations of the former, such as chorioretinitis or intracranial calcifications, are present. A strongly positive CMV-specific IgM during early infancy is suggestive of congenital CMV infection, but IgM antibody assays vary in accuracy for the identification of primary infection.

Question 7. How Should You Monitor the Response to Treatment?

Neonatal HSV Disease

The primary measure of responsiveness to therapy is clinical improvement in the patient. All patients with CNS HSV involvement should have a repeat lumbar puncture at the end of intravenous acyclovir therapy to determine that the CSF specimen is PCR-negative in a reliable laboratory, and to document the end of therapy CSF indices.[30] Those persons who remain PCR-positive should continue to receive intravenous antiviral therapy until PCR-negativity is achieved.[30,73] There are no data correlating clearance or persistence of HSV DNA in blood with clinical outcomes. Therefore, serial blood PCR measurements of HSV DNA in blood are not recommended to establish response to antiviral therapy or guide determinations regarding the appropriate time to discontinue therapy.

Congenital CMV Infection

The only published controlled data on the treatment of congenital CMV disease involved use of intravenous ganciclovir for 6 weeks in babies with symptomatic disease involving the central nervous system.[74] Although there is a great deal of work being performed in the area, at the current time there are no biomarkers that are clearly established for predicting audiologic outcomes.[55,56,81-84] Therefore, treatment duration should be based upon the period established in the controlled study (namely, 6 weeks) rather than on other measures of possible response to therapy such as serial blood PCR measurements of CMV DNA.

Question 8. What Are the Biggest Gaps in Our Current Understanding of the Natural History, Diagnosis, and Management of these Infections?

Neonatal HSV Disease

The duration of parenteral therapy for neonatal HSV disease is well established at 14 (SEM disease) or 21 (CNS or disseminated disease) days. Whether to follow parenteral treatment of the acute disease with prolonged oral antiviral suppressive therapy is the most important gap in our current knowledge base. Antiviral oral suppressive therapy following parenteral treatment of acute disease has been under investigation by the CASG for many years. Two CASG studies evaluating oral suppressive therapy in babies who had neonatal HSV disease have been completed.

Results are being finalized and will be reported soon. Additional gaps in our knowledge of neonatal HSV disease relate to detection of HSV DNA in whole blood, both for diagnosis of infection and for assessment of treatment efficacy over time. Groups in Utah and other centers are actively evaluating these deficiencies at this time.

Congenital CMV Infection

Six weeks of antiviral therapy improves audiologic outcomes in babies with symptomatic congenital CMV disease involving the CNS. Whether longer term therapy improves outcomes to a greater extent is a major gap in our current knowledge base. This question of duration of antiviral treatment is being evaluated in a CASG study of oral valganciclovir. All subjects have symptomatic congenital CMV disease, and are receiving either 6 weeks of antiviral therapy or 6 months of antiviral therapy. Accrual is almost complete, and the impact of longer therapy on hearing and developmental outcomes will be available by 2013. Another area where there is a tremendous unmet need is in the identification of biomarkers (either host or virus) that will predict who is at highest risk of sequelae from congenital CMV infection, especially asymptomatic infection. Without the availability of such data to inform the selection of populations at highest risk, treatment studies in babies with asymptomatic congenital CMV infection will be very challenging to justify given the toxicities of the currently available antiviral agents.

Conclusions

An impressive amount of knowledge has been amassed over the past 3 decades about the pathogenesis, diagnosis, and treatment of congenital CMV infection and neonatal HSV disease. Management recommendations have been standardized and broadly implemented. As has been the case with other areas of medicine, however, as new information is learned new questions arise. Frontiers will continue to be advanced and new therapeutic options and modalities identified.

References

1. Whitley RJ, Roizman B. Herpes simplex virus infections. *Lancet*. 2001;357:1513-1518.
2. Schopfer K, Lauber E, Krech U. Congenital cytomegalovirus infection in newborn infants of mothers infected before pregnancy. *Arch Dis Child*. 1978;53:536-539.
3. Stagno S, Reynolds DW, Huang ES, et al. Congenital cytomegalovirus infection. *N Engl J Med*. 1977;296:1254-1258.
4. Boppana SB, Rivera LB, Fowler KB, et al. Intrauterine transmission of cytomegalovirus to infants of women with preconceptional immunity. *N Engl J Med*. 2001;344:1366-1371.
5. Stagno S, Pass RF, Dworsky ME, et al. Maternal cytomegalovirus infection and perinatal transmission. *Clin Obstet Gynecol*. 1982;25:563-576.
6. Brown ZA, Benedetti J, Ashley R, et al. Neonatal herpes simplex virus infection in relation to asymptomatic maternal infection at the time of labor. *N Engl J Med*. 1991;324:1247-1252.
7. Brown ZA, Vontver LA, Benedetti J, et al. Effects on infants of a first episode of genital herpes during pregnancy. *N Engl J Med*. 1987;317:1246-1251.
8. Corey L, Wald A. Genital herpes. In: Holmes KK, Sparling PF, Mardh PA, et al, eds. *Sexually Transmitted Diseases*. 3rd ed. New York: McGraw-Hill; 1999:285-312.
9. Nahmias AJ, Josey WE, Naib ZM, et al. Perinatal risk associated with maternal genital herpes simplex virus infection. *Am J Obstet Gynecol*. 1971;110:825-837.
10. Brown ZA, Wald A, Morrow RA, et al. Effect of serologic status and cesarean delivery on transmission rates of herpes simplex virus from mother to infant. *JAMA*. 2003;289:203-209.
11. Yeager AS, Arvin AM. Reasons for the absence of a history of recurrent genital infections in mothers of neonates infected with herpes simplex virus. *Pediatrics*. 1984;73:188-193.
12. Prober CG, Sullender WM, Yasukawa LL, et al. Low risk of herpes simplex virus infections in neonates exposed to the virus at the time of vaginal delivery to mothers with recurrent genital herpes simplex virus infections. *N Engl J Med*. 1987;316:240-244.
13. Yeager AS, Arvin AM, Urbani LJ, et al. Relationship of antibody to outcome in neonatal herpes simplex virus infections. *Infect Immun*. 1980;29:532-538.
14. Parvey LS, Ch'ien LT. Neonatal herpes simplex virus infection introduced by fetal-monitor scalp electrodes. *Pediatrics*. 1980;65:1150-1153.
15. Kaye EM, Dooling EC. Neonatal herpes simplex meningoencephalitis associated with fetal monitor scalp electrodes. *Neurology*. 1981;31:1045-1047.
16. Whitley RJ. Herpes simplex viruses. In: Fields BN, Knipe DM, Howley PM, et al, eds. *Fields Virology*. 3rd ed. Philadelphia: Lippincott-Raven; 1996:2297-2342.

17. Anonymous. ACOG practice bulletin. Management of herpes in pregnancy. Number 8 October 1999. Clinical management guidelines for obstetrician-gynecologists. *Int J Gynaecol Obstet.* 2000;68: 165-173.
18. Whitley RJ, Corey L, Arvin A, et al. Changing presentation of herpes simplex virus infection in neonates. *J Infect Dis.* 1988;158:109-116.
19. Peng J, Krause PJ, Kresch M. Neonatal herpes simplex virus infection after cesarean section with intact amniotic membranes. *J Perinatol.* 1996;16:397-399.
20. Taber LH, Frank AL, Yow MD, et al. Acquisition of cytomegaloviral infections in families with young children: a serological study. *J Infect Dis.* 1985;151:948-952.
21. Pass RF, August AM, Dworsky M, et al. Cytomegalovirus infection in day-care center. *N Engl J Med.* 1982;307:477-479.
22. Pass RF, Hutto C, Ricks R, et al. Increased rate of cytomegalovirus infection among parents of children attending day-care centers. *N Engl J Med.* 1986;314:1414-1418.
23. Adler SP. The molecular epidemiology of cytomegalovirus transmission among children attending a day care center. *J Infect Dis.* 1985;152:760-768.
24. Hutto C, Ricks R, Garvie M, et al. Epidemiology of cytomegalovirus infections in young children: day care vs. home care. *Pediatr Infect Dis.* 1985;4:149-152.
25. Pass RF, Little EA, Stagno S, et al. Young children as a probable source of maternal and congenital cytomegalovirus infection. *N Engl J Med.* 1987;316:1366-1370.
26. Hutto C, Little EA, Ricks R, et al. Isolation of cytomegalovirus from toys and hands in a day care center. *J Infect Dis.* 1986;154:527-530.
27. Faix RG. Survival of cytomegalovirus on environmental surfaces. *J Pediatr.* 1985;106:649-652.
28. Stagno S, Reynolds DW, Pass RF, et al. Breast milk and the risk of cytomegalovirus infection. *N Engl J Med.* 1980;302:1073-1076.
29. Kimberlin DW, Lin CY, Jacobs RF, et al. Safety and efficacy of high-dose intravenous acyclovir in the management of neonatal herpes simplex virus infections. *Pediatrics.* 2001;108:230-238.
30. Kimberlin DW, Lin CY, Jacobs RF, et al. Natural history of neonatal herpes simplex virus infections in the acyclovir era. *Pediatrics.* 2001;108:223-229.
31. Whitley R, Arvin A, Prober C, et al. A controlled trial comparing vidarabine with acyclovir in neonatal herpes simplex virus infection. *N Engl J Med.* 1991;324:444-449.
32. Whitley R, Arvin A, Prober C, et al. Predictors of morbidity and mortality in neonates with herpes simplex virus infections. *N Engl J Med.* 1991;324:450-454.
33. Whitley RJ, Nahmias AJ, Soong SJ, et al. Vidarabine therapy of neonatal herpes simplex virus infection. *Pediatrics.* 1980;66:495-501.
34. Whitley RJ. Herpes simplex virus infections. In: Remington JS, Klein JO, eds. *Infectious Diseases of the Fetus and Newborn Infants.* 3rd ed. Philadelphia: W.B. Saunders Company; 1990:282-305
35. Sullivan-Bolyai JZ, Hull HF, Wilson C, et al. Presentation of neonatal herpes simplex virus infections: implications for a change in therapeutic strategy. *Pediatr Infect Dis.* 1986;5:309-314.
36. Arvin AM, Yeager AS, Bruhn FW, et al. Neonatal herpes simplex infection in the absence of mucocutaneous lesions. *J Pediatr.* 1982;100:715-721.
37. Elek SD, Stern H. Development of a vaccine against mental retardation caused by cytomegalovirus infection in utero. *Lancet.* 1974;1(7845):1-5.
38. Fowler KB, McCollister FP, Dahle AJ, et al. Progressive and fluctuating sensorineural hearing loss in children with asymptomatic congenital cytomegalovirus infection. *J Pediatr.* 1997;130:624-630.
39. Harris S, Ahlfors K, Ivarsson S, et al. Congenital cytomegalovirus infection and sensorineural hearing loss. *Ear Hearing.* 1984;5:352-355.
40. Fowler KB, Dahle AJ, Boppana SB, et al. Newborn hearing screening: will children with hearing loss caused by congenital cytomegalovirus infection be missed? *J Pediatr.* 1999;135:60-64.
41. Demmler GJ. Infectious Diseases Society of America and Centers for Disease Control. Summary of a workshop on surveillance for congenital cytomegalovirus disease. *Rev Infect Dis.* 1991;13: 315-329.
42. Stagno S, Whitley RJ. Herpesvirus infections of pregnancy. Part I: Cytomegalovirus and Epstein-Barr virus infections. *N Engl J Med.* 1985;313:1270-1274.
43. McCracken GH Jr, Shinefield HM, Cobb K, et al. Congenital cytomegalic inclusion disease. A longitudinal study of 20 patients. *Am J Dis Child.* 1969;117:522-539.
44. Pass RF, Stagno S, Myers GJ, et al. Outcome of symptomatic congenital cytomegalovirus infection: results of long-term longitudinal follow-up. *Pediatrics.* 1980;66:758-762.
45. Weller TH. The cytomegaloviruses: ubiquitous agents with protean clinical manifestations. I. *N Engl J Med.* 1971;285:203-214.
46. Weller TH, Hanshaw JB. Virologic and clinical observations on cytomegalic inclusion disease. *N Engl J Med.* 1962;266:1233-1244.
47. Conboy TJ, Pass RF, Stagno S, et al. Early clinical manifestations and intellectual outcome in children with symptomatic congenital cytomegalovirus infection. *J Pediatr.* 1987;111:343-348.
48. Ahlfors K, Ivarsson SA, Harris S. Report on a long-term study of maternal and congenital cytomegalovirus infection in Sweden. Review of prospective studies available in the literature. *Scand J Infect Dis.* 1999;31:443-457.
49. Dahle AJ, Fowler KB, Wright JD, et al. Longitudinal investigation of hearing disorders in children with congenital cytomegalovirus. *J Am Acad Audiol.* 2000;11:283-290.
50. Williamson WD, Desmond MM, LaFevers N, et al. Symptomatic congenital cytomegalovirus. Disorders of language, learning, and hearing. *Am J Dis Child.* 1982;136:902-905.

12

51. Williamson WD, Percy AK, Yow MD, et al. Asymptomatic congenital cytomegalovirus infection. Audiologic, neuroradiologic, and neurodevelopmental abnormalities during the first year. *Am J Dis Child*. 1990;144:1365-1368.

52. Morton CC, Nance WE. Newborn hearing screening—a silent revolution. *N Engl J Med*. 2006;354: 2151-2164.

53. Boppana SB, Fowler KB, Vaid Y, et al. Neuroradiographic findings in the newborn period and long-term outcome in children with symptomatic congenital cytomegalovirus infection. *Pediatrics*. 1997; 99:409-414.

54. Boppana SB, Pass RF, Britt WJ, et al. Symptomatic congenital cytomegalovirus infection: neonatal morbidity and mortality. *Pediatr Infect Dis J*. 1992;11:93-99.

55. Fowler KB, Boppana SB. Congenital cytomegalovirus (CMV) infection and hearing deficit. *J Clin Virol*. 2006;35:226-231.

56. Rivera LB, Boppana SB, Fowler KB, et al. Predictors of hearing loss in children with symptomatic congenital cytomegalovirus infection. *Pediatrics*. 2002;110:762-767.

57. Stronati M, Lombardi G, Di Comite A, et al. Breastfeeding and cytomegalovirus infections. *J Chemother*. 2007;19(Suppl 2):49-51.

58. Vochem M, Hamprecht K, Jahn G, et al. Transmission of cytomegalovirus to preterm infants through breast milk. *Pediatr Infect Dis J*. 1998;17:53-58.

59. Maschmann J, Hamprecht K, Dietz K, et al. Cytomegalovirus infection of extremely low-birth weight infants via breast milk. *Clin Infect Dis*. 2001;33:1998-2003.

60. Takahashi R, Tagawa M, Sanjo M, et al. Severe postnatal cytomegalovirus infection in a very premature infant. *Neonatology*. 2007;92:236-239.

61. Vancikova Z, Kucerova T, Pelikan L, et al. Perinatal cytomegalovirus hepatitis: to treat or not to treat with ganciclovir. *J Paediatr Child Health*. 2004;40:444-448.

62. Bradshaw JH, Moore PP. Perinatal cytomegalovirus infection associated with lung cysts. *J Paediatr Child Health*. 2003;39:563-566.

63. Hsu ML, Cheng SN, Huang CF, et al. Perinatal cytomegalovirus infection complicated with pneumonitis and adrenalitis in a premature infant. *J Microbiol Immunol Infect*. 2001;34:297-300.

64. Neuberger P, Hamprecht K, Vochem M, et al. Case-control study of symptoms and neonatal outcome of human milk-transmitted cytomegalovirus infection in premature infants. *J Pediatr*. 2006;148: 326-331.

65. Kothari A, Ramachandran VG, Gupta P. Cytomegalovirus infection in neonates following exchange transfusion. *Ind J Pediatr*. 2006;73:519-521.

66. Mussi-Pinhata MM, Yamamoto AY, do Carmo Rego MA, et al. Perinatal or early-postnatal cytomegalovirus infection in preterm infants under 34 weeks gestation born to CMV-seropositive mothers within a high-seroprevalence population. *J Pediatr*. 2004;145:685-688.

67. Yasuda A, Kimura H, Hayakawa M, et al. Evaluation of cytomegalovirus infections transmitted via breast milk in preterm infants with a real-time polymerase chain reaction assay. *Pediatrics*. 2003;111: 1333-1336.

68. Vollmer B, Seibold-Weiger K, Schmitz-Salue C, et al. Postnatally acquired cytomegalovirus infection via breast milk: effects on hearing and development in preterm infants. *Pediatr Infect Dis J*. 2004;23: 322-327.

69. Hamprecht K, Maschmann J, Jahn G, et al. Cytomegalovirus transmission to preterm infants during lactation. *J Clin Virol*. 2008;41:198-205.

70. Whitley RJ, Yeager A, Kartus P, et al. Neonatal herpes simplex virus infection: follow-up evaluation of vidarabine therapy. *Pediatrics*. 1983;72:778-785.

71. American Academy of Pediatrics. Herpes simplex. In: Pickering LK, Baker CJ, Long SS, Kimberlin DW, eds. *Red Book: 2009 Report of the Committee on Infectious Diseases*. 28th ed. Elk Grove Village, IL: American Academy of Pediatrics; 2009:363-373

72. Englund JA, Fletcher CV, Balfour Jr HH. Acyclovir therapy in neonates. *J Pediatr*. 1991;119: 129-135.

73. Kimberlin DW, Lakeman FD, Arvin AM, et al. Application of the polymerase chain reaction to the diagnosis and management of neonatal herpes simplex virus disease. *J Infect Dis*. 1996;174: 1162-1167.

74. Kimberlin DW, Lin CY, Sanchez PJ, et al. Effect of ganciclovir therapy on hearing in symptomatic congenital cytomegalovirus disease involving the central nervous system: a randomized, controlled trial. *J Pediatr*. 2003;143:16-25.

75. Berg FS. Characteristics of the target population. In: Berg FS, Blair JC, Viehweg SH, Wilson-Vlotman A, eds. *Educational Audiology for the Hard of Hearing Child*. Orlando, FL: Grune & Stratton; 1986.

76. Habilitation and rehabilitation. In: Northern JL, ed. *Hearing Disorders*. Boston: Little, Brown, and Company; 1976.

77. Oliver SE, Cloud GA, Sanchez PJ, et al. Neurodevelopmental outcomes following ganciclovir therapy in symptomatic congenital cytomegalovirus infections involving the central nervous system. *J Clin Virol*. 2009;46(Suppl 4):S22-S26.

78. Kimberlin DW, Acosta EP, Sanchez PJ, et al. Pharmacokinetic and pharmacodynamic assessment of oral valganciclovir in the treatment of symptomatic congenital cytomegalovirus disease. *J Infect Dis*. 2008;197:836-845.

79. American Academy of Pediatrics. Cytomegalovirus infection. In: Pickering LK, Baker CJ, Long SS, Kimberlin DW, eds. *Red Book: 2009 Report of the Committee on Infectious Diseases*. 28th ed. Elk Grove Village, IL: American Academy of Pediatrics; 2009:275-280.

80. Boppana SB, Ross SA, Novak Z, et al. Dried blood spot real-time polymerase chain reaction assays to screen newborns for congenital cytomegalovirus infection. *JAMA*. 2010;303:1375-1382.
81. Noyola DE, Demmler GJ, Williamson WD, et al. Cytomegalovirus urinary excretion and long term outcome in children with congenital cytomegalovirus infection. Congenital CMV Longitudinal Study Group. *Pediatr Infect Dis J*. 2000;19:505-510.
82. Rosenthal LS, Fowler KB, Boppana SB, et al. Cytomegalovirus shedding and delayed sensorineural hearing loss: results from longitudinal follow-up of children with congenital infection. *Pediatr Infect Dis J*. 2009;28:515-520.
83. Boppana SB, Fowler KB, Pass RF, et al. Congenital cytomegalovirus infection: association between virus burden in infancy and hearing loss. *J Pediatr*. 2005;146:817-823.
84. Ross SA, Novak Z, Fowler KB, et al. Cytomegalovirus blood viral load and hearing loss in young children with congenital infection. *Pediatr Infect Dis J*. 2009;28:588-592.

12

CHAPTER 13

Pain and Stress: Potential Impact on the Developing Brain

Lisa Eiland, MD

- Pain Circuits
- Development of Pain Circuits
- Long-Term Consequences of Early Pain Exposure
- Stress
- Long-Term Consequences of Early Stress Exposure
- Conclusions

CASE HISTORY

Baby N is a 25-week-gestation male infant born to a 37-year-old gravida 4 para 0 woman. His mother presented in preterm labor with premature rupture of membranes. Baby N was delivered vaginally within 2 hours of his mother's admission. Secondary to poor respiratory effort, resuscitation included positive-pressure ventilation and, ultimately, intubation. Apgar scores were 4 and 7 at 1 and 5 minutes, respectively. The birth weight was 834 g. Upon admission to the neonatal intensive care unit (NICU), the patient was started on a ventilator with moderate support settings. An orogastric tube (OGT), peripheral intravenous catheter, umbilical arterial catheter (UAC), and umbilical venous catheter (UVC) were placed. A sepsis workup was undertaken, and antibiotics started. The patient's NICU stay was notable for the following: both umbilical catheters were discontinued on the third day of life (DOL 3), and a peripherally inserted central catheter (PICC) line was placed. He was extubated to nasal continuous positive airway pressure (CPAP) on DOL 7. The patient remained on CPAP until DOL 49. Trophic feedings were started on DOL 3, and full enteral feeds were achieved on DOL 12. The patient began nippling feeds on DOL 56, and the OGT was discontinued on DOL 90. The patient was discharged home on DOL 95. From the viewpoint of the medical and nursing staff, the patient had an unremarkable NICU stay. From the viewpoint of the patient, his stay was quite remarkable. During his NICU hospitalization, the patient had 468 procedures that caused discomfort or pain, and he was subjected to stressors for 95 consecutive days (Table 13-1).

In 1981, Robinson and Gregory[1] provided the first evidence that premature infants could tolerate analgesia during invasive surgery. Subsequent work demonstrated that analgesia not only was safe but also improved the postoperative outcome of preterm infants.[2] These pioneering works brought well-deserved attention to the need to better understand and treat neonatal pain, even among premature infants. Unfortunately, the current knowledge about neonatal pain processes remains incomplete and too often the pain is undertreated. The experiences of infants receiving neonatal

Table 13-1 SUMMARY OF PROCEDURES PERFORMED ON BABY N DURING NICU HOSPITALIZATION

Respiratory:	
Intubation without sedation or anesthesia	1 time
Suctioning via endotracheal tube	56 times
Suction of oropharynx	235 times
Orogastric tube placement	107 times
Noise stress	Daily × 95 days
Cold stress	Daily × 95 days
Heel lancing	63 times
Retinopathy of prematurity examination	6 times
Circumcision	1 time

intensive care highlights many of these inadequacies, because inherent in the contemporary delivery of neonatal intensive care is repeated exposure to pain and other stressful stimuli. The goal of this chapter is to present the current understanding of neonatal pain and stress and in particular the potential long-term effects of early exposure to them. Special attention is given to premature infants, because they account for the majority of infants receiving prolonged intensive care.

The current knowledge regarding neonatal pain and stress has relied heavily on experimental research involving rodent models. In particular, rat pups have been used to model preterm infants. At birth, the developmental maturity of the central nervous system (CNS) of the rat pup parallels that of a 24-week-gestation preterm infant, and the 12-day-old rat pup approximates a term infant.[3,4] Of course, these developmental parallels are not exact, because different components of the CNS develop at different times. Although this model is not perfect, rodent research has greatly increased our understanding of neonatal pain and stress.

Finally, it should be noted that the forthcoming descriptions of both pain and stress circuits are presented to yield basic understanding to those involved in the delivery of neonatal intensive care and are in no way meant to convey that the circuits themselves are simplistic and straightforward. The pathways that integrate pain and stress are exceedingly complex, and the current knowledge of these processes remains limited.

Pain Circuits

The International Association for the Study of Pain defines pain as an unpleasant sensory and emotional experience associated with objective or potential tissue damage.[5] Transmission of pain involves the activation of nociceptors in the periphery. Signals from nociceptors are transmitted via three types of primary afferents: Aβ, Aδ, and C fibers. The A fibers are myelinated and rapidly carry well-localized pain signals to the cortical regions of the brain. Aβ fibers convey touch, pressure, and proprioception, whereas smaller Aδ fibers convey touch, heat, and pain. In contrast to A fibers, C fibers are unmyelinated and slowly conduct poorly localized aching and burning sensations to the subcortical regions of the brain. All three fiber types have cell bodies located adjacent to the vertebral column in dorsal root ganglia that project to the dorsal horn of the spinal cord. Within the dorsal horn, afferent nociceptive signals are amplified or attenuated by a range of substances produced by primary afferents. These substances are summarized in Table 13-2.

From the dorsal horn, most nociceptive signals are carried by axons that cross and ascend in the contralateral spinal cord via the spinothalamic tract. Conveying pain, cold, warmth, and touch, the spinothalamic tract is the most important tract for ascending nociceptor fibers.[6] This tract ascends to ventroposterior and medial

Table 13-2 NEUROCHEMISTRY OF PRIMARY AFFERENTS

Excitatory amino acids	Glutamate
	Aspartate
Neuropeptides	Tachykinin substance P
	Calcitonin gene–related peptide
	Adenosine triphosphate
	Nitric oxide
	Prostaglandins
Neurotrophins	Nerve growth factor
	Brain-derived neurotrophic factor
	Neurotrophin-3

thalamic nuclei and then to associative and somatosensory areas. These cortical areas mediate discriminative and localizing aspects of pain. A second ascending tract is the spinomesencephalic tract, and these projections terminate in nuclei of the midbrain such as the periaqueductal gray (PAG) and the cuneiform nucleus. Periaqueductal gray projections contribute to avoidance behavior and activate the structure's descending analgesia system. A third ascending tract is the spinoreticular tract. Spinoreticular neurons project to the limbic system and mediate pain-associated arousal, activate endogenous analgesia systems, and trigger affective, neuroendocrine, and autonomic responses to pain.[6,7] Nociceptive signals that do not ascend the spinal tract are processed as spinal reflexes. These afferent fibers enter the dorsal horn from the periphery, but instead of ascending, they synapse on interneurons in the dorsal horn. In turn, these interneurons synapse on ventral horn motor neurons. This nociceptive circuit results in reflex muscle contraction and withdrawal from noxious stimuli. This circuit does not involve conscious perception of pain but prevents tissue injury. Figure 13-1 provides a schematic overview of pain circuitry.

Development of Pain Circuits

As shown in Figure 13-2, nociceptive circuits appear as early as the 7th week of gestation, with cutaneous peripheral receptors appearing in the perioral region of the fetus. By the 11th week, receptors spread to include the face, palms of hands, and soles of feet. By 15 weeks, receptors are found in the trunk and proximal parts of the arms and legs. By 20 weeks, receptors encompass all cutaneous and mucous surfaces.[8,9] The afferent fibers connecting these peripheral receptors with the dorsal horn also develop early in gestation, appearing during the 8th week of gestation.[10] During the 13th week, the afferent system of the dorsal horn's substantia gelatinosa is developing.[9,10] The substantia gelatinosa neurons play a role in integrating and modulating input of Aδ and C fiber afferents. The dorsal horn of the newborn contains large peripheral receptive fields that decrease in size with maturation. Spinothalamic connections develop around the 14th week and are complete by the 20th week. Finally, thalamocortical connections begin to appear during the 17th week and are complete by the 26th to 30th week.[11]

Theoretically, starting by the 16th week, pain transmission from a peripheral receptor to the cortex is possible; however, not until at least the 26th week are the components of the full circuit in place.[12] Importantly, once pain circuits are formed, it is the critical fine-tuning of these circuits that occurs late in gestation and throughout the postnatal period that gives this system functionality.

Developmental Fine-Tuning of Pain Circuits
Influence of Neurotrophins

The exact mechanisms leading to the establishment and pruning of synaptic connections in pain circuits remain unknown. Most of what is known about the processes that fine-tune developing pain circuitry is derived from rodent models.

13

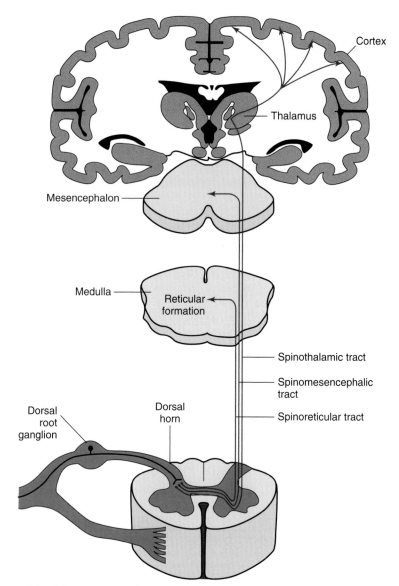

Figure 13-1 Schematic view of nociceptive circuits. (From Abram SE. *Pain medicine: The requisites in anesthesiology.* Philadelphia: Mosby; 2006.)

Overall, these processes appear to be neurotrophin and activity dependent.[13] As is true for neurons throughout the nervous system, neurotrophins play a key role in development of nociceptive neurons. Competitive interactions of neurotrophins likely play a role in establishing the different proportions of nociceptor subtypes. For example, the differentiation of Aδ fiber high-threshold mechanoreceptors and C fiber nociceptors is regulated by neurotrophin-3 (NT3) and nerve growth factor (NGF).[13,14] Aside from its role in nociceptor differentiation, nerve growth factor also plays a role in the ability of nociceptors to respond to noxious heat stimuli and regulates the density of nociceptors in the skin.[15-17] Given the importance of neurotrophins in the development of nociceptors, it is not surprising that imbalances of neurotrophins during development can lead to long-term aberrant pain perception. Thus environmental stimuli such as early injury can modulate neurotrophin balance—for example, by increasing nerve growth factor and producing long-term hyperinnervation of skin.[18,19] This alteration in nerve density can influence long-term pain perception.

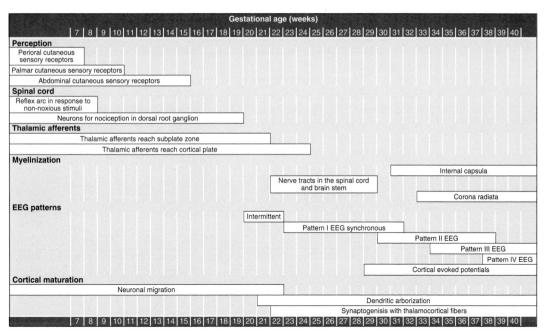

Figure 13-2 Anatomical and functional development related to pain perception. (From Simons SHP, Tibboel D: Pain perception development and maturation. *Semin Fetal Neonatal Med.* 2006;11:227.)

Influence of Excitatory and Inhibitory Synaptic Connections

Another critical modulator of pain circuit function is synaptic connectivity. Throughout development, there is fine-tuning of excitatory and inhibitory circuits. Excitatory synapse transmission is modulated by three receptor types: α-amino-3-hydroxy-5-methyl-4-isoxazolepropionic acid receptors (AMPARs), kainate receptors (KARs), and N-methyl-D-aspartate receptors (NMDARs). These receptors are localized on various postsynaptic neurons in the dorsal horn and presynaptically on primary afferents.[6] AMPARs are highly expressed in the dorsal horn of newborns, and their expression declines throughout development. Indeed newborn AMPAR levels are five times greater than adult levels.[20] In addition to the overall decline there is redistribution of receptor subtypes, which likely has functional implications. AMPAR subtypes GluR1, GluR2, and GluR4 are more prevalent in adults, and the ratio of GluR2 to GluR1, GluR3 and GluR4 is lower than that of newborns.[20] Because GluR2 reduces calcium permeability of the AMPARs,[21] higher GluR2 expression early in development could account for greater AMPAR-dependent calcium influx in neonates. The latter is thought to influence synaptic plasticity and efficacy.[13,22]

A second class of receptors important in excitatory transmissions are kainate receptors, which mediate excitatory glutamatergic C-fiber transmission[23] by dampening AMPAR- and NMDAR-mediated currents.[24,25] Kainate receptor expression also decreases with maturation and is absent in adult spinal cord.[26]

The third class of excitatory receptors are NMDARs, which follow the same pattern of expression as AMPARs and kainate receptors—that is, they are highly expressed in the neonatal dorsal horn and their expression declines with maturation.[27] NMDARs are expressed in all laminae in the spinal cord early in development, but they are restricted to lamina II in adults.[27] Functionally, this redistribution of NMDAR subtypes influences signal transduction. Specifically, decreases in the proportion of the NR2A subtype results in an increase in the decay rate of excitatory postsynaptic currents.[28] Overall, the developmental patterns of excitatory inputs yield a more excitable circuit in the newborn than exists in the adult.

Inhibitory circuits found in spinal cord are mediated by glycine receptors (GlyRs) and γ-aminobutyric acid receptors (GABARs). Glycine is evident earlier in

13

development and provides faster inhibition than GABA. Despite this early expression, the ability of GlyR activation to produce miniature inhibitory postsynaptic currents (mIPSCs) occurs much later in development than for GABARs.[29] This delayed functionality in GlyR is the basis for the predominance of GABA-mediated inhibition in the newborn. The latter provides slow inhibition via mIPSCs in lamina II. GABA-inhibitory synapses increase in number during the newborn period but then decline with maturation.[30] The frequency of GABA-mediated mIPSCs in the newborn is low in comparison with adults, but the decay time is prolonged. This prolonged decay time occurs secondary to the production of 5α-reduced neurosteroids in the dorsal horn of newborns,[30] which are not produced in the adult spinal cord.

Another factor unique to the newborn inhibitory circuitry is high intracellular concentration of chloride ions (Cl^-). As a consequence, activation of GABARs early in development is depolarizing rather than hyperpolarizing. Thus activation of the GABARs is not inhibitory. The developmental appearance of the potassium chloride co-transporter, KCC2, decreases intracellular chloride concentration such that activation of GABARs becomes hyperpolarizing and inhibitory with time.[31] Overall, increased GABAR expression coupled with prolonged decay times of mIPSCs increases GABA-mediated drive in newborns. These developmental differences in inhibitory circuits also contribute to higher excitatory tone in newborns.

Influence of Descending Pathways

Aside from influences of the local milieu and synaptic connections on development of nociceptive pathways, brainstem input modulates nociceptive circuits. In the adult, descending brainstem pathways provide a prominent mechanism in controlling pain transmission.[32,33] Brainstem fibers containing noradrenergic input reach the spinal cord gray matter prior to birth, and fibers containing serotonin input appear at about the time of birth.[34] The onset of functionality of these circuits remains unclear. Studies in rats show that noradrenergic fibers peak during the second week of life[35] and at this time are functionally capable of suppressing C fiber potentials.[36] Serotonergic fibers do not seem to have inhibitory input until nearly the third week of life, when their density and distribution mirror adult patterns.[37] Overall, in the newborn, brainstem input to newborn pain circuitry is weak and poorly targeted.

In summary strong and abundant A fiber input, immature GABA and glycine signaling, and weak inhibitory brainstem input render increased excitatory tone to neonatal nociceptive pathways (Fig. 13-3).

Secondary to this increased excitatory tone in neonatal nociceptive pathways, noxious stimulation often results in prolonged circuit discharge and likely contributes to the diffuse and exaggerated reflex behavior that characterizes the developmentally immature circuitry. The abdominal skin reflex provides an example of developmental differences in neurosensory responses to stimulation. Thus the developmentally immature demonstrate diffuse activation, whereas a more specific response is evoked with maturity.[38] Specifically, stimulation of abdominal skin in infants younger than 36 weeks of gestation produces not only contraction of abdominal musculature but also either unilateral or bilateral hip flexion. From 36 to 52 weeks of gestation, bilateral hip flexion ceases but unilateral hip flexion persists. It is not until after 52 weeks that reflex radiation ceases and abdominal skin stimulation produces isolated activation of abdominal musculature. Maturity produces a more refined response to sensory stimulation.

Neonatal Pain Reflex Versus Pain Experience

Exaggerated reflex behavior has prompted the question of whether premature infants and neonates experience greater pain. Pain experiences, however, by definition must involve the cerebral cortex and cognitive brain function, so pain-induced reflex behavior cannot be equated as pain experience.[39] Some studies examining pain responses in preterm infants with and without brain injury seem to suggest that in the immature brain, there is not significant supraspinal pain processing. Specifically, Oberlander and associates[40] compared the biobehavioral responses with pain in preterm infants having significant brain injury (cystic periventricular leukomalacia and/or grade 4 intraventricular hemorrhage [IVH]) with those in preterm infants

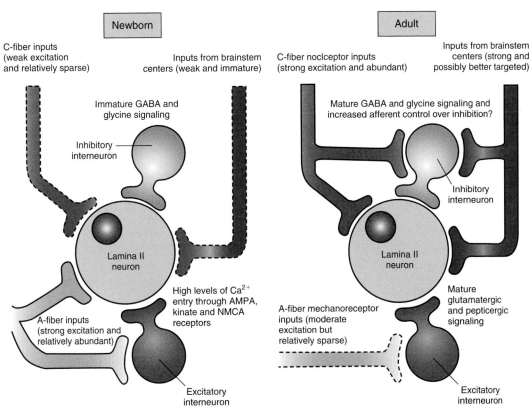

Figure 13-3 Excitatory and inhibitory inputs of neonatal nociceptive pathways. *AMPA,* α-Amino-3-hydroxy-5-methyl-4-isoxazolepropionic acid; *GABA,* γ-aminobutyric acid; *NMDA,* N-methyl-D-aspartate. (From Fitzgerald M. The development of nociceptive circuits. *Nat Rev Neurosci.* 2005;6:507-520.)

with less significant brain injury (minimal or no intraventricular hemorrhage). Infants born at 26 weeks of gestation were studied at 32 weeks, and no differences were found between the two groups in the biobehavioral responses to pain. The researchers interpreted these results to imply that pain responses in the immature brain are mediated below the level of the midbrain. An alternative interpretation is that without bilateral injury, supraspinal pain circuitry remains intact.

Later research, however, supports the hypothesis that the immature brain processes painful stimuli. Near-infrared spectroscopy has been used to demonstrate cortical activation during heelsticks in infants ranging from 24 weeks of gestation to term.[41,42] In these studies, changes in cortical hemodynamics were interpreted as changes in cortical activity. In all infants studied, activation of the contralateral somatosensory cortex occurred almost immediately following a heelstick. The magnitude of the cortical responses to heelsticks increased with postmenstrual age, a pattern that likely relates to maturation of cortical pathways. By contrast, the latency in response, which ranged from 2 to 19 seconds, was negatively correlated with postmenstrual age, a finding that likely relates to low conduction velocity and slow synaptic response in the more immature circuits. Interestingly, males exhibited greater cortical activation than females. Finally, both studies demonstrated a quiescent somatosensory cortex with non-noxious tactile stimulation. Together these findings suggest that the very premature infant is quite capable of experiencing pain; that is, premature infants reliably demonstrate cortical activation following noxious stimuli.

Long-Term Consequences of Early Pain Exposure

Given the cumulative evidence suggesting that neonates are capable of processing noxious stimuli and experiencing pain, attention must be given to the potential long-term sequelae of repeated early pain exposure. Infants receiving intensive care may experience anywhere from 2 to 62 procedures a day that cause pain or discomfort.[43-46] Of greater note, an epidemiologic study of neonatal procedural pain revealed that more than 90% of painful or uncomfortable procedures in neonates are conducted without preprocedural analgesia.[43] The consequences of early pain exposure have been explored in humans, but most evidence regarding the long-term effects of early pain exposure is drawn from rodent models.

Evidence from Rodent Models

Animal research aimed at delineating the long-term consequences of neonatal pain attempt to model three clinical scenarios. The first is acute pain such as that resulting from needlesticks. The second is inflammatory pain, such as that resulting from intravenous fluid infiltration. The third is tissue injury, such as that resulting from chest tube insertion. The long-term effects of acute pain and tissue injury are consistent, whereas the long-term effects of inflammatory pain are variable. In regard to acute pain, repetitive needlesticks during the neonatal period decrease pain thresholds and produce anxiety-like behavior in mature animals.[47,48] It should be noted, however, that repetitive needlesticks may lead to tissue injury and inflammatory changes, and the long-term effects of these injuries are distinct from those of acute injury. The long-term effect of neonatal inflammation on pain perception has been reported as no effect,[49] increased sensitivity,[50-52] and decreased sensitivity.[53,54] This inconsistency is likely a consequence of several factors, such as different modes of inflammatory injury, different strains of rodents, and different ages of injury, as well as different ages of assessment of sequelae. Finally, in regard to neonatal tissue injury, data regarding its long-term anatomic effects are quite consistent; it results in abnormal sprouting of primary afferents, hyperinnervation, and hyperexcitability of dorsal root ganglia.[13,55,56] Overall, rodent model data suggest that painful neonatal procedures can lead to long-term aberrant sensory processing.

Evidence in Humans

Studies designed to investigate the long-term sequelae of neonatal pain in humans are limited by ethical considerations. The majority of studies rely on pain exposures that are inherent to neonatal intensive care unit (NICU) care, and because it is difficult to standardize patient care, these studies are limited by numerous confounding factors. As was the case in rodent models, the available data regarding long-term effects of early pain exposure in humans yield inconsistent results.[57-60] First, in a small study of 17 infants, Fitzgerald and colleagues[57] showed that preterm infants, aged 27 to 32 weeks of gestation, demonstrated hyperalgesia in response to repeated heel lancing during the first month of life. Specifically, thresholds of the flexion reflex were lowered in repeatedly injured heels and were approximately 50% of those of uninjured heels. Functionally, these results suggest that injured heels become more sensitive to subsequent sensory inputs. Further, this group demonstrated that the application of EMLA cream prior to heel lancing restored flexion threshold levels in injured heels to those of uninjured sites. Overall, these finding suggest that minimally noxious stimuli in areas previously exposed to repeated noxious stimuli are likely to be interpreted as painful stimuli and that the use of an anesthetic may prevent this sensitization.

Second and in contrast, Grunau and associates[58] demonstrated that pain reactivity during heel lancing in very low-birth-weight infants at 32 weeks' postconceptual age was dampened in comparison with term controls. This desensitization was correlated with previous exposure to a high number of skin-breaking procedures, low gestational age, and postnatal dexamethasone exposure, whereas previous exposure to morphine appeared to normalize pain reactivity. This group assessed pain using the Neonatal Facial Coding System and power spectral estimates of heart rate, whereas Fitzgerald and colleagues[57] used von Frey hairs to assess sensory thresholds. Perhaps the different methodologies account for the seemingly contrasting results.

Third, the work of Herman and coworkers[59] suggests that both peripheral and supraspinal pain processes are altered by NICU experiences. These researchers used the thenar eminence of the nondominant hand to test peripheral pain processes and the right maxillaris muscle to evaluate supraspinal/trigeminal nerve processing. Former preterm infants (25- to 32-week infants) and term infants who had spent at least 7 days in hospital were tested between 9 and 14 years of age. The NICU-exposed children demonstrated greater perceptual sensitization to tonic heat (a state in which temperature is held constant once the heat threshold is reached) and a higher heat pain threshold than age-matched controls. In contrast, no differences in mechanical stimulation perception or pain thresholds were found. This work conflicts with that of Fitzgerald and colleagues,[57] because no differences were found in mechanical stimulation perception, yet the finding of higher heat pain thresholds seems to concur with the desensitization reported by Grunau and associates.[58]

Fourth, a long-term follow-up study by Buskila and colleagues[60] assessed tenderness thresholds in former very low-birth-weight preterm infants and comparison term controls at 11 to 18 years of age. They showed that the very low-birth-weight infants exhibited more tender points and lower tenderness thresholds. There was a significant correlation between birth weight and tenderness thresholds.

In summary, both rodent models and human studies demonstrate that early noxious stimuli exposure can significantly alter long-term sensory processing.

Stress

Stress can be defined in many ways. The American Academy of Pediatrics, in its latest policy statement on "Prevention and Management of Pain and Stress in the Neonate," defines stress as "a physical, chemical or emotional factor that causes bodily or mental tension and may be a factor in disease causation."[61] Key brain regions and organ systems orchestrate the stress response.

The Stress Axis

The hypothalamic-pituitary-adrenal (HPA) axis plays a key role in stress responses and, as such, is often referred to as the "stress axis." The HPA axis operates in concert with and is modulated by brain regions like the hippocampus, prefrontal cortex, and amygdala.

The Stress Response

When humans are exposed to stress, the medial paraventricular nucleus (PVN) of the hypothalamus secretes corticotropin-releasing hormone (CRH) and arginine vasopressin (AVP). These peptides stimulate the anterior pituitary to release adrenocorticotropic hormone (ACTH). In turn, ACTH stimulates the adrenal glands to synthesize and release glucocorticoids and catecholamines. Glucocorticoids and catecholamines act on organ systems, mobilizing and preparing the organism to deal with the inciting stressor. The following discussion focuses on the role of glucocorticoids in the stress response (Fig. 13-4).

In general, the stress response is governed by feedback loops at multiple levels. This feedback system serves to amplify or dampen the stress response, depending on the type, duration, and intensity of the stressor. Within the brain, the hippocampus serves to shut down the stress response and the amygdala activates the stress axis. On the other hand, the prefrontal cortex, which is important in gathering and integrating sensory information and controlling the emotional state, has both stimulatory and inhibitory effects on the HPA axis. The rudimentary components of the feedback loops involved in the regulation of the HPA axis are discussed in the next section as the development of this system is described.

Development of the Stress Axis

The fetal HPA axis is important in maintaining intrauterine homeostasis and driving the maturation of organ systems.[62-64] Elements of this axis begin to appear as early as the fourth week of gestation, and basic functionality, such as steroidogenesis, is evident by the eighth week.[65] A developmental time frame for appearance of key elements of the stress axis is outlined in Table 13-3. Although the fetal HPA axis is primarily regulated by the placenta, its function can be modulated by a number of

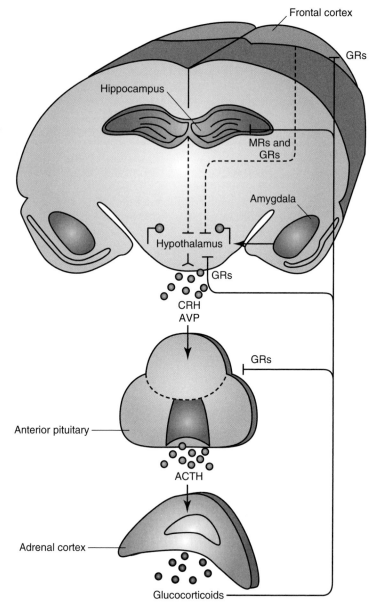

Figure 13-4 Schematic overview of the stress axis. *ACTH,* Adreno-coticortropic hormone; *AVP,* arginine vasopressin; *CRH,* corticotropin-releasing factor; *GR,* glucocorticoid receptor; *MR,* mineralocorticoid receptor. (From Lupien SJ, McEwen BS, Gunnar MR, et al. Effects of stress throughout the lifespan on the brain, behaviour and cognition. *Nat Rev Neurosci.* 2009;10:434-445.)

other factors. It is stimulated by hypoxia, hypotension, hemorrhage, psychological stress, noxious stimuli, and neuropeptides and is inhibited by glucocorticoids and vagal stimulation.[62]

Corticotropin-Releasing Hormone

The fetal hypothalamus is capable of producing CRH, but during intrauterine life, the placenta serves as the more important source of CRH for the fetus. In utero, CRH regulates adrenocortical differentiation, anterior pituitary corticotropic cell maturation, and expression of pro-opiomelanocortin (POMC), a prohormone that can be cleaved to produce ACTH.

Arginine Vasopressin

In addition to the production of CRH, the fetal hypothalamus produces AVP, which acts synergistically with CRH on the anterior pituitary to stimulate ACTH release. AVP, however, has less of a role in influencing basal levels of ACTH, but functions primarily to influence stress-induced ACTH secretion.

Table 13-3 DEVELOPMENTAL APPEARANCE OF KEY ELEMENTS OF THE STRESS AXIS

	Time of Appearance (in Gestation)	Source*
Hypothalamus	7 wk	Brosnan, 2001
Corticotropin-releasing hormone fibers	16 wk	Bresson, 1985
Arginine vasopressin fibers	11 wk	Swaab, 1995
Portal system connecting hypothalamus to pituitary	11.5 wk	Thliveris, 1980
Anterior pituitary	6 wk; matures by 8 wk	Brosnan, 2001
Corticotropes	7 wk	Baker, 1975
Adrenocorticotropic hormone secretion	8 wk	Asa, 1986
Adrenal cortex (prenatal)	4 wk; at 8 wk has zones; at 10 wk there is rapid growth of fetal zone; at 20-30 wk, remodeling begins so as to resemble adult cortex	Mesiano, 1997 and Sucheston, 1968
Adrenal cortex (postnatal): Fetal zone degeneration	Immediate	Keene, 1927
Zona fasciculata maturation	Within 3 wk	Keene, 1927
Cortisol	10-20 wk using progesterone de novo late gestation (third trimester)	Baulieu, 1963; Macnaughton, 1977; Mesiano, 1997; and Seron-Ferre, 1978
Glucocorticoid receptor messenger RNA	<24 wk	Noorlander, 2006

From Bolt RJ, van Weissenbruch MM, Lafeber HN, Delemarre-van de Waal HA. Development of the hypothalamic-pituitary-adrenal axis in the fetus and preterm infant. *J Pediatr Endocrinol Metab.* 2002;15:759-769. Figure 3.
*Sources for Table 13-3 can be found following the reference list at the end of this chapter.

Adrenocorticotropic Hormone

During development, ACTH controls adrenocortical growth, differentiation, and steroidogenesis. The influence of ACTH on adrenal growth and differentiation seems to be most significant during the second half of gestation. Adrenal gland development in the absence of ACTH, as occurs in anencephalic fetuses, progresses normally until the 15th to 20th week of gestation. Involution of the adrenal glands in anencephalic infants does not occur until after midgestation.[66,67] In regard to its role in steroidogenesis, ACTH stimulates cell surface receptors in the adrenal cortex, leading to the production and secretion of dehydroepiandrosterone sulfate (DHEAS) and cortisol. Dehydroepiandrosterone sulfate provides substrates for estrogen synthesis and thus indirectly influences the fetal HPA axis—that is, the conversion of cortisol to biologically inactive cortisone by estrogens.

Cortisol

Although at low levels throughout most of gestation (see Table 13-3), cortisol significantly contributes to the maturation of organ systems, such as the lungs, gastrointestinal tract, liver, and central nervous system. During intrauterine life, the placenta is the most important source of cortisol for the fetus. Postnatally, cortisol is involved in a wide variety of processes, including immune modulation, gluconeogenesis, and metabolism of substrate like proteins and carbohydrates. This chapter focuses on cortisol's role as a key effector of the stress axis. Most cortisol is bound to serum proteins, namely corticotropin-binding protein and albumin.[68] Protein-bound cortisol is physiologically inactive, whereas free cortisol binds primarily to cytosolic glucocorticoid and mineralocorticoid receptors (GRs and MRs) in the CNS and periphery. Once bound, corticosteroid receptors translocate to the nucleus, where they influence gene expression. Within brain regions, such as the hippocampus, binding of cortisol to glucocorticoid receptors provides negative feedback to the hypothalamus to decrease CRH secretion and eventually turns off the stress response. Overall, feedback loops throughout the stress axis terminate the stress response, and there is return to baseline function after stress exposure.

Allostasis

More than 3 decades ago, Sterling and Eyer coined the term *allostasis* to describe the active adaptive processes that function to maintain homeostasis during the stress response.[69] When these processes are overwhelmed by either severe or repeated stress, the effects can be detrimental effects. Allostatic load refers to maladaptive stress responses that can result from inadequate activation of the stress axis, repeated activation of the stress axis, or failure to terminate the stress response.[70] This dysregulated allostasis results in disease.[71]

Long-Term Consequences of Early Stress Exposure

There is substantial evidence from animals and increasing evidence from humans that exposure of the developing brain to stress can lead to dysregulated allostasis. A commonly applied model of chronic early life stress is the rodent model of maternal separation,[72] which involves removing rat pups from their dams early in the postnatal period. The most frequently used period of separation is 3 hours daily over the first 2 weeks of life. Separation from the dam is a potent stimulator of the HPA axis in rats.[73-75] At postnatal day 2, a rat pup's brain developmentally parallels that of a 24-week-gestation infant, and at postnatal day 12 it parallels that of a term infant. Thus, stress exposure in the rat pup during the first 2 weeks of life parallels the clinical scenario of a preterm infant exposed to NICU stressors from birth at 24th weeks of gestation to discharge at term.

Effect of Early Stress on Stress Reactivity

Experimental Observations

Adult rats exposed to maternal separation as neonates (MS rats) exhibit long-term alterations in stress reactivity. Specifically, key mediators of the stress response are altered. First, CRH levels are significantly increased in the hippocampus[76] and hypothalamus.[77] Second, although basal levels of ACTH are not altered, stress-induced levels of ACTH are significantly increased.[72,78,79] Finally, as might be predicted on the basis of altered CRH and ACTH levels, adult MS rats exhibit altered corticosterone levels. Specifically, there is no change in basal corticosterone levels, but stress-induced corticosterone levels are significantly increased.[75,79,80] Aside from the influence of CRH and ACTH levels, significantly decreased levels of hippocampal glucocorticoid receptors in adult MS rats likely contribute to exaggerated stress-induced corticosterone levels.[79] Overall, these early life stress-induced perturbations in stress axis mediators lead to exaggerated physiologic responses to stress. These changes produce allostatic load, a risk factor in disease development.

Human Observations

Similar perturbations have been found in preterm infants who have been exposed to NICU stress. Grunau and colleagues[81] compared the stress reactivity of term infants with that of extremely low-gestational-age (ELGA) infants (born between 23 and 28 weeks of gestation) and very low-gestational-age infants (VLGA) infants (born between 29 and 32 weeks of gestation). In a series of studies, starting at 32 weeks postconceptional age (PCA) and extending through 18 months corrected chronologic age, cortisol and ACTH levels in ELGA and VLGA infants were examined. The two stressors examined were a series of nursing care procedures and blood collection by heel lancing. At 32 weeks PCA, ELGA infants exhibit lower stress-induced cortisol secretion than term infants.[81] This blunted cortisol secretion was significantly related to the number of skin-breaking procedures experienced during NICU stay. In a subsequent study, this same group of researchers found no differences in basal or stress-induced ACTH and cortisol levels in a separate cohort of ELGA and VLGA infants tested at 32 weeks PCA.[82] In this instance, clustered nursing care was used as a stressor. What accounts for this difference in results from the initial study is not clear. Perhaps differences in stressor severity contributed to differences in outcome measures. At 3 months corrected age, ELGA and VLGA infants continue to exhibit lower basal cortisol levels.[83] It is not until 8 months corrected age that the patterns of cortisol secretion change, in that ELGA and VLGA infants exhibit higher basal and novelty-induced salivary cortisol levels than term infants.[83,84] As was the case at 32 weeks PCA and 3 months corrected age, cortisol levels were significantly associated with the number of skin-breaking neonatal procedures experienced. At 18 months corrected age, ELGA infants continue to exhibit higher basal levels of cortisol.[83]

In their latest study, Grunau and associates[85] examined cortisol responses to 4-month vaccinations. In this cohort of ELGA and VLGA infants, only the stress reactivity of male infants differed significantly from the responses of term controls. Thus they exhibited significantly lower cortisol levels at baseline and after vaccination stress.[85] This agrees with previous studies that found lower stress-induced cortisol levels at 32 weeks and 3 months PCA. Exaggerated stress reactivity does not seem to occur until at least 8 months of age. This study raises important questions regarding gender-specific effects, in that male infants were affected but female infants were not. Unfortunately, in previous studies from this group, the influence of gender was not determined. Overall, what seems consistent is that cortisol responses in ELGA and VLGA infants are significantly associated with the number of skin-breaking procedures experienced during NICU hospitalization. Given the common nature of skin-breaking procedures in NICU patients, it is not difficult to imagine that such patients are at increased risk for long-term alteration of HPA axis reactivity. Again, perturbations of HPA axis reactivity are associated with allostatic load and, as such, are risk factors for disease development.

Effect of Early Stress on Cognition

Animal studies have demonstrated long-term alterations in cognition associated with early life stress. Specifically, during adulthood, MS rats consistently demonstrate deficits in hippocampus-dependent spatial memory.[75,86-89] In humans it is very difficult to design a study forming a causal link between early life stress and cognitive deficits. We can only infer that stress may play a role in producing cognitive deficits in those exposed to early stress. Consider that a significant proportion of preterm infants exhibit cognitive deficits without radiologic evidence of brain injury.[90-94] However, such cognitive deficits have been associated with regional volumetric differences in the brain.[95] For example, smaller hippocampal volumes are significantly associated with long-term working memory impairment.[96] This result may seem inconsistent with findings in adults, in whom the prefrontal cortex plays a more important role in working memory. However, in developing brain, on the basis of its functional connectivity to the prefrontal cortex, the hippocampus appears to play a critically important role in working memory. Specifically, evidence suggests that early hippocampal injury may create a functional abnormality of the prefrontal cortex.[97,98] Because working memory contributes to cognitive functioning, deficits in working memory in preterm infants may form the basis of difficulty in language development, literacy, writing skills, mathematical abilities,[99-103] and executive functions, such as planning and organization.[104,105] What is the evidence linking stress to volumetric changes in the hippocampus? In adults chronic stress is associated with hippocampal volumetric atrophy.[106-110] It is plausible that chronic stress exposure contributes to the long-term hippocampal volumetric atrophy in the preterm infant that has been associated with deficits in working memory.

Effect of Early Stress on Affect and Behavior

In the MS rodent model of early life stress, long-term alterations in affect have been well documented. Specifically, MS rats exhibit anxiety-like and depressive-like behavior. In regard to humans, there are two lines of evidence suggesting that early life stress increases the risk for psychopathologies like depression and anxiety disorders. First, adults with a history of early life adversity are at increased risk for depression during adulthood.[111-114] Early life adversity in these studies was child abuse, including neglect and physical or sexual abuse. Interestingly, those with a history of early life adversity who suffer from depression are more likely to exhibit reduced hippocampal volume and exaggerated HPA axis reactivity.[111,115] Infants receiving intensive care are clearly subjected to severe and prolonged adversity. The second line of evidence suggesting an association between early stress and affect disorders comes from former preterm infants. In comparison with term peers, former preterm infants have more than twice the risk for development of depression.[116,117] There is no direct evidence that this increased risk of depression is related to NICU stressor exposure, but on the basis of animal and human data on early life adversity, it is certainly plausible that NICU stressors contribute to a higher risk of depression.

Overall, there is strong evidence from animal models implicating early life stress in long-term exaggerated stress reactivity, impaired cognition, and increased anxiety-like and depression-like behavior. Human data is limited by confounding factors, but this evidence also suggests that early stress produces similar long-term adverse outcomes.

Conclusions

The experiences of infants exposed to neonatal intensive care are marked by repeated exposure to pain and stress. There is convincing evidence from animal models that exposure to early adversity has long-term deleterious effects. Multiple studies of former preterm infants also suggest that noxious exposures early in development have far-reaching undesirable consequences. Providers involved in the delivery of neonatal intensive care are called upon to prevent where possible and alleviate where unavoidable the pain, stress, and discomfort of those vulnerable infants. The goal should be to direct as much attention to signs of discomfort as is given to clinical signs such as hypoxia and infection. Indeed, discomfort is the most prevalent clinical condition experienced by patients in the NICU. Ultimately, making the comfort of such patients a priority provides a feasible means of significantly decreasing near- and long-term morbidities as well as improving lifelong health.

References

1. Robinson S, Gregory GA. Fentanyl-air-oxygen anesthesia for ligation of patent ductus arteriosus in preterm infants. *Anesth Analg.* 1981;60:331-334.
2. Anand KJ, Sippell WG, Aynsley-Green A. Randomised trial of fentanyl anaesthesia in preterm babies undergoing surgery: effects on the stress response. *Lancet.* 1987;1:243-248.
3. Avishai-Eliner S, Brunson KL, Sandman CA, Baram TZ. Stressed-out, or in (utero)? *Trends Neurosci.* 2002;25:518-524.
4. Rice D, Barone Jr S. Critical periods of vulnerability for the developing nervous system: evidence from humans and animal models. *Environ Health Perspect.* 2000;108(Suppl 3):511-533.
5. Merskey H, Bogduk N; International Association for the Study of Pain, Task Force on Taxonomy. *Classification of chronic pain: descriptions of chronic pain syndromes and definitions of pain terms.* 2nd ed. Seattle: IASP Press; 1994.
6. Abram SE. *Pain medicine: the requisites in anesthesiology.* Philadelphia: Mosby/Elsevier; 2006.
7. Anand KJ, Carr DB. The neuroanatomy, neurophysiology, and neurochemistry of pain, stress, and analgesia in newborns and children. *Pediatr Clin North Am.* 1989;36:795-822.
8. Vanhatalo S, van Nieuwenhuizen O. Fetal pain? *Brain Dev.* 2000;22:145-150.
9. Bijlani V, Rizvi TA, Wadhwa S. Development of spinal substrate for nociception in man. *NIDA Res Monogr.* 1988;87:167-179.
10. Okado N. Onset of synapse formation in the human spinal cord. *J Comp Neurol.* 1981;201:211-219.
11. Kostovic I, Goldman-Rakic PS. Transient cholinesterase staining in the mediodorsal nucleus of the thalamus and its connections in the developing human and monkey brain. *J Comp Neurol.* 1983;219:431-447.
12. Van de Velde M, Jani J, De Buck F, Deprest J. Fetal pain perception and pain management. *Semin Fetal Neonatal Med.* 2006;11:232-236.
13. Fitzgerald M. The development of nociceptive circuits. *Nat Rev Neurosci.* 2005;6:507-520.
14. Lewin GR. Neurotrophins and the specification of neuronal phenotype. *Philos Trans R Soc Lond B Biol Sci.* 1996;351:405-411.
15. Lewin GR, Mendell LM. Regulation of cutaneous C-fiber heat nociceptors by nerve growth factor in the developing rat. *J Neurophysiol.* 1994;71:941-949.
16. Ritter AM, Lewin GR, Kremer NE, Mendell LM. Requirement for nerve growth factor in the development of myelinated nociceptors in vivo. *Nature.* 1991;350:500-502.
17. Albers KM, Wright DE, Davis BM. Overexpression of nerve growth factor in epidermis of transgenic mice causes hypertrophy of the peripheral nervous system. *J Neurosci.* 1994;14:1422-1432.

18. Reynolds ML, Fitzgerald M. Long-term sensory hyperinnervation following neonatal skin wounds. *J Comp Neurol*. 1995;358:487-498.
19. Constantinou J, Reynolds ML, Woolf CJ, et al. Nerve growth factor levels in developing rat skin: upregulation following skin wounding. *Neuroreport*. 1994;5:2281-2284.
20. Jakowec MW, Fox AJ, Martin LJ, Kalb RG. Quantitative and qualitative changes in AMPA receptor expression during spinal cord development. *Neuroscience*. 1995;67:893-907.
21. Burnashev N, Khodorova A, Jonas P, et al. Calcium-permeable AMPA-kainate receptors in fusiform cerebellar glial cells. *Science*. 1992;256:1566-1570.
22. Liu SJ, Zukin RS. Ca2+-permeable AMPA receptors in synaptic plasticity and neuronal death. *Trends Neurosci*. 2007;30:126-134.
23. Li P, Wilding TJ, Kim SJ, et al. Kainate-receptor-mediated sensory synaptic transmission in mammalian spinal cord. *Nature*. 1999;397:161-164.
24. Agrawal SG, Evans RH. The primary afferent depolarizing action of kainate in the rat. *Br J Pharmacol*. 1986;87:345-355.
25. Kerchner GA, Wilding TJ, Li P, et al. Presynaptic kainate receptors regulate spinal sensory transmission. *J Neurosci*. 2001;21:59-66.
26. Stegenga SL, Kalb RG. Developmental regulation of N-methyl-D-aspartate- and kainate-type glutamate receptor expression in the rat spinal cord. *Neuroscience*. 2001;105:499-507.
27. Gonzalez DL, Fuchs JL, Droge MH. Distribution of NMDA receptor binding in developing mouse spinal cord. *Neurosci Lett*. 1993;151:134-137.
28. Bardoni R, Magherini PC, MacDermott AB. NMDA EPSCs at glutamatergic synapses in the spinal cord dorsal horn of the postnatal rat. *J Neurosci*. 1998;18:6558-6567.
29. Baccei ML, Fitzgerald M. Development of GABAergic and glycinergic transmission in the neonatal rat dorsal horn. *J Neurosci*. 2004;24:4749-4757.
30. Schaffner AE, Behar T, Nadi S, et al. Quantitative analysis of transient GABA expression in embryonic and early postnatal rat spinal cord neurons. *Brain Res Dev Brain Res*. 1993;72:265-276.
31. Ben-Ari Y. Excitatory actions of GABA during development: the nature of the nurture. *Nat Rev Neurosci*. 2002;3:728-739.
32. Gebhart GF. Descending modulation of pain. *Neurosci Biobehav Rev*. 2004;27:729-737.
33. Dubner R, Ren K. Brainstem mechanisms of persistent pain following injury. *J Orofac Pain*. 2004;18: 299-305.
34. Rajaofetra N, Sandillon F, Geffard M, Privat A. Pre- and post-natal ontogeny of serotonergic projections to the rat spinal cord. *J Neurosci Res*. 1989;22:305-321.
35. Millan MJ. Descending control of pain. *Prog Neurobiol*. 2002;66:355-474.
36. Kendig JJ, Savola MK, Woodley SJ, Maze M. Alpha 2-adrenoceptors inhibit a nociceptive response in neonatal rat spinal cord. *Eur J Pharmacol*. 1991;192:293-300.
37. Bregman BS. Development of serotonin immunoreactivity in the rat spinal cord and its plasticity after neonatal spinal cord lesions. *Brain Res*. 1987;431:245-263.
38. Andrews KA, Desai D, Dhillon HK, et al. Abdominal sensitivity in the first year of life: comparison of infants with and without prenatally diagnosed unilateral hydronephrosis. *Pain*. 2002;100: 35-46.
39. Anand KJS, Stevens BJ, McGrath PJ. *Pain in neonates and infants*. 3rd ed. New York: Elsevier, Edinburgh; 2007.
40. Oberlander TF, Grunau RE, Fitzgerald C, Whitfield MF. Does parenchymal brain injury affect biobehavioral pain responses in very low birth weight infants at 32 weeks' postconceptional age? *Pediatrics*. 2002;110:570-576.
41. Slater R. Cantarella A, Gallella S, et al. Cortical pain responses in human infants. *J Neurosci*. 2006;26:3662-3666.
42. Bartocci M, Bergqvist LL, Lagercrantz H, Anand KJ. Pain activates cortical areas in the preterm newborn brain. *Pain*. 2006;122:109-117.
43. Carbajal R, Rousset A, Danan C, et al. Epidemiology and treatment of painful procedures in neonates in intensive care units. *JAMA*. 2008;300:60-70.
44. Bouza H. The impact of pain in the immature brain. *J Matern Fetal Neonatal Med*. 2009;22: 722-732.
45. Lago P, Garetti E, Merazzi D, et al. Guidelines for procedural pain in the newborn. *Acta Paediatr*. 2009;98:932-939.
46. Spence K, Henderson-Smart D. Closing the evidence-practice gap for newborn pain using clinical networks. *J Paediatr Child Health*. 2011;47:92-98.
47. Johnston CC, Walker CD, Boyer K. Animal models of long-term consequences of early exposure to repetitive pain. *Clin Perinatol*. 2002;29:395-414.
48. Anand KJ, Coskun V, Thrivikraman KV, et al. Long-term behavioral effects of repetitive pain in neonatal rat pups. *Physiol Behav*. 1999;66:627-637.
49. Hohmann AG, Neely MH, Pina J, Nackley AG. Neonatal chronic hind paw inflammation alters sensitization to intradermal capsaicin in adult rats: a behavioral and immunocytochemical study. *J Pain*. 2005;6:798-808.
50. Ruda MA, Ling QD, Hohmann AG, et al. Altered nociceptive neuronal circuits after neonatal peripheral inflammation. *Science*. 2000;289:628-631.
51. Lidow MS, Song ZM, Ren K. Long-term effects of short-lasting early local inflammatory insult. *Neuroreport*. 2001;12:399-403.
52. LaPrairie JL, Murphy AZ. Long-term impact of neonatal injury in male and female rats: sex differences, mechanisms and clinical implications. *Front Neuroendocrinol*. 2010;31:193-202.

13

13

53. Bhutta AT, Rovnaghi C, Simpson PM, et al. Interactions of inflammatory pain and morphine in infant rats: long-term behavioral effects. *Physiol Behav.* 2001;73:51-58.
54. Ren K, Anseloni V, Zou SP, et al. Characterization of basal and re-inflammation-associated long-term alteration in pain responsivity following short-lasting neonatal local inflammatory insult. *Pain.* 2004;110:588-596.
55. De Lima J, Alvares D, Hatch DJ, Fitzgerald M. Sensory hyperinnervation after neonatal skin wounding: effect of bupivacaine sciatic nerve block. *Br J Anaesth.* 1999;83:662-664.
56. Reynolds M, Alvares D, Middleton J, Fitzgerald M. Neonatally wounded skin induces NGF-independent sensory neurite outgrowth in vitro. *Brain Res Dev Brain Res.* 1997;102:275-283.
57. Fitzgerald M, Millard C, McIntosh N. Cutaneous hypersensitivity following peripheral tissue damage in newborn infants and its reversal with topical anaesthesia. *Pain.* 1989;39:31-36.
58. Grunau RE, Oberlander TF, Whitfield MF, et al. Demographic and therapeutic determinants of pain reactivity in very low birth weight neonates at 32 weeks' postconceptional Age. *Pediatrics.* 2001;107:105-112.
59. Hermann C, Hohmeister J, Demirakca S, et al. Long-term alteration of pain sensitivity in school-aged children with early pain experiences. *Pain.* 2006;125:278-285.
60. Buskila D, Neumann L, Zmora E, et al. Pain sensitivity in prematurely born adolescents. *Arch Pediatr Adolesc Med.* 2003;157:1079-1082.
61. Prevention and management of pain and stress in the neonate. American Academy of Pediatrics. Committee on Fetus and Newborn. Committee on Drugs. Section on Anesthesiology. Section on Surgery. Canadian Paediatric Society. Fetus and Newborn Committee. *Pediatrics.* 2000;105:454-461.
62. Ng PC. The fetal and neonatal hypothalamic-pituitary-adrenal axis. *Arch Dis Child Fetal Neonatal Ed.* 2000;82:F250-F254.
63. Mesiano S, Jaffe RB. Developmental and functional biology of the primate fetal adrenal cortex. *Endocr Rev.* 1997;18:378-403.
64. Tegethoff M, Pryce C, Meinlschmidt G. Effects of intrauterine exposure to synthetic glucocorticoids on fetal, newborn, and infant hypothalamic-pituitary-adrenal axis function in humans: a systematic review. *Endocr Rev.* 2009;30:753-789.
65. Bolt RJ, van Weissenbruch MM, Lafeber HN, Delemarre-van de Waal HA. Development of the hypothalamic-pituitary-adrenal axis in the fetus and preterm infant. *J Pediatr Endocrinol Metab.* 2002;15:759-769.
66. Carr BR, Parker CR Jr, Porter JC, et al. Regulation of steroid secretion by adrenal tissue of a human anencephalic fetus. *J Clin Endocrinol Metab.* 1980;50:870-873.
67. Pansky B. *Review of medical embryology.* New York: Macmillan; 1982.
68. Gayrard V, Alvinerie M, Toutain PL. Interspecies variations of corticosteroid-binding globulin parameters. *Domest Anim Endocrinol.* 1996;13:35-45.
69. Fisher S, Reason JT. *Handbook of life stress, cognition, and health.* New York: Wiley, Chichester; 1988.
70. McEwen BS, Stellar E. Stress and the individual. Mechanisms leading to disease. *Arch Intern Med.* 1993;153:2093-2101.
71. McEwen BS. Central effects of stress hormones in health and disease: understanding the protective and damaging effects of stress and stress mediators. *Eur J Pharmacol.* 2008;583:174-185.
72. Ladd CO, Huot RL, Thrivikraman KV, et al. Long-term behavioral and neuroendocrine adaptations to adverse early experience. *Prog Brain Res.* 2000;122:81-103.
73. Haltmeyer GC, Denenberg VH, Thatcher J, Zarrow MX. Response of the adrenal cortex of the neonatal rat after subjection to stress. *Nature.* 1966;212:1371-1373.
74. Schoenfeld NM, Leathem JH, Rabii J. Maturation of adrenal stress responsiveness in the rat. *Neuroendocrinology.* 1980;31:101-105.
75. Huot RL, Plotsky PM, Lenox RH, McNamara RK. Neonatal maternal separation reduces hippocampal mossy fiber density in adult Long Evans rats. *Brain Res.* 2002;950:52-63.
76. Ivy AS, Rex CS, Chen Y, et al. Hippocampal dysfunction and cognitive impairments provoked by chronic early-life stress involve excessive activation of CRH receptors. *J Neurosci.* 2010;30:13005-13015.
77. Plotsky PM, Meaney MJ. Early, postnatal experience alters hypothalamic corticotropin-releasing factor (CRF) mRNA, median eminence CRF content and stress-induced release in adult rats. *Brain Res Mol Brain Res.* 1993;18:195-200.
78. Lippmann M, Bress A, Nemeroff CB, et al. Long-term behavioural and molecular alterations associated with maternal separation in rats. *Eur J Neurosci.* 2007;25:3091-3098.
79. Ladd CO, Huot RL, Thrivikraman KV, et al. Long-term adaptations in glucocorticoid receptor and mineralocorticoid receptor mRNA and negative feedback on the hypothalamo-pituitary-adrenal axis following neonatal maternal separation. *Biol Psychiatry.* 2004;55:367-375.
80. Uchida S, Hara K, Kobayashi A, et al. Early life stress enhances behavioral vulnerability to stress through the activation of REST4-mediated gene transcription in the medial prefrontal cortex of rodents. *J Neurosci.* 2010;30:15007-15018.
81. Grunau RE, Holsti L, Haley DW, et al. Neonatal procedural pain exposure predicts lower cortisol and behavioral reactivity in preterm infants in the NICU. *Pain.* 2005;113:293-300.
82. Holsti L, Weinberg J, Whitfield MF, Grunau RE. Relationships between adrenocorticotropic hormone and cortisol are altered during clustered nursing care in preterm infants born at extremely low gestational age. *Early Hum Dev.* 2007;83:341-348.
83. Grunau RE, Haley DW, Whitfield MF, et al. Altered basal cortisol levels at 3, 6, 8 and 18 months in infants born at extremely low gestational age. *J Pediatr.* 2007;150:151-156.

84. Grunau RE, Weinberg J, Whitfield MF. Neonatal procedural pain and preterm infant cortisol response to novelty at 8 months. *Pediatrics*. 2004;114:e77-e84.

85. Grunau RE, Tu MT, Whitfield MF, et al. Cortisol, behavior, and heart rate reactivity to immunization pain at 4 months corrected age in infants born very preterm. *Clin J Pain*. 2010;26:698-704.

86. Eiland L, McEwen BS. Early life stress followed by subsequent adult chronic stress potentiates anxiety and blunts hippocampal structural remodeling. *Hippocampus*. 2010;22:82-91.

87. Aisa B, Tordera R, Lasheras B, et al. Cognitive impairment associated to HPA axis hyperactivity after maternal separation in rats. *Psychoneuroendocrinology*. 2007;32:256-266.

88. Aisa B, Elizalde N, Tordera R, et al. Effects of neonatal stress on markers of synaptic plasticity in the hippocampus: implications for spatial memory. *Hippocampus*. 2009;19:1222-1231.

89. Uysal N, Ozdemir D, Dayi A, et al. Effects of maternal deprivation on melatonin production and cognition in adolescent male and female rats. *Neuro Endocrinol Lett*. 2005;26:555-560.

90. Bhutta AT, Cleves MA, Casey PH, et al. Cognitive and behavioral outcomes of school-aged children who were born preterm: a meta-analysis. *JAMA*. 2002;288:728-737.

91. Woodward LJ, Anderson PJ, Austin NC, et al. Neonatal MRI to predict neurodevelopmental outcomes in preterm infants. *N Engl J Med*. 2006;355:685-694.

92. Nongena P, Ederies A, Azzopardi DV, Edwards AD. Confidence in the prediction of neurodevelopmental outcome by cranial ultrasound and MRI in preterm infants. *Arch Dis Child Fetal Neonatal Ed*. 2010;95:F388-F390.

93. O'Shea TM, Counsell SJ, Bartels DB, Dammann O. Magnetic resonance and ultrasound brain imaging in preterm infants. *Early Hum Dev*. 2005;81:263-271.

94. Rademaker KJ, Uiterwaal CS, Beek FJ, et al. Neonatal cranial ultrasound versus MRI and neurodevelopmental outcome at school age in children born preterm. *Arch Dis Child Fetal Neonatal Ed*. 2005;90:F489-F493.

95. Peterson BS Vohr B, Staib LH, et al. Regional brain volume abnormalities and long-term cognitive outcome in preterm infants. *JAMA*. 2000;284:1939-1947.

96. Beauchamp MH, Thompson DK, Howard K, et al. Preterm infant hippocampal volumes correlate with later working memory deficits. *Brain*. 2008;131:2986-2994.

97. Wood GK, Quirion R, Srivastava LK. Early environment contributes to developmental disruption of MPFC after neonatal ventral hippocampal lesions in rats. *Synapse*. 2003;50:223-232.

98. Tseng KY, Amin F, Lewis BL, O'Donnell P. Altered prefrontal cortical metabolic response to mesocortical activation in adult animals with a neonatal ventral hippocampal lesion. *Biol Psychiatry*. 2006;60:585-590.

99. Rudner M, Ronnberg J. The role of the episodic buffer in working memory for language processing. *Cogn Process*. 2008;9:19-28.

100. Gathercole SE, Alloway TP, Willis C, Adams AM. Working memory in children with reading disabilities. *J Exp Child Psychol*. 2006;93:265-281.

101. Gersten R., Jordan NC, Flojo JR. Early identification and interventions for students with mathematics difficulties. *J Learn Disabil*. 2005;38:293-304.

102. Andersson U. Working memory as a predictor of written arithmetical skills in children: the importance of central executive functions. *Br J Educ Psychol*. 2008;78:181-203.

103. Lundberg I, Sterner G. Reading, arithmetic, and task orientation—how are they related? *Ann Dyslexia*. 2006;56:361-377.

104. Lyon GR, Krasnegor NA. *Attention, memory, and executive function*. Baltimore: Brookes; 1996.

105. Proctor A, Wilson B, Sanchez C, Wesley E. Executive function and verbal working memory in adolescents with closed head injury (CHI). *Brain Inj*. 2000;14:633-647.

106. Czeh B, Abumaria N, Rygula R, Fuchs E. Quantitative changes in hippocampal microvasculature of chronically stressed rats: no effect of fluoxetine treatment. *Hippocampus*. 2010;20:174-185.

107. Donohue HS, Gabbott PL, Davies HA, et al. Chronic restraint stress induces changes in synapse morphology in stratum lacunosum-moleculare CA1 rat hippocampus: a stereological and three-dimensional ultrastructural study. *Neuroscience*. 2006;140:597-606.

108. McEwen BS. Physiology and neurobiology of stress and adaptation: central role of the brain. *Physiol Rev*. 2007;87:873-904.

109. Bremner JD. Stress and brain atrophy. *CNS Neurol Disord Drug Targets*. 2006;5:503-512.

110. Gianaros PJ, Jennings JR, Sheu LK, et al. Prospective reports of chronic life stress predict decreased grey matter volume in the hippocampus. *Neuroimage*. 2007;35:795-803.

111. Heim C, Newport DJ, Mletzko T, et al. The link between childhood trauma and depression: insights from HPA axis studies in humans. *Psychoneuroendocrinology*. 2008;33:693-710.

112. Bradley RG, Binder EB, Epstein MP, et al. Influence of child abuse on adult depression: moderation by the corticotropin-releasing hormone receptor gene. *Arch Gen Psychiatry*. 2008;65:190-200.

113. Andersen SL, Teicher MH. Stress, sensitive periods and maturational events in adolescent depression. *Trends Neurosci*. 2008;31:183-191.

114. Chapman DP, Whitfield CL, Felitti VJ, et al. Adverse childhood experiences and the risk of depressive disorders in adulthood. *J Affect Disord*. 2004;82:217-225.

115. Vythilingam M, Heim C, Newport J, et al. Childhood trauma associated with smaller hippocampal volume in women with major depression. *Am J Psychiatry*. 2002;159:2072-2080.

116. Conrad AL, Richman L, Lindgren S, Nopoulos P. Biological and environmental predictors of behavioral sequelae in children born preterm. *Pediatrics*. 2010;125:e83-e89.

117. Hack M, Youngstrom EA, Cartar L, et al. Behavioral outcomes and evidence of psychopathology among very low birth weight infants at age 20 years. *Pediatrics*. 2004;114:932-940.

13

Sources for Table 13-3

Asa SL, Kovacs K, Laszlo FA, et al. Human fetal adenohypophysis. Histologic and immunocytochemical analysis. *Neuroendocrinology*. 1986;43:308-316.

Baker BL, Jaffe RB. The genesis of cell types in the adenohypophysis of the human fetus as observed with immunocytochemistry. *Am J Anat*. 1975;143:137-161.

Baulieu EE, Dray F. Conversion of H3-Dehydroisoandrosterone (3beta-Hydroxy-Delta5-Androsten-17-One) Sulfate to H3-Estrogens in Normal Pregnant Women. *J Clin Endocrinol Metab*. 1963;23: 1298-1301.

Bresson JL, Clavequin MC, Fellmann D, Bugnon C. Anatomical and ontogenetic studies of the human paraventriculo-infundibular corticoliberin system. *Neuroscience*. 1985;14:1077-1090.

Brosnan PG. The hypothalamic pituitary axis in the fetus and newborn. *Semin Perinatol*. 2001;25: 371-384.

Keene MF. Observations on the Development of the Human Suprarenal Gland. *J Anat*. 1927;61: 302-324.

Macnaughton MC, Taylor T, McNally EM, Coutts JR. The effect of synthetic ACTH on the metabolism of [4-14C]-progesterone by the previable human fetus. *J Steroid Biochem*. 1977;8:499-504.

Mesiano S, Jaffe RB. Developmental and functional biology of the primate fetal adrenal cortex. *Endocr Rev*. 1997;18:378-403.

Noorlander CW, De Graan PN, Middeldorp J, et al. Ontogeny of hippocampal corticosteroid receptors: effects of antenatal glucocorticoids in human and mouse. *J Comp Neurol*. 2006;499:924-932.

Seron-Ferre M, Lawrence CC, Siiteri PK, Jaffe RB. Steroid production by definitive and fetal zones of the human fetal adrenal gland. *J Clin Endocrinol Metab*. 1978;47:603-609.

Sucheston ME, Cannon MS. Development of zonular patterns in the human adrenal gland. *J Morphol*. 1968;126:477-491.

Swaab DF. Development of the human hypothalamus. *Neurochem Res*. 1995;20:509-519.

Thliveris JA, Currie RW. Observations on the hypothalamo-hypophyseal portal vasculature in the developing human fetus. *Am J Anat*. 1980;157:441-444.

CHAPTER 14

Neonatal Hypotonia and Neuromuscular Disorders

Jahannaz Dastgir, DO, Keung-kit Chan, MBBS, MRCPCH, and
Basil T. Darras, MD

- ● Definition of Hypotonia
- ● Physical Examination and Assessment of a Hypotonic Child
- ● Differential Anatomic Diagnosis of Hypotonia
- ● Common Neuromuscular Disorders Manifesting Principally with Hypotonia
- ● Approach to Hypotonia

Neonatal hypotonia, often referred to as the "floppy infant syndrome," is the main presenting clinical feature of most neuromuscular diseases of early life.[1] However, disorders of the central nervous system may also manifest with hypotonia. In this chapter, we (1) define hypotonia, (2) discuss the physical examination and assessment of the hypotonic infant, (3) discuss the differential anatomic diagnosis of hypotonia, (4) summarize the most common neuromuscular disorders manifesting principally with hypotonia, and (5) present our stepwise diagnostic approach to the investigation of neonatal hypotonia.

Definition of Hypotonia

Two types of muscle tone can be assessed clinically: postural and phasic. Postural (antigravity) tone is a sustained, low-intensity muscle contraction in response to gravity. It is mediated by both gamma and alpha motor neuron systems in the spinal cord, and it is assessed clinically by passive manipulation of the limbs. Phasic tone is a brief contraction in response to a high-intensity stretch. It is mediated by the alpha motor neuron system only and is examined clinically by elicitation of the muscle stretch reflexes. Hypotonia is defined as reduction in postural tone, with or without a change in phasic tone. When postural tone is depressed, the trunk and limbs cannot overcome gravity and the child appears hypotonic or floppy.

An approximate caudal-rostral progression in the development of muscle tone has been described by Sainte-Anne Dargassies.[2] At postconceptional age 28 weeks, there is minimal resistance to passive manipulation in all limbs; by 32 weeks, flexor tone can be appreciated in the lower extremities; and by 36 weeks, flexor tone is also present in the upper limbs. By term, strong flexor tone in all four limbs can be demonstrated with passive movements.

Physical Examination and Assessment of a Hypotonic Child

Volpe[3] describes the physical examination of a hypotonic infant in detail. Following a careful general physical examination, the neurologic assessment should include an evaluation of primary neonatal reflexes, a sensory examination, and, most importantly, a motor examination (Box 14-1). General physical examination may reveal organomegaly, skin changes, dysmorphic features, contractures, abnormalities of the

---

Box 14-1 HYPOTONIA: PHYSICAL EXAMINATION

- General physical examination
- Appearance/posture (flaccid)
- Passive manipulation of the limbs
- Mobility and muscle power
- Muscle stretch reflexes
- Primary neonatal reflexes
- Sensation
- Traction response (head lag)
- Vertical suspension (slip through)
- Horizontal suspension (drapes over)
- Scarf sign, heel to ear or chin

---

genitalia, respiratory rate or pattern irregularities, or evidence of traumatic injury (e.g., bruising, petechiae). Abnormal primary neonatal reflexes refers to their persistence. In normal infants, the Moro reflex disappears by 6 months of age,[4,5] the palmar grasp becomes less obvious after 2 months of age, and the tonic neck response should diminish by 6 to 7 months of age.[4-6] Sensation can be tested by withdrawal from a stimulus (e.g., touching the infant with a small brush), and abnormalities in sensation may suggest the presence of a congenital neuropathy (e.g. hereditary motor-sensory or sensory-autonomic neuropathies), but admittedly, this is difficult to assess in infants.

The motor examination includes assessment of posture, muscle tone, mobility, muscle power, and muscle stretch reflexes. When muscle tone is assessed, the infant's head should be placed in the midline in order to eliminate the effect of the tonic neck response. Minimal resistance to passive manipulation of arms or legs is an important clinical feature of hypotonia. Weak cry, poor suck, and poor respiratory effort may be noted in an otherwise very alert infant. Most hypotonic infants demonstrate a classic froglike posture: full abduction and external rotation of the legs as well as a flaccid extension or flexion of the arms. Congenital dislocation of the hips may be noted because poor muscle tone in utero failed to maintain the femoral head in the acetabulum. Spontaneous antigravity movements of limbs may be absent or decreased. In a full-term newborn or older infant, passive movement of the infant's elbow across the midline produces a scarf sign. Similarly, a positive heel ear test is readily demonstrated by opposing the heel to the ear. Finally, muscle stretch reflexes may be normal, brisk, or hypoactive (i.e., absent or decreased).

Muscle tone can be evaluated further by performing the traction response, vertical suspension, and horizontal suspension maneuvers.[7]

Traction Response

To elicit the traction response, the examiner grasps the infant's hands and wrists and slowly raises the infant from the supine to a seated position. The normal infant's head is maintained at midline, or at least for a few seconds, when the seated position is reached. However, the hypotonic infant tends to have significant head lag when pulled to the seated position and does not keep the head erect when sitting.

Vertical Suspension

To perform the vertical suspension maneuver, the examiner places both hands beneath the infant's armpits and lifts the infant straight up. In a normal infant, the shoulder muscles press down against the examiner's hands and enable the infant to suspend vertically without falling. When the normal infant is in vertical suspension, the head is maintained in the midline, and hips, knees, and ankles are in flexion. When this maneuver is performed in the hypotonic infant, the infant slips through the examiner's hands with both legs usually extended.

> **Box 14-2** HYPOTONIA: DIFFERENTIAL ANATOMIC DIAGNOSIS
>
> - Brain
> - Spinal cord
> - Anterior horn cell
> - Peripheral nerve
> - Neuromuscular junction
> - Muscle

Horizontal Suspension

In the horizontal suspension maneuver, the examiner uses one hand to support the infant's trunk in a prone position and observes the resulting posture. A normal infant flexes or fully extends the limbs, straightens the back, and keeps the head in the midline position for at least a few seconds. The hypotonic infant's head and limbs hang loosely, and the trunk drapes over the examiner's hand.

Some clinicians use signs borrowed from the premature infant examination (described previously), such as the scarf sign (i.e., approximation of elbow to opposite shoulder) and heel to ear or chin, in an effort to quantitate muscle tone. We do not use these routinely in the assessment of tone but have found them useful in the diagnosis of congenital laxity of ligaments.

Differential Anatomic Diagnosis of Hypotonia

Neonatal hypotonia may be the manifestation of pathology involving the central nervous system (CNS), the peripheral nervous system (i.e., lower motor unit), or both (Box 14-2). In infants with cerebral or central hypotonia, nearly two thirds of cases, the perinatal or prenatal history may suggest a CNS insult. There may also be associated global (rather than an isolated gross motor) developmental delay, occasionally seizures, microcephaly, dysmorphic features, and/or malformation of the brain and/or other organs. Central hypotonia may be associated with brisk and/or persistent primitive reflexes and normal to brisk muscle stretch reflexes. The degree of weakness noted in infants with central hypotonia is usually less than the degree of hypotonia (nonparalytic hypotonia) (Table 14-1). In lower motor unit hypotonia or peripheral hypotonia, developmental delay is primarily gross motor and is associated with absent or depressed muscle stretch reflexes and/or muscle atrophy and fasciculations of the tongue. In general, antigravity limb movements are decreased and cannot be elicited via postural reflexes. In infants with this condition, the degree of weakness is proportional or in excess of the degree of hypotonia (paralytic hypotonia) (see Table 14-1). Trauma to the high cervical cord due to traction in breech or cervical presentation may also initially manifest as flaccid paralysis, which may be asymmetric, and absence of muscle stretch reflexes; later on, however, upper motor neuron signs develop.

Because muscle tone is also determined by the viscoelastic properties of muscles and joints, connective tissue disorders such as Marfan's and Ehlers-Danlos syndromes, osteogenesis imperfecta, and also benign laxity of the ligaments can manifest as hypotonia. In addition, there is combined cerebral and lower motor unit hypotonia seen in infants and older children with congenital myotonic dystrophy, some congenital muscular dystrophies, peroxisomal disorders, mitochondrial encephalomyopathies, neuroaxonal dystrophy, leukodystrophies (e.g., globoid cell leukodystrophy), familial dysautonomia, and asphyxia secondary to motor unit disease (Box 14-3). Further, hypotonia without significant weakness may be a feature of systemic diseases such as sepsis, congenital heart disease, hypothyroidism, rickets, and renal tubular acidosis.

Neuromuscular diseases in infancy manifest primarily with hypotonia and weakness; however, infants with severe hypotonia, and only marginal weakness,

Table 14-1 CEREBRAL (CENTRAL) VERSUS LOWER MOTOR UNIT (PERIPHERAL) HYPOTONIA

	Cerebral (Central) Hypotonia	Lower Motor Unit (Peripheral) Hypotonia
History	Consistent with central nervous system insult; seizures	Decreased fetal movements; contractures; torticollis; hip dysplasia
Developmental delay	Decreased level of alertness; global developmental delay	Alert look; no global delay; delayed gross motor development
General physical examination	Microcephaly, dysmorphic features	Muscle atrophy, fasciculations, joint contractures; weak cry; weak suck
Other organ involvement	Malformation of other organs	No abnormalities of other organs besides musculoskeletal
Weakness	Weakness less than degree of hypotonia (nonparalytic hypotonia)	Weakness in proportion with or excess to degree of hypotonia (paralytic hypotonia)
Postural reflexes	Movement through postural reflexes (e.g., tonic neck response)	Failure of movement with postural reflexes
Muscle stretch reflexes	Normal or brisk, clonus, Babinski sign	Absent or depressed
Other	Brisk and/or persistent infantile reflexes (e.g., Moro, palmar grasp)	Decreased antigravity limb movements

usually do not have a disorder of the lower motor unit (anterior horn cell, peripheral and cranial nerves, neuromuscular junction, and muscle). These infants may have genetic conditions, metabolic disturbances, or systemic disorders (e.g., congenital heart disease, renal failure). Early on, neonates with CNS pathology may present with profound hypotonia, decreased reflexes, and moderate to severe but transient weakness; however, they also tend to have seizures, obtundation, cranial nerve abnormalities, and/or a history of perinatal asphyxia. With recovery, they gradually develop better strength, increased muscle stretch reflexes, and muscle tone often distal to proximal. This picture is in contrast to that of asphyxiated infants with disorders of the lower motor unit in whom the weakness, hypotonia, and hyporeflexia persist. Alternatively, profound weakness and hypotonia without signs of CNS involvement occur in newborn infants with isolated neuromuscular disease and no history of perinatal asphyxia. Muscle stretch reflexes vary depending on the anatomic level of pathology along the motor unit (i.e., prominent hyporeflexia or total areflexia in anterior horn cell disorders and neuropathies, reduced reflexes in proportion to the degree of weakness in myopathies, and often normal reflexes in disorders of the neuromuscular junction). Again, approximately two thirds of patients with neonatal hypotonia have cerebral etiologies, and one third have lower motor unit diseases.[8]

Box 14-3 COMBINED CEREBRAL AND MOTOR UNIT HYPOTONIA

- Congenital myotonic dystrophy
- Congenital muscular dystrophies
- Peroxisomal disorders
- Leukodystrophies
- Mitochondrial encephalomyopathies
- Neuroaxonal dystrophy
- Familial dysautonomia
- Asphyxia secondary to motor unit disease

Box 14-4 CEREBRAL (CENTRAL) HYPOTONIA

- Chromosomal disorders
- Other genetic defects
- Acute hemorrhagic and other brain injury
- Hypoxic/ischemic encephalopathy
- Chronic nonprogressive encephalopathies
- Peroxisomal disorders (e.g., Zellweger syndrome, neonatal adrenoleukodystrophy)
- Metabolic defects
- Drug intoxication
- Benign congenital hypotonia

Box 14-4 lists the most common causes of cerebral (central) hypotonia. Prasad and Prasad[9] review the metabolic and genetic disorders manifesting with hypotonia and suggest a diagnostic algorithm.

Common Neuromuscular Disorders Manifesting Principally with Hypotonia

This chapter reviews the most common genetic and acquired disorders of the lower motor unit (Table 14-2). Most of these conditions manifest with hypotonia.

Anterior Horn Cell and Peripheral Nerve Disorders
Spinal Muscular Atrophies

The following three clinical variants of spinal muscular atrophy (SMA) based on the rate of progression and age at onset of the disease have been described: (1) acute SMA, or SMA type I, or Werdnig-Hoffmann disease; (2) intermediate SMA, or SMA type II; and (3) chronic SMA, or SMA type III, or Kugelberg-Welander disease.[10,11] Here, we discuss primarily SMA type I, which may be seen clinically during infancy.

Table 14-2 NEUROMUSCULAR DISEASES IN THE HYPOTONIC INFANT AND CHILD

Anterior horn cell or peripheral nerve	Spinal muscular atrophies Hypoxic-ischemic myelopathy Traumatic myelopathy Neurogenic arthrogryposis Congenital neuropathies: axonal Hypomyelinating Dejerine-Sottas Hereditary sensory and autonomic neuropathy Giant axonal neuropathy Metabolic inflammatory
Neuromuscular junction	Transient neonatal myasthenia gravis Congenital myasthenic syndromes Hypermagnesemia Aminoglycoside toxicity Infantile botulism
Muscle	Congenital muscular dystrophies Congenital myotonic dystrophy Infantile facioscapulohumeral muscular dystrophy Congenital myopathies Metabolic myopathies Mitochondrial myopathies

14

SMA Type I, or Werdnig-Hoffmann Disease

Generalized hypotonia and weakness may be noted shortly after birth in infants with SMA type I, and in 95% of cases, before age 4 months. Prenatal onset (known as SMA, type 0) has been described, and may be experienced by the mother as weakening of fetal movements during the last trimester of the pregnancy. At birth or in the first 6 months of life, weak sucking, difficulty with swallowing, labored breathing, extreme hypotonia, severe weakness, and hyperabduction of the hips (frog legs) become apparent. Arthrogryposis multiplex congenita is uncommon in SMA type I but, nonetheless, has been observed rarely. Patients with type I SMA never sit unsupported.[10,12] Examination shows hypotonia, areflexia, and weakness, typically affecting the lower extremities earlier and more severely than the upper extremities and the proximal muscles more often than the distal ones. The anterior-posterior diameter of the thorax is decreased, and there may be pectus excavatum with paradoxical respirations. As the disease advances, there is paralysis of the bulbar muscles, loss of the cough reflex, and an inaudible cry. Wasting and fasciculations of the tongue may be observed during wakefulness and sleep but they can be easily confused with simple tongue tremors. Death usually occurs in the first year or, less often, in the second year of life, most commonly related to aspiration pneumonia. An unusual variety of SMA type I related to diaphragmatic paralysis (spinal muscular atrophy with respiratory distress type I, SMARDI) has been described, manifesting primarily with respiratory distress in the first 2 months of life, before any skeletal muscle involvement. In classic SMA type I, the respiratory insufficiency is due to intercostal rather than diaphragmatic paralysis.[13]

Electromyography (EMG) may reveal excessive spontaneous activity during the first 3 months of life consisting of multiple discharges that occur at frequency 5 to 15 Hz in relaxed muscles and persist during sleep. Motor unit potentials are increased in duration, and many are polyphasic and poorly recruited by voluntary activation. Muscle biopsy examination demonstrates small- and large-group atrophy, with intermixed groups of hypertrophic fibers. The hypertrophic fibers are histochemically type I fibers, whereas the atrophic fibers are type I and type II.[10] Postmortem histologic examination of the spinal cord shows loss of anterior horn cells. Serum creatine phosphokinase (CPK) concentration can be mildly to moderate elevated, usually up to five times the upper limit of normal. Given the availability of genetic diagnosis, EMG and muscle biopsy are used only rarely in the diagnosis of SMA.

In 1990, all three types of autosomal recessive SMA were mapped to a single locus on chromosome 5q11.2-13.3.[14] Subsequently, in 1995, two groups reported the preferential deletion of two genes, the survival motor neuron (SMN)[15,16] and the neuronal apoptosis inhibitory protein gene (NAIP),[17] in patients with SMA. Homozygous deletions of the telomeric copy of the SMN gene (SMN1) can be detected in 90% to 95% of patients with SMA, regardless of severity (types I, II, and III).[15] Most of the remaining patients have deletion of SMN1 in one allele and a point mutation in the other; a very small fraction of the deletion-negative patients have rare non–chromosome 5 types of SMA. A commercially available assay for the homozygous loss of telomeric exon 7 and/or 8 of the SMN gene thus provides a highly correlated marker for the prenatal and postnatal diagnoses of SMA type I. NAIP deletions are seen in more than 45% of patients with type I SMA and in less than 20% of those with type II and type III .[17] Despite the occurrence of NAIP deletions, NAIP has not been proven to be important in the pathogenesis of SMA.

SMA Types II and III

Most patients with SMA types II and III are normal at birth. In a series of 19 infants who were later classified as having SMA type II, all were found to be normal at birth.[18] The onset of the disease, however, is before the age of 18 months.[19] Patients can sit unsupported but never stand. Survival to ages 5 and 25 years are 98.5% and 68.5%, respectively. Many patients with SMA type III achieve normal gross motor milestones early on and often into later childhood. The onset of symptoms is usually after age 18 months, and patients can stand alone; lifespan is almost normal. The SMA phenotype is determined, at least in part, by the number of copies of the centromeric copy of the SMN gene, known as SMN2 (which produces a small amount [≈10%] of full-length SMN protein); patients with milder phenotypes tend to have more copies of SMN2. Most patients with SMA type I have one or two copies of SMN2 (80%), most patients with SMA type II have two or three copies (82% have 3 copies), and the vast majority (96%) of patients with SMA type III have three or four copies of SMN2.[20]

Congenital Neuropathies

Congenital Hypomyelinating and Axonal Neuropathies

Sladky[21] reviewed 14 infants with neuropathy. He described 9 infants with demyelinating neuropathy, including 4 with hypomyelination, 3 with steroid-responsive chronic inflammatory demyelinating polyneuropathy (CIDP), and 2 with a leukodystrophy. Four of five axonal neuropathies in the same sibship were X-linked, and one was a sporadic case. Neonates with congenital neuropathies usually manifest with severe hypotonia, weakness, and hyporeflexia or areflexia, closely resembling SMA type I. However, cerebrospinal fluid protein is elevated in most infants with congenital neuropathies, not a finding in SMA type I. EMG and nerve conduction studies (NCSs) not only are important for confirming the diagnosis and distinguishing between neuropathies and SMA type 1, but also help identify whether there are demyelinating or axonal features. Nevertheless, electrophysiologic studies may be unable to differentiate between inherited noninflammatory and acquired inflammatory neuropathies. Although nerve biopsy may be helpful in establishing the diagnosis, it may not exclude chronic inflammatory demyelinating polyneuropathy. A number of infants with congenital neuropathies may also have the early onset of hereditary motor and sensory neuropathies (HMSNs) such as Charcot-Marie-Tooth disease type 1A (CMT1A) or CMT1B (known as Dejerine-Sottas disease, CMT 4E (neonatal hypotonia and arthrogryposis), a metabolic disease such as mitochondrial cytopathy or a leukodystrophy, hereditary sensory and autonomic neuropathy (e.g., Riley-Day syndrome), or giant axonal neuropathy.

Disturbances of Neuromuscular Transmission

Transient Neonatal Myasthenia Gravis

Transient neonatal myasthenia gravis results from the transplacental transfer of circulating anti–acetylcholine receptor antibodies from a myasthenic mother. It develops in about 10% to 20% of infants born to myasthenic mothers. The syndrome usually manifests within hours of birth but may be delayed for up to 3 days; the main features are feeding difficulties (87%), generalized weakness (69%), respiratory difficulties (65%), weak cry (60%), facial diplegia (54%), ptosis (50%), and sometimes external ophthalmoplegia. Respiratory failure is uncommon but it may occur. The presence of arthrogryposis, pulmonary hypoplasia, polyhydramnios, weak fetal movements, or stillbirth signify onset in utero. The severity of the disease in infants correlates poorly with clinical severity in mothers and with maternal antibody titer; however, falling antibody titers correlate with clinical improvement. Infants with transient neonatal myasthenia gravis (TNMG) are born to mothers with a relatively high ratio of antibodies directed against the fetal acetylcholine receptor (AChR) to those against the adult AChR. Transient neonatal myasthenia gravis may rarely occur in infants born to seronegative mothers and may rarely be secondary to anti-MuSK antibodies.[22] The mean duration of symptoms is 18 days, with a range of 5 days to 3 months. The diagnosis is confirmed by demonstration of a high serum concentration of acetylcholine receptor antibody in newborn infants. Although it is less frequently utilized, diagnosis may also be confirmed via reversal of the symptoms with edrophonium chloride (Tensilon), given either as an intramuscular or subcutaneous injection of 0.04 to 0.15 mg/kg or as 0.1 mg/kg body weight intravenously delivered in fractional amounts over a number of minutes after a test dose of 0.01 mg/kg.

Clinical improvement becomes apparent in a few minutes after the intravenous administration of edrophonium chloride and may last for 10 to 15 minutes. Given the possibility of cardiac bradyarrhythmias subsequent to the intravenous use of edrophonium chloride, however, the intramuscular and subcutaneous routes are preferable in newborn infants. In severely compromised neonates, an exchange transfusion should be attempted. For infants with only feeding and swallowing problems, a longer lasting effect (1 to 3 hours) may be achieved with the intramuscular or subcutaneous injection of about 0.05 mg/kg per dose neostigmine methyl sulfate 15 to 30 minutes before each feeding, although this agent may induce increased tracheal secretions. The same medication can also be administered through a nasogastric tube at 10 times the parenteral dose (0.5 mg/kg/dose) 45 to 60 minutes prior to feeding.

Acquired Autoimmune Myasthenia Gravis

Only minor differences exist between acquired autoimmune myasthenia gravis in children and that in adults, but the onset of symptoms is always after age 6 months and in most cases after 2 years.

Congenital Myasthenic Syndromes

Congenital myasthenic syndromes can be classified according to the site of the defect—that is, presynaptic, postsynaptic, synaptic, or mixed.[23] These are defects of neuromuscular transmission, and the classification and main features of the most common forms are shown in Table 14-3. Congenital myasthenic syndromes usually manifest in infancy with generalized hypotonia and fluctuating weakness, weak cry

Table 14-3 CONGENITAL MYASTHENIC SYNDROMES

Defect	Inheritance	Clinical Features	Tensilon Test	Treatment
Article I: Presynaptic				
Familial infantile myasthenia with episodic apnea (choline acetyltransferase mutations)	AR	Hypotonia Ptosis Apnea No ophthalmoparesis Generalized weakness	+	AChE inhibitors
Article II: Postsynaptic or Synaptic				
Congenital end-plate AChE deficiency	AR	Asymmetric ptosis Ophthalmoparesis Distal weakness Delayed pupillary constriction to light	–	No response to AChE inhibitors
Classic slow channel syndrome	AD	Ophthalmoparesis Fluctuating ptosis Head and wrist extensor weakness	–	No response to AChE inhibitors
Congenital AChR deficiency (rapsyn or ε-subunit mutations)	AR	Hypotonia Ptosis Ophthalmoplegia (ε-subunit) Strabismus (rapsyn) Respiratory failure (rapsyn) Feeding difficulties Arthrogryposis (rapsyn)	+	AChE inhibitors
Dok-7 myasthenia	AR	Proximal weakness Ptosis Facial weakness Respiratory failure	–	Poor response to AchE inhibitors

AChE, Acetylcholinesterase; *AChR,* acetylcholine receptor; *AD,* autosomal dominant; *AR,* autosomal recessive.

and suck, respiratory distress, apnea, and feeding difficulties. Fluctuating ptosis, ophthalmoparesis, and abnormal fatigability on exertion may be present during infancy and childhood. Later on, delayed motor milestones may be noted and will, in some cases, progress during adolescence and adulthood. Testing for anti–acetylcholine receptor antibodies is negative. The diagnosis is based on clinical history and examination, family history (if present), EMG findings, and the clinical response to acetylcholinesterase inhibitors. Results of edrophonium chloride testing, although less frequently in use today, are positive in most types of congenital myasthenic syndromes, except in the classic slow channel syndrome and in congenital end-plate acetylcholinesterase deficiency (see Table 14-3). If a clinical response to edrophonium chloride occurs, long-term treatment with neostigmine or pyridostigmine is needed. In most cases, however, detailed EMG studies as well as in vitro microphysiologic, ultrastructural, and histochemical studies of intercostal muscle biopsy specimens are required to establish the diagnosis.

Infantile Botulism

Patients in whom botulism develops in infancy are normal at birth but between the age of 10 days and 12 months (median age at presentation is 10 weeks) demonstrate acutely severe weakness, dysphagia, constipation, weak cry, severe hypotonia, and respiratory insufficiency.[24] On examination, there is diffuse hypotonia and weakness, ptosis, ophthalmoplegia with pupillary involvement (mydriasis) in some cases, reduced gag reflex, and usually preservation of muscle stretch reflexes.[25] Affected infants tend to deteriorate if given aminoglycosides or other neuromuscular blocking agents. On EMG examination, the compound motor unit potential amplitude is low at rest; repetitive stimulation at 2 to 5 Hz typically produces decrement, but with 20- to 50-Hz stimulation, facilitation of 125% to 3000% is seen in almost all cases. To demonstrate the increment, however, a prolonged period of stimulation (10 to 20 seconds) may be required.[26] During infancy the pathogenesis of botulism is different. The *Clostridium botulinum* is ingested, colonizes the intestinal tract, and produces toxin in situ. This process is in contrast to that in older children and adults, in whom the disease is related to ingestion of food contaminated by preformed exotoxin.[27] The diagnosis in infants is confirmed by isolation of the organism in stool. Infantile botulism is a self-limited disease; the period of profound hypotonia can last from 2 to 6 weeks, however, so the infant should be observed in the intensive care unit and should be supported if respiratory failure occurs. Botulinum immune globulin (BIG) seems to be safe and reduces the duration of the disease, the cost of the hospitalization, and the severity of illness.[28]

Magnesium Intoxication

Generalized weakness, hypotonia, and mental status changes may be seen in infants born to mothers treated with high doses of magnesium sulfate for eclampsia. Because this is a self-limited condition brought about by elevated magnesium values that impair neuromuscular transmission, specialized testing (e.g., EMG, NCSs) is not necessary. These infants may have depressed deep tendon reflexes, abdominal distention secondary to ileus, and irregularities of cardiac rhythm.

Muscle Disorders

The muscle disorders reviewed in this chapter usually manifest with hypotonia and weakness during infancy; however, a later onset may occur. They are listed in Box 14-5.

Congenital Muscular Dystrophies

In congenital muscular dystrophies (CMDs) the muscle biopsy findings are abnormal (showing features often seen in the major muscular dystrophies of later onset), but there are no unique identifying features.

CMDs can be classified into two major groups depending on the association with structural brain abnormalities on neuroimaging studies or autopsy examination.[29] The CMDs without structural CNS anomalies, also known as classic or

---

Box 14-5   MUSCLE DISORDERS IN THE HYPOTONIC INFANT

Congenital muscular dystrophies
Congenital myotonic dystrophy
Infantile facioscapulohumeral muscular dystrophy
Congenital myopathies:
  Nemaline myopathy
  Central core disease
  Centronuclear/myotubular myopathy
  Congenital fiber type disproportion
  Minicore disease
  Other congenital myopathies
Metabolic myopathies
  Acid maltase deficiency
  Mitochondrial myopathies
    Cytochrome C oxidase deficiency
    Fatty acid oxidation defects
  Non-lysosomal glycogenoses

---

occidental CMD, form a heterogenous group of disorders. In the second group—that is, those with associated structural CNS abnormalities—concomitant eye involvement and clinical evidence of significant neurologic dysfunction may be evident. The latter group includes Fukuyama muscular dystrophy (FMD), Walker-Warburg syndrome (WWS), and muscle-eye-brain disease (MEBD) (Table 14-4). A biochemical classification has been proposed as well (Table 14-5).

Congenital Muscular Dystrophies Without Structural CNS Anomalies

The CMDs without structural CNS anomalies can be subclassified now on the basis of merosin (laminin α_2 chain gene mutation) staining results of their muscle biopsy specimens into merosin-deficient and merosin-positive CMDs (see Box 14-5). Both subgroups can manifest in early infancy with hypotonia, weakness, elevated serum CPK, and joint contractures. Major feeding and respiratory difficulties are not common. The diagnosis in this group of CMDs rests on head magnetic resonance imaging (MRI), EMG or NCSs, CPK testing, and muscle biopsy histology, histochemistry, and merosin immunostaining.

Merosin-Deficient Classic Congenital Muscular Dystrophy (MDC1A). All patients with merosin-deficient CMD who are studied with cranial MRI have abnormalities of the white matter on T2-weighted images that were not seen in the group with merosin-positive CMD.[29] Given the expression of merosin in peripheral nerve and brain, slowing of motor nerve conduction velocities[30] as well as delayed somatosensory evoked potentials have been found. Of interest, both the peripheral nervous system and the CNS involvement become more pronounced with age and may be only minimal early in the course of the disease. The subgroup of patients with merosin-negative CMD is quite unique because of the associated hypomyelination of brain white matter detected by head MRI, the involvement of peripheral nerves,[30] and the somewhat severe clinical involvement.[31,32] Despite the white matter changes, most of these patients do not exhibit major neurologic deficits on standard evaluation; nonetheless, patients with seizures have been described. In general, the merosin-deficient subgroup comprises a more severe neuromuscular phenotype with relatively high serum CPK concentrations.[33] Most patients are unable to stand or walk, in contrast to the merosin-positive patients, most of whom will walk independently.[34] The phenotype of merosin-deficient CMD seems to be broadening, however. On the one hand, there are patients with mild phenotype who function well into adulthood, but on the other hand, a few patients have also demonstrated evidence of focal cortical dysgenesis (10% occipital agyria) or cerebellar hypoplasia (20%) on

Table 14-4 GENETIC LOCI FOR CONGENITAL MUSCULAR DYSTROPHY IDENTIFIED TO DATE

Disease	Mode of Inheritance	Gene Location	Symbol (Gene Product)	Alternative Disease Symbol
Classic CMD*				
Primary merosin deficiency (MDC1A)	AR	6q22-q23	*LAMA2* (laminin α_2 chain of merosin)	
Secondary merosin deficiency (MDC1B)	AR	1q42	?	
Secondary merosin deficiency (MDC1C)	AR	19q13.3	*FKRP* (fukutin-related protein)	MDDGB5
Rigid spine syndrome (RSMD)	AR	1p35-p36	*RSMD1* (selenoprotein N)	
Ullrich muscular dystrophy (UCMD)	AR AD	21q22.3	*COL6A1* (collagen VI α_1 chain)	
Bethlem myopathy				
	AD AR	21q22.3	*COL6A2* (collagen VI α_2 chain)	
	AD AR	2q37	*COL6A3* (collagen VI α_3 chain)	
Lamin A-related congenital muscular dystrophy (L-CMD)	AD	1q21.2	*LMNA*	
Integrin α_7 deficiency	AR	12q13	Integrin α_7	
CMD-Dystroglycanopathy with CNS Abnormalities and/or Mental Retardation				
Fukuyama CMD	AR	9q31-33	*FCMD* (fukutin)	MDDGA4
Muscle-eye-brain (MEB) disease or Walker-Warburg syndrome (WWS)	AR	1p33-p34	*POMGnT1* (glycosyl-transferase)	MDDGA3
	AR	9q34.1	*POMT1* (O-mannosyltransferase)	MDDGA1
	AR	9q31-q33	*FCMD* (fukutin)	MDDGA4
	AR	19q13.3	*FKRP* (fukutin-related protein)	MDDGA5
	AR	14q24.3	*POMT2* (mannosyltransferase)	MDDGA2
LARGE-related CMDs (MDC1D) (WWS-MEB)	AR	22q12.3	*LARGE* (putative glycosyl-transferase)	MDDGA6 MDDGB6

Adapted with permission from Jones K, North K. The congenital muscular dystrophies. In: Jones HR, De Vivo DC, Darras BT, eds. *Neuromuscular disorders of infancy, childhood, and adolescence: A clinician's approach.* Philadelphia: Butterworth Heinemann; 2003:633; and from *Online Mendelian Inheritance in Man* (OMIM). <http://www.ncbi.nlm.nih.gov/omim>.
Alternative citation:
Modified from Darras BT. Facioscapulohumeral, oculopharyngeal, distal, and congenital muscular dystrophies. *UpToDate.* 2011;19.3.
AR, Autosomal recessive; CMD, congenital muscular dystrophy; CNS, central nervous system; MDDG, muscular dystrophy-dystroglycanopathy.
*Structural CNS abnormalities have been described in some patients with classic CMD.

brain imaging. An intermediate phenotype, with incomplete deficiency and later onset in achievement of ambulation, has also been described. Further, two siblings from a consanguineous family with an internally deleted laminin α_2-chain gene as a result of a splice site mutation in the *LAMA2* gene have been reported; interestingly, these patients appear more mildly affected than others who completely lack this protein.[35] Secondary merosin-deficient CMDs such as FKRP-related CMD (MDC1C), are listed in Table 14-4.

Table 14-5 BIOCHEMICAL CLASSIFICATION OF CONGENITAL MUSCULAR
DYSTROPHIES (CMDS)

Conditions affecting the endoplasmic reticulum	Selenoprotein N1 (SEPN1) (rigid spine syndrome 1 [RSMD1])
Conditions involving the extracellular matrix	Laminin α_2 (MDC1A)
	Integrin α_7 (CMD)
	Integrin α_9 (CMD)
	Collagen VI (Ullrich syndrome)
Conditions affecting the glycosylation of proteins	Fukutin (Fukuyama congenital muscular dystrophy [FCMD])
	Fukutin-related protein (FKRP) (MDC1C)
	LARGE (MDC1D)
	POMT1 (WWS)
	POMT2 (WWS)
	POMGnT1 (muscle-eye-brain disease)
	Congenital disorder of glycosylation (CDG) type 1 (*N*-glycosylation disorder)*
Other	Conditions affecting nuclear envelope proteins: severe laminopathies

*Lefeber DJ, Schonberger J, Morava E, et al. Deficiency of Dol-P-Man synthase subunit DPM3 bridges the congenital disorders of glycosylation with the dystroglycanopathies. *Am J Hum Genet.* 2009;85:76-86.
MDC, Muscular dystrophy, congenital; *WWS*, Walker-Warburg syndrome.

Merosin-Positive Classic Congenital Muscular Dystrophy. The group of patients with classic CMD who are merosin-positive may well be quite heterogeneous genetically. As alluded to earlier in the comparative studies with the merosin-deficient patients, it has become apparent that the prognosis for ambulation, for the most part, appears to be much better in the merosin-positive patients.[33,36-38] However, delayed deterioration has been described in a large study from Japan.[39] This finding would indicate that the underlying dystrophic process is progressive, albeit so slowly that initial motor development outpaces this deterioration. Various merosin-positive CMDs such as rigid spine syndrome and Ullrich muscular dystrophy are listed in Table 14-4.

Congenital Muscular Dystrophies with Structural CNS Anomalies and/or Mental Retardation

Fukuyama Muscular Dystrophy. Of the CMDs with structural CNS anomalies, FMD is a major representative.[40] Described in 1960, FMD is the second most prevalent form of muscular dystrophy in Japan, after Duchenne muscular dystrophy (DMD), with a DMD-to-FMD prevalence ratio of 2.1 : 1. FMD has been described in non–Japanese Americans and Europeans but, overall, is rare outside Japan. The FMD gene locus has been mapped to chromosome 9q31-33[41,42]; it appears to be inherited as an autosomal recessive trait; and the defective gene has been isolated and the respective protein product has been named fukutin.[39]

FMD manifests with generalized weakness and hypotonia at birth, joint contractures, and depressed muscle stretch reflexes. Other clinical features include microcephaly and delayed psychomotor development. Convulsions occur in 50% of cases. CPK value is usually significantly elevated (10-50 times the upper limit of normal). Muscle biopsy shows myopathic changes consisting of endomysial and perimysial fibrosis, rounded muscle fibers with involvement of both type I and type II fibers, and increased numbers of type IIC fibers. Head MRI and autopsy studies usually show diffuse cerebral pachygyria, cerebral and cerebellar polymicrogyria, hydrocephalus ex vacuo, subpial gliosis, and heterotopias. Polymicrogyria is found consistently in the cerebellum. Death usually occurs by 10 years of age.

Walker-Warburg Syndrome. WWS also seems to be inherited as an autosomal recessive trait. Although a case of WWS has been described in a family with FMD, linkage to the FMD locus on 9q31-33 has been excluded in at least a number of families. The major features are a severe neonatal phenotype with weakness, hypotonia, hydrocephalus, macrocephaly, and eye abnormalities.[43] The muscle biopsy findings are indistinguishable from those in other disorders in this group; there are major myopathic changes, albeit nonspecific. Deficient laminin α_2-chain and α-dystroglycan staining has been described.[44]

The neuropathologic features detected by head MRI and autopsy examination vary little from case to case and include hydrocephalus (communicating or ex vacuo), type II (cobblestone) lissencephaly[45] with or without polymicrogyria, cerebellar hypoplasia, Dandy-Walker malformation, small optic nerves and olfactory tracts, absence of corpus callosum, colpocephaly, encephalocele(s), and heterotopias. The cortex is composed of two layers separated by an irregular plain layer containing glial fibers and axons. All cerebellar cortical layers can be seen, however. The pathologic changes affecting the eye include optic nerve hypoplasia, retinal detachment and dysplasia, microphthalmia, anterior segment abnormalities, cataract formation, corneal opacities, and shallow anterior chamber. Most patients with WWS die in early infancy. A fraction of patients (20%) with WWS have mutations in the gene coding for POMT1 (mannosyltransferase) on chromosome 9q34.1 (see Table 14-4) but they also may have mutations in the fukutin, fukutin-related protein, POMT2, POMGnT1, and LARGE genes.[44,46-48]

Muscle-Eye-Brain Disease (Santavuori Congenital Muscular Dystrophy). The clinical features of MEBD have been described in a number of Finnish families,[49] some with a history of consanguinity, suggesting autosomal recessive inheritance. The 9q31-q33 locus of FMD has been excluded in a number of Finnish pedigrees, and although the muscle, eye, and brain findings resemble those in WWS, the phenotype is much milder. Affected patients can usually sit, stand, and walk, but subsequent development of spasticity (usually by age 5 years) leads to loss of gross motor skills. There is hypotonia early in life, slow gross motor development, hydrocephalus, seizures probably related to cortical dysplasia (pachygyria and polymicrogyria),[50] and eye involvement with optic atrophy, retinal dysplasia, high myopia, progressive failure of vision, and abnormal results on the electroretinogram (ERG) and visual evoked potentials (VEPs). In the Santavuori variety of CMD, eye involvement is usually not obvious in the newborn period. In fact, the electroretinogram findings may remain normal until 7 years of age. Visual evoked potentials become delayed and increased in amplitude. Patients survive beyond age 3 years, but death usually occurs between 6 and 16 years. Haltia and colleagues[50] reported weak immunostaining for merosin with normal laminin β_2 chain staining in muscle from patients with MEBD. α-Dystroglycan immunostaining is reduced in MEBD. The gene mutated in MEBD is a glycosyltransferase (POMGnT1) gene and has been mapped at 1p32-p34.[51] Fukutin, LARGE, POMT1, POMT2 and POMGnT1 are putative glucotransferases involved in the glycosylation of α-dystroglycan (see Table 14-4); mutations in these genes can also result in an MEB phenotype.

Congenital Myotonic Dystrophy

Myotonic dystrophy, a multisystem disease originally described by Steinert in 1909, is the most prevalent form of muscular dystrophy. The congenital form of the disease occurs in 15% to 25% of infants born to affected mothers. The pregnancy is usually complicated by poor fetal movements and polyhydramnios. Clinical features include hypotonia at birth, respiratory distress, clubfoot, poor suck and swallow, and myopathic facies. The weakness of facial and jaw muscles produces a tented upper lip. At birth respiratory distress is a common occurrence, but myotonia is not present

14

during the neonatal period. In fact, myotonia may not be present until age 5 to 8 years. As the child gets older, cognitive impairment becomes apparent in most cases. Congenital myotonic dystrophy is always transmitted through an affected mother, who may be asymptomatic or only mildly symptomatic.

In congenital myotonic dystrophy, the CPK value is usually normal. Although the infant's EMG may fail to show myotonia, the maternal EMG findings are always abnormal. Muscle biopsy shows nonspecific abnormalities consisting of increased variability in fiber size with type I fiber atrophy in some cases. The genetic defect in myotonic dystrophy has been identified as an expansion of a trinucleotide CTG repeat located in the 3′ untranslated region of a gene, which codes for a serine-threonine protein kinase, also known as myotonin protein kinase.[52,53] Normal individuals contain between 4 and 49 copies of the CTG repeat. Normal individuals with 38 to 49 copies of the repeat are classified as having a borderline category (premutation) because of the small possibility of expansion of the CTG repeat in their offspring.[54] Mildly affected individuals, or asymptomatic mutation carriers, have 50 to 80 CTG repeats, whereas affected subjects have between 100 and 2000 or more copies (full mutation). Infants with congenital myotonic dystrophy usually have more than 750 copies. The CTG copy number increases during successive generations, explaining the phenomenon of genetic anticipation (increasing severity of the disease phenotype and/or earlier onset in successive generations) in families with myotonic dystrophy.[55] Although for a given number of repeats (>100) a wide range in disease severity may be observed, infants with severe congenital myotonic dystrophy and their mothers tend to have a greater number of CTG repeats. The greater the CTG repeat expansion in the mother, the higher the probability that her offspring will be affected with the congenital form of the illness. Unfortunately, these findings do not explain the exclusive maternal inheritance in cases of congenital myotonic dystrophy. Genomic imprinting or the presence of a maternal intrauterine factor has been proposed as possible mechanisms.

If myotonic dystrophy is suspected in a hypotonic neonate, the mother should be examined, even if she is thought to be asymptomatic, and the examiner should look closely for evidence of myotonia or weakness of distal muscles and also neck flexors. Currently, the most sensitive way to confirm the diagnosis in an infant is blood testing for the CTG repeat expansion utilizing polymerase chain reaction (PCR) and/or Southern blot analysis.[56] If the diagnosis of myotonic dystrophy cannot be established in the mother on the basis of clinical presentation and physical examination, EMG sampling of multiple muscles may be necessary to identify myotonia.

Infantile Facioscapulohumeral Muscular Dystrophy

Facioscapulohumeral dystrophy (FSHD) is an autosomal dominant dystrophy with a distinct phenotype.[57,58] To date, the precise genetic defect in this major form of FSH has yet to be identified. However, the diagnosis in FSHD can be suspected and/or easily made clinically in most patients with this disorder. Typically, the children have prominent facial as well as scapulohumeral muscle weakness; striking asymmetry of muscle involvement is a typical feature of FSH muscular dystrophy.

The infantile variety of FSHD, which is often sporadic in inheritance, has a very early onset (usually within the first few years of life) and is rapidly progressive, with wheelchair confinement by age 9 to 10 years in most cases.[58] There is profound facial weakness, with an inability to close the eyes in sleep, to smile, and to show any evidence of facial expression. The weakness rapidly involves the shoulder and hip girdles with lumbar lordosis, resulting in pronounced forward pelvic tilt, and hyperextension of the knees and the head upon walking. Marked weakness of the wrist extensors may result in a wristdrop. Young children with early-onset FSHD and a very small number of chromosome 4q35 repeats often have epilepsy, cognitive impairment, and severe sensorineural hearing loss.[59]

A commercial DNA test is now available for FSH muscular dystrophy.[60] Most patients with classic FSHD, for whom detailed molecular studies have been done, carry a chromosomal rearrangement within the subtelomere of chromosome 4q (4q35).[61] A tandem array of 3.3-kb repeated DNA elements (D4Z4) is deleted in patients with FSHD.[62] In the general population, the number of repeat units varies from 11 to more than 100; in patients with FSHD, an allele of 1 to 10 residual units is observed because of the deletion of an integral number of these units.[63] Most infants with FSHD have only one to three copies of the repeat unit. This new diagnostic test is positive in 95% of typical FSH cases.[64] Nonetheless, the sensitivity of the genetic test for atypical cases remains uncertain.[65] In patients with typical cases, there is no value in performing a muscle biopsy.

Congenital Myopathies

Shy and Magee[66] introduced the term *congenital myopathy* to describe central core disease and any myopathy present at birth excluding muscular dystrophy. Unfortunately, inclusion of conditions like nemaline myopathy and centronuclear myopathy, which may be progressive and in some cases lethal, blurred the clinical distinction from the muscular dystrophies. These conditions are, however, distinct at a pathologic level. In congenital muscular dystrophies the muscle biopsy findings are dystrophic and nonspecific, whereas in congenital myopathies there are distinct myopathologic features without significant fibrosis, muscle fiber degeneration, and replacement with adipose tissue. In congenital myopathies, the specificity of distinguishing pathologic features has declined with the inclusion of conditions with similar but not identical histologic features, such as multicore or minicore disease.

Hypotonia and weakness are the major clinical features. However, other characteristic features of congenital myopathy, like scoliosis, ptosis, and ophthalmoplegia, may not be apparent at birth. Therefore, despite the frequent history of infantile hypotonia, diagnosis may be delayed until gross motor developmental delay and associated weakness develop in late infancy or early childhood. In the congenital myopathies, EMG findings may be normal or indicate myopathy, with small polyphasic motor unit potentials, normal nerve conduction studies, normal repetitive nerve stimulation, and absence of abnormal spontaneous activity. The CPK level is usually normal or slightly elevated. This is a helpful distinction from congenital muscular dystrophies, in which CPK levels are usually moderately to markedly elevated. The diagnosis of congenital myopathies is heavily dependent on the muscle biopsy, which reveals the characteristic features for which the disorder has been named.[67] Table 14-6 summarizes the genetics and main clinical features of congenital myopathies.

Nemaline Myopathy

The term *nemaline* has been used to characterize the presence of rods or threadlike structures (Greek *nema*, thread) seen in the muscle biopsy specimens of patients with this type of congenital myopathy.[68] Of the three different types (neonatal, late infantile/early childhood, late childhood/adult), the neonatal type is the most severe, presenting with hypotonia, diminished spontaneous activity, history of poor fetal movements, and early respiratory distress.[69] More commonly, presentation is delayed until after the newborn period, when gross motor delay with proximal weakness develops.

Serum CPK value is usually normal or slightly elevated and the EMG findings may be normal, myopathic, neuropathic, or mixed. The diagnosis is made by finding of the characteristic nemaline bodies on muscle biopsy. These bodies originate from the Z disks and tend to cluster under the sarcolemma. Frequently type I fiber predominance is present. Histochemically, α-actinin, myosin, and actin have been detected in nemaline bodies.[70] In a large Australian family characterized by relatively late-onset and predominantly distal muscle involvement, close linkage to the 1q22-q23 region[71] was found with subsequent detection of mutations in the tropomyosin-3 gene.[72] In this family the inheritance was autosomal dominant. This form has been named NEM1. A second type of the autosomal recessive form of the disease (NEM2) has been linked to a locus on chromosome 2q21.2-q22, where the nebulin gene has been mapped; mutations in this gene have now been identified in patients with nemaline myopathy. In the autosomal dominant families there is a curious female predominance.[73] To date, six genes have been involved in the pathogenesis of

Table 14-6 CONGENITAL MYOPATHIES

Disease	Genes	Proteins	Onset	Weakness	Cardiac	Respiratory	Facial	Oculo-motor	Prognosis
Myotubular myopathy (centronuclear myopathy, X-linked)	MTM1	Myotubularin	Prenatal-congenital	+++	−	++	+++	+++	Death during infancy; some survive to adulthood
Centronuclear myopathy: Classic	?	?	Late infancy-early childhood	+	−	++	++	++	Ambulation until adolescence
Adult	DNM2 BIN1 RYR1	Dynamin 2 Amphiphysin Ryanodine receptor	Infancy, childhood, 2nd-3rd decade	+	−	−	+	+/−	Slowly progressive
Nemaline myopathy: Severe (congenital)	ACTA1 NEB TPM3 TNNT1	α-Actin Nebulin Tropomyosin 3 Troponin T type 1	Birth	+++	−	++	+++	−	Death in neonatal period
Typical (congenital)	ACTA1 NEB TPM3 TPM2 CFL2	α-Actin Nebulin Tropomyosin 3 Tropomyosin 2 Cofilin 2	1st year	++	+/−	+	+++	−	Many survive to adulthood

Disease	Gene	Protein	Age at onset						Prognosis
Childhood	ACTA1, NEB, TPM3	α-actin, Nebulin, Tropomyosin 3	Prepubertal	+	−	−	−	−	Many survive to adulthood
Adult	ACTA1, NEB	α-actin, Nebulin	3rd-6th decade	+	+	+/−	++	−	Adulthood
Central core, classic	RYR1	Ryanodine receptor	Infancy	+	Rare	−	+	−	Adulthood?
Multiminicore disease	SEPN1	Selenoprotein N1	Infancy to early childhood	++	Rare	++	++	Rare	Variable
Congenital myopathy and fatal cardiomyopathy	TTN	Titin	Infancy to childhood	+++	+++	?	−	−	?
Congenital fiber-type disproportion	ACTA1, SEPN1, TPM3, RYR1	α-actin, Selenoprotein N1, α-tropomyosin, Ryanodine receptor	1st year	+ to +++	Rare	+ to +++ (30%)	+	+/−	Variable
Actin myopathy (non-nemaline)	ACTA1	α-actin	Congenital	+++	+	+++	++	?	High mortality
Hyaline body myopathy	MYH7	Slow β-cardiac myosin heavy chain	Congenital-adult						
Reducing body myopathy	FHL-1	Four and a half LIM domain-1 protein	Congenital-adult	+++ to +	+			+; ptosis	

Courtesy Dr. Peter Kang, Neuromuscular Program, Children's Hospital, Boston.
+++, Severe; ++, moderate; +, mild; +/−, mild or absent; −, not reported so far.

14

nemaline myopathy (α-tropomyosin, nebulin, α-actin, β-tropomyosin, troponin T type I, and cofilin 2).

Central Core Disease

The vast majority of patients with central core disease (CCD) present with hypotonia in early infancy and childhood and a subsequent delay in motor milestones.[74] Rarely, severe hypotonia and marked contractures are present at birth. More commonly, skeletal abnormalities are present, particularly congenital dislocation of the hips, flat feet, pes cavus, clubfoot, and kyphoscoliosis. The clinical course varies from non-progressive to slowly progressive. An association between CCD and malignant hyperthermia has been observed.[75] The diagnosis is based primarily on the histologic finding of central cores on muscle biopsy. The cores appear to be packed with myo-fiber material and depleted of organelles.

CCD is transmitted by autosomal dominant inheritance.[76] Linkage analysis in four families with CCD has resulted in mapping of the locus to chromosome 19q12-13.2 and more specifically to the 19q13.1[77] segment, where the ryanodine receptor-1 gene (RYR1) is located. Mutations of the ryanodine receptor-1 gene have been detected in families with susceptibility to malignant hyperthermia and patients with CCD.[78] It appears that at least some forms of CCD and malignant hyperthermia are allelic disorders of the same genetic defect. Therefore, the expression of CCD may be related to some additional as yet unidentified factor.

Centronuclear/Myotubular Myopathy

The mode of inheritance of the centronuclear/myotubular myopathy has been debated. Two major forms of inheritance have emerged, an X-linked form seen primarily in congenital, severely affected cases and an autosomal dominant late-onset form. In some early-onset cases, the inheritance appears to be autosomal recessive. Early-onset cases are the most common form of centronuclear/myotubular myopathy and manifest with severe hypotonia, weakness and respiratory distress. Affected infants are very weak and have major feeding difficulties, facial diplegia, bilateral ptosis, and limitation of eye movements (external ophthalmoplegia). Fre-quently, dysmorphic features are evident, such as pectus carinatum, micrognathia, simian creases, high-arched palate, and talipes equinovarus.[79] The chest radiograph always shows slender ribs. Despite intensive respiratory support, infants with this disorder rarely survive and improve their motor function. Survivors have a mar-fanoid appearance. Focal or generalized seizures, albeit uncommon, have been reported. The muscle biopsy shows central nuclei present in many muscle fibers and type 1 fiber predominance.[80] A radial pattern of staining is noted with oxida-tive enzyme stains. The gene defect in the X-linked recessive variety (MTM1) was mapped to Xq28[81] and subsequently isolated. The protein product was designated myotubularin.[82] The myotubularin gene is highly conserved in evolution (expressed in yeast) and is ubiquitously expressed in human tissue despite the fact that the disease shows muscle specificity. No specific treatment is available, and most patients with the neonatal form require intensive respiratory support and gastric feeding. Although some improvement is usually noted with maturation, most neonates remain ventilator dependent. Dynamin 2, amphiphysin (B1N1), and also RYR1 (see Table 14-4) mutations have also been described in patients with centronuclear myopathy.[83]

Congenital Fiber Type Disproportion

Congenital fiber type disproportion (CFTD) typically manifests with hypotonia and weakness at birth or in the neonatal period.[84] Contractures of the hands and feet and skeletal abnormalities are common. There is delay in acquisition of motor mile-stones.[85] The CPK value is normal, and EMG findings may be normal or myopathic. The muscle biopsy shows type I fiber atrophy, which is a nonspecific finding noted in other clinically diverse conditions. Therefore, the existence of CFTD as an entity has been debated. A group of patients with hypotonia and type 1 fiber predominance has been described in whom decrease in the size of type 1 fibers is not observed.

Type 1 fiber predominance is another nonspecific feature of many myopathies. Despite the debate over the specificity of CFTD, it is not unusual to find type 1 fiber atrophy and type 1 fiber predominance in muscle biopsy specimens of hypotonic infants. Although these findings do not reliably predict an improving course, many of these infants have a good outcome and, as such, deserve supportive measures. α-Actin (*ACTA1*), *RYR1*, α-tropomyosin, and selenoprotein N (*SEPN1*) mutations have been described in patients with CFTD.[86,87]

Minicore Myopathy

Minicore myopathy [multiminicore disease (MmD)] is a recessive congenital myopathy characterized by multiple areas of loss of oxidative activity in muscle biopsy specimens. Its onset is usually at birth or during infancy and sometimes in childhood. It manifests with predominantly axial and proximal weakness, hypotonia, and arthrogryposis. Two thirds of affected children have scoliosis and respiratory difficulties. The presence of minicores has been linked to the following four clinical phenotypes: (1) classic phenotype with significant axial weakness, early respiratory impairment, and severe scoliosis; (2) predominantly hip girdle weakness sometimes associated with arthrogryposis at birth; (3) classic phenotype with associated external ophthalmoplegia; and (4) marked distal atrophy and weakness affecting primarily the upper extremities.

Patients with the classic axial presentation of multiminicore disease have recessive mutations in the selenoprotein N (*SEPN1*) gene, which also causes congenital muscular dystrophy with rigidity of the spine (RSMD1). The multiminicore disease phenotype with predominant hip girdle weakness and the one with distal atrophy and weakness have been linked to mutations in the skeletal muscle ryanodine receptor (*RYR1*) gene. Recently, *RYR1* gene recessive mutations were also identified in the subset of patients with multiminicore disease and external ophthalmoplegia.[88]

Other Congenital Myopathies

In addition to the four most common congenital myopathies described previously, there are uncommon types of congenital myopathies characterized by hypotonia, weakness, delay in motor milestones, and a less well-defined pattern of inheritance. Their names, which reflect their myopathologic features, include the following: (1) actin myopathy (nonnemaline); (2) fingerprint body myopathy; (3) sarcotubular myopathy; (4) hyaline body myopathy; (5) reducing body myopathy; (6) cytoplasmic body myopathy; (7) myopathy with myotubular aggregates; (8) zebra body myopathy; and (9) trilaminar myopathy. The mutated genes are known in some of them (see Table 14-6), but in all of these conditions, the diagnosis is made by muscle biopsy, underscoring the significance of this procedure in the evaluation of newborns with weakness and hypotonia unrelated to CNS dysfunction or systemic disease.

Metabolic Myopathies

Acid Maltase Deficiency (Glycogen Storage Disease II)

Acid maltase is a lysosomal α-1,4-glucosidase that releases glucose from glycogen, oligosaccharides and maltose. Acid maltase deficiency (AMD) is separated into three major groups: infantile, childhood, and adult. All types are transmitted by autosomal recessive inheritance.

Infantile Acid Maltase Deficiency (Pompe's Disease). Infantile AMD may present in the newborn period, but the onset is usually during the second or third month of life. The presentation usually consists of rapidly progressive weakness, hypotonia, and enlargement of the heart, tongue, and liver. Storage of glycogen in the brain and spinal cord results in CNS dysfunction with diminished alertness and hyporeflexia. Respiratory and feeding difficulties are common, and death, usually from cardiorespiratory failure, commonly occurs before the age 2 years. The electrocardiogram (ECG) shows a short PR interval, high QRS amplitude, and left ventricular hypertrophy.[89] In one infant a Wolff-Parkinson-White syndrome was noted. The diagnosis is supported by an increased CPK value, generally less than 10 times the upper limit of normal, and myopathic EMG findings, with abundant myotonic discharges and occasionally with fibrillation potentials and positive waves. Acid maltase activity is deficient in muscle, liver, heart, leukocytes, and cultured fibroblasts. To confirm the diagnosis the enzyme is usually assayed in lymphocytes and/or muscle tissue, and sometimes in urine.[90] The muscle biopsy shows large vacuoles with a high glycogen content (periodic acid–Schiff [PAS]-positive) and strong reactivity for acid phosphatase, identifying them as secondary lysosomes. Despite the detection of numerous mutations in the acid α-1,4-glucosidase gene on chromosome 17q23,[91] DNA testing is not yet routinely available. In the past, aside from supportive management of the cardiorespiratory insufficiency, there was no effective treatment for infantile AMD. Enzyme replacement therapy has now become available and has good results.[92]

Mitochondrial Myopathies

Cytochrome c Oxidase Deficiency

Fatal Infantile Myopathy. Fatal infantile myopathy manifests soon after birth with severe lactic acidosis, profound hypotonia and weakness, feeding difficulties, and respiratory insufficiency. In some cases, myopathy with or without an associated cardiomyopathy may be the only manifestation. More commonly, however, there is an associated renal deToni-Fanconi-Debre syndrome. Most of the infants with this myopathy die from cardiorespiratory insufficiency before 1 year of age. Muscle biopsy shows ragged-red fibers with accumulation of glycogen and lipid in most but not all cases. Histochemical staining for cytochrome c oxidase (COX) activity is undetectable, and biochemical analysis of skeletal muscle tissue shows virtual absence of COX activity.[93] A severe depletion of mitochondrial DNA (mtDNA) has been detected in patients with fatal infantile myopathy.

Benign Infantile Myopathy. The benign variety of infantile myopathy manifests at or soon after birth with generalized weakness and hypotonia, respiratory and feeding difficulties, and severe lactic acidosis.[94] Unlike the fatal form, this condition is confined to the skeletal muscle. Infants with this disease tend to improve spontaneously during the first year of life and are normal by age 3 years. Muscle histochemistry and/or standard biochemical assays show almost undetectable COX activity. With age this enzyme activity recovers. Ragged-red fibers have been observed in early muscle biopsy specimens but disappear during childhood. The benign variety is distinguished from the fatal form by the immunologic detection (immunotitration by enzyme-linked immunosorbent assay [ELISA]) of the enzyme in muscle tissue.[95] In the fatal type of COX deficiency, the enzyme protein is undetectable by ELISA.[96] Most cases have been sporadic. This condition is thought to result from mutations in a tissue-specific and developmentally regulated fetal COX isoform. Because the enzymatic deficiency is reversible, aggressive support is advised in infants with COX deficiency.

Fatty Acid Oxidation Defects

This group of disorders known as the fatty acid oxidation defects includes the following: (1) the carnitine deficiency syndromes; (2) defects in carnitine palmitoyltransferases CPT I and CPT II as well as in translocase; and (3) defects of fatty acid β-oxidation enzymes. Most of these conditions manifest in infancy with hypotonia, generalized weakness, and in some cases cardiomegaly and/or hepatic failure. There may be associated nonketotic or hypoketotic hypoglycemia, hyperammonemia, reduced total and/or free carnitine (rarely, increased free and total carnitine) values, elevated serum acylcarnitine values, and abnormal urine dicarboxylic acids and acylglycines. The serum CPK value may be normal or highly elevated. Affected newborns may be lethargic and/or comatose. Muscle biopsy may reveal accumulation of lipid, primarily in type I fibers. The diagnosis requires detection of the enzymatic deficiency in cultured skin fibroblasts and/or muscle tissue. In cases of true primary muscle carnitine deficiency, the clinical response to carnitine supplementation may be dramatic. Therefore, a trial of carnitine supplementation is warranted in infants with carnitine transport defects. *Organic acidurias* may also manifest with weakness, hypotonia, cardiomyopathy, and liver enlargement, probably due to secondary carnitine deficiency. In the secondary syndromes, the muscle biopsy shows lipid but not glycogen accumulation. Abnormal organic acids and acylcarnitines can be demonstrated by the appropriate testing of urine and serum.

Nonlysosomal Glycogenoses

Phosphorylase Deficiency

Phosphorylase deficiency may manifest in early infancy with severe generalized weakness and hypotonia, feeding difficulties, and respiratory insufficiency.[97] Areflexia or hyporeflexia is usually present but the child remains alert without evidence of encephalopathy.[98] The serum CPK concentration is elevated, and the muscle biopsy is diagnostic, showing myopathic changes with subsarcolemmal and intermyofibrillar deposits of glycogen. Phosphorylase activity is undetectable in muscle tissue by either histochemistry or enzymatic methods.

Phosphofructokinase Deficiency

A neonatal variety of phosphofructokinase (PFK) deficiency has been described, manifesting with congenital weakness, hypotonia, swollen joints, multiple contractures, and, in some cases, seizures, cortical blindness, and corneal opacifications.[99] There may be evidence of cardiomyopathy, but hemolysis develops in none of the infantile cases. CPK values and uric acid are increased in most patients. The muscle biopsy shows accumulation of glycogen under the sarcolemma and between myofibrils. The diagnosis is confirmed by the immunohistochemical demonstration of absence of PFK staining in muscle, and diminished muscle PFK activity on enzymatic assay. In infants with PFK deficiency, the enzyme is present in red blood cells in normal amounts. The biochemical basis of the infantile variety of PFK deficiency is not clear and is probably heterogeneous.

Approach to Hypotonia

Our stepwise approach to the diagnostic investigation of infantile hypotonia is as follows (Fig. 14-1):

1. Conduct a detailed history (history of polyhydraminios, intrauterine growth retardation, reduced fetal movement), and physical examination (as described previously), including tests of muscle stretch reflexes, antigravity limb movements, and contractures.[100]
2. Exclude systemic illness and congenital laxity of ligaments.
3. If central hypotonia is suspected, conduct MRI or MR spectroscopy studies, metabolic studies, and genetic testing for Prader-Willi syndrome (deletion of 15q11-13) and Down syndrome (trisomy 21). Also test for very-long-chain fatty acids and/or perform other peroxisomal tests. Consider lumbar puncture for measurement of cerebrospinal fluid lactate, glucose, and protein and, if indicated, cerebrospinal fluid neurotransmitter testing.
4. If peripheral hypotonia is suspected, first examine the mother. If she has signs of myotonic dystrophy, perform a DNA test for 19qCTG repeat expansion in the child. Elicit any history of autoimmune myasthenia gravis in the mother
   a. Consider electromyography and nerve conduction studies to evaluate for myasthenia, botulism, neuropathy or anterior horn cell disease, and myopathy. Consider performing a Tensilon test if myasthenic syndrome is suspected.
   b. Measure the child's electrolytes, CPK, lactate, pyruvate, carnitine, and/or other biochemical markers:
      (1) If CPK/EMG results are normal, conduct a DNA test for Prader-Willi syndrome.

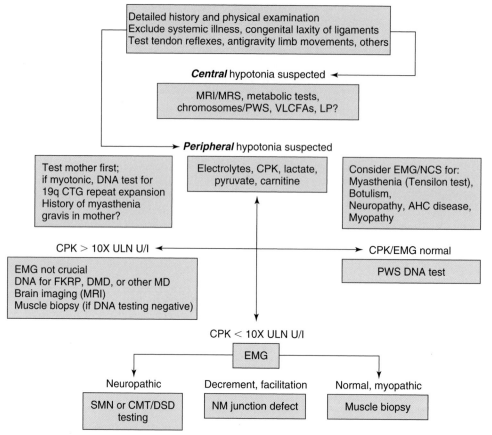

Figure 14-1 Stepwise approach to hypotonia. *CMT*, Charcot-Marie-Tooth neuropathy; *CPK*, creatine phosphokinase; *DMD*, Duchenne muscular dystrophy; EMG, electromyography; *FKRP*, fukutin-related protein; *MD*, muscular dystrophy; *MRI*, magnetic resonance imaging; *MRS*, magnetic resonance spectroscopy; *NCS*, nerve conduction study; *NM*, neuromuscular; *SMN*, survival motor neuron; *VLCFAs*, very-long-chain fatty acids.

(2) If CPK concentration is more than 10 times the upper limit of normal, EMG is not crucial. Perform DNA tests for FKRP (fukutin-related protein) gene mutations, and/or other muscular dystrophies. Consider brain imaging (MRI). If DNA testing results are negative, conduct a muscle biopsy.

(3) If CPK is elevated less than 10 times the upper limit of normal, conduct EMG. If the electromyogram findings indicate neurogenic changes, order genetic testing for survival motor neuron (SMN) gene or Charcot-Marie-Tooth/Dejerine-Sottas disease. An electromyogram showing decrement or facilitation indicates a neuromuscular junction defect. If the electromyographic findings are normal or indicate myopathy, conduct a muscle biopsy (EMG findings may be normal in certain myopathies).

References

1. Volpe JJ. *Neurology of the Newborn.* 5th ed. Philadelphia: WB Saunders; 2008.
2. Sainte-Anne Dargassies S. *Neurological Development in the Full-Term and Premature Neonate.* New York: Elsevier North Holland; 1979.
3. Volpe JJ. Neonatal hypotonia. In: Jones HR Jr, De Vivo DC, Darras BT, eds. *Neuromuscular Disorders of Infancy, Childhood, and Adolescence: A Clinician's Approach.* Philadelphia: Butterworth Heinemann; 2003:113-122.
4. Gingold MK, Jaynes ME, Bodensteiner JB, et al. The rise and fall of the plantar response in infancy. *J Pediatr.* 1998;133:568.

5. Paine RS, Brazelton TB, Donovan DE, et al. Evolution of postural reflexes in normal infants and in the presence of chronic brain syndromes. *Neurology*. 1964;14:1036.
6. Futagi Y, Tagawa T, Otani K. Primitive reflex profiles in infants: differences based on categories of neurological abnormality. *Brain Dev*. 1992;14:294.
7. Fenichel GM. The hypotonic infant. In: *Clinical pediatric neurology, a signs and symptoms approach*. 5th ed. Philadelphia: Elsevier Saunders; 2005:149-169.
8. Richer LP, Shevell MI, Miller SP. Diagnostic profile of neonatal hypotonia: an 11-year study. *Pediatr Neurol*. 2001;25:32.
9. Prasad AN, Prasad C. Genetic evaluation of the floppy infant. *Semin Fetal Neonatal Med*. 2011; 16:99.
10. Dubowitz V. Disorders of the lower motor neurone: the spinal muscular atrophies. In: Dubowitz V, ed. *Muscle Disorders in Childhood*. London: Saunders; 1995:325-369.
11. Morrison KE, Harding AE. Disorders of the motor neuron. In: Harding AE, ed. *Genetics and Neurology*. London: Bailliere Tindall; 1994:431-445.
12. Bundey S. Spinal muscular atrophies (SMAs). In: Bundey S, ed. *Genetics and neurology*. Edinburgh: Churchill Livingstone; 1985:172-193.
13. Grohmann K, Varon R, Stolz P, et al. Infantile spinal muscular atrophy with respiratory distress type 1 (SMARD1). *Ann Neurol*. 2003;54:719.
14. Gilliam TC, Brzustowicz LM. The molecular basis of the spinal muscular atrophies. In: Rosenberg RN, Pruisner SB, DiMauro S, et al. eds. *The molecular and genetic basis of neurological disease*. Philadelphia: Butterworth Heinemann; 1993:883-887.
15. Hahnen E, Forkert R, Marke C, et al. Molecular analysis of candidate genes on 5q13 in autosomal recessive spinal muscular atrophy: evidence of homozygous deletions of the SMN gene in unaffected individuals. *Hum Mol Genet*. 1995;4:1927.
16. Lefebvre S, Burglen L, Reboullet S, et al. Identification and characterization of a spinal muscular atrophy-determining gene. *Cell*. 1995;80:155.
17. Roy N, Mahadevan MS, McLean M. The gene for neuronal apoptosis inhibitor protein (NAIP), a novel protein with homology to baculoviral inhibitors of apoptosis is partially deleted in individuals with type I, II, and III spinal muscular atrophy (SMA). *Cell*. 1995;80:167.
18. Byers RK, Banker BQ. Infantile muscular atrophy. *Arch Neurol*. 1961;5:140.
19. Munsat TL. Workshop report. International SMA collaboration. *Neuromusc Disord*. 1991;1:81.
20. Feldkotter M, Schwarzer V, Wirth R, et al. Quantitative analyses of SMN1 and SMN2 based on real-time lightCycler PCR: fast and highly reliable carrier testing and prediction of severity of spinal muscular atrophy. *Am J Hum Genet*. 2002;70:358.
21. Sladky JT. Chronic sensory-motor neuropathies in children. Paper presented at: Annual Meeting of the American Association of Electrodiagnostic Medicine Course A. LA: New Orleans; 1993.
22. Behin A, Mayer M, Kassis-Makhoul B, et al. Severe neonatal myasthenia due to maternal anti-MuSK antibodies. *Neuromuscul Disord*. 2008;18:443.
23. Engel AG, Ohno K, Harper CM. Congenital myasthenic syndromes. In: Jones Jr HR, De Vivo DC, Darras BT, eds. *Neuromuscular disorders of infancy, childhood, and adolescence: a clinician's Approach*. Philadelphia: Butterworth Heinemann; 2003:555-574.
24. Gutmann L, Pratt L. Pathophysiologic aspects of human botulism. *Arch Neurol*. 1976;33:175.
25. Cherington M. Botulism: clinical, electrical and therapeutic considerations. In: Lewis GE, ed. *Biomedical aspects of botulism*. New York: Academic; 1981:327-330.
26. Cornblath DR, Sladky JT, Sumner AJ. Clinical electrophysiology of infantile botulism. *Muscle Nerve*. 1983;6:448.
27. Sunada Y, Bernier SM, Utani A, et al. Identification of a novel mutant transcript of laminin alpha 2 chain gene responsible for muscular dystrophy and dysmyelination in dy2J mice. *Hum Mol Genet*. 1995;4:1055.
28. Arnon SS, Schechter R, Maslanka SE, et al. Human botulism immune globulin for the treatment of infant botulism. *N Engl J Med*. 2006;354:462.
29. Dubowitz V. 41st ENMC international workshop on congenital muscular dystrophy. *Neuromuscul Disord*. 1996;6:295.
30. Shorer Z, Philpot J, Muntoni F, et al. Demyelinating peripheral neuropathy in merosin-deficient congenital muscular dystrophy. *J Child Neurol*. 1995;10:472.
31. Helbling-Leclerc A, Zhang X, Topaloglu H, et al. Mutations in the laminin alpha 2-chain gene (LAMA2) cause merosin-deficient congenital muscular dystrophy. *Nat Genet*. 1995;11:216.
32. Tome FM, Evangelista T, Leclerc A, et al. Congenital muscular dystrophy with merosin deficiency. *C R Acad Sci III*. 1994;317:351.
33. Philpot J, Sewry C, Pennock J, et al. Clinical phenotype in congenital muscular dystrophy: correlation with expression of merosin in skeletal muscle. *Neuromuscul Disord*. 1995;5:301.
34. Kobayashi O, Hayashi Y, Arahata K, et al. Congenital muscular dystrophy: clinical and pathologic study of 50 patients with the classical (Occidental) merosin-positive form. *Neurology*. 1996;46:815.
35. Allamand V, Sunada Y, Salih MAM, et al. Mild congenital muscular dystrophy in two patients with an internally deleted laminin α2-chain. *Hum Mol Genet*. 1997;6:747.
36. Vainzof M, Marie SKN, Reed UC, et al. Deficiency of merosin (laminin M or α2) in congenital muscular dystrophy associated with cerebral white matter alterations. *Neuropediatrics*. 1995;26:293.
37. Connolly AM, Pestronk A, Planer GJ, et al. Congenital muscular dystrophy syndromes distinguished by alkaline and acid phosphatase, merosin, and dystrophin staining. *Neurology*. 1996;46:810.
38. North KN, Specht LA, Sethi RK, et al. Congenital muscular dystrophy associated with merosin deficiency. *Neurol*. 1996;11:291.

14

39. Kobayashi K, Nakahori Y, Miyake M, et al. An ancient retrotransposal insertion causes Fukuyama-type congenital muscular dystrophy. *Nature*. 1998;394:388.
40. Fukuyama Y, Osawa M, Suzuki H. Congenital progressive muscular dystrophy of the Fukuyama type: clinical, genetic and pathological considerations. *Brain Dev*. 1981;3:1.
41. Toda T, Segawa M, Nomura Y, et al. Localization of a gene for Fukuyama type congenital muscular dystrophy to chromosome 9q31-33. *Nat Genet*. 1993;5:283.
42. Yoshioka M, Kuroki S. Clinical spectrum and genetic studies of Fukuyama congenital muscular dystrophy. *Am J Med Genet*. 1994;53:245.
43. Dobyns WB, Pagon RA, Armstrong D, et al. Diagnostic criteria for Walker-Warburg syndrome. *Am J Med Genet*. 1989;32:195.
44. Beltran-Valero de Bernabe D, Currier S, Steinbrecher A, et al. Mutations in the O-mannosyltransferase gene POMT1 give rise to the severe neuronal migration disorder Walker-Warburg syndrome. *Am J Hum Genet*. 2002;71:1033.
45. Dobyns WB, Truwit CL. Lissencephaly and other malformations of cortical development: 1995 update. *Neuropediatrics*. 1995;26:132.
46. de Bernabe DB, van Bokhoven H, van Beusekom E, et al. A homozygous nonsense mutation in the fukutin gene causes a Walker-Warburg syndrome phenotype. *J Med Genet*. 2003;40:845.
47. Beltran-Valero de Bernabe D, Voit T, Longman C, et al. Mutations in the FKRP gene can cause muscle-eye-brain disease and Walker-Warburg syndrome. *J Med Genet*. 2004;41:e61.
48. van Reeuwijk J, Janssen M, van den Elzen C, et al. POMT2 mutations cause alpha-dystroglycan hypoglycosylation and Walker-Warburg syndrome. *J Med Genet*. 2005;42:907.
49. Santavuori P, Somer H, Sainio K, et al. Muscle-eye brain disease (MEB). *Brain Dev*. 1989;11:147.
50. Haltia M, Leivo I, Sorne RH, et al. Muscle-eye-brain disease: a neuropathological study. *Ann Neurol*. 1997;41:173.
51. Yoshida A, Kobayashi K, Manya H, et al. Muscular dystrophy and neuronal migration disorder caused by mutations in a glycosyltransferase, POMGnT1. *Dev Cell*. 2001;1:717.
52. Aslanidis C, Jansen G, Amemiya C, et al. Cloning of the essential myotonic dystrophy region and mapping of the putative defect. *Nature*. 1992;355:548.
53. Brook JD, McCurrach ME, Harley HG, et al. Molecular basis of myotonic dystrophy: expansion of a trinucleotide (CTG) repeat at the 3′ end of a transcript encoding a protein kinase family member. *Cell*. 1992;68:799.
54. Harley HG, Rundle SA, Reardon W. Unstable DNA sequence in myotonic dystrophy. *Lancet*. 1992;339:1125.
55. Suthers GK, Huson SM, Davies KE. Instability versus predictability: the molecular diagnosis of myotonic dystrophy. *J Med Genet*. 1992;29:761.
56. Brunner HG, Nillesen W, van Oost BA. Presymptomatic diagnosis of myotonic dystrophy. *J Med Genet*. 1992;29:780.
57. Munsat TL, Piper D, Cancilla P, et al. Inflammatory myopathy with facioscapulohumeral distribution. *Neurology*. 1972;22:335.
58. Taylor DA, Carroll JE, Smith ME, et al. Facioscapulohumeral dystrophy associated with hearing loss and Coats syndrome. *Ann Neurol*. 1982;12:395.
59. Funakoshi M, Goto K, Arahata K. Epilepsy and mental retardation in a subset of early onset 4q35-facioscapulohumeral muscular dystrophy. *Neurology*. 1998;50:1791.
60. Kohler J, Rohrig D, Bathke KD, et al. Evaluation of the facioscapulohumeral muscular dystrophy (FSHD1) phenotype in correlation to the concurrence of 4q35 and 10q26 fragments. *Clin Genet*. 1999;55:88.
61. Griggs RC, Tawil R, Storvick D, et al. Genetics of facioscapulohumeral muscular dystrophy: new mutations in sporadic cases. *Neurology*. 1993;43:2369.
62. Hewitt JE, Lyle R, Clark LN, et al. Analysis of the tandem repeat locus D4Z4 associated with facioscapulohumeral muscular dystrophy. *Hum Mol Genet*. 1994;3:1287.
63. Tawil R, Figlewicz DA, Griggs RC, et al. Facioscapulohumeral dystrophy: a distinct regional myopathy with a novel molecular pathogenesis. FSH Consortium. *Ann Neurol*. 1998;43:279.
64. Ricci E, Galluzzi G, Deidda G, et al. Progress in the molecular diagnosis of facioscapulohumeral muscular dystrophy and correlation between the number of KpnI repeats at the 4q35 locus and clinical phenotype. *Ann Neurol*. 1999;45:751.
65. Vitelli F, Villanova M, Malandrini A, et al. Inheritance of a 38-kb fragment in apparently sporadic facioscapulohumeral muscular dystrophy. *Muscle Nerve*. 1999;22:1437.
66. Shy GM, Magee KR. A new congenital non-progressive myopathy. *Brain*. 1956;79:610.
67. Sewry CA. Pathological defects in congenital myopathies. *J Muscle Res Cell Motil*. 2008;29:231.
68. Shy GM, Engel WK, Somers JE, et al. Nemaline myopathy: a new congenital myopathy. *Brain*. 1963;86:793.
69. Shafig SA, Dubowitz V, Peterson H, et al. Nemaline myopathy: report of a fatal case with histochemical and electron microscopic studies. *Brain*. 1967;90:817.
70. Wallgren-Pettersson C, Arjomaa P, Holmberg C. Alpha-actinin and myosin light chains in congenital nemaline myopathy. *Pediatr Neurol*. 1990;6:171.
71. Laing NG, Majda BT, Akkari PA, et al. Assignment of a gene (NEMI) for autosomal dominant nemaline myopathy to chromosome I. *Am J Hum Genet*. 1992;50:576.
72. Laing NG, Wilton SD, Akkari PA, et al. A mutation in the alpha tropomyosin gene TPM3 associated with autosomal dominant nemaline myopathy. *Nat Genet*. 1995;9:75.
73. Scarlato G, Pellegrini G, Moggio M. Familial nemaline myopathy. *Neuropediatrics*. 1982;13:211.
74. Engel WK, Foster JB, Hughes BP. Central core disease—an investigation of a rare muscle cell abnormality. *Brain*. 1961;84 167.

14

75. Denborough MA, Dennett XK, Anderson RM. Central core disease and malignant hyperthermia. *Br Med J*. 1973;1:272.

76. Byrne E, Blumbergs PC, Hallpike JF. Central core disease. Study of a family with five affected generations. *J Neurol Sci*. 1982;53:77.

77. Haan EA, Freemantle CJ, McCure JA, et al. Assignment of the gene for central core disease to chromosome 19. *Hum Genet*. 1990;86:187.

78. Zhang Y, Chen HS, Khanna VK. A mutation in the human ryanodine receptor gene associated with central core disease. *Nature Genet*. 1993;5:46.

79. Kinoshita M, Cadman TE. Myotubular myopathy. *Arch Neurol*. 1968;18:265.

80. Spiro AJ, Shy GM, Gonatas NK. Myotubular myopathy: persistence of fetal muscle in an adolescent boy. *Arch Neurol*. 1966;14:1.

81. Thomas NST, Sarfarazi M, Roberts K, et al. X-linked myotubular myopathy (MTM1) evidence for linkage to Xq28 DNA marker loci. *J Med Genet*. 1990;27:284.

82. Laporte J, Hu LJ, Kretz C, et al. A gene mutated in X-linked myotubular myopathy defines a new putative tyrosine phosphatase family conserved in yeast. *Nature Genet*. 1996;13:175.

83. Bitoun M, Maugenre S, Jeannet PY, et al. Mutations in dynamin 2 cause dominant centronuclear myopathy. *Nat Genet*. 2005;37:1207.

84. Brooke MH. Congenital fiber type disproportion. In: Kakulas BA, ed. *Clinical studies in myology*. International Congress Series Vol 295. Amsterdam: Excerpta Medica ICS; 1973:147.

85. Lenard HG, Goebel HH. Congenital fibre type disproportion. *Neuropediatrics*. 1975;6:220.

86. Laing NG, Clarke NF, Dye DE, et al. Actin mutations are one cause of congenital fibre type disproportion. *Ann Neurol*. 2004;56:689.

87. Clarke NF, Kidson W, Quijano-Roy S, et al. SEPN1: associated with congenital fiber-type disproportion and insulin resistance. *Ann Neurol*. 2006;59:546.

88. Jungbluth H, Zhou H, Hartley L, et al. Minicore myopathy with ophthalmoplegia caused by mutations in the ryanodine receptor type 1 gene. *Neurology*. 2005;65:1930.

89. Bulkley BH, Hutchins GM. Pompe's disease presenting as hypertrophic myocardiopathy with Wolff-Parkinson-White syndrome. *Am Heart J*. 1978;92:246.

90. Salafsky IS, Nadler HL. Deficiency of acid alpha glucosidase in the urine of patients with Pompe disease. *J Pediatr*. 1973;82:294.

91. Zhong N, Martiniuk F, Tzall S, et al. Identification of a missense mutation in one allele of a patient with Pompe disease, and use of endonuclease digestion of PCR-amplified RNA to demonstrate lack of mRNA expression from the second allele. *Am J Hum Genet*. 1991;49:635.

92. Kishnani PS, Nicolino M, Voit T, et al. Chinese hamster ovary cell-derived recombinant human acid alpha-glucosidase in infantile-onset Pompe disease. *J Pediatr*. 2006;149:89.

93. Rimoldi M, Bottacchi E, Rossi L. Cytochrome-c-oxidase deficiency in muscle of a floppy infant without mitochondrial myopathy. *J Neurol*. 1982;227:201.

94. Zeviani M, Peterson P, Servidei S. Benign reversible muscle cytochrome c oxidase deficiency: a second case. *Neurology*. 1987;37:64.

95. Tritschler HJ, Bonilla E, Lombes A, et al. Differential diagnosis of fatal and benign cytochrome c oxidase-deficient myopathies of infancy: an immunohistochemical approach. *Neurology*. 1991;41:300.

96. Bresolin N, Zeviani M, Bonilla E. Molecular defects in cytochrome c oxidase deficiency: decrease of immunologically detectable enzyme in muscle. *Neurology*. 1985;35:802.

97. DiMauro S, Hartlage P. Fatal infantile form of muscle phosphorylase deficiency. *Neurology*. 1978;28:1124.

98. Milstein J, Herron T, Haas J. Fatal infantile muscle phosphorylase deficiency. *J Child Neurol*. 1989;4:186.

99. Servidei S, Bonilla E, Diedrich RG. Fatal infantile form of muscle phosphofructokinase deficiency. *Neurology*. 1986;36:1465.

100. Vasta I, Kinali M, Messina S, et al. Can clinical signs identify newborns with neuromuscular disorders? *J Pediatr*. 2005;146:73.

14

CHAPTER 15

Amplitude-Integrated EEG and Its Potential Role in Augmenting Management Within the NICU

Mona C. Toet, MD, PhD, and Linda S. de Vries, MD, PhD

15

- **Amplitude-Integrated EEG**
- **Assessment of aEEG Background Pattern**
- **Comparison with Standard EEG**
- **Pitfalls and Artifacts**
- **Gaps in Knowledge**
- **Conclusion**

Interest in the neonatal brain has increased considerably during the last few decades. This is in part due to better diagnostic methods in the acute and subacute stages. The presence and extent of structural lesions of the brain is provided by imaging techniques such as ultrasound and magnetic resonance imaging (MRI). Information about cerebral metabolism can also be obtained during the same examination using MR spectroscopy. Near-infrared spectroscopy (NIRS) allows noninvasive monitoring of brain oxygenation and cerebral hemodynamics.

Electroencephalography (EEG) or amplitude-integrated EEG (aEEG) provides information about brain function. It may detect epileptic discharges and changes in background activity following hypoxia-ischemia. aEEG is now used routinely in an increasing number of neonatal intensive care units (NICUs). In a 2010 paper, the extent of EEG monitoring in NICUs was evaluated through analysis of 210 surveys (124 from Europe and 54 from the United States).[1] Ninety percent of the respondents had access to either EEG or aEEG monitoring; 51% had both. The EEG was mainly interpreted by neurophysiologists (72%), whereas aEEG was usually interpreted by the neonatologist (80%). As many as 31% of the respondents reported that they were not confident in their ability to interpret aEEG/EEG.

Amplitude-Integrated EEG

Maynard[2] originally constructed the cerebral function monitor (CFM) in the late 1960s for continuous monitoring. Prior[2a,2b] developed the clinical application, mainly for adult patients, during anesthesia and intensive care, after cardiac arrest, during status epilepticus, and after heart surgery.

The term *aEEG* is currently preferred to denote a method for encephalographic monitoring whereas CFM is used to refer to a specific type of equipment. The EEG signal for the single-channel aEEG is usually recorded from one pair of parietally placed electrodes (corresponding to P3 and P4 according to the international EEG 10-20 classification, ground Fz). Using two channels (F3-P3 and F4-P4 or C3-P3 and C4-P4, ground Fz according to the international EEG 10-20 classification) will provide information about hemispheric asymmetry, which may be especially helpful in children with a unilateral brain lesion.[3] In the two-channel recording the F3-P3 and F4-P4 position is preferred, opposed to the short electrode distance of the P3-C3 and P4-C4 position, which will affect background patterns.

263

The signal is amplified and passed through an asymmetric band-pass filter that strongly prefers higher frequencies over lower ones and suppresses activity below 2 Hz and above 15 Hz in order to minimize artifacts from such sources as sweating, movement, muscle activity, and electrical interference. Additional processing includes semilogarithmic amplitude presentation, rectification, smoothing, and considerable time compression. The signal is displayed on a semilogarithmic scale at slow speed (6 cm/hour). A second tracing continuously displays the original EEG from either one or two channels. The electrode impedance is continuously recorded but not necessarily displayed, but there will be an alarm when the impedance is high, often because of a loose electrode. The bandwidth in the output reflects variations in minimum and maximum EEG amplitude, both of which depend on the maturity and severity of illness of the newborn infant. Owing to the semilogarithmic scale used to plot the output, changes in background activity of very low amplitude (<5 µV) are enhanced. The information in the aEEG trace can be enhanced by modifying the gray scale so that a particular spot is determined by the length of time spent at that spot. This feature is useful when defining the lower border of the trace (Fig. 15-1) and analyzing changes caused by ictal periods.

Assessment of aEEG Background Pattern

The aEEG traces are assessed visually on the basis of pattern recognition and classified into the five following categories in full-term infants[4]:

- The continuous normal voltage (CNV) pattern is a continuous trace with a voltage of 10-25 (−50) µV (see Figs. 15-8A and 15-9C).
- Discontinuous normal voltage (DNV) pattern is a discontinuous trace, in which the low voltage is predominantly above 5 µV (no burst suppression) (see Fig. 15-9B).

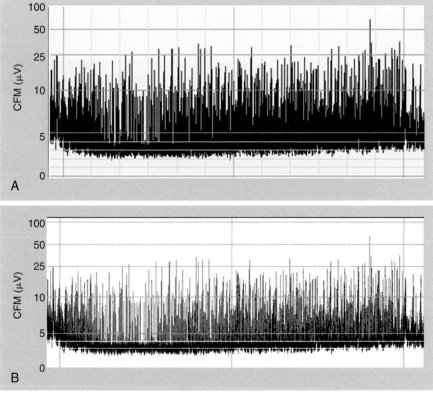

Figure 15-1 A, Burst suppression (BS) pattern without gray scale. **B,** BS pattern with grayscale.

- Discontinuous background pattern (burst suppression [BS]); periods of low voltage (inactivity) intermixed with bursts of higher amplitude (see Fig. 15-3C).
- Continuous background pattern of very low voltage (around or below 5 µV) (CLV).
- Very low voltage, mainly inactive tracing with activity below 5 µV (flat trace [FT]).

The classification offered by Al Naqeeb and colleagues[5] uses absolute values for background patterns, as follows:

Normal: upper margin >10 µV; lower margin >5 µV.

Moderately abnormal: upper margin >10 µV; lower margin <5 µV.

Severely abnormal: upper margin <10 µV; lower margin <5 µV.

We prefer the pattern recognition criteria because the background pattern may be influenced by the drift of the baseline, as described in the following case history. This drift is especially common in tracings from infants with very poor background activity, in which the lower margin is lifted upward by an electrocardiography (ECG) signal. (See also Toet and associates.[6])

CASE HISTORY 1

Patient 1 was born at term via emergency cesarean section because of a sinusoidal pattern on cardiotocography (CTG). The umbilical artery pH was 6.70. The first-measured arterial lactate value was 30 mmol/L. The aEEG showed a drift of the baseline with seizures (Fig. 15-2). As the lower margin was >5 µV, the question was raised whether cooling was indicated. A loading dose of lidocaine was given.

When the two aEEG scoring systems, pattern recognition and background values, were compared in the same dataset containing comparable normothermia and hypothermia-treated infants,[7] it was noted that the pattern recognition method was superior for early outcome prediction in a subgroup of patients with hypoxic-ischemic encephalopathy (HIE). The appearance of the aEEG trace is influenced by several factors, including interference from the electrocardiogram, muscle activity, and interelectrode distance.[8] Interobserver variability was slightly lower with voltage classification than with pattern recognition, although the two methods are equally good when compared with the real EEG.[9] The voltage classification is easier to use for clinicians with little experience in reading aEEG, but one should always try to

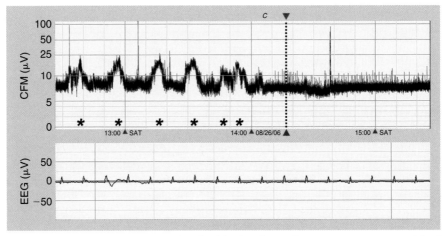

Figure 15-2 Patient 1. *Upper panel,* Drift of the baseline with seizures (*). *Lower panel,* Real EEG to electrocardiography (EEG:ECG) artifact. Loading dose of lidocaine given at C.

assess the underlying pattern. It has been shown that a BS pattern may be read as a normal voltage pattern when a drift of the baseline is bringing the lower margin above 5 μV.[10] When this artifact is not recognized, hypothermia may not be offered to eligible infants. Having access to the raw EEG may help the clinician recognize this artifact, because the ECG artifact that tends to be the cause of the drift of the baseline can be seen superimposed on the EEG.

Comparison with Standard EEG

Background Pattern

There have been several studies in which aEEG and standard EEG were performed simultaneously to compare the two techniques. Overall there appeared to be a good correlation between the aEEG and EEG background patterns in the full-term infant with moderate to severe neonatal encephalopathy.[11,12]

Prognostic Value of aEEG in HIE: Noncooled Situation

The value of the background pattern in the prediction of neurodevelopmental outcome was already well established with the use of the standard EEG. A poor background pattern, which persists beyond the first 12 to 24 hours after birth (BS, low voltage, and FT) are well known to carry a poor prognosis. A later study by Murray and colleagues[13] described the evolution of EEG changes after an hypoxic-ischemic insult. They recorded continuous, multichannel, video EEG from 6 hours to 72 hours after delivery, and then assessed neurologic outcome at 24 months in 44 infants. Of those, 20 (45%) had abnormal outcomes. The best predictive ability was seen at 6 hours of age—area under the receiver operator characteristic curve: 0.958 (95% confidence interval [CI] 0.88-1.04; $P = 0.000$). EEG features that were associated with abnormal outcomes were background amplitude less than 30 μV, interburst interval (IBI) longer than 30 seconds, electrographic seizures, and absence of sleep-wake cycling at 48 hours.

The prognostic value of early (within 72 hours after birth) severely abnormal aEEG background activity (BS, CLV, or FT) in HIE is described in the meta-analysis of eight studies by Spitzmiller and coworkers.[14] A sensitivity of 91% (CI 87%-95%) and a negative likelihood ratio of 0.09 for aEEG tracings was found to accurately predict poor outcome. The relationship between aEEG amplitude measures, Sarnat grades, and MRI abnormality scores has also been reported. The relationship was strongest for the minimum amplitude measures in both hemispheres. The presence of a minimum amplitude less than 4 μV was associated with the presence of severe MRI abnormalities.[15]

Both positive and negative predictive values were slightly lower when aEEG was assessed at 3 instead of 6 hours after birth, but they were still considered sufficiently high to use this technique for early selection of candidates for hypothermia or other intervention studies. Combining a neurologic examination with aEEG performed less than 12 hours after birth further increased predictive accuracy from 75% to 85%.[16]

Recovery of the background pattern within 24 hours after perinatal asphyxia with a poor background activity (BS, FT, CLV) has been reported in 20% of cases in another study.[17] Of these infants, 60% survived with a mild disability or were normal at follow-up. The patients who did not recover either died in the neonatal period or survived with a severe disability.

Another way of looking at recovery of the background pattern is to assess the presence, quality, and time of onset of sleep-wake cycling (SWC) (see Figs. 15-8A and 15-9C). The presence, time of onset, and quality of SWC reflects the severity of the hypoxic-ischemic insult to which the newborn has been exposed. The time of onset of SWC was shown to predict neurodevelopmental outcome on the basis of whether SWC returned before 36 hours (good outcome) or after 36 hours (bad outcome). Therefore we recommend continuous monitoring for at least 48 hours or until a normal SWC pattern is established.[18]

In infants with hypoxia-ischemia, we recommend continuous aEEG monitoring for a minimum period of 48 to 72 hours, or beyond rewarming in those receiving hypothermia (see later discussion), to allow enough time for recovery of the background activity and to assess time of onset of SWC. In those who are treated with antiepileptic drugs (AEDs), we would recommend continuation of monitoring until epileptic discharges have stopped and medication (except for possible maintenance medication) has been tailed off.

Prognostic Value of aEEG in HIE: Cooled Situation

CASE HISTORY 2

Patient 2 was born at 40 weeks of gestation and weighing 4000 g. Emergency cesarean section was performed for vaginal blood loss. Apgar scores were 0 (1 min), 2 (5 min), and 4 (10 min). The infant was resuscitated for 8 minutes with three injections of epinephrine. Another episode of bradycardia needing epinephrine and cardiac massage occurred at 20 minutes. Umbilical cord pH was not measured. The first arterial blood specimen yielded the following values: lactate 23 mmol/L, Hb 3.9 mmol/L. The infant underwent cooling for 72 hours at 33.5° C. Seizures were treated with phenobarbital, midazolam, and lidocaine. Midazolam blood levels were 0.80 mg/L at 56 hours (strongly elevated) and within the normal range at 75 hours (Fig. 15-3). MRI on day 4 showed discrete white matter abnormalities. MRI on day 9 demonstrated normal myelination of the posterior limb of the internal capsule and white matter. Follow-up at 24 months included evaluation with Bayley Scales of Intellectual Development, 3rd version (BSID/III), which yielded a Mental Developmental Index (MDI) of 90 and a Psychomotor Development Index (PDI) of 107.

The first study describing the prognostic value of aEEG in infants with HIE treated with hypothermia was by Hallberg and coworkers.[19] In their study 26 infants fulfilled the criteria for hypothermia treatment (0.9 /1000), of whom 23 were treated with hypothermia, and all of these infants had available aEEG data. Normal 1-year outcome was found in 10 of 15 infants with severely abnormal BS pattern or worse at 6 hours of age. Severe abnormalities were found to be significantly predictive for abnormal outcome after 36 hours. These investigators concluded that among asphyxiated infants treated with hypothermia, only those who had aEEG abnormalities persisting at and beyond 24 hours after birth have a poor neurologic outcome at 1 year.

In a study by Thoresen and colleagues,[7] the predictive value of aEEG at 6 hours on outcomes was evaluated in normothermia-treated infants and hypothermia-treated infants. The background activity was assessed by pattern analysis and voltage analysis. The best outcome predictor was investigated. In total 74 infants were recruited by using the Cool-Cap entry criteria, and their outcomes were assessed by using the Bayley Scales of Infant Development II at 18 months.[20] Time to normal aEEG was a better predictor than time to SWC. Never achieving SWC always predicted poor outcome. The researchers concluded that early aEEG patterns can be used to predict outcome for infants treated with normothermia but not hypothermia. Infants with good outcome had normalized background patterns by 24 hours when treated with normothermia and by 48 hours when treated with hypothermia. They also concluded that the pattern recognition method in combination with evaluation of the real EEG trace is superior to the voltage criteria method. The appearance of SWC in cooled infants with HIE was also addressed in a paper by Tachenouchi and coworkers.[20a] They found that although onset of SWC is markedly delayed in term neonates with moderate to severe HIE who are treated with hypothermia, approximately 65% who acquire SWC have a normal outcome. Therefore SWC is an important additional tool for assessing recovery in term infants with moderate to severe HIE treated with hypothermia.

Care should be taken when AEDs are given for seizures in infants who have not recovered the background pattern within 24 to 48 hours (see Fig. 15-3). High

15

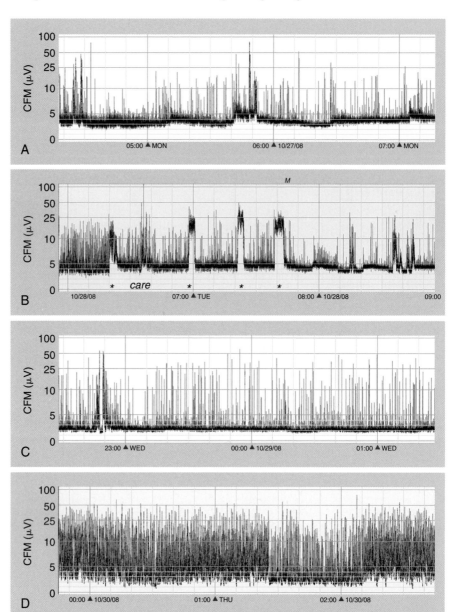

Figure 15-3 Patient 2. **A,** Start of cooling (severe burst suppression [BS] pattern, almost FT). **B,** 32 hours after birth during cooling. BS pattern with seizures (*). *M*, Midazolam. **C,** 48 hours after birth (cooled). BS pattern. **D,** 72 hours after birth. Discontinuous normal voltage (DNV) and BS patterns.

blood levels of AEDs (with may be altered metabolism due to cooling) may influence background pattern of aEEG (see Fig. 15-3C). Filippi and colleagues[21] already showed that phenobarbital administered to newborns undergoing whole-body hypothermia results in higher plasma concentrations and longer half-lives than expected in normothermic newborns.

aEEG and Seizures

Seizure Detection

Ray[22] reviewed five studies to answer the question whether aEEG is as accurate as conventional EEG in the detection of seizures. Because of the nature of the aEEG technique, it is not surprising that very brief seizure activity as well as focal seizure activity may be missed. This problem was also shown by Shellhaas and colleagues[23] in a large dataset of 125 conventional EEGs with 851 neonatal seizures. They reported that 94% of the conventional EEGs detected one or more seizures on the C3-C4 channel. Thus, conventional EEG remains the gold standard for quantification of seizure burden.

Detection of individual seizures using aEEG has been found in two studies to be difficult (rate 12%-38%) without access to the real EEG, especially when the seizures were infrequent, brief, or of low amplitude.[24,25] There were no false-positive results among control records. Infants with focal seizures, however, tend to have more widespread ictal discharges during the continuous registration, which will be identified. In addition, 81% of the neonatal seizures originated from central temporal or midline vertex electrodes, which can potentially be picked up by the aEEG electrodes.[11] An important study was that by Shah and colleagues,[26] who showed that the combination of two-channel aEEG with the real EEG signal detected the majority (76%) of electrical seizures in at-risk newborn infants. aEEG in combination with the real EEG signal was clearly better in seizure detection than aEEG alone (27% vs. 44%). In a review by Evans and colleagues,[12] 44 studies with aEEG and simultaneous conventional EEG were analyzed. Sensitivity for the presence of seizures by aEEG was 80%, and specificity was 50%. A number of seizures were overdiagnosed by aEEG as well as by standard EEG (63% vs. 45.5 %, respectively). The specificity of aEEG for seizure detection was higher in neonates undergoing EEG for suspected seizures. On the other hand, monitoring for seizures with limited channel aEEG (two channels with access to the real EEG) can be accurately interpreted, compares favorably with conventional EEG, and is associated with a trend toward reduced seizure burden.[27]

Sometimes the aEEG is suspicious of a seizure pattern but the real EEG is not conclusive. This could represent multifocal epileptiform activity. The only way to verify this is to perform a full EEG, as described in the next case history.

CASE HISTORY 3

The pregnancy that produced patient 3 was complicated during the last few weeks by hypertension and pre-eclampsia. At term a 3620-g boy was born by ventouse delivery. Apgar scores were 4 (1 min) and 9 (5 min). He started to have seizures within 1 to 2 hours after birth (Fig. 15-4A), which were treated initially with phenobarbital, and he was transferred to the NICU. He subsequently needed ventilatory support and was given phenobarbital, midazolam, lidocaine, clonazepam, and pyridoxine because of refractory seizures. Cranial ultrasound performed within 24 hours after birth showed diffuse echogenicities in the subcortical white matter and basal ganglia. MRI demonstrated massive areas of subcortical abnormalities in the left hemisphere and extensive bilateral cortical injury, seen as high signal intensity on DWI (Fig. 15-4B). The infant died on day 7. Cardiac and metabolic evaluation showed no abnormalities. Postmortem examination of the brain revealed changes compatible with severe hypoxic-ischemic injury.

Seizure burden is known to be very high in encephalopathic neonates. A video conventional EEG study by Murray and colleagues[28] showed that only one third of neonatal EEG seizures display clinical signs on simultaneous video recordings. Two thirds of these clinical manifestations were not recognized or were misinterpreted by experienced neonatal staff, with very low interobserver agreement.[29] Clinical diagnosis is therefore not sufficient for the recognition and management of neonatal seizures.

A rapid rise of both the lower and the upper margins of the aEEG tracing is suggestive of an ictal discharge (see Fig. 15-3B). Seizures can be recognized as single

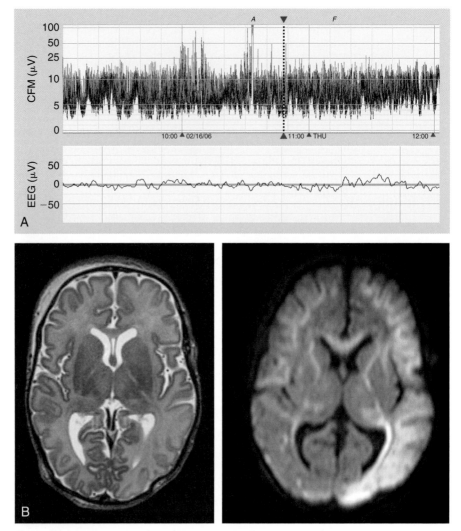

Figure 15-4   Patient 3. **A,** The aEEG (*upper panel*) at 17 hours after birth was suspicious for seizures, but the one-channel real EEG (*lower panel*) was not conclusive. A standard EEG (between *A* and *F*) showed a multifocal status epilepticus, especially in the central areas. **B,** The MRI-T2 sequence (a) performed on day 6 showed increased signal intensity and loss of the cortical ribbon, especially in the left parieto-occipital region while the DWI (b) showed extensive bilateral cortical involvement.

seizures, repetitive seizures, and status epilepticus (see Fig. 15-10C). The last usually has a sawtooth pattern. Correct interpretation is greatly improved by simultaneous real EEG recording, which is available on digital devices (see Fig. 15-9A), and the gray scale software available on some of the newer machines also helps make the correct diagnosis.

Since the increased use of continuous monitoring, it has become apparent that subclinical seizures are common and occur especially following administration of the first AED. This so-called uncoupling or electroclinical dissociation has been reported by several groups and was found in 50% to 60% of the children studied. The aEEG can play an important role in the detection of these subclinical seizures.[30,31]

Even status epilepticus is not uncommon, occurring in 18% of 56 full-term infants admitted with neonatal seizures recorded with aEEG in one study.[32] The duration of status epilepticus may influence prognosis as well. In a group of 48 infants with HIE and aEEG-detected status epilepticus, there was a significant difference in background pattern, as well as in duration of the status epilepticus, between infants with poor outcome and those with good outcome. The background pattern at the onset of status epilepticus appeared to be the main predictor of outcome in all neonates with status epilepticus.

Whether the use of two channels (or more) for aEEG is indicated in all infants is still under debate. It seems to be better to use two channels instead of one channel (cross-cerebral) in children with unilateral brain lesions.[3] Although some ictal discharges arose from the affected hemisphere, the discharge could usually be recognized on the cross-cerebral recording. In general there was good agreement with regard to classification of the background pattern between the one-channel and two-channel recordings.

Should Subclinical Seizures Be Treated?

There is no consensus on whether clinical events without an EEG correlate should be treated or how aggressively to treat electrographic-only seizures (see also Chapter 8).[33,34] Although human data are scarce, several studies do suggest an adverse effect of both clinical and subclinical seizures on neurodevelopmental outcome.[35-37] Neonatal seizures have been reported to predispose patients to later problems with regard to cognition, behavior, and development of postneonatal epilepsy.[35-37] Two previous aEEG studies showed that infants treated for both clinical and subclinical seizures had a lower incidence of postneonatal epilepsy (8%-9%), compared with those treated only for clinical seizures (20%-50%).[38-41] It was of interest that in the study by Brunquell and colleagues,[37] the infants with subtle seizures and generalized tonic seizures had a significantly higher prevalence of postneonatal epilepsy ($P = 0.04$ and $P = 0.01$, respectively), mental retardation ($P = 0.02$ and $P = 0.007$), and cerebral palsy ($P = 0.03$ and $P = 0.002$) in comparison with patients with other seizure types. Subtle seizures were, in addition, more likely to be associated with abnormalities on the neurologic examination at follow-up ($P = 0.03$). Prolonged seizures can raise brain temperature and thus increase metabolic demands.[42] Prolonged seizures cause progressive cerebral hypoxia and increase local cerebral blood flow and may steal perfusion from injured brain regions.[43] In a study by Miller and coworkers[36] of term newborns with HIE, brain injury was independently associated with the severity of seizures. This group performed MRI and proton magnetic resonance spectroscopy (MRS) in 90 full-term infants. Thirty-three (37%) demonstrated EEG-confirmed seizures, which were rated with their score, on the basis of frequency and severity, EEG findings, and AED use. Multivariable linear regression tested the independent association of seizure severity with impaired cerebral metabolism measured by lactate/choline and compromised neuronal integrity measured by N-acetylaspartate/choline in the basal nuclei and intervascular boundary zones. Seizure severity was associated with increased lactate/choline in both the intervascular boundary zone ($P < 0.001$) and the basal nuclei ($P < 0.011$) when data were controlled for the potential confounders MRI abnormalities and amount of resuscitation at birth. Seizure severity was independently associated with diminished N-acetylaspartate choline in the intervascular boundary zone ($P < 0.034$).

The same group was also able to show an independent effect of clinical neonatal seizures and their treatment on neurodevelopment in 77 children who were born at term, were at risk for hypoxic-ischemic brain injury, and had undergone MRI in the newborn period.[44] About one third of the children (25/77) had clinically detected neonatal seizures. The neonatal MRI findings were classified for anatomic distribution and severity of acute injury. The severity of brain injury was assessed with high-resolution newborn MRI, and outcome was assessed at age 4 years with use of the Full-Scale Intelligence Quotient (FSIQ) of the Wechsler Preschool and Primary Scale of Intelligence–Revised as well as a neuromotor score. After data were controlled for severity of injury on MRI, the children with neonatal seizures had worse motor and cognitive outcomes than those without seizures. The children with severe seizures had a lower FSIQ than those with mild or moderate seizures ($P < 0.0001$). The major limitation of these two important studies is the reliance on clinical evaluation for classification of seizure diagnosis and severity.

In the randomized controlled trial performed by van Rooij and coworkers,[45] the seizure burden was very high in both groups (treatment of subclinical seizures vs. treatment of clinical seizures only) but was higher in the group undergoing treatment of clinical seizures only. It was of interest to see that there was a significant correlation between the duration of seizure patterns and the severity of brain injury on MRI in the group treated for seizures only, but not in the group treated for clinical as well as subclinical seizures.

aEEG in Preterm Infants

CASE HISTORY 4

> Patient 4 was born by emergency cesarean section because of fetal bradycardia, at 25+2 weeks of gestation and a birth weight of 860 g. Apgar scores were 5 (1 min) and 8 (5 min). The newborn, a boy, was supported with nasal continuous positive airway pressure (CPAP) and received caffeine during the first few days after delivery. The cranial ultrasound results were normal. On day 3, aEEG already showed an immature cycling pattern (Fig. 15-5).

In parallel with multichannel EEG, aEEG background activity is more discontinuous in preterm infants. Normative values for aEEG background activity at different gestational ages have been published.[46] A scoring system for evaluation of brain maturation in preterm infants has also been developed.[47] Zhang and colleagues[48] described reference values for aEEG amplitude, obtained for infants with a wide range of postmenstrual ages (30-55 weeks) in 274 infants. The normative amplitudes of aEEG margins, especially of the lower margin in quiet sleep, were

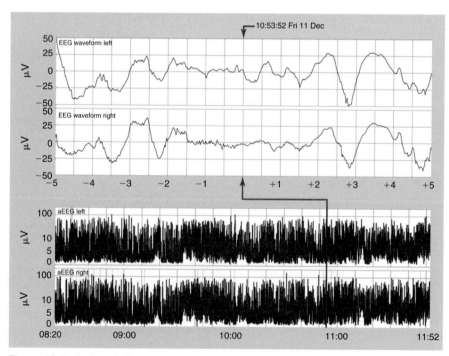

Figure 15-5 Patient 4. Day 3, two-channel aEEG recording. This is a normal background pattern for this gestation (25 wks) with an immature cycling pattern.

recommended as a source of reference data for the identification of potentially abnormal aEEG results. The upper and lower margins of the aEEGs in both active and quiet sleep clearly rose in infants after the neonatal period. The bandwidth defined as the graphic distance decreased almost monotonically throughout the postmenstrual age range from 30 to 55 weeks. The lower margin of the aEEG was positively correlated with postmenstrual age, with a larger rank correlation coefficient during quiet sleep ($r = 0.89$) than during active sleep ($r = 0.49$).

Also, studies with automated quantification of aEEG characteristics in premature infants through the use of digital equipment have been reported. Niemarkt and colleagues[49] described a method whereby the upper margin amplitude (UMA), lower margin amplitude (LMA), and bandwidth (BW) were quantitatively calculated by means of a special software system. In addition, the relative duration of discontinuous background pattern (discontinuous background defined as activity with LMA <5 μV, expressed as a percentage) was calculated. Analyses of the first week recordings demonstrated a strong positive correlation between gestational age and LMA, whereas the percentage of discontinuous pattern decreased significantly. Longitudinally, all infants showed an increase of LMA. This group found that gestational age and postnatal age (PA) both contributed independently and equally to LMA and the percentage of discontinuous pattern. They also found a strong correlation between postmenstrual age (gestational age + postnatal age) and LMA and the percentage of discontinuous pattern, respectively. They concluded that LMA and percentage of discontinuous pattern are simple quantitative measures of neurophysiologic development and may be used to evaluate neurodevelopment in infants.

Other groups looked at IBI duration or burst duration as a measure of discontinuity (or maturation). Palmu and colleagues[50] described the characteristics of activity bursts in the early preterm EEG, to assess interrater agreement of burst detection by visual inspection, and to determine the performance of an automated burst detector that uses a nonlinear energy operator (NLEO). They concluded that visual detection of bursts from the early preterm EEG is comparable albeit not identical between raters. The original automated detector underestimates the amount of burst occurrence but can be readily improved to yield results comparable to visual detection. Further clinical studies are warranted to assess the optimal descriptors of burst detection for monitoring and prognostication. Validation of a burst detector may offer an evidence-based platform for further development of brain monitors in very preterm babies.

Sleep-wake cycling can be clearly identified in the aEEG from around 30 weeks of gestation, but also at 25 to 26 weeks gestational age, a cyclical pattern resembling SWC can be seen in stable infants (see Fig. 15-5). Effects from some common medications, such as surfactant, morphine, and diazepam, can be readily seen in the aEEG of preterm infants.[51,52]

Early prediction of outcome from aEEG is a more complicated issue in preterm infants than in full-term infants. A mainly discontinuous background pattern can be considered normal in most infants younger than 30 weeks of gestation. In the most immature infants, factors other than initial brain function may influence long-term neurodevelopmental outcome, such as bronchopulmonary dysplasia and late-onset sepsis, making prediction of outcome from the early EEG less certain. Nevertheless, several EEG and aEEG studies have shown early background depression to correlate with the severity of a periventricular-intraventricular hemorrhage.[53] Klebermass and colleagues[54] assessed the prognostic values of aEEG and cranial ultrasound in premature infants. Specificity was 73% for assessment within the first and increased to 95% in the second week of life, whereas sensitivity stayed nearly the same, at 87% (first week) to 83% (second week). Cranial ultrasound showed a specificity of 86% within the first and second week; sensitivity also stayed nearly the same (74% and 75%). These researchers concluded that the aEEG also has a predictive value for later outcome in preterm infants and can be used as an early prognostic tool. West and colleagues[55] evaluated infants born before 29 weeks of gestation very early in life with two-channel EEG. Seventy-six infants had an EEG within 48 hours of delivery and a developmental assessment (Bayley II at 18 months corrected age). The analyzed segments of the EEG were obtained at 24 (3-48) hours of age (median [range]). The neurophysiologist's assessment was a better predictor of adverse outcome than the continuity measures: positive predictive value 95% CI 75 (54% to 96%) versus 41 (22% to 60%) at 25 μV threshold, negative predictive value 88% (80% to 96%) versus 84% (74% to 94%), and positive likelihood ratio 9.0 (3.2 to 24.6) versus 2.0 (1.2 to 3.6)). All infants with definite seizures identified by the neurophysiologist had poor outcomes. The investigators concluded that modified bedside EEG has the potential to assist with identification of extremely preterm infants at risk for adverse neurodevelopmental outcomes. However, analysis by a neurophysiologist performed better than the currently available continuity analyses.

In an analogy of amplitude depression after severe asphyxia in term infants, ter Horst and coworkers[56] related neonatal acute physiology score (Score for Neonatal Acute Physiology II [SNAP-II] as an acute reflection of severity of illness) in preterm infants with aEEG scores. The aEEGs were assessed by pattern recognition, by calculating a Burdjalov score, and by calculating the mean values of the 5th, 50th, and 95th percentiles of the aEEG amplitudes. Illness severity was determined within the first 24 hours of life. These researchers recorded aEEGs in 38 infants with a mean gestational age of 29.7 weeks (26.0-31.8 weeks) during the first 5 days of life. They found that severity of illness as measured by the SNAP-II and low blood pressure had a negative effect on the aEEG findings in of preterm infants.

Epileptic seizure activity in preterm infants can be identified in a similar way as in full-term infants. Epileptic seizure activity, often without clinical symptoms, is very common in the aEEG during development of intracerebral hemorrhages. Identifying seizure activity on a discontinuous background pattern can be very difficult. With access to the real EEG on digital devices, this problem can be handled more easily, especially with the new seizure detection algorithm on some devices.

CASE HISTORY 5

Patient 5, a girl, was born at 29 weeks of gestation with a birth weight of 1200 g after premature rupture of membranes and an intrauterine infection. Apgar scores were 8 (1 min) and 9 (5 min). The cranial ultrasound scan revealed a bilateral grade 2 intraventricular hemorrhage. Therefore a two-channel aEEG recording was obtained (Fig. 15-6). Clinically the infant was stable while receiving nasal CPAP. She had no clinical seizures. The aEEG at 48 hours after birth showed subclinical seizures, which were recognized by the seizure detection algorithm but were difficult to recognize visually. She was given a single loading dose (20 mg/kg) of phenobarbital. At 36 months of age, she had a developmental quotient (DQ) of 99 when evaluated with the Griffiths Developmental Scales.

Pitfalls and Artifacts

The simultaneous recording of the real EEG, present on the newer digital devices, may help in the identification of artifacts in aEEG[57] that are quite common during long-term recordings. Hagmann and colleagues[58] have shown that 12% of their 200 hours of recording was affected by artifacts. This effect was due to electrical interference in 55% of cases, which could be either ECG artifact (39%) or fast activity (>50 Hz, 61%) and to movement artifact in the remaining 45%. They stated that the dual facility (aEEG with simultaneous real EEG) is crucial for the correct interpretation of the aEEG. Simultaneous recording of the real EEG appears to be especially important in the preterm infant. One study found that 60% of the recordings in preterm infants consisted of artifacts.[59] In this study, frontal electrodes were used, possibly explaining some of the artifacts.

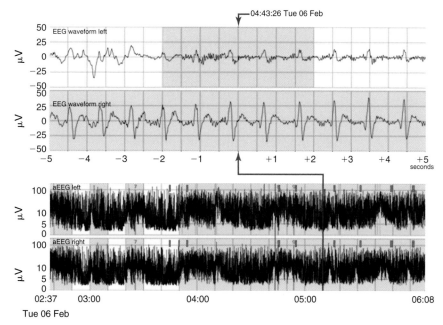

15

Figure 15-6   Patient 5. Cycling pattern at 29 weeks of gestation, day 2. Subclinical seizures recognized by the seizure detection algorithm (*pink lines*).

Inappropriate electrode position can also lead to aEEG recordings with artifact or drift of the baseline, as described in Case History 1. Some apparently normal aEEGs in severely encephalopathic babies have ECG artifacts, which could explain a drift of a severely depressed baseline to a baseline within the normal voltage range (see Fig. 15-2). It is very important to recognize this drift of the baseline, because the interpretation of aEEG background patterns may be used for intervention studies. In a study by Sarkar and colleagues,[60] 54 infants with moderate or severe HIE were evaluated with aEEG for selection for hypothermic neuroprotection. Seven encephalopathic infants with normal aEEGs who did not undergo hypothermia were subsequently shown to have abnormalities on MRI. The researchers concluded that there was a poor correlation between early aEEG and short-term adverse outcomes, with a sensitivity of 54.8% and a negative predictive value of only 44%. All of these normal aEEGs, however, had ECG artifacts, which could explain the drift of the baseline (Personal Communication, J. Barks, MD). Retrospectively, these patients would have been eligible for the cooling study on the basis of their background pattern.

Medication can also affect the background pattern. AEDs can cause a temporary decrease in amplitude on the aEEG recording, although this decrease did not influence prognosis.[15,18] Other drugs can also have this effect, as was shown by a case report of an overdose of morphine.[61] We therefore recommend the use of pattern recognition, taking the values of upper and lower margins into account as well.

Seizure-Like Artifacts

Any movement or handling of the baby, such as a ventilation artifact, which causes a sudden increase of the baseline of the aEEG recording, can also mimic seizure activity on the aEEG, as described in the following case history (Fig. 15-7). The simultaneously recorded single-channel real EEG signal can help with more accurate interpretation of aEEG traces.[57] In addition, marking of events on the aEEG recording by nursing staff is very important.

CASE HISTORY 6

Patient 6 was born at 31 weeks of gestation with a birth weight of 1500 g. The infant was ventilated because of infant respiratory distress syndrome (IRDS) complicated by a pneumothorax. The patient received morphine continuously (0.25 mg/kg/day), and findings of a cranial ultrasound examination were normal.

aEEG in Other Clinical Conditions

Another clinical condition in neonates for which continuous monitoring of EEG is useful is congenital heart disease (CHD), especially after surgery with deep hypothermic cardiac arrest.[62] Only a few studies describe the role of the aEEG in this condition, some in combination with near-infrared spectroscopy.[63] In one study,[64] the aEEG data obtained before surgery were described in neonates with CHD. The first 72 hours after the start of prostaglandin E1 therapy were used for analysis. The background patterns were mildly abnormal in 45% of the infants and severely abnormal at some point during the recording in 14% of the infants. A severely abnormal aEEG and epileptiform activity were associated with more profound acidosis. The researchers of this study concluded that the majority of infants with CHD had an abnormal aEEG before surgery. aEEG helped identify epileptiform activity and was a useful tool to evaluate brain function prior to surgery in infants with CHD.

The same group also studied aEEG during neonatal sepsis with or without meningitis.[65] Their aim was to investigate the longitudinal course and prognostic value of aEEG in infants with neonatal sepsis or meningitis and a gestation of 34 to 42 weeks. They found that a low-voltage background pattern, SWC, and epileptiform activity on the aEEG are helpful to predict neurologic outcome in infants with neonatal sepsis or meningitis. Others looked at the effect of sepsis on the aEEG in extremely premature infants.[66] Monthly aEEG was performed from 28 weeks until 36 weeks postmenstrual age in 108 premature infants born before 28 weeks of

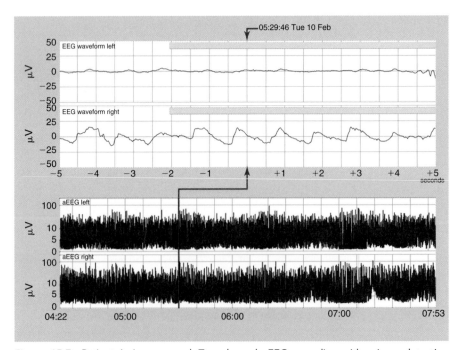

Figure 15-7 Patient 6. *Lower panel,* Two-channel aEEG recording with seizure detection alert because of a rhythmic pattern. This turned out to be an artifact, because the waveform pattern on the real EEG (*upper panel*) synchronizes with the ventilator settings. Background pattern is slightly depressed for this age, owing to morphine medication.

gestation. Additional aEEG recordings were performed during the infants first episode of sepsis. These investigators found that sepsis was associated with acute EEG changes, as indicated by BS, but not with a decreased rate of brain wave maturation.

A sudden rise in arterial $PaCO_2$ levels can result in a sudden drop in aEEG amplitude, as described in the following case history.

CASE HISTORY 7

Patient 7, a full-term infant, was sent home after a normal vaginal delivery and good Apgar scores. She was admitted to the NICU on the second day after birth because of septicemia, which turned out to be a group B streptococcal infection. She needed high-frequency oscillation because of pulmonary hypertension and blood pressure support. On day 7, aEEG showed a sudden drop in amplitude (Fig. 15-8), which was accompanied clinically by a rise in PCO_2 that was found to be caused by a blocked tube. When the PCO_2 returned to normal, so did the aEEG amplitude.

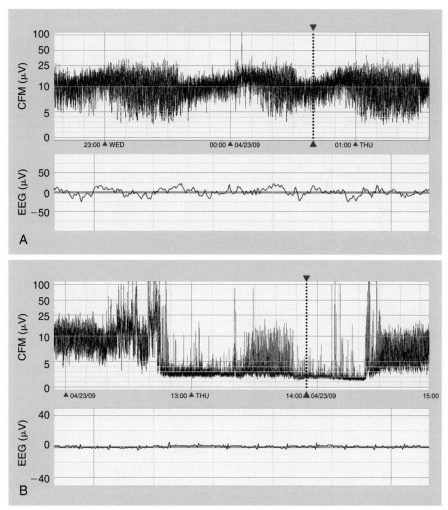

Figure 15-8 Patient 7. aEEG tracings from day 7. **A,** Normal background pattern with clear sleep-wake cycling (CNV SWC). **B,** Sudden drop in amplitude to an almost flat trace. During this period of low amplitude, there was a sudden rise in PCO_2 up to 130 mm Hg because of a blocked tube. The aEEG pattern returned to normal when the PCO_2 normalized.

Wikström and colleagues[67] performed an observational study in 32 infants with a gestational age of 22 to 27 weeks. They performed simultaneous single-channel EEG and repeated blood gas and plasma glucose analyses during the first 3 days (n = 247 blood samples with corresponding EEG). Interburst intervals (IBIs) and EEG power were averaged at the time of each blood sample. The researchers found a linear relationship between $PaCO_2$ and IBI; increasing $PaCO_2$ was associated with longer IBI. One day after birth, a 1-kPa increase in $PaCO_2$ was associated with a 16% increase in IBI in infants who survived the first week without severe brain injury. EEG power was highest at a $PaCO_2$ value of 5.1 kPa and was attenuated at both higher and lower $PaCO_2$ values. In addition, the group found that plasma glucose levels, corrected for carbon dioxide effects, were also associated with IBI. Lowest IBIs appeared at a plasma glucose level of 4.0 mmol/L, and there was a U-shaped relationship between plasma glucose level and EEG with increasing discontinuity at glucose concentrations above and below 4.0 mmol/L. Both carbon dioxide and plasma glucose levels influenced EEG activity in extremely preterm infants, and values considered to be within normal physiologic ranges were associated with the best EEG background. Increasing EEG discontinuity occurred at $PaCO_2$ levels frequently applied in lung protection strategies; in addition, moderate hyperglycemia was associated with measurable EEG changes showing longer IBIs. Hyperglycemia is considered a marker of illness severity and has now been identified as a risk factor for death and for reduction in white matter volume at term equivalent age.[68] The long-term effects of changes in $PaCO_2$ and blood glucose values on brain function are not known.

Severe hyperbilirubinemia may also lead to aEEG background depression with or without seizures. One EEG study showed a transient effect on background activity.[69] aEEG can be used in congenital metabolic disorders that may lead to hyperammonemia and seizures. Deterioration of background patterns, abnormal SWC patterns, and seizures have been described and can be recognized in various metabolic diseases.[70]

CASE HISTORY 8

Patient 8 was a male infant of Chinese origin who was born at 37+2 weeks of gestation. Severe hyperbilirubinemia developed with a blood bilirubin level of 588 μmol/L on day 5. The infant had seizures at a referring hospital, where aEEG monitoring was begun (Fig. 15-9). Following a loading dose of phenobarbital (20 mg/kg), he was referred to our NICU. The brainstem auditory evoked potentials were abnormal, and MRI showed clear signal intensity changes in the globus pallidum. The infant was treated with an exchange transfusion and received phototherapy. Further evaluation revealed a glucose-6-phosphate dehydrogenase (G6PD) deficiency. At 23 months, evaluation with the Griffiths Developmental Scales yielded a developmental quotient (DQ) of 98, and the patient only showed a mild auditory neuropathy.

CASE HISTORY 9

Patient 9, a term infant, was born at home after an uncomplicated pregnancy and delivery. He was admitted to the hospital on day 2 because of a low temperature and an incident after oral feeding. In the hospital, a sepsis workup was done. He demonstrated seizures (Fig. 15-10) with apnea and needed ventilation. He was referred to our NICU. The patient was treated with phenobarbital, midazolam, lidocaine, and pyridoxine because of refractory seizures. The serum ammonia value was elevated right at admission and demonstrated a subsequent linear increase (1245→3293→3293→ 8700 μmol/L). He was subsequently diagnosed to have urea cycle defect (ornithine transcarbamylase deficiency) and died on day 4.

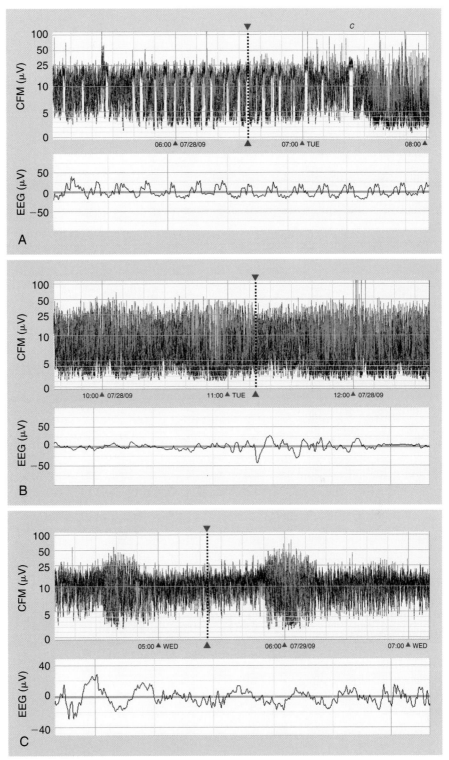

Figure 15-9 Patient 8. **A,** Epileptiform activity at the referring hospital on aEEG (*top panel*), and epileptiform activity on the real EEG (*lower panel*). A loading dose of phenobarbital was given at C. **B,** Day 5 on admission (after phenobarbital). Discontinuous normal voltage (DNV) pattern without seizures. **C,** Day 6 (one day after admission). Continuous normal voltage (CNV) pattern with sleep-wake cycling (SWC).

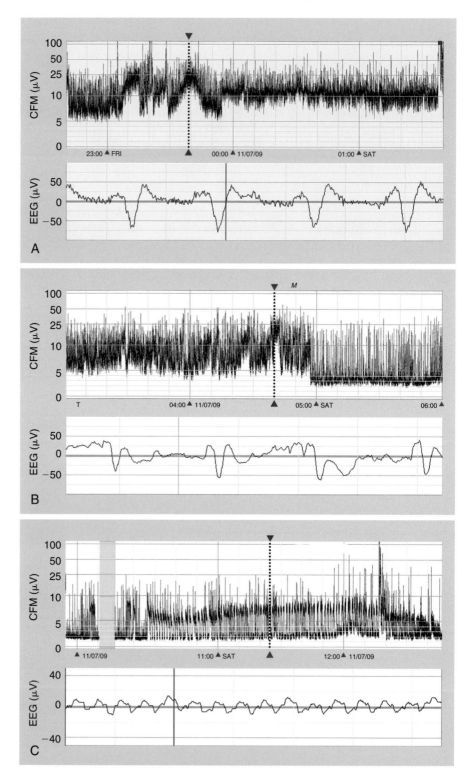

Figure 15-10   Patient 9. **A,** On admission, the patient was documented on aEEG to have seizures. **B,** Day after admission, repetitive seizures occurred. Following a loading dose of midazolam (at M), a sparse burst suppression (BS) pattern was shown. **C,** Several hours after tracing in **B,** status epilepticus on a flat background pattern could be seen.

Gaps in Knowledge

As with all (new) techniques, there is a learning curve. As Boylan and colleagues[1] reported, aEEG is mainly assessed by neonatologists, and 30% of them are not confident in their ability to interpret it. Therefore, training is essential. EEG remains the golden standard, so if one is not sure about the assessment of the aEEG, one should perform a full EEG. Therefore it is very important for clinicians to have a good relationship with the neurophysiology department of the hospital. Furthermore, we advise performing a full EEG during office hours at least once during the aEEG recording of several days.

The aEEG assessment of a preterm infant is very different from and harder to interpret than that of a term infant. The preterm population appears to be especially at risk for artifacts during the recording, and simultaneous assessment of the real EEG is therefore important.[59] Now, with the advent of digital equipment, other techniques may become available and important as well, such as interburst interval and the automated burst detector that uses a nonlinear energy operator (NLEO).[50] Much more research should be done in this field.

Conclusion

aEEG monitoring is increasingly considered to be the standard of care in the neonatal unit, not only in infants suffering from hypoxic-ischemic encephalopathy or infants with seizures but also in infants who are seriously ill with CHD, sepsis with or without meningitis, and metabolic diseases. Clinicians should therefore be aware not only of the advantages of aEEG monitoring but also of its pitfalls.

References

1. Boylan GB, Burgoyne L, Moore C, et al. An international survey of EEG use in the neonatal intensive care unit. *Acta Paediatr.* 2010;99:1150-1155.
2. Maynard DE. EEG analysis using an analogue frequency analyser and a digital computer. *Electroencephalogr Clin Neurophysiol.* 1967;23:487.
2a. Prior PF. EEG monitoring and evoked potentials in brain ischaemia. *Br J Anaesth.* 1985;57:63-81.
2b. Prior PF, Maynard DE. *Monitoring cerebral function. Long-term recordings of cerebral electrical activity and evoked potentials.* Amsterdam: Elsevier; 1986:1-441.
3. van Rooij LG, de Vries LS, van Huffelen AC, Toet MC. Comparison of 2-ch and 1-ch aEEG with respect to seizure-activity and background pattern *Arch Dis Child Fetal Neonatal Ed.* 2010;95:F160-F168.
4. Hellström-Westas L, Rosén I, de Vries LS, Greisen G. Amplitude-integrated EEG classification and interpretation in preterm and term infants. *Neonatal Rev.* 2006;7:e76-e86.
5. Al Naqeeb N, Edwards AD, Cowan F, Azzopardi D. Assessment of neonatal encephalopathy by amplitude integrated electroencephalography. *Pediatrics.* 1999;103:1263-1271.
6. Toet MC, van Rooij GM, de Vries LS. The use of amplitude integrated EEG for assessing neonatal injury. *Clin Perinatol.* 2008;35:665-678.
7. Thoresen M, Hellström-Westas L, Liu X, de Vries LS. Effect of hypothermia on amplitude-integrated electroencephalogram in infants with asphyxia. *Pediatrics.* 2010;126:e131-e139.
8. Quigg M, Leiner D. Engineering aspects of the quantified amplitude-integrated electroencephalogram in neonatal cerebral monitoring. *J Clin Neurophysiol.* 2009;26:145-149.
9. Shellhaas RA, Gallagher PR, Clancy RR. Assessment of neonatal electroencephalography (EEG) background by conventional and two amplitude-integrated EEG classification systems. *J Pediatr.* 2008;153:369-374.
10. de Vries LS, Toet MC. How to assess the aEEG background. *J Pediatr.* 2009;154:625-626.
11. Toet MC, van der Meij W, de Vries LS, van Huffelen AC. Comparison between simultaneously recorded amplitude integrated EEG (cerebral function monitor) and standard EEG in neonates. *Pediatrics.* 2002;109:772-779.
12. Evans E, Koh S, Lerner J, et al. Accuracy of amplitude integrated EEG in a neonatal cohort. *Arch Dis Child.* 2010;95:F169-F173.
13. Murray DM, Boylan GB, Ryan CA, Connolly S. Early EEG Findings in Hypoxic-Ischemic Encephalopathy Predict Outcomes at 2 Years. *Pediatrics.* 2009;124:e459-e467.
14. Spitzmiller E, Phillips T, Meinzen-Derr J, Hoath SB. Amplitude-integrated EEG is useful predicting neurodevelopmental outcome in full-term infants with hypoxic-ischaemic encephalopathy: a meta-analysis. *J Child Neurology.* 2007;22:1069-1078.
15. Shah DK, Lavery S, Doyle LW, et al. Use of 2- channel bedside electroencephalogram monitoring in term-born encephalopathic infants related to cerebral injury defined by Magnetic Resonance Imaging. *Pediatrics.* 2006;118:47-55.

15

16. Shalak LF, Laptook AR, Velaphi SC, Perlman JM. Amplitude-integrated electroencephalography coupled with an early neurologic examination enhances prediction of term infants at risk for persistent encephalopathy. *Pediatrics*. 2003;111:351-357.
17. van Rooij LG, Toet MC, Osredkar D, et al. Recovery of amplitude integrated electroencephalographic background patterns within 24 hours of perinatal asphyxia. *Arch Dis Child Fetal Neonatal Ed*. 2005;90:F245-F251.
18. Osredkar D, Toet MC, van Rooij LGM, et al. Sleep-wake cycling on amplitude-integrated EEG in full-term newborns with hypoxic-ischemic encephalopathy. *Pediatrics*. 2005;115:327-332.
19. Hallberg B, Grossmann K, Bartocci M, Blennow M. The prognostic value of early aEEG in asphyxiated infants undergoing systemic hypothermia treatment. *Acta Pædiatrica*. 2010;99:531-536.
20. Gunn AJ, Wyatt JS, Whitelaw A, et al. Therapeutic hypothermia changes the prognostic value of clinical evaluation of neonatal encephalopathy. *J Pediatr*. 2008;152:55-58.
20a. Takenouchi T, Rubens EO, Yap VL, et al. Delayed Onset of Sleep-Wake Cycling with Favorable Outcome in Hypothermic-Treated Neonates with Encephalopathy. *J Pediatr*. 2011;159:232-237.
21. Filippi L, La Marca G, Cavallaro G, et al. Phenobarbital for neonatal seizures in ischemic encephalopathy: A pharmacokinetic study during whole body hypothermia. *Epilepsia*. 2011;52:794-801.
22. Ray S. Question 1. Is aEEG as accurate as conventional EEG in the detection of seizures? *Arch Dis Child*. 2011;96:314-316.
23. Shellhaas RA, Clancy RR. Characterization of neonatal seizures by conventional EEG and single-channel EEG. *Clin Neurophysiol*. 2007;118:2156-2216.
24. Shellhaas RA, Soaita AI, Clancy RR. Sensitivity of amplitude-integrated electroencephalography for neonatal seizure detection. *Pediatrics*. 2007;120:770-777.
25. Bourez-Swart MD, van Rooij L, Rizzo C, et al. Detection of subclinical electroencephalographic seizure patterns with multichannel amplitude-integrated EEG in full-term neonates. *Clin Neurophysiol*. 2009;120:1916-1922.
26. Shah DK, Mackay MT, Lavery S, et al. The Accuracy of Bedside EEG Monitoring as Compared with Simultaneous Continuous Conventional EEG for Seizure Detection in Term Infants. *Pediatrics*. 2008;121:1146-1154.
27. Lawrence R, Mathur A. Nguyen The Tich S,Zempel J, Inder TE. A pilot study of continuous limited-channel aEEG in term infants with encephalopathy. *J Pediatr*. 2009;154:835-841.
28. Murray DM, Boylan GB, Ali I, et al. Defining the gap between electrographic seizure burden, clinical expression, and staff recognition of neonatal seizures. *Arch Dis Child Fetal Neonatal Ed*. 2008;93:F187-F191.
29. Malone A, Ryan CA, Fitzgerald A, et al. Interobserver agreement in neonatal seizure identification. *Epilepsia*. 2009;50:2097-2101.
30. Boylan GB, Rennie JM, Pressler RM, et al. Phenobarbitone, neonatal seizures, and video-EEG. *Arch Dis Child Fetal Neonatal Ed*. 2002;86:F165-F170.
31. Scher MS, Alvin J, Gaus L, et al. Uncoupling of EEG-clinical neonatal seizures after antiepileptic drug use. *Pediatr Neurol*. 2003;28:277-280.
32. van Rooij LGM, de Vries LS, Handryastuti S, et al. Neurodevelopmental outcome in Term Infants with Status Epilepticus detected with amplitude-integrated electroencephalography. *Pediatrics*. 2007;120:e354-e363.
33. Shankar R, Painter MJ. Neonatal seizures: after all these years we still love what doesn't work. *Neurology*. 2005;64:776-777.
34. Silverstein FS, Jensen FE. Neonatal seizures. *Ann Neurol*. 2007;62:112-120.
35. McBride MC, Laroia N, Guillet R. Electrographic seizures in neonates correlate with poor neurodevelopmental outcome. *Neurology*. 2000;55:506-513.
36. Miller SP, Weiss J, Barnwell A, et al. Seizure-associated brain injury in term newborns with perinatal asphyxia. *Neurology*. 2002;58:542-548.
37. Brunquell PJ, Glennon CS, Dimario FJ, et al. Prediction of outcome based on clinical seizure type in newborn infants. *J Pediatr*. 2002;140:707-712.
38. Hellström-Westas L, Blennow G, Lindroth M, et al. Low risk of seizure recurrence after early withdrawal of anti-epileptic treatment in the neonatal period. *Arch Dis Child*. 1995;72:F97-F101.
39. Toet MC, Groenendaal F, Osredkar D, et al. Postneonatal epilepsy following amplitude-integrated EEG-detected neonatal seizures. Pediatric *Neurol*. 2005;32:241-247.
40. Clancy RR, Legido A. Postnatal epilepsy after EEG-confirmed neonatal seizures. *Epilepsia*. 1991;32:69-76.
41. Ronen GM, Buckley D, Penney S, Streiner DL. Long-term prognosis in children with neonatal seizures: a population-based study. *Neurology*. 2007;69:1816-1822.
42. Yager JY, Armstrong EA, Jaharus C, et al. Preventing hyperthermia decreases brain damage following neonatal hypoxic-ischemic seizures. *Brain Res*. 2004;1011:48-55.
43. Boylan GB, Panerai RB, Rennie JM, et al. Cerebral blood flow velocity during neonatal seizures. *Arch Dis Child Fetal Neonatal Ed*. 1999;80:F105-F110.
44. Glass HC, Glidden D, Jeremy RJ, et al. Clinical Neonatal Seizures are Independently Associated with Outcome in Infants at Risk for Hypoxic-Ischemic Brain Injury. *J Pediatr*. 2009;155:318-323.
45. van Rooij LG, Toet MC, van Huffelen AC, et al; Effect of treatment of Subclinical Neonatal Seizures Detected with aEEG:. Randomized Controlled trial. *Pediatrics*. 2010;125:e358-e366.
46. Olishar M, Klebermass K, Kuhle S, et al. Reference values for amplitude integrated electroencephalographic activity in preterm infants younger than 30 weeks' gestational age. *Pediatrics*. 2004;113:e61-e66.
47. Burdjalov VF, Baumgart S, Spitzer AR. Cerebral function monitoring: a new scoring system for evaluation of brain maturation in neonates. *Pediatrics*. 2003;112:855-861.

15

48. Zhang D, Liu Y, Hou X, et al. Reference Values for Amplitude-Integrated EEGs in Infants From Preterm to 3.5 Months of Age. *Pediatrics*. 2011;127:e1280-e1287.
49. Niemarkt HJ, Andriessen P, Peters CHL, et al. Quantitative Analysis of Amplitude-Integrated Electroencephalogram Patterns in Stable Preterm Infants, with Normal Neurological Development at One Year. *Neonatology*. 2010;97:175-182.
50. Palmu K, Wikstrom S, Eero Hippelainen E, Boylan G. Detection of "EEG bursts" in the early preterm EEG: visual vs. automated detection. *Clin Neurophysiol*. 2010;121:1015-1022.
51. Hellstrom-Westas L, Bell AH, Skov L, et al. Cerebroelectrical depression following surfactant treatment in preterm neonates. *Pediatrics*. 1992;89:643-647.
52. Bell AH, Greisen G, Pryds O. Comparison of the effects of phenobarbitone and morphine administration on EEG activity in preterm babies. *Acta Paediatr*. 1993;82:35-39.
53. Hellström-Westas L, Klette H, Thorngren-Jerneck K, Rósen I. Early prediction of outcome with aEEG in preterm infants with large intraventricular hemorrhages. *Neuropediatrics*. 2001;32:319-324.
54. Klebermass K, Olischar M, Waldhoer T, et al. Ampliude-integrated EEG pattern predicts further outcome in preterm infants. *Pediatr Res*. 2011;70:102-108.
55. West CR, Harding JE, Williams CE, et al. Cot-side electroencephalography for outcome prediction in preterm infants: observational study. *Arch Dis Child Fetal Neonatal Ed*. 2011;96:F108-F113.
56. ter Horst HJ, Jongbloed-Pereboom M, van Eykern LA, Bos AF. Amplitude-integrated electroencephalographic activity is suppressed in preterm infants with high scores on illness severity, *Early Hum Dev*. 2011;87:385-390.
57. de Vries NKS, ter Horst HJ, Bos AF. The added value of simultaneous EEG and Amplitude-integrated EEG recordings in Three Newborn Infants. *Neonatology*. 2007;91:212-216.
58. Hagmann CF, Robertson NJ, Azzopardi D. Artifacts on electroencephalograms may influence amplitude-integrated EEG classification: a Qualitative Analysis in neonatal encephalopathy. *Pediatrics*. 2006;118:2552-2554.
59. Suk D, Krauss AN, Engel M, Perlman JM. Amplitude-integrated electroencephalography in the NICU: frequent artifacts in premature infants may limit its utility as a monitoring device. *Pediatrics*. 2009; 123:e328-e332.
60. Sarkar S, Barks JD, Donn SM. Should amplitude-integrated electroencephalography be used to indentify infants suitable for hypothermic neuroprotection? *J Perinatol*. 2008;28:117-122.
61. Niemarkt NJ, Halbertsma FJJ, Andriessen P, et al. Amplitude-integrated electroencephalographic changes in a newborn induced by overdose of morphine and corrected with naloxone. *Acta Paediatr*. 2008;97:127-134.
62. Clancy RR, Sharif U, Ichord R, et al. Electrographic neonatal seizures after infant heart surgery. *Epilepsia*. 2005;46:84-90.
63. Toet MC, Flinterman A, Laar I, et al. Cerebral oxygen saturation and electrical brain activity before, during, and up to 36 hours after arterial switch procedure in neonates without pre-existing brain damage: its relationship to neurodevelopmental outcome. *Exp Brain Res*. 2005;165:343-350.
64. ter Horst HJ, Mud M, Roofthooft MTR, Bos AF. Amplitude integrated electroencephalographic activity in infants with congenital heart disease before surgery. *Early Hum Dev*. 2010;86:759-764.
65. ter Horst HJ, van Olffen M, Remmelts HJ, et al. The prognostic value of amplitude integrated EEG in neonatal sepsis and/or meningitis. *Acta Paediatr*. 2010;99:194-200.
66. Helderman JB, Welch CD, Leng X, O'Shea MT. Sepsis-associated electroencephalographic changes in extremely low gestational age neonates. *Early Hum Dev*. 2010;86:509-513.
67. Wikström S, Lundin F, Ley D, et al. Carbon Dioxide and Glucose Affect Electrocortical Background in Extremely Preterm Infants. *Pediatrics*. 2011;127:e1028-1034.
68. Alexandrou G, Skiöld B, Karlén J, et al. Early hyperglycemia is a risk factor for death and white matter reduction in preterm infants. *Pediatrics*. 2010;125:e584-e591.
69. Gürses D, Kiliç I, Sahiner T. Effects of hyperbilirubinemia on cerebrocortical electrical activity in newborns. *Pediatr Res*. 2002;52:125-130.
70. Theda C. Use of amplitude integrated electroencephalography (aEEG) in patients with inborn errors of metabolism—a new tool for the metabolic geneticist. *Mol Genet Metab*. 2010;100:S42-S48.

15

CHAPTER 16

Magnetic Resonance Imaging's Role in the Care of the Infant at Risk for Brain Injury

Gregory A. Lodygensky, MD, Caroline C. Menache, MD, and Petra S. Hüppi, MD

- ● **The Term Newborn**
- ● **The Preterm Infant**
- ● **Advanced Quantitative MRI with Image Analysis Tools**

Despite marked improvements in antenatal and perinatal care, perinatal brain injury remains one of the most important medical complications in the newborn resulting in significant handicap later in life. Remarkable experimental advances have helped the understanding of many of the cellular and vascular mechanisms of perinatal brain damage, showing a correlation between the nature of the injury and the maturation of the brain. Early identification of brain injury and appropriate prognostication, however, remain major challenges to neonatal care. New diagnostic tools have emerged to detect early brain injury and help predict outcome.

Magnetic resonance (MR) techniques are one of these new diagnostic tools that allow the assessment of the developing brain in detail, thanks to their resolution power and noninvasiveness. The capacity of such techniques to provide detailed structural as well as metabolic and functional information without the use of ionizing radiation is unique.

Conventional MR imaging (MRI) is therefore now widely used for identifying normal and pathologic brain morphology, giving objective information about the structure of the neonatal brain during development. Diffusion-weighted imaging (DWI),[1] MR spectroscopy (MRS),[2] and functional MRI (fMRI; blood oxygenation level–dependent [BOLD] imaging)[3] are newer techniques that complement conventional MRI and can indicate some of the pathophysiologic mechanisms occurring during brain injury in the newborn and the postinjury plasticity. This chapter focuses on the role of the different MR techniques in the study of perinatal brain injury. The specific patterns of brain injury identified by different imaging techniques are illustrated by case presentations, each followed by the discussion of pathophysiologic and neurodevelopmental outcome associated with the described brain lesion. This approach should allow the reader to make the right choice of imaging method at the right time to decide on intervention and withdrawal of care as well as to accurately predict the range of neurofunctional outcome.

The Term Newborn

Neonatal brain injury in the term infant is most frequently related to hypoperfusion and/or hypoxemia followed by reperfusion as the infant is resuscitated, typically shortly after delivery. This experience is summarized in the term *asphyxia*, progressive hypoxemia and hypercapnia with significant metabolic acidosis occurring both antenatally, intrapartum, and neonatally.[4] Perinatal asphyxia may lead to hypoxic-ischemic encephalopathy (HIE), which is the clinically defined condition of disturbed neurologic function in the term newborn, characterized by insufficient respiration, depression of tone and reflexes, altered level of consciousness, and, often, seizures.[5] The subsequent neurologic deficits of concern are grouped together under the term *cerebral palsy* (CD)[6,7] but include different motor deficits, such as spasticity, choreoathetosis, dystonia, and ataxia. Further cognitive deficits and seizures might also be the end result of neonatal HIE.

The major neuropathologic subtypes associated with neonatal HIE include selective neuronal necrosis, the most common injury observed, and which is necrosis of neurons in a characteristic, although often widespread, distribution. The four basic patterns of the topography of the neuronal injury depend on the severity and temporal characteristics of the insult, and on the gestational age of the neonate. Thus, pontosubicular necrosis occurs more frequently in premature than in term infants and the basal ganglia neurons of the putamen are more likely to be affected in term infants, whereas neurons within globus pallidus are more frequently affected in premature infants.[8]

The reasons why a particular term infant with ischemia may have one of the various patterns of selective neuronal necrosis or primarily parasagittal cerebral injury is not entirely clear. It might be related to a brainstem- and basal ganglia–sparing reflex,[9,10] whereby the blood flow is redirected to basal ganglia, the brainstem, and the cerebellum in cases of mild to moderate asphyxia, a process that does not occur in case of severe abrupt hypoperfusion, such as uterine rupture or cord compression. Prenatal or postnatal generalized systemic circulatory insufficiency can also generate focal or multifocal ischemic necrosis. However, other etiologies occurring without HIE are also common for this type of focal lesion (see later).

The occurrence of a neonatal neurologic syndrome is one of the important considerations for considering an intrapartum insult as a likely cause for the brain injury. The neurologic symptoms of severe HIE are described in Table 16-1. Important systemic abnormalities (renal, cardiac, hepatic) related to ischemia accompany the neurologic manifestations in most cases.[11]

Clinicopathologic correlations can be made for the different neuropathologic varieties of neonatal HIE in the term infant and are summarized in Box 16-1.

The following five cases of term perinatal asphyxia exemplify the clinical course, the neuroimaging characteristics, and the subsequent neurodevelopmental outcome and illustrate the role and appropriate timing of MRI in the evaluation of the term newborn after perinatal asphyxia.

Table 16-1 NEUROLOGIC SYNDROME OF SEVERE HYPOXIC-ISCHEMIC ENCEPHALOPATHY

Birth to 12 hours	Deep stupor or coma Periodic breathing or respiratory failure Intact pupillary and oculomotor response Hypotonia and minimal movements/rarely hypertonia Seizures
12-24 hours	Variable change in alertness More seizures Apneic spells Jitteriness Weakness (upper limbs in terms; lower limbs in preterms)
24-72 hours	Stupor or coma Respiratory arrest Oculomotor and pupillary changes
After 72 hours	Persistent but diminished stupor Disturbed sucking, swallowing, gag and tongue movements Hypotonia > hypertonia Weakness (upper limbs in terms; lower limbs in prematures)

Modified from Volpe J. *Neurology of the newborn.* 5th ed. Philadelphia: Saunders; 2008.

Box 16-1 ETIOLOGIES OF FOCAL AND MULTIFOCAL ISCHEMIC LESIONS

Idiopathic (majority of cases)
Vascular maldevelopment
Vasculopathy
Vasospasm (e.g., with cocaine use)
Vascular distortion (obstetric trauma to head and neck)
Vascular manipulation-ligation (e.g., for extracorporeal membrane oxygenation)
Embolus:
 • Placental thrombosis or tissue fragments (twin pregnancy with death of co-twin)
 • Involuting fetal vessels (thrombi)
 • Catheterized vessels (thrombi or air)
 • Cardiac: myxoma or rhabdomyoma, right-to-left shunt, patent foramen ovale
Thrombus:
 • Meningitis with arteritis or phlebitis
 • Trauma
 • Disseminated intravascular coagulation
 • Polycythemia
 • Hypercoagulable state: protein C, protein S, or antithrombin III deficiency,
   antiphospholipid antibodies, factor V Leiden mutation
 • Hypernatremia-dehydration

Modified from Volpe J. *Neurology of the newborn.* 5th ed. Philadelphia: Saunders; 2008.

CASE 1

HISTORY

Term pregnancy with signs of fetal distress, cesarean section, low Apgar score, perinatal acidosis (pH 6.99). On day 1, general hypotonia, tonic deviations of eyes, sucking, smacking subtle seizures. Normalization of the neurologic findings on day 10.

NEUROIMAGING STUDIES

Results of neonatal head ultrasound scan performed on day 1 were normal (Fig. 16-1). MRI on day 3 revealed no significant signal abnormalities on T2-weighted images but some signal hyperintensities on T1-weighted images, especially in the central cortex. DWI showed abnormal signal intensities with reduced apparent diffusion coefficients (ADCs) bilaterally in the thalamus and internal capsule. Some discrete areas of reduced ADCs could be seen in the cortex. On a follow-up study on day 10 (Fig. 16-2), the thalami appeared hyperintense on T2-weighted images.

CLINICAL CORRELATES IN THE NEONATAL PERIOD

This child exhibited signs of moderately severe impairment of bilateral hemispheres, which characteristically results in diffuse hypotonia. He also presented with neonatal seizures of the subtle type, which are thought to result from diffuse cortical injury and could reflect the discrete areas of reduced ADC seen in the cortex. The normalization of the neurologic findings at 10 days of life is a good prognostic sign.

LONG-TERM CLINICAL CORRELATES

Ultimately, this child showed signs of moderate spasticity, especially in the upper limbs, but was able to walk unaided at age 3 years with a certain degree of truncal hypotonia. His fine motor skills were delayed because of dystonic movements of the arms. Dystonia appeared around age 12 months and became more prominent with time. He had no major cognitive deficits. The mild spasticity was explained by the involvement of the central white matter (seen best on DWI at day 3), and the dystonia was the result of the thalamoputaminal lesions.

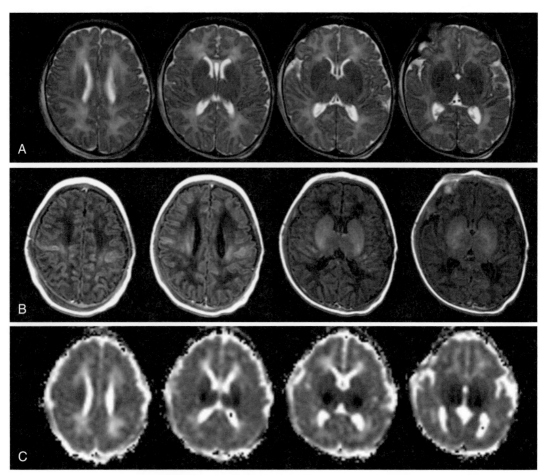

Figure 16-1 Case 1: Perinatal asphyxia and MRI at day 3 of life. **A,** T2-weighted images with slight T2 hyper-intensity of the thalami, no striking signal abnormalities. **B,** T1-weighted images show abnormal high signal intensities in several cortical areas, specifically in the depth of sulci. Thalamic area is slightly hypointense. **C,** Diffusion-weighted images show striking lesions *(dark)* with ADC reduction in bilateral thalami and in some discrete central cortical areas.

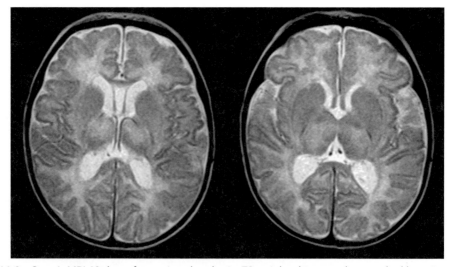

Figure 16-2 Case 1: MRI 10 days after perinatal asphyxia. T2-weighted images show marked hyperintensities in bilateral thalami involving in part the internal capsule and mild ventricular dilation.

CASE 2

HISTORY

Term pregnancy with signs of fetal distress, emergency cesarean section for uterine rupture, meconium aspiration, low Apgar scores (1 [1 min], 3 [5 min], 5 [10 min]), perinatal acidosis (pH 6.84). Initial general hypotonia, then hypertonicity, no seizures.

NEUROIMAGING STUDIES

Results of neonatal head ultrasound scan performed on day 1 were normal. MRI on day 1 revealed no significant signal abnormalities on T2-, T1- and diffusion-weighted images. Single-voxel proton MRS (^{1}H-MRS) obtained on basal ganglia showed elevated lactate (Lac) resonance at 1.3 ppm with no loss of N-acetylaspartate (NAA) (Fig. 16-3). Follow-up MRI at day 10 demonstrated bilateral thalami and putamen, which appeared hyperintense on T2-weighted images with clear distinction on proton density images with no cortical signal abnormalities (see Fig. 16-3). On T1-weighted images, hyperintensities in this region can be confounded with hyperintensities due to myelination (Figs. 16-3 and 16-4). ^{1}H-MRS on day 10 now shows normalization of lactate and reduction of NAA resonances (see Fig. 16-4).

CLINICAL CORRELATES IN THE NEONATAL PERIOD

After a brief period of hypotonia, corresponding most likely to the bilateral involvement of the reticular activating system in the diencephalon, this child rapidly demonstrated the characteristic hypertonia associated with basal ganglia lesions caused by the involvement of the extrapyramidal system. It was interesting to note that no clinical seizures were observed, most likely in relation to the fact that there were no cortical lesions. However, electrographic seizures could not be excluded.

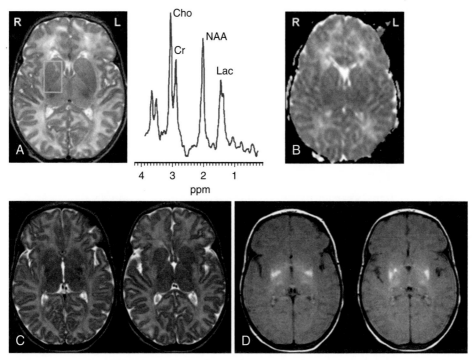

Figure 16-3 Case 2: MRI examination obtained at 12 hours (**A** and **B**) and 10 days (**C** and **D**) after perinatal asphyxia. **A,** Axial T2-weighted image *(left)* shows no signal abnormalities, and single-voxel ^{1}H-MR spectroscopy performed over the right basal ganglia *(right)* shows markedly increased lactate (Lac) resonance with preserved N-acetylaspartate (NAA), creatine (Cr), and choline (Cho) resonances. **B,** Diffusion-weighted image with axial apparent diffusion coefficient (ADC) map shows no diffusion abnormalities. **C,** Axial T2-weighted images show areas of high and low signal intensity in the putamen and thalamus, representing clear ischemohemorrhagic lesions. **D,** Axial proton density images demonstrate prominent detection of the lesion's extension.

Figure 16-4 Case 2: Coronal and axial inversion recovery sequences with T1-weighted contrast at 10 days after perinatal asphyxia. T1 hyperintensities appear irregular (**A** and **C**) compared with the regular distribution of beginning myelination in **B**. **D**, ¹H-MR spectroscopy shows normalization of lactate (Lac) and reduction of N-acetylaspartate (NAA) in comparison with results on day 1 (see Fig. 16-3B). *Cho,* Choline; *Cr,* creatine.

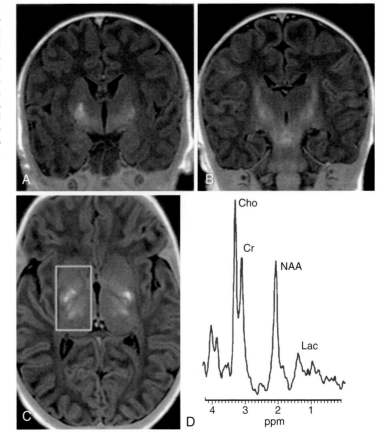

LONG-TERM CLINICAL CORRELATES

Striking truncal hypotonia and severe dystonic posturing of the upper extremities developed in this child, severely limiting her motor development, although there was no spasticity. She was unable to walk unaided at age 3 years. Her cognitive functions were, however, preserved. The diagnosis was severe CP of the dystonic type.

CASE 3

HISTORY

Term pregnancy with intrauterine growth restriction, fetal distress, cesarean section, meconium aspiration, perinatal acidosis (pH 7.08), persistent pulmonary hypertension.

NEUROIMAGING STUDIES

Results of neonatal head ultrasound performed on day 1 were normal. MRI on day 1 revealed no significant signal abnormalities on T2- and T1-weighted images, and standard DWI showed no striking signal abnormality (Fig. 16-5). ADC values measured in the right basal ganglia (ADC 0.8 mm²/ms) and central white matter (ADC 0.8 mm²/ms), respectively, were markedly lower than those in normal term neonates (1.0-1.2/1.4 mm²/ms).[12] ¹H-MRS performed on basal ganglia reveals elevated lactate resonance at 1.3 ppm with no loss of NAA. Follow-up MRI showed marked T2 signal abnormalities in the basal ganglia with involvement of the left internal capsule and extension into the central white matter in a parasagittal distribution (Fig. 16-6).

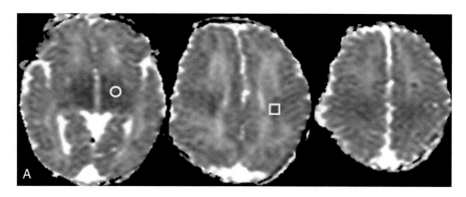

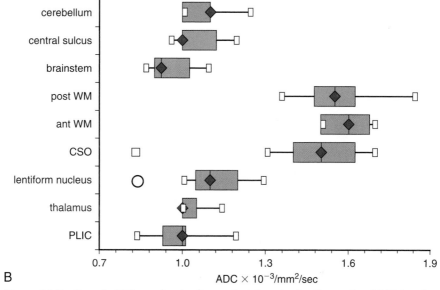

Figure 16-5 Case 3: MRI on day 1 after perinatal asphyxia. Conventional MR imaging revealed no signal abnormalities *(not shown)*. **A,** Diffusion-weighted imaging shows no overt lesions, but ADC values measured in the left basal ganglia (ADC 0.8 mm²/ms) *(circle)* and central white matter (ADC 0.8 mm²/ms) *(square)*, respectively, reveal markedly lower ADC values than seen in normal term neonates. **B** shows box plots of ADC distribution in normal full-term newborns in different regions of the brain. *ant,* Anterior; *CSO,* centrum semi ovale; *PLIC,* posterior limb of the internal capsule; *post,* posterior; *WM,* white matter. (From Rutherford M, Counsell S, Allsop J, et al. Diffusion-weighted magnetic resonance imaging in term perinatal brain injury: a comparison with site of lesion and time from birth. *Pediatrics.* 2004;114: 1004-1014.)

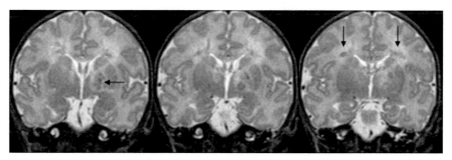

Figure 16-6 Case 3: MRI 7 days after perinatal asphyxia. Coronal T2-weighted images show T2 hypointensities and hyperintensities in the central white matter with additional left-sided lesions in the internal capsule and lateral thalamus *(arrows).*

CLINICAL CORRELATES IN THE NEONATAL PERIOD

This infant did not have striking neurologic abnormalities in the neonatal period. The only symptoms were a moderate hypotonia along with some weakness in the upper extremities.

LONG-TERM CLINICAL CORRELATES

Development of marked right upper extremity palsy at the age of 6 months. The child did not reach for objects with the right hand and exhibited a spastic position of the right arm during leg movements. In the ventral position, she was unable to elevate her right arm. These impairments reflected involvement of the left internal capsule. At age 18 months, she showed signs of hyper-reflexia of the deep tendon reflexes, presumably related to the bilateral white matter lesions, but spasticity predominated on the right side. Her cognitive performances were mildly delayed. She was able to walk unaided at age 2 years. The diagnosis is spastic CP predominantly involving the right side.

CASE 4

HISTORY

Term pregnancy with uterine rupture at delivery. Delivery room resuscitation with Apgar scores of 0 (1 min), 0 (5 min), and 3 (10 min) and severe peri-natal acidosis. On day 1, development of moderate HIE with lethargy and hypotonia was coupled with intermittent hypertonia and jitteriness. Sponta-neous movements were diminished. Convulsions appeared early.

NEUROIMAGING STUDIES

Results of neonatal head ultrasound performed on day 1 were normal. MRI on day 2 revealed no significant signal abnormalities on T2- and T1-weighted images. Diffusion-weighted images revealed reduced ADC bilaterally in the putamen and thalami (Fig. 16-7). ^{1}H-MRS performed on the basal ganglia showed elevated lactate resonance at 1.3 ppm with no loss of NAA resonance. Follow-up MRI at 17 days showed marked T2 signal abnormalities in the basal ganglia and alteration of the perirolandic cortex bilaterally, visible on proton density images as well as on T2-weighted images (see Fig. 16-7). At 2 months of age, additional atrophy and delay in myelination were present (Fig. 16-8).

CLINICAL CORRELATES IN THE NEONATAL PERIOD

The infant presented with neonatal seizures and a disturbed level of con-sciousness, which reflected the bilateral cortical lesions.

LONG-TERM CLINICAL CORRELATES

The child demonstrated a severe spastic quadriplegia consistent with the bilateral parasagittal lesions. Additionally, dystonia started around the age of 12 to 18 months. This extrapyramidal syndrome was a consequence of the basal ganglia lesions. The child was severely disabled and unable to walk unaided. Cognitive impairment was mild.

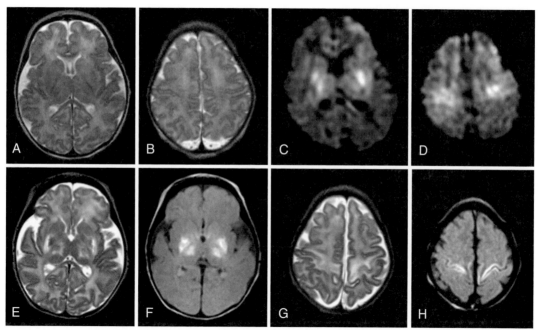

Figure 16-7   Case 4: MRI at day 2 **(A to D)** and day 10 **(E to H)** after perinatal asphyxia. **A** and **B,** Conventional T2-weighted images at the level of the basal ganglia and the high centrum semiovale show no signal abnormalities. Diffusion-weighted images show striking hyperintensities in the bilateral putamen and thalamus **(C)** and some high signal in the central cortex **(D)**. MRI at 10 days after insults confirms distribution of lesions with hyperintensities and hypointensities on T2-weighted images **(E)** and typical high signal intensity with good lesion definition in proton density images **(F)**. the perirolandic cortex has typical hyperintensities on T2-weighted **(G)** and proton density **(H)** images.

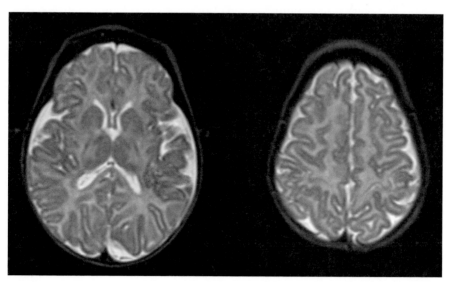

Figure 16-8   Case 4: MRI at 2 months of age reveals the same lesions with marked atrophy and delayed myelination.

16

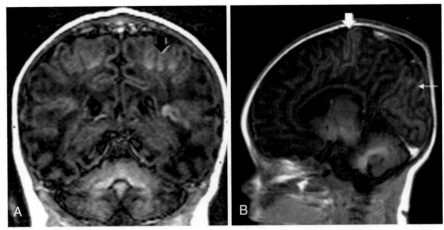

Figure 16-9 **A** and **B,** Typical parasagittal distribution of T1 hyperintensities in cortical neuronal necrosis of deep sulcal cortex of another patient with acute perinatal asphyxia.

CASE 5

HISTORY

Term pregnancy with persistent signs of fetal distress, cesarean section, low Apgar score with meconium aspiration and cardiorespiratory resuscitation.

On day 1 general hypotonia, tonic deviations of eyes, sucking, smacking subtle seizures, and electroencephalographic status epilepticus were observed.

NEUROIMAGING STUDIES

Neonatal head ultrasound performed on day 1 showed small ventricles and increased parenchymal echogenicity. MRI performed on day 5 demonstrated extensive edema with the cortex roughly isointense with white matter on T2- and T1-weighted images and apparent sparing of the basal ganglia. On DWI, markedly decreased ADCs can be seen in the cortex, white matter, and basal ganglia (Fig. 16-9 A and B). Follow-up MRI demonstrated evolution into multicystic encephalopathy with loss of both hemispheric gray and white matter and severe ex vacuo hydrocephaly (Fig. 16-9 C and D).

CLINICAL CORRELATES IN THE NEONATAL PERIOD

The generalized hypotonia and the seizures reflected the bilateral extensive cortical injury. The status epilepticus, which is not uncommon in full-term asphyxia, was consistent with the severity of the insult.

LONG-TERM CLINICAL CORRELATES

The child went on to exhibit severe spastic quadriplegia with mental retardation and microcephaly. Spasticity was a major issue. The seizure disorder persisted during the first months of life. The electroencephalography (EEG) signal remained severely depressed, indicating diffuse cortical necrosis. The diagnosis was severe spastic CP.

Cranial Ultrasonography for the Evaluation of HIE

Ultrasonography is still the only bedside technique available to image the neonatal brain. In term perinatal asphyxia and evolving HIE, the most typical findings in the acute phase are represented by poor differentiation of cortical sulci and diffuse increase of parenchymal echogenicity and slitlike ventricles.[13] These features can be primarily related to diffuse cerebral edema. Hemorrhagic necrosis in the basal ganglia can lead to hyperechogenic basal ganglia, which have been shown to be predictive of poor outcome,[14,15] and an echolucent line running through the basal ganglia region corresponding to the posterior limb of the internal capsule.[16] However, the findings of many early ultrasound scans in neonates with HIE lesions are normal or nonspecific, as illustrated in images for the cases shown here. Ultrasound examination can be considered a first-step technique that excludes significant hemorrhage, periventricular calcifications, overt brain malformation, and signs of well-established injury dating the insult before birth. However, accurate assessment of brain injury should be made with an MRI study.

MR Techniques in the Evaluation of Perinatal Asphyxia or HIE

MRI has become the technique of choice to evaluate the ischemic brain both in adults and in the newborn.[17] The use of advanced MRI techniques, such as DWI and MRS spectroscopy, has further improved MRI's capability to investigate the neonatal brain. Generally, to increase the signal-to-noise ratio, a higher field magnet (1.5 T) should be used, allowing for high-resolution imaging and increased sensitivity for spectroscopy.[18,19]

Conventional MRI Sequences and Features in HIE

The basic information in conventional MRI is represented by T1- and T2-weighted images. Proton density and fluid attenuation inversion recovery (FLAIR) images help illustrate brain lesions with slightly different contrast from those seen in T1- and T2-weighted images. A neonatal MRI protocol should provide good quality T1- and T2-weighted images with a maximum field of view of 16 to 18 cm and a slice thickness of 3 mm or less. Because of the higher water content of the neonatal brain with longer T1 and T2 relaxation times, the repetition time should be increased in both the T1- and T2-weighted imaging sequences. Typically sequence parameters for T1-weighted images should include an increased TR to 800 ms. T2-weighted imaging should have a TR above 5000 ms with a TE of 125 to 150 ms.[17,20] To compensate for a long TR the echo train length can be increased.

Selective Neuronal Necrosis after Perinatal Asphyxia

As shown in the first four cases, selective involvement of areas with advanced maturation and higher energy demands—the putamen, lateral thalami, and perirolandic cortex—are particularly susceptible to injury. Characteristic changes representing selective neuronal necrosis in these areas on T1-weighted images are T1 hyperintensities, which become apparent 3 to 7 days after the insult. These T1 hyperintensities might represent cellular reaction of glial cells and macrophages containing lipid droplets and/or some mineralization of necrotic cells. Some difficulties identifying these lesions arise from the fact that early myelination shows the same image characteristics.[21] T1 hyperintensities in the internal capsule due to beginning myelination need to be differentiated from lateral thalamic lesions and lesions in the putamen. Often the posterior limb appears swollen and has lost its normal T1 hyperintensity/T2 hypointensity, a feature with a bad prognostic value because it is associated with spastic hemiplegia.[22] On T2-weighted images, the thalami might appear slightly hyperintense in the acute phase (see Case 1), but these signal changes tend to be very difficult to detect. T2 hyperintensities become more apparent in later stages, illustrated also by well-defined lesions on proton density images (see Case 2). Evolution of these lesions is marked by progressive atrophy of the involved area (e.g., putamen, thalami, rolandic cortex) with persistent T2 hyperintensity and possible cavitation.[23]

Of note, similar lesions in the bilateral thalami, lenticular nucleus, and globus pallidum can be detected also in premature infants with documented severe anoxic insults, most frequently in association with the typical periventricular white matter injuries.[8]

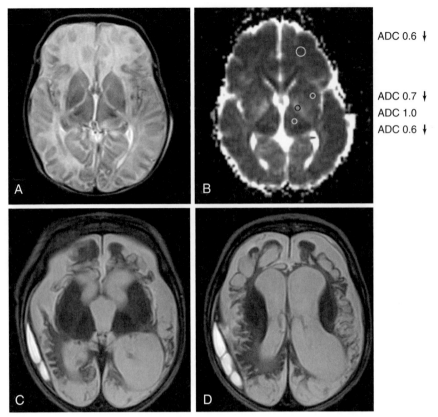

ADC 0.6 ↓

ADC 0.7 ↓
ADC 1.0
ADC 0.6 ↓

Figure 16-10 Case 5: **A,** Axial T2-weighted image on day 2 shows diffuse T2 hyperintensities with loss of gray-white matter differentiation. **B,** Diffusion-weighted image has markedly reduced ADC (ADC <1.0 mm²/ms) values throughout the brain, indicating ongoing necrosis. **C** and **D,** Chronic-stage T2-weighted images show multicystic encephalopathy and massive ventricular dilatation.

Parasagittal Cerebral Injury

Isolated parasagittal injury refers to a lesion of the cerebral cortex and the subcortical white matter with a defined distribution—that is, parasagittal superomedial aspects of the cortical convexities, usually bilateral but often asymmetric in its extension.[24] During the acute phase the cortex might show increased T1-weighted signal intensity or little abnormality on conventional MRI (Fig. 16-10). Chronic changes involve cortical thinning and atrophy.

Multicystic Encephalomalacia

Case 5 shows another form of brain injury associated with HIE. Early on (<2 days), conventional MRI findings are characterized by a diffuse T1 hypointensity and T2 hyperintensity involving both the cortex and the subcortical white matter but sparing the cerebellum and the more basal structures of the medulla (see Fig 16-9). Late intrauterine generalized prolonged systemic circulatory insufficiency is probably at the origin of these lesions, which evolve into severe cortical atrophy with cavitation and are invariably associated with a severe neurologic syndrome.

Diffusion-Weighted Imaging Sequences and Features in HIE

DWI measures the self-diffusion of water. The two primary pieces of information available from DWI studies, water ADC and diffusion anisotropy measures, change dramatically during development, reflecting underlying changes in tissue water content and cytoarchitecture.[1,25] ADC is a quantitative measure (velocity) of overall water diffusion in tissue, and anisotropy is a measure of directionality of water diffusion in a given tissue. The developing human brain presents several challenges for the application of DWI. Values for the water diffusion parameters differ markedly between neonatal brain and adult brain and vary with age. As a result, much of the knowledge about DWI, which is derived from studies of the mature, adult human brain, is not directly applicable to the developing brain.

For DWI, the optimum b value required to make the measurement has to be optimized, because it differs between newborn and adult brains. In general, a b value corresponding to approximately 1.1/ADC provides the greatest contrast-to-noise ratio for such a measurement.[26] In neonatal brain, the high b value is typically on the order of 700 to 1000 mm^2/s. DWI parameters also change in response to brain injury. The decrease in water diffusion associated with injury was initially described for animals[27,28] and adult human stroke,[29] and was subsequently confirmed for human infants.[12] Cases 1 and 4 clearly show the marked reduction of ADC in the basal ganglia with only slight hyperintensities on T2-weighted images, which can be easily missed. DWI in this case detects the lesion more reliably.

There is still debate about the precise mechanism for the decrease in ADC associated with injury. Changes in ADC following injury are dynamic. ADC values are initially decreased but subsequently increase, so that they are greater than normal and remain so in the chronic phase of injury. During the transition between decreased and increased values, there is a brief period during which values are normal, a process referred to as pseudonormalization. Pseudonormalization takes place roughly 2 days after stroke in a rat model[30] and at approximately 9 days after injury in adult human stroke.[31] Preliminary data indicate that the timing of pseudonormalization in the human newborn follows more closely that in the adult human than that in rodents, taking place at roughly 7 days after injury.[32] Interpretation of ADC values to detect acute brain injury in the developing brain needs to be adjusted for the regional differences in ADC values according to age (see Fig.16-5).[12] Case 3 shows that without numeric measurement of ADC, acute tissue alteration on diffusion maps can be missed. Case 2 illustrates that DWI performed very early in the human newborn (<24 hours) might also miss ischemic injury, which has been reported in several studies.[32-34]

From these studies the current role of DWI in the evaluation of the term newborn with HIE can be summarized as follows:

1. DWI performed less than 24 hours after injury may demonstrate focal abnormalities when ADC values are measured and compared with regional age–corresponding values; however, the full extent of lesions might not be detected.
2. DWI with ADC measurements obtained between days 2 and 4 may detect lesions not detected by conventional MRI.
3. DWI at 7 to 10 days is less sensitive then conventional MRI because of pseudonormalization.

Magnetic Resonance Spectroscopy in HIE

^{1}H-MRS has also entered the clinical arena of MR techniques routinely used for the evaluation of the brain; it permits the noninvasive study of metabolic alterations in the brain tissue. The physiologist is usually interested in the intracellular concentration of a chemical species in a particular cell type. It must be noted, though, that the in vivo human MR measurement in single-voxel MRS is an average (over the sensitive volume) of all tissue types. In the brain, therefore, we generally assess a combination of glial and neuronal cells with different extracellular space, depending on how much white matter, gray matter, or cerebrospinal fluid the volume of interest contains.

When oxidative phosphorylation is impaired, energy metabolism follows the alternative route of anaerobic glycolysis and produces lactic acid. Lactate has a chemical shift of 1.3 ppm and presents as a doublet peak in in vivo ^{1}H-MRS because of coupling effects. Groenendal and colleagues[35] first described markedly elevated lactate values in five infants with severe perinatal asphyxia. The five patients died during the neonatal period. ¹H-MRS data have been generated that demonstrate regional differences in lactate elevation after hypoxic-ischemic events in newborns. Single voxel ¹H-MRS point-resolved spectroscopy technique used in newborns with asphyxia showed greater increase of the Lac/NAA ratio in the basal ganglia than in the occipitoparietal cerebrum.[36] This finding corresponds to the signal abnormalities observed with early DWI after term hypoxia-ischemia. Case 2 illustrates the typical changes in ¹H-MRS after term perinatal hypoxia-ischemia.

Early spectroscopy (<18 hours after the event) and measurement of high Lac/Cr ratio in ¹H-MRS correlated well with neurodevelopmental outcome at 1 year.[37] This acute-phase lactic acidosis is followed by persistently elevated lactate values not associated with acidosis from 1 or 2 several weeks after the hypoxic-ischemic event.[38-40] However, ¹H-MRS performed in the first 24 hours after the insult is sensitive to the presence of hypoxic-ischemic brain injury and seems to be suitable for the detection of brain injury on the first day, when conventional MRI and DWI might not yet detect the injury. Early MRS has been shown to predict outcome more accurately than very early DWI alone.[41]

As markers of cell integrity, other metabolites visible on ¹H-MRS can be used for the assessment of hypoxic-ischemic encephalopathy. Ratios of NAA to choline (Cho) and NAA to creatine (Cr) have been used to assess cellular metabolic integrity in neonatal brain injury.[2,42-44] Studies using ¹H-MRS at a distance (>1 to 2 weeks) from the hypoxic-ischemic event showed good correlation between reduced NAA ratios with adverse neurodevelopmental outcome,[40,43-45] whereas in early (acute-stage) disease, ¹H-MRS ratios of NAA with other metabolites were not correlated with outcome.

From these studies, the current role of ¹H-MRS in the evaluation of the term newborn with HIE can be summarized as follows:

1. ¹H-MRS can play an important role in the assessment of encephalopathic term infants. Elevated lactate-to-NAA, lactate-to-creatine, and lactate-to-choline ratios or elevated absolute concentrations of lactate at less than 24 hours reliably indicate cellular injury.

2. ¹H-MRS might therefore be more useful than DWI techniques in identifying infants who would benefit from early therapeutic interventions.

CASE 6

HISTORY

Term pregnancy with signs of fetal distress, cesarean section after failed forceps attempt, thick meconium, Apgar scores of 1 (1 min) and 6 (5 min), and perinatal acidosis (pH 6.93). Initial lethargy, with very few spontaneous movements, no spontaneous eye opening, frank axial and distal hypotonia, diminished reflexes of the upper and lower limbs, no grasping, no suction, Moro reflex barely present. Onset of seizures by 8 hours of life requiring phenobarbital.

NEUROIMAGING STUDIES

MRI on day 2 revealed restrictive diffusion with a low ADC in the internal part of the temporal lobe, the centrum semiovale bilaterally, and the parietal cortex predominantly on the left, with no restrictive diffusion identified in the basal ganglia (Fig. 16-11). Proton spectroscopy showed a minimal lactate peak in the basal ganglia and a clear one in the occipital white matter (Fig. 16-12). ADC in the MRI on day 6 revealed wide areas of restrictive diffusion, with a low ADC affecting mostly the white matter in both occipital lobes, in the parietal and temporal lobe predominantly on the left, and in the frontal lobes predominantly on the right, as well as the corpus callosum. Proton spectroscopy on day 6 with a voxel in the basal ganglia showed a comparable NAA peak with a clear increase in the lactate peak equally present in the occipital white matter. MRI performed at 5 months of age revealed significant ventricular dilation in the setting of widespread atrophy, sequelae of the posterior parietal ischemic brain injury, and thinning of the corpus callosum.

CLINICAL CORRELATES IN THE NEONATAL PERIOD

This child manifested initial signs of severe impairment with persistent seizures requiring additional antiepileptic therapies. These seizures can potentially be explained by the left temporal injury seen on MRI, with significant increase in size on the second MRI and cortical involvement (see Fig. 16-12). The anticonvulsant therapies were discontinued on the sixth day of life with no recurrence of seizures. His discharge neurologic findings at 19 days of life revealed a child able to follow gaze with a normal distal tone, a mild axial hypotonia, and normal archaic reflexes.

LONG-TERM CLINICAL CORRELATES

He later had infantile spasms, which were treated successfully by vigabatrin until 8 months of age. At his last visit at 8 months, he had normal axial and distal tone with normal strength and normal reflexes of the upper and lower limbs.

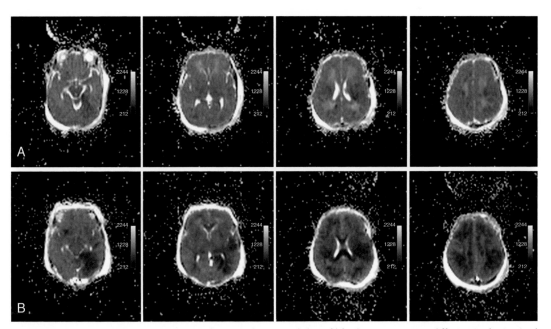

Figure 16-11   Case 6: **A,** First ADC map done on the second day of life shows restrictive diffusion in the internal part of the temporal lobe, the centrum semiovale, bilaterally. **B,** Second ADC map obtained on the sixth day of life shows areas of restrictive diffusion with low ADC values affecting mostly the white matter in both occipital lobes, in the parietal and temporal lobe predominantly on the left, and in the frontal lobes predominantly on the right as well as the corpus callosum.

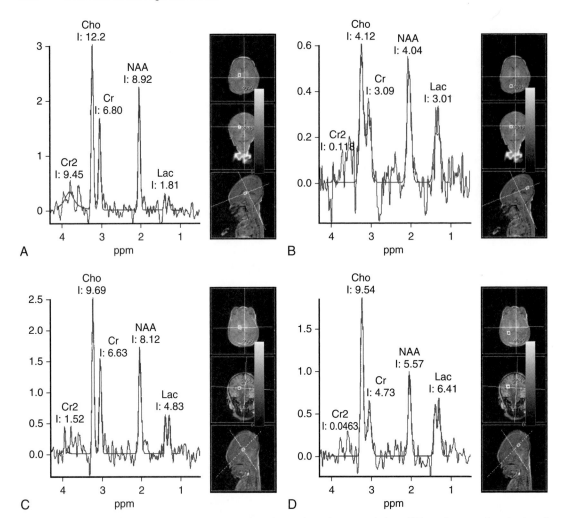

Figure 16-12 Case 6: First proton spectroscopy performed on the second day of life with a voxel in the basal ganglia (**A**), showing a minimal lactate peak, and a voxel in the occipital white matter (**B**), showing a clear lactate (Lac) peak at 1.3 ppm. Second proton spectroscopy on sixth day of life with a voxel in the basal ganglia (**C**), showing a comparable *N*-acetylaspartate (NAA) peak, with a clear increase in the lactate peak equally present in the occipital white matter (**D**). *Cho,* Choline; *Cr2,* creatine.

MRI in the Settings of Therapeutic Neonatal Hypothermia

Mild therapeutic hypothermia is now recognized as the only available treatment after hypoxic-ischemic neonatal brain injury (see Chapter 5). In such an acute context, thorough assessment of brain integrity is mandatory for managing the patient and helping the family. Estimating the severity of neonatal resuscitation, determining the neurologic status according to the Sarnat classification, and assessing the electroencephalographic trace are so far the only available bedside tools. Cerebral ultrasonography, unfortunately, has limited predictive value in the setting of acute neonatal brain injury. MRI, which in this setting requires close collaboration among the neonatologists, nursing staff, and neuroradiologist, will give a thorough assessment of brain integrity and map out the extent of injury following asphyxia and might guide neurointerventions such as hypothermia. To date few studies have addressed the question of how MRI can be used in the assessment of newborns either while they are undergoing therapeutic hypothermia or after the completion of therapeutic hypothermia.

MRI During Hypothermia

The rationale of performing an MRI during hypothermia is to determine whether there is massive brain injury, which would lead to questions about ongoing medical treatment with possible withdrawal of life-sustaining therapies and eventually whether this is a significant well-established injury dating the time of insult to before birth. It is possible also that MRI might be used in the future to monitor and tailor the length of hypothermia.

The question then becomes the following: What is known of the validity of neonatal cerebral MRI during hypothermia? What are the effects of hypothermia on proton spectroscopy? On DWI?

The ADC has a biphasic evolution following hypoxic-ischemic injury in newborns in conditions of normothermia. Animal data have shown that ADC corresponds to cytotoxic edema with ongoing cell death and that its measure correlates with caspase-3 activation[46,47] as well as with the neurodevelopmental outcome.[48] There are no data to date showing the nature of the ADC evolution during therapeutic hypothermia in human newborns. Is the biphasic evolution identical both in its time course and in its amplitude for a comparable injury? The measurement of ADC is directly influenced by temperature, with a calculated 6% reduction of the ADC at 33.5° C. In light of the normative data established by Rutherford and associates[12] in conditions of normothermia, the measurement of ADC in normal uninjured tissue might give falsely decreased measures, although the hypoxic-ischemic brain regions express generally a much higher reduction, of 35% or more. Moreover, the direct effect of localized cortical cooling in rhesus monkeys has been shown to induce a measurable decrease in ADC only with temperatures as low as 20° C.[49] The question remains whether the ADC in this setting is a reliable biomarker of injury. In a small prospective cohort, qualitative analysis of MRI during hypothermia was performed on days 1, 2, and 10 of life.[50] Restricted ADC regions could be identified in brain injury. As in normothermic conditions, significant injury was better defined on an ADC map on day 2 than within the first 24 hours of life.

Phosphorus spectroscopy has been studied during hypothermia in an animal model, with a seminal publication showing that therapeutic hypothermia reduced the degree of second energy failure after hypoxic-ischemic injury.[51] Temperature changes induce minimal chemical shift of the water peak, which can be used to quantify temperature when studied in relation to the temperature-independent shift of the neighboring metabolites[52,53] and should not affect the magnitude of metabolic peak of lactate or NAA. Clinical experience and data published by Wintermark and colleagues[50] showed that spectroscopy remains a reliable tool to assess brain integrity during hypothermia. Interestingly, the second evaluation on day 2 showed greater increase in lactate than the evaluation performed within a few hours of birth.

MRI Performed after Hypothermia

The rational of performing a MRI after the completion of therapeutic hypothermia is to establish the extent of brain injury. When is the best time to perform the examination? Is MRI valid?

Conventional T1- and T2-weighted images obtained after completion of hypothermia (8 days of life) have been demonstrated to have the same predictive ability as those in noncooled newborn infants.[54] Unfortunately, the Total Body Hypothermia for Neonatal Encephalopathy (TOBY) Study did not include early predetermined timing for MRI with the precise analysis of the ADC. Massaro and colleagues[55] found that T2 hyperintensity quantification of the putamen and the thalamus when it was adjusted to the ocular vitreous signal intensity had better predictive value than T1-weighted or ADC analysis. In this study MRI was performed during the second week of life, explaining why the ADC had limited value, because injury can produce an ADC value within the pseudonormalization time frame. Further studies are needed to define lesion evolution by MRI in neonatal HIE and hypothermia treatment.

Focal and Multifocal Ischemic Brain Necrosis without Asphyxia

As mentioned previously, focal and multifocal ischemic brain necrosis can also occur without HIE, and the sole presence of these brain lesions also places neonates in the high-risk infant category even if they have not suffered asphyxia. These lesions occur within the distribution of single or multiple major blood vessels. Almost 90% of the infarcts are unilateral, and of these lesions nearly all involve the middle cerebral artery (MCA), 75% of them involving the distribution of the left middle cerebral artery for a yet unexplained reason.

The major etiologies of these infarcts occurring without significant asphyxia are presented in Box 16-1. The neonatal and long-term clinical correlates are described in Table 16-2.

Table 16-2 NEONATAL AND LONG-TERM CLINICAL CORRELATES OF THE DIFFERENT VARIETIES OF HYPOXIC-ISCHEMIC ENCEPHALOPATHY

Topography of the Major Injury	Neonatal Correlates	Long-Term Correlates
Selective neuronal necrosis of the diffuse type	Stupor and coma (cortical injury) Seizures (cortical injury) often of the subtle type Hypotonia (cortical or anterior horn injury) Oculomotor disturbance (cranial nerve nuclei injury) Disturbed sucking, swallowing (brainstem involvement)	Intellectual retardation (cortical injury) Spastic quadriparesis (cortical injury) Seizure disorders (10%-30%) (cortical injury) Impairment of cortical visual function Precocious puberty (10%) (hypothalamus) Impairment of sucking, swallowing, drooling, fixed facial expression (bulbar or pseudobulbar palsy) Hearing deficits (cochlear neurons) Atonic cerebral palsy (rare) (anterior horn cells)
Selective neuronal necrosis of cortical–deep nuclear type	Same symptoms except that the tone is usually increased, especially with stimulation	Same symptoms Additionally: delayed onset of dystonia (6-12 months and even as late as 7-14 years of age)
Selective neuronal necrosis of deep nuclear–brainstem type	Same symptoms as above Additionally: ptosis, facial paresis, ventilatory disturbances	Prolonged difficulties with feeding Normal cognition in 50%
Parasagittal cerebral injury	Proximal weakness predominant in the upper limbs Seizures (variable) Disturbed level of alertness (variable)	Possible spastic quadriparesis Intellectual deficits (often specific)
Focal and multifocal brain necrosis (cortical and subcortical)	Seizures, usually focal Hemiparesis or quadriparesis if bilateral	Spastic hemiparesis or quadriparesis Cognitive deficits Seizure disorder

Modified from Volpe J. *Neurology of the newborn.* 5th ed. Philadelphia: Saunders; 2008.

Neonatal seizures occur in 80% to 85% of patients and are in most cases focal, with clonic movements contralateral to the lesion. Regarding long-term correlates, hemiparesis occurs only in 25% of patients with unilateral lesions. The likelihood of hemiparesis depends on the extent of the lesion, on the involvement, even if not severe, of the contralateral hemisphere, or both.[56] Thus hemiparesis is almost certain if the distribution of the stem of the middle cerebral artery is affected, or if there are bilateral lesions. However, if only a cortical branch or lenticulostriate vessels are affected, the likelihood of hemiparesis is around 10%. This relatively good outcome in unilateral lesions is probably related to the ability of the opposite hemisphere to reestablish ipsilateral corticospinal tract innervation (brain plasticity). Seizure disorders occur in 10% to 50% of infants, depending on the study.[57] Cognitive function is impaired if lesions are bilateral. Only 20% to 25% of infants with unilateral lesions have cognitive problems.

CASE 7

The pregnancy was uneventful. During spontaneous labor, the cardiotocogram showed variable decelerations with signs of fetal distress, and emergency cesarean section was performed for acute fetal bradycardia. The Apgar scores were 5 (1 min), 9 (5 min), and 9 (10 min). The infant was transferred to the neonatal unit for surveillance. On day 3 of life, the infant had apneic attacks, and convulsions were noted with head deviation.

NEUROIMAGING STUDIES

MRI on day 4 revealed significant signal abnormalities on ADC maps and diffusion-weighted images during the acute phase. DWI showed a striking reduction of diffusivity and ADC in the left temporoparieto-occipital region, with involvement also of the basal ganglia and internal capsule, consistent with an acute infarction (Fig. 16-13). Thus, the mean value for ADC in the intact right hemisphere was $1.68 \pm 0.12 \ \mu m^2/ms$, whereas in the corresponding left hemisphere, the ADC was $0.60 \pm 0.04 \ \mu m^2/ms$, reflecting the dramatic decline in ADC values during acute ischemic injury. MR angiography showed permeable vessels on both sides. On day 8 of life, mean ADC values were $1.69 \pm 0.09 \ \mu m^2/ms$ in the right hemisphere and $0.93 \pm 0.19 \ \mu m^2/ms$ in the left hemisphere. The MRI at 6 weeks of age showed tissue dissolution in the left posterior cerebral region with increased ADC values, $2.85 \pm 0.15 \ \mu m^2/ms$, and with normal ADC values, $1.44 \pm 0.16 \ \mu m^2/ms$, in the right hemisphere. T2-weighted images at 6 weeks of age showed that the lesion had evolved with tissue dissolution (see Fig. 16-13). At 13 weeks, diffusion tensor images showed loss of optic radiation fibers; there was also loss of cortical visual response on fMRI (not shown). At 12 and 20 months of age, diffusion tensor imaging (DTI) with fiber tracking illustrated recovery of optic radiation fibers and preserved anterior cerebral activation upon visual stimulation in the lesioned hemisphere (Fig. 16-14).

CLINICAL CORRELATES IN THE NEONATAL PERIOD

The preceding case is a typical description of focal infarct, in which the seizures start after 2 or 3 days of life, without other neurologic signs. In particular, no hypotonia or lethargy was described. In this situation the seizures are the result of a focal cortical lesion and not due to diffuse cortical impairment.

LONG-TERM CLINICAL CORRELATES

This child demonstrated hemiplegia contralaterally to the side of the lesion, which was expected because of the extent of the lesion. Alteration of the visual field in the area of the infarct also occurred. Some degree of intellectual impairment developed as well, which was predictable from the size of the lesion.

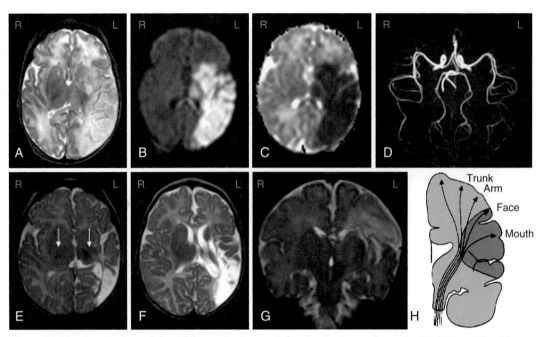

Figure 16-13 Case 7: Acute left middle cerebral artery infarction in the newborn. **A,** Axial T2-weighted image where infarction appears as missed cortex with absence of cortical-subcortical differentiation due to acute edema. Diffusion-weighted image **(B)** and ADC map **(C)** with clear demarcation of ischemic zone. **D,** MR angiography shows reperfused middle cerebral artery on the left. **E** and **F,** Axial T2-weighted images in the chronic phase of infarction show cystic transformation of the initial ischemic zone and absence of left-sided myelination in the posterior limb of the internal capsule *(arrows)*. **G,** Coronal T2-weighted image corresponding to the diagram representing corticospinal tracts and innervation **(H)**. (From Volpe J. *Neurology of the newborn.* 5th ed. Philadelphia: Saunders; 2008.)

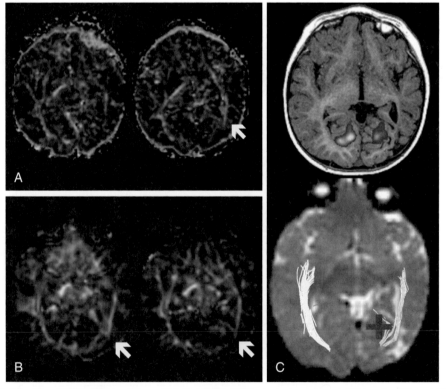

Figure 16-14 Case 7: On diffusion tensor imaging (DTI) with anisotropy maps at 12 months **(A)** and 20 months **(B)**, *arrows* indicate recovery of optic radiation fibers visualized by DTI. **C,** Functional MRI response to visual stimulation at 20 months of age shows recovery of cortical vision in the area of tract recovery. (Adapted from Seghier ML, Lazeyras F, Zimine S, et al. Visual recovery after perinatal stroke evidenced by functional and diffusion MRI: case report. *BMC Neurol.* 2005;5:17.)

MR Techniques in the Evaluation of Focal Ischemic Infarction in the Term Newborn

MRI is the technique of choice for evaluating focal neonatal cerebral infarctions because ultrasonography shows only ill-defined, slight hyperechogenicity, the peripheral cortical extension of which is difficult to evaluate.

Conventional MRI shows loss of corticosubcortical differentiation on both T1- and T2-weighted images because of the increase in T2 signal intensity in the edematous cortex, which thus approaches the intensity of the unmyelinated white matter. This sign is also called the disappeared cortex sign. The best modality to identify a focal ischemic infarct is DWI, which shows striking reduction of ADC in the acute phase and tissue dissolution thereafter, which results in a porencephalic cyst with T2 characteristics of cerebrospinal fluid (CSF).

As outlined in the clinical description, focal ischemic infarction may have less severe neurologic sequelae probably owing to the brain's potential for plasticity.[56,58]

Advanced MR techniques, such as diffusion tensor imaging and fMRI, have been shown to be of use in the study of postinjury plasticity.[59] The geometric nature of the diffusion tensor can be used to display the architecture of the brain white matter fiber tracts, illustrating them by vector images. fMRI can illustrate functional brain activation by measuring changes in local perfusion on the basis of the blood oxygenation level–dependent contrast. In a case of perinatal middle cerebral artery stroke (Case 6) at 20 months of age, event-related fMRI showed significant activation in the visual cortex of the injured left hemisphere that was not observed at 3 months of age.[60] DTI vector maps suggest recovery of the optic radiation in the vicinity of the lesion. Optic radiations in the injured hemisphere were more prominent in DTI at 20 months of age than in DTI at 12 months of age, indicating that functional cortical recovery is supported by structural modifications that involve major pathways of the visual system.

Traumatic Brain Lesions of the Posterior Fossa

Intracranial hemorrhage as such is another important brain lesion in the neonatal period, particularly affecting the preterm infant but also occurring in the full-term infant in certain situations. In particular, traumatic brain lesions of the posterior fossa in the term newborn associated with massive hemorrhage can have serious neurologic sequelae. One mechanism responsible for this lesion is occipital osteodiastasis. This consists of traumatic separation of the cartilaginous joint between the squamous and lateral portions of the occipital bone. In the most severe forms, the dura and the occipital sinus are torn, resulting in massive subdural hemorrhage in the posterior fossa and cerebellar laceration. Risk factors for this condition are breech delivery, vacuum extraction, primiparity, and fetomaternal disproportion.

Clinical manifestations in the most severe cases are immediate signs of brainstem compression (stupor or coma, oculomotor and pupillary abnormalities, nuchal rigidity with opisthotonos, respiratory abnormalities, bradycardia, and then respiratory arrest), and this syndrome is rapidly lethal. In less severe forms, neurologic signs can be absent in the first hours; then symptoms of increased intracranial pressure develop owing to ventricular dilation (block of the CSF flow in the posterior fossa). The signs of brainstem compression due to the posterior fossa hematoma appear later. In addition, seizures occur in the majority of patients, most likely because of the accompanying subarachnoid blood. Long-term outcome is poor in severe occipital diastasis. If the posterior fossa hemorrhage is less pronounced, the outcome is more variable, depending on the rate of rapidity of diagnosis and intervention. With extension of the hemorrhage into the cerebellum, cerebellar deficits due to destruction of the cerebellar tissue are almost invariably present (intention tremor, dysmetria, truncal ataxia, and hypotonia). Hydrocephalus requiring ventriculoperitoneal shunts occur in 50% of cases. Cognitive deficits are also variably present.

CASE 8

HISTORY

Term pregnancy with vaginal delivery instrumented by vacuum for nonprogression of labor; Apgar scores were 9 (1 min), 9 (5 min), and 10 (10 min), with a pH of 7.23. On day 1, general hypotonia, tonic-clonic seizures, and subsequent tonic seizures appeared.

NEUROIMAGING STUDIES

Neonatal head ultrasound performed on day 2 showed posterior fossa hemorrhage with enlarged ventricles. MRI on day 2 revealed a large T2-hypointense lesion in the posterior fossa involving the cerebellar vermis with concomitant ventricular dilation. On the sagittal images the vein of Galen could be identified. MR angiography demonstrated no arterial or venous malformation. Tonsillar herniation of the cerebellum was present. On follow-up T2-weighted images, marked cerebellar lesions were apparent (Fig. 16-15).

CLINICAL CORRELATES IN THE NEONATAL PERIOD

This child presented with hypotonia, which could be due to brainstem compression, and seizures due to cortical irritation by the subarachnoid blood. The brainstem compression signs that are common in this situation were not clinically apparent when the diagnosis was made, in part because of the occurrence of seizures, which resulted in the emergency neuroimaging. Surgical removal of the hematoma was then undertaken. The child had a cardiac arrest during surgery secondary to the massive blood loss and was immediately resuscitated, with success.

LONG-TERM CLINICAL CORRELATES

The patient presented with severe truncal hypotonia and truncal ataxia with delayed spontaneous walking. This child also experienced mild spasticity in the lower extremities. Her cognitive function was normal at age 5 years. However cerebellar deficits, such as intention tremor, dysmetria, and truncal ataxia, persisted.

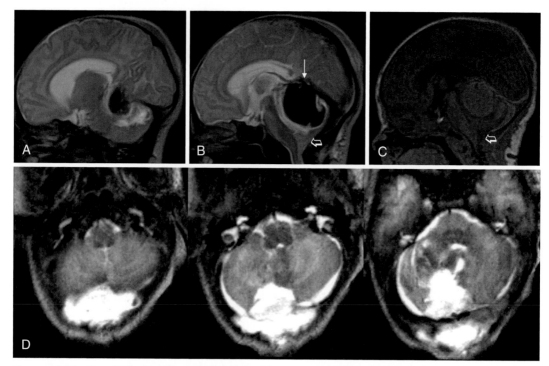

Figure 16-15 Case 8: Sagittal T1- and T2-weighted images acquired on day 2 reveal a large T2-hypointense lesion in the posterior fossa involving the cerebellum with concomitant ventricular dilation (**A** and **B**). The vein of Galen can be identified (**B**, *small arrow*), and tonsillar herniation of the cerebellum is present (**B** and **C**, *large arrows*). **C,** Sagittal T-1 weighted image with hemorrhagic lesion isointense compatible with acute bleeding. **D,** Axial T2-weighted images show residual cerebellar lesion.

MR Techniques in the Evaluation of Traumatic Brain Injury in the Term Newborn

Because the posterior fossa is the primary site of subdural hemorrhage after traumatic birth, cranial ultrasound through the anterior fontanelle has limited capacity to detect the extent of posterior fossa lesions. The MRI appearance of blood depends on the oxidative state of hemoglobin and its environment. Acute hemorrhage (3 hours to 10 days) therefore shows isointense to slight hyperintense on T1-weighted images (gradient-echo sequences preferred) and low signal intensity on T2-weighted images (see Fig. 16-15) with evolution to high signal intensity on T2-weighted images between 10 days and 3 weeks after the hemorrhage (see Fig. 16-15). MR angiography can exclude vein of Galen malformations and sinus thrombosis. Sagittal image planes are necessary to look for cerebellar tonsillar herniation in the presence of posterior fossa hemorrhage.

The Preterm Infant

MR Techniques in the Evaluation of the Preterm Infant

Brain injury in the premature infant is composed of multiple lesions, principally described as germinal matrix intraventricular hemorrhage (IVH), venous hemorrhagic infarction, posthemorrhagic hydrocephalus, and periventricular leukomalacia (PVL). Importantly, many preterm infants show neurodevelopmental delay without having been diagnosed with any of these typical perinatal brain injuries (see Chapters 3 and 17).

The site of origin of IVH is the subependymal germinal matrix, which is a very cellular, gelatinous, highly vascularized region. The exact site of the hemorrhage seems to be the capillary-venule or small venule level.[61] In 80% of cases, the blood then enters the lateral ventricles and spreads through the ventricular system. The presence of blood may create an obliterative arachnoiditis over days to weeks with obstruction of CSF flow. The blood clot can also lead to impaired CSF circulation at the aqueduct of Sylvius and the arachnoid villi. One of the possible consequences of this phenomenon is the development of progressive ventricular dilation and hydrocephalus, which may require shunting. Posthemorrhagic hydrocephalus may happen in an acute, subacute, or chronic way (see Chapter 4). Approximately 15% of infants also have a characteristic parenchymal lesion, with a triangular shape, in the white matter situated dorsally and laterally to the external angle of the lateral ventricle. This lesion corresponds to a hemorrhagic infarction.[62] The time of onset of IVH is the first day of life in 50% of cases and the first 3 days of life in 90% of cases. The neonatal clinical correlates vary from a catastrophic neurologic deterioration in minutes to hours, if the IVH is massive, to a clinically silent syndrome. The long-term neurologic prognosis is mostly dictated by the extent of the intraparenchymal lesion. Neurologic sequelae mostly consist of spastic hemiparesis or asymmetric quadriparesis with cognitive deficits. Posthemorrhagic hydrocephalus is more likely if the IVH is severe and can contribute to the neurologic sequelae in some cases.

PVL has classically been described as a disorder characterized by multifocal areas of necrosis, forming cysts in the deep periventricular cerebral white matter, which are often symmetric and occur adjacent to the lateral ventricles. The earliest neuropathologic changes are those of coagulation necrosis of all cellular elements with loss of cytoarchitecture and tissue vacuolation.[63] Axonal swelling and intense activated microglial reactivity and proliferation are observed as early as 3 hours after insult.[64,65] In addition, in the periphery of these focal lesions, a marked astrocytic and vascular endothelial hyperplasia characterizes the brain tissue reaction at the end of the first week. After 1 to 2 weeks macrophage activity, with characteristic lipid-laden macrophages, predominates over the astrocytic reactivity, with progressive cavitation of the tissue and cyst formation thereafter. During subacute and chronic stages of PVL, swollen axons calcify, accumulate iron, and degenerate, particularly at the periphery of the injured zone. The deep focal necrotic lesions of PVL occur in areas that are considered arterial end zones. The state of development of the periventricular vessels is a function of gestational age, and the degree of ischemia required to produce these focal lesions may vary with the state of development of these vessel and thus with gestational age.[66]

These focal necrotic lesions correlate well with the development of spastic CP in very low-birth-weight (VLBW) infants, whereas the increasingly large number of very low-birth-weight infants with mild motor impairment and cognitive and behavioral deficits[67] may relate to a more diffuse injury to the developing white matter that has only recently been recognized. Diffuse white matter damage is macroscopically characterized by a paucity of white matter, thinning of the corpus callosum, and, in later stages, ventriculomegaly and delayed myelination.

The pathogenesis of the more diffuse lesions may relate in part to the development of the penetrating vessels more peripherally. These diffuse lesions also seem to be related to less severe ischemia than the focal ones. In sick premature infants, the cerebral circulation tends to become pressure passive—that is, when blood pressure falls, so does the cerebral blood flow. This mechanism adds to ischemia in the pathogenesis of cerebral white matter injury. Neuropathologic findings of the diffuse type of cerebral injury in the preterm infant further includes preferential death of preoligodendrocytes,[68,69] axonal damage,[65] and death of the transitory subplate neurons[70] through mechanisms of oxidative injury, glutamate toxicity, and presence of cytotoxic cytokines produced by infection and inflammation. The injury of the white matter secondary to cytotoxic cytokines has been shown to occur prenatally in the setting of chorioamnionitis[71-73] or postnatally in the setting of sepsis or necrotizing enterocolitis. These inflammatory factors are likely to be more important in the pathogenesis of the more diffuse-type PVL. Diffuse neuronal loss, especially in lower cortical layers, the hippocampus, and the cerebellar Purkinje cell layer is described in preterm brain neuropathologic studies.[74] The clinical correlates of PVL are described in Table 16-3.

At least some of the cognitive deficits associated with PVL may be due to subsequent disturbance of cortical neuronal organization because of injury to subplate neurons, to late migrating astrocytes, or to axons with retrograde disturbances in dendritic development.[70,75-79]

The role of MRI in the diagnosis and prognosis of these lesions is illustrated in the next four cases.

CASE 9

HISTORY

Premature infant born at 27 weeks of gestation, with hyaline membrane disease, pneumothorax, and neonatal sepsis.

NEUROIMAGING STUDIES

Neonatal head ultrasound performed on day 5 showed bilaterally increased periventricular echodensities (Fig 16-16A). On day 10, persistent periventricular echodensities with appearance of small echolucencies can bee seen (see Fig. 16-16B). MRI at term shows periventricular cysts surrounded by hyperintense areas on T1-weighted images, consistent with gliosis. The lateral ventricles are enlarged and irregularly shaped. There is overall volume reduction of the white matter, especially posteriorly (Fig. 16-17).

CLINICAL CORRELATES IN THE NEONATAL PERIOD

There was no definite neurologic syndrome in the neonatal period.

LONG-TERM CLINICAL CORRELATES

The child demonstrated spastic diplegia as a sequela of the bilateral PVL. This is a good example of a PVL occurring in the setting of hemodynamic alterations but also inflammation due to the neonatal sepsis. The spastic diplegia was severe, so the child was unable to walk without help by age 3 years. There was mild intellectual impairment. The child also presented with a strabismus.

Table 16-3   CLINICAL CORRELATES OF PERIVENTRICULAR LEUKOMALACIA

Topography of the injury	Periventricular white matter (descending motor fibers, optic radiations, and association fibers)
Neonatal correlates	Lower limb weakness may be seen.
Long-term correlates	Spastic diplegia Visual deficits In the more severe forms: involvement of upper extremities and intellectual impairment Epilepsy in 3% Intellectual and visual deficits can also occur in infants without motor deficits in the more diffuse form of PVL.

Modified from Volpe J. *Neurology of the newborn.* 5th ed. Philadelphia: Saunders; 2008.

16

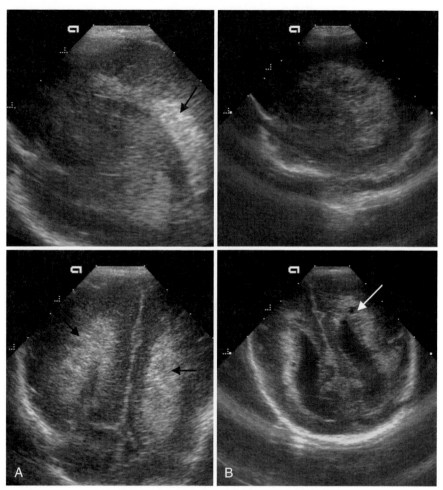

Figure 16-16   Case 9: **A,** Head ultrasound scan on day 5 of life shows an increased and slightly irregular periventricular hyperechogenicity *(black arrows).* **B,** Head ultrasound scan at day 10 demonstrates persisting periventricular hyperechogenicity and the appearance of echolucencies *(white arrow).* These are typical ultrasound images of evolving periventricular leukomalacia.

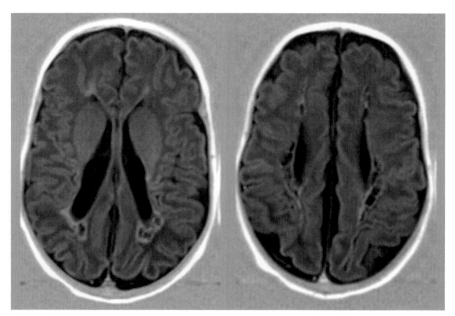

Figure 16-17 Case 9: MRI at term age with inversion recovery sequence optimized for T1-weighted contrast, illustrating the periventricular cysts surrounded by hyperintense areas consistent with gliosis. The lateral ventricles are enlarged and irregularly shaped with squared-off posterior horns. There seems to be overall volume reduction of the white matter, especially posteriorly. These findings are typical for late-stage periventricular leukomalacia.

CASE 10

HISTORY

Preterm infant born at 29 weeks of gestation by emergency cesarean section because of signs of placental abruption; primary resuscitation, perinatal acidosis, respiratory distress syndrome.

NEUROIMAGING STUDIES

Neonatal head ultrasound performed on day 2 shows bilateral IVHs with mild ventricular dilation and local extension into frontal white matter indicative of periventricular venous infarction. MRI on day 2 confirms IVH, with unilateral venous infarction and large T2 hypointense ventricles and T2 hypointensity adjacent to the ventricle with typical flaring pattern (Fig. 16-18 A and B). The rest of the white matter parenchyma shows no focal T2 abnormalities, but DWI measurements reveal abnormal low ADC values (0.8 μm^2/ms) in the periventricular white matter (see Fig. 16-18C). Follow-up MRI 3 weeks later shows tissue dissolution in the peripheral white matter with T2 signal similar to CSF, residual IVH illustrated by T2 hypointensities, and hydrocephalus (Fig. 16-19).

CLINICAL CORRELATES IN THE NEONATAL PERIOD

There was no major neurologic syndrome in the neonatal period.

LONG-TERM CLINICAL CORRELATES

This child had a very poor outcome, with severe spastic quadriplegia, epilepsy, and visual and cognitive impairments. All these sequelae are due to the severe bilateral cystic leukomalacia and not to the bilateral IVH or the unilateral PVHI. This is a good example of early leukomalacia detectable only by ADC measurements, which clearly changes neurologic prognosis early on. The hydrocephalus in this case is due to tissue loss surrounding the ventricles (ex vacuo hydrocephalus).

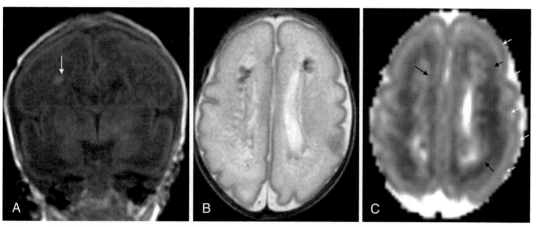

Figure 16-18   Case 10: MRI in early-evolving periventricular leukomalacia. **A,** Coronal T1-weighted conventional image shows small hyperintense lesion *(arrow)* in the periventricular white matter, representing a small hemorrhagic component that was seen as hypointensities on the T2-weighted images **(B)**. **B,** Axial T2-weighted image shows diffuse hyperintensities of the white matter that are difficult to interpret in the immature brain. **C,** Axial ADC map shows diffuse restriction of water diffusion with ADC values measured<1 mm²/ms in the periventricular white matter *(white arrows)* and areas of increased ADC *(black arrows)* representing areas of beginning liquefaction.

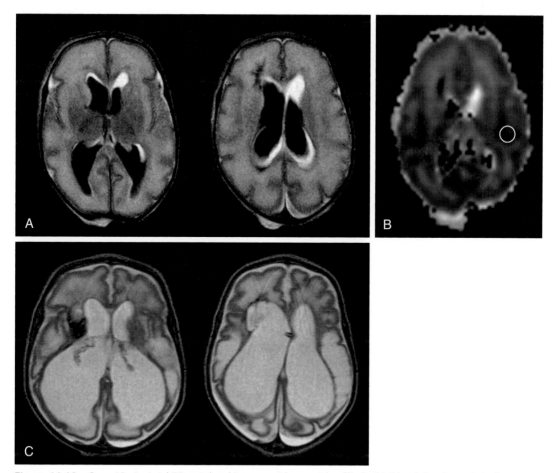

Figure 16-19   Case 10: **A,** Axial T2-weighted images with ventricles filled with blood (low intensity) of an acute intraventricular hemorrhage with periventricular hemorrhagic infarction into frontal parenchyma *(arrows)* with normal-appearing adjacent white matter. **B,** Diffusion-weighted image shows reduced ADC values (0.8 mm²/ms) *(circle)* in the parietal white matter. **C,** Evolution after 3 weeks shows as multicystic encephalopathy with marked hydrocephalus on axial T2-weighted images.

CASE 11

HISTORY

Triplet pregnancy with moderate preterm labor at 24 to26 weeks of gestation and premature rupture of membranes at 30 weeks of gestation. Reduced growth of one triplet and alteration of umbilical Doppler measurements leads to cesarean section at 33 weeks of gestation. Triplet 1 is small-for-gestational age with normal Apgar scores.

NEUROIMAGING STUDIES

Neonatal ultrasonography on day 2 illustrates bilateral periventricular hyperechogenicity (Fig. 16-20). Conventional MRI at term reveals multiple areas of diffuse T2 hyperintensities in the white matter and subcortical white matter cysts as well as some T2 hypotensities/T1 hypotensities corresponding to gliotic changes in the periventricular white matter (Fig. 16-21). Figure 16-22 illustrates the delay in brain maturation observed at term, with a delay in the myelination of the posterior limb of the internal capsule.

CLINICAL CORRELATES IN THE NEONATAL PERIOD

There was no major neurologic syndrome in the neonatal period.

LONG-TERM CLINICAL CORRELATES

This patient demonstrated increased tone in the four extremities, but predominantly involving the lower limbs with hyperreflexia and moderate spasticity of both legs, in relation to the white matter cysts visualized on neuroimaging. She was, however, able to walk without help at age 2 years. Her intellectual performances were markedly delayed, most likely as a sequela of the more diffuse white matter alterations. This case illustrates the fact that white matter injuries of both types (cystic and diffuse) can also happen prenatally as a sequela of poor perfusion and/or inflammation.

CASE 12

HISTORY

Preterm infant with gestational age at birth of 25 weeks, birth weight 650 g. Neonatal course significant for respiratory distress syndrome with subsequent chronic lung disease, ligation of patent ductus arteriosus, necrotizing enterocolitis, and nosocomial sepsis.

NEUROIMAGING STUDIES

Neonatal ultrasound findings were normal throughout the neonatal period. Conventional MRI at term revealed diffuse T2 hyperintensities and T1 hypointensities in the white matter with poor cortical gyrification, and on DWI, markedly elevated ADC values (ADC >1.8 mm^2/ms throughout the central white matter) (Fig. 16-23).

CLINICAL CORRELATES IN THE NEONATAL PERIOD

There was no major neurologic syndrome in the neonatal period.

LONG-TERM CLINICAL CORRELATES

General neurodevelopmental delay was noted on follow-up, with increased tone in all four extremities and poor fine motor performance. The child had a motor development level of 16 months at 24 months corrected age. There was marked delay in cognitive development, with a developmental age of 15 months at 24 months corrected age and poor attention control. He had received special neurodevelopmental interventions since birth. This case is a good illustration of diffuse white matter alteration that was not visualized by cranial ultrasound scanning.

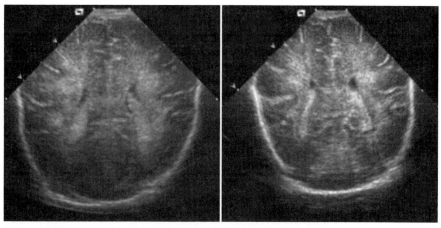

Figure 16-20   Case 11: Cranial ultrasound scans acquired in the first week of life showing mild diffuse white matter hyperechogenicity.

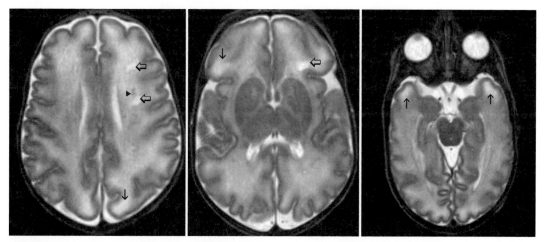

Figure 16-21   Case 11: MRI at term. Axial T2-weighted images show diffuse excessive hyperintense white matter (DEHSI) *(small arrows)* with some small cystic lesions *(large arrows)* in periventricular white matter, which also contains small punctate hypointense lesions *(triangle)*.

Cranial Ultrasonography in the Preterm Infant

Neonatal ultrasonography is the one major bedside technique to image the neonatal brain. Leviton and associates[80] postulated in 1990 that ultrasonographic white matter echodensities and echolucencies in low-birth-weight infants predicted later handicap more accurately than any other antecedent. Unlike IVH, damage to the white matter can have different appearances, and depending on the timing of the injury, the imaging characteristics can be nonspecific with generally an increase in echogenicity in the acute phase of the injury (see Figs. 16-16 and 16-20). In clinical practice, at least in the older preterm infant, the condition of white matter is judged from its echogenic potential in comparison with the choroid plexus. Generally the echogenicity found in early PVL is similar in intensity to that of the choroid plexus, with a bilateral but slightly asymmetric appearance, which can be sharply delineated and may have nodular components. This appearance has to be differentiated from normal peritrigonal flaring, which is perfectly symmetric and has a radial appearance. Evolution of such hyperechogenicity can be twofold, either completely disappearing or evolving into cysts and/or ventricular dilation. Cyst formation in analog to neuropathology is a process typical for the second week (10-40 days) after the

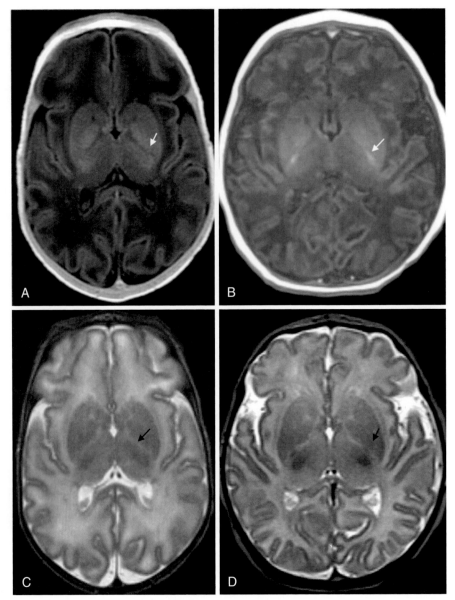

Figure 16-22   MRI in a preterm at term age **(A** and **C)** and in a full-term newborn **(B** and **D)**; axial inversion recovery sequence with T1-weighted contrast showing absence of myelination in the posterior limb of the internal capsule **(A)**, compared with full-term infant **(B)**, with typical T1 hyperintensity in the posterior limb of the internal capsule. Axial T2-weighted images of Case 11 with absence of T2 hypointensity in the posterior limb of the internal capsule **(C)**, compared with presence of T2 hypointensities in the full-term infant **(D)**. Note also the difference in complexity of cortical folding between the preterm infant at term and the full-term newborn.

insult. DeVries and colleagues[81] postulated an ultrasound-based classification for PVL of four grades, with higher grades being associated with increasing neurodevelopmental handicap. Grade I is transient (>7 days) periventricular densities without cyst formation. If cysts develop and are few in number and localized primarily in frontal and frontoparietal white matter, PVL is grade II. When the densities are widespread and extend into the parieto-occipital region, grade III PVL is present; they may grow and gradually disappear leaving an irregularly dilated lateral ventricle. If cysts are present all the way into the subcortical area, resembling porencephaly, grade IV PVL is present (Table 16-4).

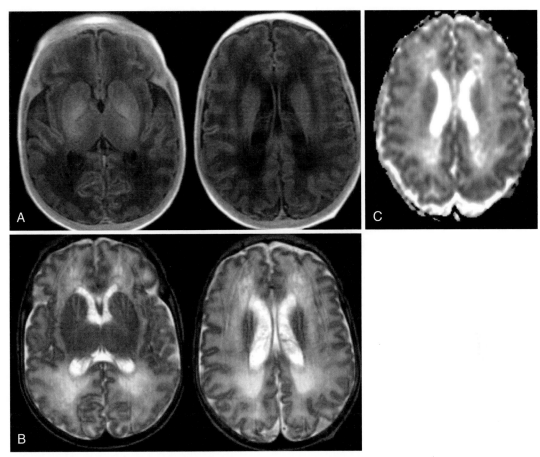

Figure 16-23 Case 12. MRI examination at term of a preterm infant born at 25 weeks of gestation. Cranial ultrasound findings were throughout the perinatal period. Axial inversion recovery sequence with T1-weighted contrast shows low signal intensity in the white matter **(A)**, which corresponds in the T2-weighted images to high signal intensity throughout the white matter with moderately dilated ventricles and poor cortical folding **(B)**. **C,** ADC values of the central white matter are diffusely elevated with values >1.8 mm²/ms. Also note the poor cortical gyrification with simple gyri that most likely represents secondary rather than tertiary sulci.

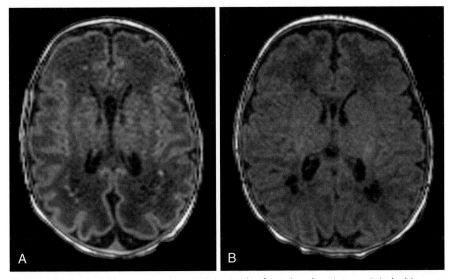

Figure 16-24 **A,** White matter abnormalities in the frontal and parieto-occipital white matter characterized by chainlike T1 hyperintensities in a 31⅔-week preterm infant with small adjacent cysts on axial T1-weighted images at 2 weeks of life. **B,** The cysts have evolved on the second MRI at term-equivalent age into significant bilateral periventricular cysts consistent with cystic periventricular leukomalacia.

Table 16-4 ULTRASOUND CASSIFICATION OF PERIVENTRICULAR LEUKOMALACIA *

Grade I	Transient periventricular echodensities (PVEs) (>7 days)
Grade II	PVES evolving into localized frontoparietal cystic lesions
Grade III	PVES evolving into extensive periventricular cystic lesions
Grade IV	Echodensities evolving into extensive periventricular and subcortical cysts

Modified from DeVries L, Eken P, Dubowitz L. The spectrum of leukomalacia using cranial ultrasound. *Behav Brain Res.* 1992;49:1-6.
*Classification needs longitudinal assessment with daily to weekly ultrasound evaluations.

Ultrasound can be regarded as the ideal mode of imaging to detect cystic PVL, but it has very limited value for detecting diffuse white matter injury, as shown in studies comparing neonatal sonography with MRI.[82-86]

Conventional MRI in the Preterm Infant

Conventional MRI features of chronic white matter injury in the immature brain are characterized either by cysts similar to those seen on ultrasound or, more importantly, by a persistent high signal intensity of the white matter in T2-weighted images representing diffuse white matter injury (see Figs. 16-18 and 16-21; Fig. 16-22).[87] This imaging characteristic is later associated with the thinning of the corpus callosum and loss of white matter volume as a result (see later). In several studies involving preterm infants, brain diffuse excessive high signal intensity (DEHSI) in the cerebral white matter on T2-weighted imaging was reported to be present in 40% to 75% of low-birth-weight preterm infants imaged at term (see Fig. 16-21).[88] MRI is further ideally equipped to assess delayed myelination. The absence of myelination in the posterior limb of the internal capsule (missing T1 high signal intensity and missing low signal intensity) at term age is a good indicator of later neuromotor impairment (see Fig. 16-22).[89,90]

Conventional T1- and T2-weighted images can also show other signal abnormalities in the periventricular white matter. In the subacute phase of white matter injury, MRI detects punctate periventricular areas of T1 signal hyperintensities (Fig. 16-23). The precise neuropathologic correlate of these signal abnormalities is not completely known but may be due to some hemorrhagic components of the lesion. They most likely, however, represent the cellular reaction of glial cells and macrophages, which are known to contain lipid droplets (see earlier neuropathology description), which explain perfectly the high signal intensity on T1-weighted images.[91] These localized T1 hyperintensities are less prominent at term[92a] instead, widened ventricles or periventricular cysts may appear, such as in Figures 16-24 and 16-25. Punctate T1 hyperintensities can also be transitory (related to hemorrhages) and, if not associated with ventricular dilation or white matter cysts (Fig. 16-26), be associated with normal neurodevelopmental outcome.

Cortical differentiation can be qualitatively appreciated on conventional MRI, and preterm infants with diffuse white matter abnormalities often show poor cortical gyrification at term with simple-appearing gyri and sulci compared with the complex tertiary sulci seen in full-term infants (see Figs. 16-22 and 16-24). Quantification of these changes can be assessed by three-dimensional MRI techniques described later.

DWI in the Preterm Infant

Early assessment of periventricular white matter in preterm infants with DWI can reveal bilateral periventricular diffusion restriction similar to the typical distribution of PVL when ultrasound and conventional MRI show no or nonspecific abnormalities (see Fig. 16-18).[92b] Reduced ADC values in an otherwise normal preterm brain are considered an early indicator of white matter damage (just as reduced ADC values are seen shortly after the onset of an acute cerebral ischemic lesion in the full-term newborn). The typical histologic changes in the acute phase of PVL outlined previously, such as cellular and axonal swelling and astrocytic hyperplasia, are characterized by some of the same mechanisms leading to restriction of water

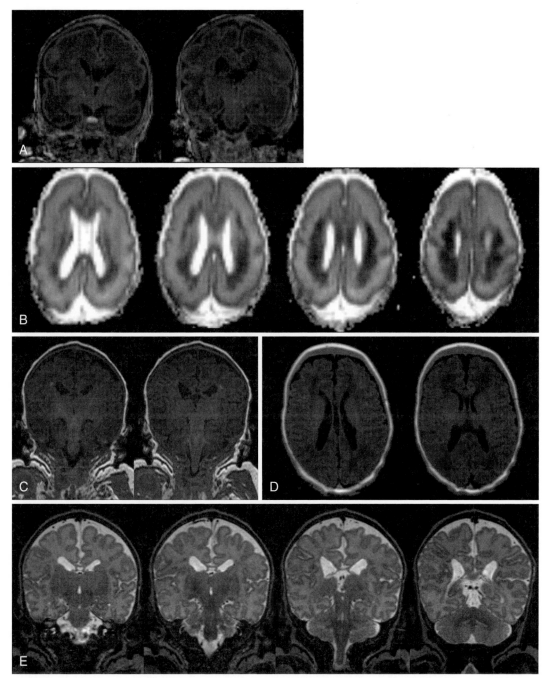

Figure 16-25   MRI on day 5 of life of a preterm infant born at 28 weeks of gestation with a birth weight of 1260 g. **A,** T1-weighted images demonstrate periventricular T1 hyperintensities. **B,** ADC maps show bilateral extensive diffusion restriction in the periventricular white matter. **C,** T1-weighted MR images at term show some punctate lesions (T1 hyperintense) with loss of white matter and reduced T1 hypersignal in the internal capsule. **D,** Axial inversion recovery images showing squared-off dilated ventricles. **E,** Coronal T2-weighted images demonstrate dilated asymmetric ventricles, loss of periventricular white matter. At 3 years of age, this child had cerebral palsy with distal predominant tetraspasticity and mild cognitive delay.

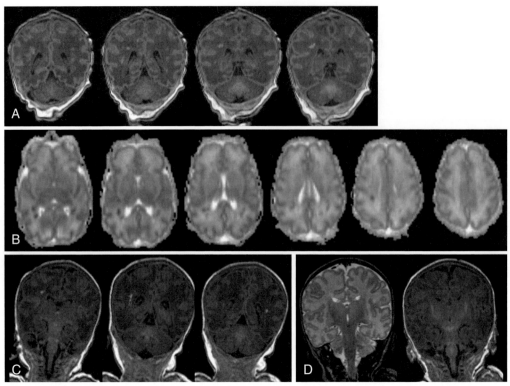

Figure 16-26 Preterm infant born at 32 weeks of gestation with signs of fetal distress. **A,** MRI at 3 days of age shows extensive periventricular punctate white matter lesions (T1 hyperintensities). **B,** ADC maps show punctate areas of restricted diffusion corresponding to T1-weighted signal abnormalities. **C,** At 10 days of life, T1-weighted images show punctate lesions in periventricular white matter with no ventricular dilation. **D,** T2-weighted *(left)* and T1-weighted image *(right)* performed at term age show no signal abnormality, no ventricular dilation, and normal myelination. Images are compatible with hemorrhagic lesions of the white matter that disappear. At 3 years of age the child showed normal neurodevelopmental outcome.

diffusivity. They considerably change the microstructure of white matter and therefore change water diffusivity.

The diffuse T2 hyperintensities of DEHSI, as indicators of the chronic phase of white matter injury, are associated with higher ADC values, confirming the locally higher tissue water content and loss of microstructure impeding water diffusion in those areas (see Fig. 16-23).[92-94] These high ADC values are similar to those seen in the very immature healthy white matter; therefore a potential explanation for the failure of ADC to decline from high levels in the extremely premature infant to lower levels in the term infant in the presence of DEHSI might be related to prior injury with destruction of normal cellular elements (e.g., preoligodendrocytes) or a delay in maturation.[95] Further quantitative measures of diffusion at term among premature infants with perinatal white matter lesions, when compared with those in preterm infants without white matter injury, showed lower anisotropy values in the area of the previous injury—that is, central periventricular white matter—but also in the underlying posterior limb of the internal capsule.[25,93] The lower anisotropy in the injured cerebral white matter suggests that white matter fiber tracts were destroyed or their subsequent development was impaired. The lower anisotropy in the internal capsule further suggests a disturbance in the development of the descending corticospinal tracts.[96] This finding might well be the basis for the reduction in myelination in the posterior limb of the internal capsule observed on conventional MRI, which was shown to be highly correlated with development of motor deficits. DTI has provided new insights into microstructural white matter development and seems to be an ideal tool to assess alteration of white matter pathways in neurologic disease.

MRS in the Preterm Infant

The biochemical characteristics of white matter damage in preterm infants have been studied in vivo using MRS.[97,98] Similar to the MRS in term asphyxia, for which it has high diagnostic value, MRS in acute-phase immature white matter injury can detect indicators of anaerobic glycolysis with increased intracerebral lactate.[36] Preliminary results show that white matter damage in the preterm infant studied around term gestational age resulted in high Lac-to-Cr and high myoinositol-to-Cr ratios.[98] The increased presence of lactate at this chronic stage was not associated with changes in pH, whereas NAA, as a marker of neuroaxonal integrity, was reduced in the damaged periventricular white matter. Astrocytes further play a variety of complex nutritive and supportive roles in relation to neuronal metabolic homeostasis. For example, astrocytes take up glutamate and convert it to glutamine; the removal of glutamate from the extracellular space protects surrounding cells from excitotoxicity due to glutamate. Glutamate uptake into astrocytes further stimulates glycolysis within the astrocyte, with production of lactate that can be used by neurons as an energy substrate.[99] Given that chronic phase white matter injury is characterized by widespread cerebral white matter astrocytosis, this change in metabolite composition might be an expression of alterations in cellular composition and substrate utilization.

Advanced Quantitative MRI with Image Analysis Tools

Three-dimensional (3D) MRI methods combined with image postprocessing techniques have been developed that allow volumetric assessment of brain development and an absolute quantitation of myelination in the newborn.[100-103] These techniques allow exact definition of brain volume and can therefore accurately monitor brain growth, measure CSF volume, and determine volume changes in white matter and cortical gray matter. 3D MRI volumetric techniques have been used to evaluate the effect on subsequent brain development of early white matter injury in premature infants. In premature infants with preceding white matter injury, the volume of myelinated white matter at term was significantly lower than in premature infants without prior white matter injury and infants born at term, measuring the degree of delay of myelination. Furthermore, this study showed a marked decrease in cortical gray matter volume in preterm infants with prior periventricular white matter injury, indicating impaired cerebral cortical development after early white matter injury.[104] In a population study, similar volumetric changes of overall brain development in preterm infants were confirmed with the finding of significantly less myelinated white matter and cortical gray matter in preterm infants than in full-term infants, with a reduction also of deep nuclear gray matter (basal ganglia) most pronounced in the lowest gestational ages.[101] Assessment of moderately preterm infants without signs of white matter injury cortical development was similar to that in full-term infants.[105] Regional assessment of white matter myelination in preterm infants further revealed particular delay in myelination in the central and posterior parts of the brain.[106] 3D MRI demonstrated significantly smaller cerebellar volume at term in preterm infants than in term infants.[107] Unilateral cerebral white matter lesions resulted in contralateral reduction of cerebellar volume, indicating the trophic interplay due to loss of cerebrocerebellar connectivity.[108]

Long-term follow-up studies of preterm infants have confirmed the permanent character of these disruptive/adaptive changes in brain development. Evaluation of preterm infants at 8 years of age with volumetric brain assessment showed persistence of cortical gray matter reduction accompanied by a reduction in the volume of the hippocampus, which correlated with cognitive scores indicating long-term functional consequences.[109] Both cortical volume and cortical thickness were shown to be reduced in 15-year-old patients who were born prematurely.[110] Voxel-based morphometry (VBM), an image analysis tool that compares brain tissue in groups after normalization to a template, has shown that adolescents and young adults born prematurely have smaller hippocampi, with a correlation with performance IQ,[111] accompanied by smaller gray matter volume in several regions of the brain than patients born at term.[112,113] Cerebral white matter was shown in voxel-based morphometry studies to be equally affected by preterm birth. Overall, white matter volume was found to be reduced in former preterm infants, with a significant impact in males born prematurely, predominantly in the cingulum, the corpus callosum, and the corticospinal tracts.[114,115]

Mathematical morphology, yet another image analysis technique, has been used to process and analyze shape to investigate primary cortical folding in the preterm brain. Poor intrauterine growth and white matter lesions result in considerable alteration of cortical surface, sulcation index, and cortical morphology.[116-119] Several reviews have summarized a vast scientific literature looking at short-term and long-term effects of prematurity on brain tissue as assessed by advanced MRI techniques.[78,120,121]

Conclusions

The main advantages of MR techniques in the evaluation of the preterm infant are as follows:

1. Abnormal signal intensities in the white matter are more reliably detected by MRI than by ultrasound.
2. More widespread non-hemorrhagic white matter injury in the presence of IVH is more readily diagnosed with MR techniques than with ultrasound in both the acute and chronic phases.
3. Diffuse white matter injury without frank cystic development can be detected by both conventional MRI (DEHSI) and DWI with measurement of ADC.
4. Myelination pattern at term, defined by inversion recovery and T1- and T2-weighted MR sequences, can predict neuromotor outcome.
5. Isolated punctate lesions identified as T1 hyperintensities without additional brain tissue alterations, such as ventricular dilation and DEHSI, are not necessarily associated with neurodevelopmental delay.
6. More advanced MRI tools such as DTI, 3D-volumetric MRI, and fMRI, can define plasticity and predict functional outcome of more complex brain functions.

Acknowledgement

Supported by Swiss National Foundation (SNF: 3200-056927/102127 32003B-113632 and SNF: 33CM30-124101).

References

1. Neil J, Miller J, Mukherjee P, Huppi PS. Diffusion tensor imaging of normal and injured developing human brain—a technical review. *NMR Biomed.* 2002;15:543-552.
2. Huppi PS, Lazeyras F. Proton magnetic resonance spectroscopy ((1)H-MRS) in neonatal brain injury. *Pediatr Res.* 2001;49:317-320.
3. Seghier ML, Lazeyras F, Huppi PS. Functional MRI of the newborn. *Semin Fetal Neonatal Med.* 2006.
4. Volpe JJ. Perinatal brain injury: from pathogenesis to neuroprotection. *Ment Retard Dev Disabil Res Rev* 2001;7:56-64.
5. Perlman JM. Summary proceedings from the neurology group on hypoxic-ischemic encephalopathy. *Pediatrics.* 2006;117:S28-S33.
6. Nelson KB, Grether JK. Potentially asphyxiating conditions and spastic cerebral palsy in infants of normal birth weight. *Am J Obstet Gynecol.* 1998;179:507-513.
7. Perlman JM. Intrapartum asphyxia and cerebral palsy: is there a link? *Clin Perinatol.* 2006;33: 335-353.
8. Barkovich A, Sargent S. Profound asphyxia in the premature infant: imaging findings. *AJNR Am J Neuroradiol.* 1995;16:1837-1846.
9. Ashwal S, Majcher JS, Vain N, Longo LD. Patterns of fetal lamb regional cerebral blood flow during and after prolonged hypoxia. *Pediatr Res.* 1980;14:1104-1110.
10. Johnson GN, Palahniuk RJ, Tweed WA, et al. Regional cerebral blood flow changes during severe fetal asphyxia produced by slow partial umbilical cord compression. *Am J Obstet Gynecol.* 1979;135:48-52.
11. Shah P, Riphagen S, Beyene J, Perlman M. Multiorgan dysfunction in infants with post-asphyxial hypoxic-ischaemic encephalopathy. *Arch Dis Child Fetal Neonatal Ed.* 2004;89:F152-F155.
12. Rutherford M, Counsell S, Allsop J, et al. Diffusion-weighted magnetic resonance imaging in term perinatal brain injury: a comparison with site of lesion and time from birth. *Pediatrics.* 2004;114:1004-1014.
13. Govaert P, de Vries LS. *An atlas of neonatal brain sonography.* Cambridge, UK: Cambridge University Press; 1997:1-363.

14. Cabanas F, Pellicer A, Perez-Higueras A, et al. Ultrasonographic findings in thalamus and basal ganglia in term asphyxiated infants. *Pediatr Neurol.* 1991;7:211-215.

15. Kashman N, Kramer U, Stavorovsky Z, et al. Prognostic significance of hyperechogenic lesions in the basal ganglia and thalamus in neonates. *J Child Neurol.* 2001;16:591-594.

16. Leijser L, Cowan F. "State of the Art" neonatal cranial ultrasound. *Ultrasound.* 2007;15:6-17.

17. Rutherford M. *MRI of the neonatal brain.* Philadelphia: WB Saunders; 2002.

18. Hüppi PS, Lazeyras F. MR spectroscopy. In: Tortori-Donati P, ed. *Pediatric neuroradiology brain.* Berlin: Springer; 2005:1049-1072.

19. Rutherford M, Malamateniou C, Zeka J, Counsell S. MR imaging of the neonatal brain at 3 Tesla. *Eur J Paediatr Neurol.* 2004;8:281-289.

20. Triulzi F, Baldoli C, Parazzini C. Neonatal MR imaging. *Magn Reson Imaging Clin N Am.* 2001;9:57-82, viii.

21. Mc Ardle CB, Richardson CJ, Nicholas DA. Developmental features of the neonatal brain: MR imaging. Part I. Gray-white matter differentiation and myelination. *Radiology.* 1987;162:223-229.

22. Rutherford MA, Pennock JM, Counsell SJ, et al. Abnormal magnetic resonance signal in the internal capsule predicts poor neurodevelopmental outcome in infants with hypoxic-ischemic encephalopathy. *Pediatrics.* 1998;102:323-328.

23. Rutherford M, Ward P, Allsop J, et al. Magnetic resonance imaging in neonatal encephalopathy. *Early Hum Dev.* 2005;81:13-25.

24. Pasternak JF. Parasagittal infarction in neonatal asphyxia. *Ann Neurol.* 1987;21:202-204.

25. Huppi PS, Dubois J. Diffusion tensor imaging of brain development. *Semin Fetal Neonatal Med.* 2006;11:489-497.

26. Conturo TE, McKinstry RC, Aronovitz JA, Neil JJ. Diffusion MRI: precision, accuracy and flow effects. *NMR Biomed.* 1995;8:307-332.

27. Moseley M, Cohen Y, Kucharczyk J, et al. Diffusion-weighted MR-imaging of anisotropic water diffusion in cat central nervous system. *Radiology.* 1990;176:439-445.

28. Rumpel H, Ferrini B, Martin E. Lasting cytotoxic edema as an indicator of irreversible brain damage: a case of neonatal stroke. *Neurosci Behav.* 1998;19:1636-1638.

29. Warach S, Chien D, Li W. Fast magnetic resonance diffusion-weighted imaging of acute human stroke. *Neurology.* 1992;42:1717-1723.

30. Li F, Han SS, Tatlisumak T, et al. Reversal of acute apparent diffusion coefficient abnormalities and delayed neuronal death following transient focal cerebral ischemia in rats. *Ann Neurol.* 1999;46:333-342.

31. Copen WA, Schwamm LH, Gonzalez RG, et al. Ischemic stroke: effects of etiology and patient age on the time course of the core apparent diffusion coefficient. *Radiology.* 2001;221:27-34.

32. McKinstry RC, Miller JH, Snyder AZ, et al. A prospective, longitudinal diffusion tensor imaging study of brain injury in newborns. *Neurology.* 2002;59:824-833.

33. Robertson R, Ben-Sira L, Barnes P, et al. MR line-scan diffusion-weighted imaging of term neonates with perinatal brain ischemia. *AJNR Am J Neuroradiol.* 1999;20:1658-1670.

34. Soul JS, Robertson RL, Tzika AA, et al. Time course of changes in diffusion-weighted magnetic resonance imaging in a case of neonatal encephalopathy with defined onset and duration of hypoxic-ischemic insult. *Pediatrics.* 2001;108:1211-1214.

35. Groenendaal F, Veehoven R, van der Grond J, et al. Cerebral lactate and N-acetylaspartate/choline ratios in asphyxiated full-term neonates demonstrated in vivo using proton magnetic resonance spectroscopy. *Pediatr Res.* 1994;35:148-151.

36. Penrice J, Cady E, Lorek A, et al. Proton magnetic resonance spectroscopy of the brain in normal preterm and term infants, and early changes after perinatal hypoxia-ischemia. *Pediatr Res.* 1996;40:6-14.

37. Hanrahan J, Cox I, Azzopardi D, et al. Relation between proton magnetic resonance spectroscopy within 18 hours of birth asphyxia and neurodevelopment at 1 year of age. *Dev Med Child Neurol.* 1999;41:76-82.

38. Hanrahan J, Cox I, Edwards A, et al. Persistent increases in cerebral lactate concentration after birth asphyxia. *Pediatr Res.* 1998;44:304-311.

39. Robertson NJ, Cowan FM, Cox IJ, Edwards AD. Brain alkaline intracellular pH after neonatal encephalopathy. *Ann Neurol.* 2002;52:732-742.

40. Robertson N, IJ C, Cowan F, et al. Cerebral intracellular lactic alkalosis persisting months after neonatal encephalopathy measured by magnetic resonance spectroscopy. *Pediatr Res.* 1999;46:287-296.

41. Zarifi MK, Astrakas LG, Poussaint TY, et al. Prediction of adverse outcome with cerebral lactate level and apparent diffusion coefficient in infants with perinatal asphyxia. *Radiology.* 2002;225:859-870.

42. Groenendaal F, Roelants-Van Rijn AM, van Der GJ, et al. Glutamate in cerebral tissue of asphyxiated neonates during the first week of life demonstrated in vivo using proton magnetic resonance spectroscopy. *Biol Neonate.* 2001;79:254-257.

43. Peden C, Rutherford M, Sargentoni J, et al. Proton spectroscopy of the neonatal brain following hypoxic-ischemic injury. *Dev Med Child Neurol.* 1993;34:285-295.

44. Roelants-Van Rijn AM, van Der GJ, de Vries LS, Groenendaal F. Value of (1)H-MRS using different echo times in neonates with cerebral hypoxia-ischemia. *Pediatr Res.* 2001;49:356-362.

45. Shu S, Ashwal S, Holshauser B, et al. Prognostic value of 1H-MRS in perinatal CNS insults. *Pediatr Neurol.* 1997;17:309-318.

16

46. Lodygensky G, West, T., Moravec MD, et al. Diffusion characteristics associated with neuronal injury and glial activation following hypoxia-ischemia in the immature brain. *Magn Reson Med.* 2011; 66:839-845.

47. Wendland MF, Faustino J, West T, et al. Early diffusion-weighted MRI as a predictor of caspase-3 activation after hypoxic-ischemic insult in neonatal rodents. *Stroke.* 2008;39:1862-1868.

48. Boichot C, Mejean N, Gouyon JB, et al. Biphasic time course of brain water ADC observed during the first month of life in term neonates with severe perinatal asphyxia is indicative of poor outcome at 3 years. *Magn Reson Imaging.* 2011;29:194-201.

49. Khachaturian MH, Arsenault J, Ekstrom LB, et al. Focal reversible deactivation of cerebral metabolism affects water diffusion. *Magn Reson Med.* 2008;60:1178-1189.

50. Wintermark P, Hansen A, Soul J, et al. Early versus late MRI in asphyxiated newborns treated with hypothermia. *Arch Dis Child Fetal Neonatal Ed.* 2011;96:F36-F44.

51. Thoresen M, Penrice J, Lorek A, et al. Mild hypothermia after severe transient hypoxia-ischemia ameliorates delayed cerebral energy failure in the newborn piglet. *Pediatr Res.* 1995;37:667-670.

52. Laptook A, Corbett R, Sterett R, et al. Modest hypothermia provides partial neuroprotection for ischemic neonatal brain. *Pediatr Res.* 1994;35:436-442.

53. Lutz NW, Kuesel AC, Hull WE. A 1H-NMR method for determining temperature in cell culture perfusion systems. *Magn Reson Med.* 1993;29:113-118.

54. Rutherford M, Ramenghi LA, Edwards AD, et al. Assessment of brain tissue injury after moderate hypothermia in neonates with hypoxic-ischaemic encephalopathy: a nested substudy of a randomised controlled trial. *Lancet Neurol.* 2010;9:39-45.

55. Massaro A, Rais-Bahrami K, Chang T, et al. Therapeutic hypothermia for neonatal encephalopathy and extracorporeal membrane oxygenation. *J Pediatr.* 2010;157:499-501.

56. Boardman JP, Ganesan V, Rutherford MA, et al. Magnetic resonance image correlates of hemiparesis after neonatal and childhood middle cerebral artery stroke. *Pediatrics.* 2005;115:321-326.

57. Golomb MR. Outcomes of perinatal arterial ischemic stroke and cerebral sinovenous thrombosis. *Semin Fetal Neonatal Med.* 2009;14:318-322.

58. de Vries LS, van Der GJ, van Haastert IC, Groenendaal F. Prediction of outcome in new-born infants with arterial ischaemic stroke using diffusion-weighted magnetic resonance imaging. *Neuropediatrics.* 2005;36:12-20.

59. Seghier ML, Lazeyras F, Zimine S, et al. Combination of event-related fMRI and diffusion tensor imaging in an infant with perinatal stroke. *Neuroimage.* 2004;21:463-472.

60. Seghier ML, Lazeyras F, Zimine S, et al. Visual recovery after perinatal stroke evidenced by functional and diffusion MRI: case report. *BMC Neurol.* 2005;5:17.

61. Ghazi-Birry HS, Brown WR, Moody DM, et al. Human germinal matrix: venous origin of hemorrhage and vascular characteristics. *AJNR Am J Neuroradiol.* 1997;18:219-229.

62. Gould SJ, Howard S, Hope PL, Reynolds EO. Periventricular intraparenchymal cerebral haemorrhage in preterm infants: the role of venous infarction. *J Pathol.* 1987;151:197-202.

63. Deguchi K, Oguchi K, Takashima S. Characteristic neuropathology of leukomalacia in extremely low birth weight infants. *Pediatr Neurol.* 1997;16:296-300.

64. Deguchi K, Oguchi K, Matsuura N, et al. Periventricular leukomalacia: relation to gestational age and axonal injury. *Pediatr Neurol.* 1999;20:370-374.

65. Hirayama A, Okoshi Y, Hachiya Y, et al. Early immunohistochemical detection of axonal damage and glial activation in extremely immature brains with periventricular leukomalacia. *Clin Neuropathol.* 2001;20:87-91.

66. Takashima S, Tanaka K. Development of cerebrovascular architecture and its relationship to periventricular leukomalacia. *Arch Neurol.* 1978;35:11-16.

67. Taylor HG, Minich N, Bangert B, et al. Long-term neuropsychological outcomes of very low birth weight: associations with early risks for periventricular brain insults. *J Int Neuropsychol Soc.* 2004;10:987-1004.

68. Back SA, Han BH, Luo NL, et al. Selective vulnerability of late oligodendrocyte progenitors to hypoxia ischemia. *J Neurosci.* 2002;22:455-463.

69. Haynes RL, Folkerth RD, Keefe RJ, et al. Nitrosative and oxidative injury to premyelinating oligodendrocytes in periventricular leukomalacia. *J Neuropathol Exp Neurol.* 2003;62:441-450.

70. McQuillen PS, Sheldon RA, Shatz CJ, Ferriero DM. Selective vulnerability of subplate neurons after early neonatal hypoxia-ischemia. *J Neurosci.* 2003;23:3308-3315.

71. Dammann O, Kuban KC, Leviton A. Perinatal infection, fetal inflammatory response, white matter damage, and cognitive limitations in children born preterm. *Ment Retard Dev Disabil Res Rev.* 2002;8:46-50.

72. Lodygensky GA, West T, Stump M, et al. In vivo MRI analysis of an inflammatory injury in the developing brain. *Brain Behav Immun.* 2010;24:759-767.

73. Shah DK, Doyle LW, Anderson PJ, et al. Adverse neurodevelopment in preterm infants with postnatal sepsis or necrotizing enterocolitis is mediated by white matter abnormalities on magnetic resonance imaging at term. *J Pediatr.* 2008;153:170-175.

74. Marin-Padilla M. Developmental neuropathology and impact of perinatal brain damage. II: white matter lesions of the neocortex. *J Neuropathol Exp Neurol.* 1997;56:219-235.

75. Folkerth RD, Trachtenberg FL, Haynes RL. Oxidative injury in the cerebral cortex and subplate neurons in periventricular leukomalacia. *J Neuropathol Exp Neurol.* 2008;67:677-686.

76. Gressens P, Richelme C, Kadhim HJ, et al. The germinative zone produces the most cortical astrocytes after neuronal migration in the developing mammalian brain. *Biol Neonate.* 1992;61:4-24.

77. Haynes RL, Billiards SS, Borenstein NS, et al. Diffuse axonal injury in periventricular leukomalacia as determined by apoptotic marker fraction. *Pediatr Res.* 2008;63:656-661.
78. Volpe JJ. Brain injury in premature infants: a complex amalgam of destructive and developmental disturbances. *Lancet Neurol.* 2009;8:110-124.
79. Volpe J. Subplate neurons—missing link in brain injury of the premature infant? *Pediatrics.* 1996;97:112-113.
80. Leviton A, Paneth N. White matter damage in preterm newborns—an epidemiologic perspective. *Early Hum Dev.* 1990;24:1-22.
81. DeVries L, Eken P, Dubowitz L. The spectrum of leukomalacia using cranial ultrasound. *Behav Brain Res.* 1992;49:1-6.
82. Childs AM, Cornette L, Ramenghi LA, et al. Magnetic resonance and cranial ultrasound characteristics of periventricular white matter abnormalities in newborn infants. *Clin Radiol.* 2001;56:647-655.
83. DeVries L, Eken P, Groenendaal F, et al. Correlation between the degree of periventricular leukomalacia diagnosed using cranial ultrasound and MRI later in infancy in children with cerebral palsy. *Neuropediatrics.* 1993;24:263-268.
84. Inder TE, Anderson NJ, Spencer C, et al. White matter injury in the premature infant: a comparison between serial cranial sonographic and MR findings at term. *AJNR Am J Neuroradiol.* 2003;24:805-809.
85. Maalouf EF, Duggan PJ, Counsell SJ, et al. Comparison of findings on cranial ultrasound and magnetic resonance imaging in preterm infants. *Pediatrics.* 2001;107:719-727.
86. Rijn AM, Groenendaal F, Beek FJ, et al. Parenchymal brain injury in the preterm infant: comparison of cranial ultrasound, MRI and neurodevelopmental outcome. *Neuropediatrics.* 2001;32:80-89.
87. Huppi PS. Advances in postnatal neuroimaging: relevance to pathogenesis and treatment of brain injury. *Clin Perinatol.* 2002;29:827-856.
88. Maalouf EF, Duggan PJ, Rutherford MA, et al. Magnetic resonance imaging of the brain in a cohort of extremely preterm infants8. *J Pediatr.* 1999;135:351-357.
89. Aida N, Nishimura G, Hachiya Y, et al. MR Imaging of perinatal brain damage: Comparison of clinical outcome with initial and follow-up findings. *Am J Neuroradiol.* 1998;19:1909-1921.
90. de Vries LS, Groenendaal F, van Haastert IC, et al. Asymmetrical myelination of the posterior limb of the internal capsule in infants with periventricular haemorrhagic infarction: an early predictor of hemiplegia. *Neuropediatrics.* 1999;30:314-319.
91. Schouman-Claeys E, Henry-Feugeas MC, Roset F, et al. Periventricular leukomalacia: correlation between MR imaging and autopsy findings during the first 2 months of life. *Radiology.* 1993;189:59-64.
92. Counsell SJ, Allsop JM, Harrison MC, et al. Diffusion-weighted imaging of the brain in preterm infants with focal and diffuse white matter abnormality. *Pediatrics.* 2003;112:1-7.
92a. Dyet LE, Kennea N, Counsell SJ, et al. Natural history of brain lesions in extremely preterm infants studied with serial magnetic resonance imaging from birth and neurodevelopmental assessment. *Pediatrics.* 2006;118:536-548.
92b. Inder TE, Huppi PS, Zientara GP, et al. Early detection of periventricular leukomalacia by diffusion-weighted magnetic resonance imaging techniques. *J Pediatr.* 1999;134:631-634.
93. Hüppi P, Murphy B, Maier S, et al. Microstructural brain development after perinatal cerebral white matter injury assessed by diffusion tensor magnetic resonance imaging. *Pediatrics.* 2001;107:455-460.
94. Miller SP, Vigneron DB, Henry RG, et al. Serial quantitative diffusion tensor MRI of the premature brain: development in newborns with and without injury. *J Magn Reson Imaging.* 2002;16:621-632.
95. Counsell SJ, Shen Y, Boardman JP, et al. Axial and radial diffusivity in preterm infants who have diffuse white matter changes on magnetic resonance imaging at term-equivalent age. *Pediatrics.* 2006;117:376-386.
96. Mazumdar A, Mukherjee P, Miller JH, et al. Diffusion-weighted imaging of acute corticospinal tract injury preceding Wallerian degeneration in the maturing human brain. *AJNR Am J Neuroradiol.* 2003;24:1057-1066.
97. Groenendaal F, van de Grond J, Eken P, et al. Early cerebral proton MRS and neurodevelopmental outcome in infants with cystic leukomalacia. *Dev Med Child Neurol.* 1997;39:373-379.
98. Robertson N, Kuint J, Counsell T, et al. Characterization of cerebral white matter damage in the preterm infant using 1H and 31P magnetic resonance spectroscopy. *J Cereb Blood Flow Metab.* 2000;20:1446-1456.
99. Pellerin L, Pellegri G, Martin J, Magistretti P. Expression of monocarboxylate transporter mRNAs in mouse brain: support for a distinct role of lactate as an energy substrate for the neonatal vs. the adult brain. *Proc Natl Acad Sci U S A.* 1998;95:3990-3995.
100. Hüppi P, Warfield S, Kikinis R, et al. Quantitative magnetic resonance imaging of brain development in premature and mature newborns. *Ann Neurol.* 1998;43:224-235.
101. Inder TE, Warfield SK, Wang H, et al. Abnormal cerebral structure is present at term in premature infants4. *Pediatrics.* 2005;115:286-294.
102. Gui L, Lisowski R, Faundez T, et al. Biomedical imaging: from nano to macro. Presented at the 2011 IEEE International Symposium on Automatic Segmentation of Newborn Brain MRI Using Mathematical Morphology. March 30 to April 2, 2011.

103. Prastawa M, Gilmore JH, Lin W, Gerig G. Automatic segmentation of MR images of the developing newborn brain. *Med Image Anal*. 2005;9:457-466.

104. Inder T, Hüppi P, Warfield S, et al. Periventricular white matter injury in the premature infant is associated with a reduction in cerebral cortical gray matter volume at term. *Ann Neurol*. 1999;46: 755-760.

105. Zacharia A, Zimine S, Lovblad KO, et al. Early assessment of brain maturation by MR imaging segmentation in neonates and premature infants. *AJNR Am J Neuroradiol*. 2006;27:972-977.

106. Mewes AU, Huppi PS, Als H, et al. Regional brain development in serial magnetic resonance imaging of low-risk preterm infants. *Pediatrics*. 2006;118:23-33.

107. Limperopoulos C, Soul JS, Gauvreau K, et al. Late gestation cerebellar growth is rapid and impeded by premature birth1. *Pediatrics*. 2005;115:688-695.

108. Limperopoulos C, Soul JS, Haidar H, et al. Impaired trophic interactions between the cerebellum and the cerebrum among preterm infants. *Pediatrics*. 2005;116:844-850.

109. Lodygensky GA, Rademaker K, Zimine S, et al. Structural and functional brain development after hydrocortisone treatment for neonatal chronic lung disease. *Pediatrics*. 2005;116:1-7.

110. Martinussen M, Fischl B, Larsson HB, et al. Cerebral cortex thickness in 15-year-old adolescents with low birth weight measured by an automated MRI-based method. *Brain*. 2005;128: 2588-2596.

111. Isaacs EB, Edmonds CJ, Chong WK, et al. Brain morphometry and IQ measurements in preterm children. *Brain*. 2004;127:2595-2607.

112. Gimenez M, Junque C, Vendrell P, et al. Abnormal orbitofrontal development due to prematurity. *Neurology*. 2006;67:1818-1822.

113. Kesler SR, Reiss AL, Vohr B, et al. Brain volume reductions within multiple cognitive systems in male preterm children at age twelve. *J Pediatr*. 2008;152:513-520.

114. Ment LR, Kesler S, Vohr B, et al. Longitudinal brain volume changes in preterm and term control subjects during late childhood and adolescence. *Pediatrics*. 2009;123:503-511.

115. Soria-Pastor S, Gimenez M, Narberhaus A, et al. Patterns of cerebral white matter damage and cognitive impairment in adolescents born very preterm. *Int J Dev Neurosci*. 2008;26:647-654.

116. Dubois J, Benders M, Borradori-Tolsa C, et al. Primary cortical folding in the human newborn: an early marker of later functional development. *Brain*. 2008;131:2028-2041.

117. Dubois J, Benders M, Cachia A, et al. Mapping the early cortical folding process in the preterm newborn brain. *Cereb Cortex*. 2007;18:1444-1454.

118. Hill J, Dierker D, Neil J, et al. A surface-based analysis of hemispheric asymmetries and folding of cerebral cortex in term-born human infants. *J Neurosci*. 2010;30:2268-2276.

119. Hill J, Inder T, Neil J, et al. Similar patterns of cortical expansion during human development and evolution. *Proc Natl Acad Sci U S A*. 2010;107:13135-13140.

120. Lodygensky GA, Vasung L, Sizonenko SV, Huppi PS. Neuroimaging of cortical development and brain connectivity in human newborns and animal models. *J Anat*. 2010;217:418-428.

121. Ment LR, Hirtz D, Huppi PS. Imaging biomarkers of outcome in the developing preterm brain. *Lancet Neurol*. 2009;8:1042-1055.

16

CHAPTER 17

Long-Term Follow-Up of Very Low-Birth-Weight Infants

Betty R. Vohr, MD

Modern neonatal intensive care has had major therapeutic advances in the past 10 years that have resulted in a dramatic improvement in survival of extremely low-birth-weight (ELBW; <1000-g) infants.[1-4] It has been most significant among infants at the limits of viability (23-24 weeks of gestation).[2,4,5] These infants have more neonatal morbidities,[6-10] more complex medical morbidities (respiratory, gastrointestinal, feeding, growth failure), and greater neurodevelopmental morbidities (neurologic, sensory, developmental, behavioral) after discharge from the neonatal intensive care unit (NICU).[7-13] There are numerous reports of neurodevelopmental abnormalities in ex-ELBW infants in early childhood, but growing evidence is accumulating of adverse outcomes and special health care needs for these patients at school age[14-18] and in young adulthood.[19-21]

The responsibilities for neonatal follow-up programs at tertiary care centers include surveillance of NICU quality indicators, research, and education of fellows and residents,[22] and, in some programs, clinical management after discharge. Important neurodevelopmental outcomes (quality indicators for a NICU) include cerebral palsy, retardation, vision impairment, hearing impairment, and behavior disorders, including autism. Communication of findings to the primary care provider and facilitation of referrals to necessary support services are important components of the clinical program. One of the challenges of follow-up is to identify the optimal age of assessment to determine the true outcome and functional ability of the child. Because of the challenges, costs, and feasibility of long-term tracking, most follow-up studies currently are short term (≤2 years), which may limit the interpretation of the neurodevelopmental outcome data. This chapter discusses four outcome ages: 18 to 24 months, 3 to 6 years, school age, and adolescent/young adult. The discussion covers two outcome areas: (1) cerebral palsy and other neurologic and sensory morbidities; and (2) developmental delays, cognitive impairments, and behavior disorders, including autism. A case report is provided for each of the four age categories to illustrate some of the challenges encountered in evaluating the neurodevelopmental outcomes of ELBW graduates of the NICU.

Outcome: Cerebral Palsy and Other Neurologic or Sensory Sequelae

An outcome of major concern for both pediatricians and parents of ELBW infants is cerebral palsy (CP). ELBW infants are at significant risk for brain injury secondary

17

to the effects of hypoxia-ischemia, inflammatory disorders including sepsis, necrotizing enterocolitis, and meningitis, and undernutrition superimposed on a vulnerable immature brain.[23-25] Radiographic evidence of brain injury—intraventricular hemorrhage (IVH),[26,27] periventricular leukomalacia (PVL),[23] and ventriculomegaly[28]—is associated with adverse neurodevelopmental outcomes, including CP. The strongest predictor of CP is periventricular leukomalacia.[29] Neonatologists use this radiographic information to provide feedback to families on the relative risk of neurodevelopmental sequelae. The sensitivity and specificity of abnormal cranial ultrasound findings, however, remain weak, and Laptook and associates[7] reported that the rate of CP among infants weighing1000 g at birth with normal cranial ultrasound findings was 9.4%. The ability to accurately predict outcome is complicated by the fact that other morbidities[7] and interventions[1,30-33] may be associated positively or negatively with neurodevelopmental sequelae. Two perinatal interventions (antenatal steroids[1] and prophylactic indomethacin[30,31]) are associated with a decreased risk of IVH. Postnatal steroid administration, which may increase the risk of CP,[32] is used therapeutically to wean premature infants with chronic lung disease from assisted ventilation. Laptook and associates[7] identified that within a cohort of ELBW infants with normal head ultrasound findings, male gender and multiple birth were independently associated with CP. Cerebral palsy, unfortunately, remains a major neurologic sequela among ELBW survivors, affecting 9% to 17% of survivors.[34-37] Prompt diagnosis of the infant with CP to ensure appropriate intervention services and supports for the child and family is paramount. There are, however, some challenges associated with recognizing the clinical signs, particularly if the disorder is mild or there are mixed findings.

An early definition of CP was published by Bax[38] in 1964. He described CP as "a disorder of movement and posture due to a defect or lesion of the immature brain." The definition used by the National Institute of Child Health and Human Development (NICHD) Network[13] at 18 to 22 months corrected age (CA) has the following three components: (1) abnormalities of tone, reflexes, coordination, and movement; (2) delay in motor milestones; and (3) aberrations in primitive reflexes (retention > 6 months) or failure of postural reflexes to emerge for more than 6 months. The traditional CP diagnosis is based on findings of abnormal tone and posture and is classified by the number of limbs involved (4 = quadriplegia, 3 = triplegia, 2 legs = diplegia, right or left arm and leg = hemiplegia, and 1 extremity = monoplegia). The classification of CP based on topology has been linked to ultimate motor prognosis.[13] Children with hemiplegia and diplegia are able to eventually attain functional mobility, whereas those with triplegia and quadriplegia often struggle with motor performance. Another classification of CP is based specifically on the tone and reflexes and has the following categories: spastic ($\uparrow$ tone and $\uparrow$ reflexes), choreoathetotic ($\pm\uparrow$ tone and $\uparrow$ reflexes), dystonic ($\pm\uparrow$ tone and stiff movements), ataxic ($\uparrow$ tone and ataxia), and mixed CP.[36] Fortunately for physicians there is a mixed category because many children's features do not fit nicely into a specific category.[39] Severity of CP may be classified as follows: (1) mild (impairment interferes with but does not prevent age-appropriate function; includes nonfluent walking), moderate (walks with assistive device or does not walk, sits independently or with support), or severe (no ambulation, no sitting, and no supported sitting)[37]; (2) nondisabling versus disabling[35]; and (3) by gross motor performance.[39,40] A Gross Motor Functional Classification System (GMFCS)[40] has been developed to systematically evaluate functional skills in prone, rolling, sitting, crawling, standing, walking, jumping, and running.[39,40] Wood and Rosenbaum[39] have shown that the GMFCS has stability over time in children with CP.

The 18- to 24-Month-Old Child

Cerebral Palsy

The majority of neurodevelopmental follow-up studies in multicenter networks evaluate infants to 18 or 24 months CA. Current understanding is that a definitive diagnosis of CP can be made at these ages in most children; an exception may be those with very mild CP. This discussion tries to analyze some of the issues that arise when one is making the diagnosis.

Drillien[41] published a classic study in 1972 of 300 infants weighing less than 1250 g at birth. She described early neurologic signs that she called "transient dystonia." There were four categories of neurologic signs: (1) irritability, increased crying, feeding difficulty; (2) jittery, easily startled; (3) increased tone, fisting, arching; and (4) standing on toes. Infants were categorized in the first year of life as having mild (one or two signs < 2 months), moderate (>two signs > 2 months), and severe (>two signs at 4 to 8 months) findings. She demonstrated that the percentage of infants with moderate to severe signs decreased with increasing age, from 46% at 2 months and 18% at 8 months to 6% at 12 months. Those infants with persistent severe findings were likely to go on to have CP; those who lost the findings were likely to not have CP. The transient presence of abnormal neurologic findings in ELBW infants in the first year of life has been observed by others.[42] Neurologic findings in ELBW infants in the first 6 to 12 months may indicate a need for early intervention services, but unless suspect or abnormal findings persist, they lack specificity relative to long-term outcome.

Other phenomena in the first year of life that aid in making the diagnosis include the fading of primitive reflexes and the emergence of postural reflexes in infants developing normally. In addition, the normality or abnormality of muscle tone often has not fully declared itself until 18 to 24 months of age because myelination continues during this time. *For these reasons, follow-up studies reported at 12 months of age or earlier do not provide reliable CP data.* Even at older ages, making a definitive diagnosis for children with mild CP may be challenging. Paneth and colleagues[43] demonstrated that pediatrician reliability in discriminating disabling CP from nondisabling CP and from no CP was weak but improved significantly when assessment of gross motor functional skills was added to the traditional neurologic examination. Therefore, for optimal clinical management and to ensure that accurate diagnoses and appropriate interventions are in place, serial comprehensive assessments of both neurologic signs and motor skills by trained observers are indicated for ELBW infants.

In a NICHD Network study of ELBW infants born from 1995 to 1998, CP was identified in 12.3% and other abnormal neurologic findings in 10.3% of ELBW infant survivors at 18 to 22 months CA. Other neurologic findings included hypertonia, hypotonia, seizure disorder, monoplegia, dyspraxia, and dystonia without a specific diagnosis of CP. The study demonstrated that ELBW children with CP are at increased risk of having other neurosensory morbidities, and children with quadriplegia are at greatest risk compared with children with other types of CP or no CP. For the 53 children with quadriplegia, 9.8% had seizures, 18.9% had shunts for hydrocephalus, 21.6% had severe visual impairment (i.e., legal blindness or vision worse than 20/200 in one or both eyes), 9.8% had severe hearing impairment (i.e., deafness or hearing loss requiring amplification in both ears), and 97.9% had a Bayley II Mental Developmental Index less than 70.

The assessment used by the NICHD Neonatal Research Network at 18 to 22 months CA consists of an interim medical history, updated social, demographic, and health data, neurologic assessment, assessment with the Gross Motor Classification System,[44] and a developmental assessment with the Bayley II Scales of Infant Development.[45] The neurologic examination at 18 to 22 months is based on the assessment of Amiel-Tison[46] and is performed by certified developmentalists who have been trained to reliability.

Visual Assessment

Assessment of vision for ELBW infants begins in the NICU with standard assessments by an ophthalmologist skilled in evaluating and treating infants with retinopathy of prematurity, and continues postdischarge. During follow-up visits, vision status information is obtained from parent history and ophthalmologist reports of postdischarge eye examinations, and a standard pediatric eye examination is

17

performed to evaluate the presence of strabismus, nystagmus, light reflex, tracking ability, and roving or disconjugate eye movements. Rates of vision impairment (glasses, strabismus, nystagmus) in ELBW infants at NICHD centers admitted to NICUs in 1993 to 1994 ranged from 9% to 20%, those of unilateral blindness ranged from none to 2%, and those of bilateral blindness ranged from none to 5%.[9]

Hearing Assessment

Currently, as regards assessment of hearing, close to 100% of neonates in NICUs in the United States are screened for hearing loss prior to discharge. It is recommended that NICU infants be screened with automated auditory brainstem responses (AABRs) or AABRs in combination with otoacoustic emissions (OAEs) so that no type of sensorineural hearing loss, including auditory dyssynchrony,[47] is missed. The current recommendation is that infants screened in the NICU have a diagnostic evaluation by an audiologist by 3 months of age and participate in appropriate early intervention services by 6 months of age.[48] Because some NICU infants may be missed because of multiple hospital transfers or illness severity and some infants who pass newborn hearing screening later demonstrate delayed-onset permanent hearing loss, follow-up of all very LBW (VLBW) infants by an audiologist skilled in assessing and treating infants and young children is indicated. Infants with in utero infections such as cytomegalovirus, herpes, rubella, syphilis, and toxoplasmosis are at increased risk of delayed-onset permanent hearing loss.[49-52] It has been demonstrated that infants with a permanent hearing loss who receive intervention services prior to 6 months of age have significantly better language outcomes than infants diagnosed after 6 months,[53,54] so hearing status should be confirmed as soon as possible after discharge. Rates of any hearing impairment, including conductive or unilateral, for ELBW infants at NICHD centers for infants born from 1993 to 1994 ranged from none to 28%, and rates of hearing impairment requiring bilateral amplification ranged from none to 9% at 18 to 22 months CA.[9]

Early Developmental Assessments

Traditional early developmental assessments divide skills into mental (precursor of cognitive) and motor (gross motor and fine motor) domains. Although major cognitive deficits can be detected in early infancy, more common subtle cognitive deficits and learning difficulties are difficult to detect. In addition, some infants fail to progress, deteriorate in level of function, or recover with increasing age.[55]

Between birth and 24 to 30 months most investigators use corrected age to evaluate development and interpret test scores. Corrected age is the sum of chronologic age in weeks minus the difference between gestational age at birth and 40 weeks of gestation. Although the duration of correction may be controversial, this correction is generally accepted until 30 months of age.[22,56,57]

Bayley Scales of Infant Development II

Most studies in the USA previously used the Bayley Scales of Infant Development II (BSID-II),[45] which includes a Mental Developmental Index (MDI), a Psychomotor Developmental Index (PDI), and a Behavior Rating Scale (BRS) to assess developmental outcomes of high-risk infants in the first 3 years of life. Within the NICHD Neonatal Network the Bayley tests are administered by certified examiners trained to reliability by gold standard examiners. Bayley scores of 100 ± 15 represent the mean ± standard deviation of population of normal infants born at term. A score lower than 70 (2 standard deviations below the mean) is used as evidence of significant developmental delay. An infant is classified as having neurodevelopmental impairment (NDI) if any of the following is present: moderate to severe CP, MDI or PDI lower than70, blindness in both eyes, or hearing impairment requiring bilateral amplification. The BSID-II has been limited by having two primary scores, the MDI and PDI. Therefore, it is unable to differentiate gross motor from fine motor delays and cognitive from language delays.

Data from the NICHD Neonatal Network on large cohorts indicate that there is significant evidence of subnormal cognitive performance among ELBW infants at

18 to 22 months CA. In the NICHD multicenter study of neurodevelopmental outcome, the center rate for a Bayley II MDI lower than 70 ranged from a low of 17% to a high of 62% for infants born weighing less than 1000 g.[9] In 2006 the new BSID-III,[58] which has five domains—receptive language, expressive language, fine motor, gross motor, and cognitive—was published, and most investigators have transitioned to the Bayley III. Mean scores have tended to be higher on the Bayley III than on the Bayley II.

CASE HISTORY 1

A 33-year-old G1P2 (gravida 1, pregnancies 2) with an in vitro fertilization (IVF) pregnancy delivered twin A (520 g) and twin B (630 g) at 23⅗ weeks. Although twin A had a milder neonatal course than twin B, he had severe bronchopulmonary dysplasia (BPD) and was discharged on oxygen. At discharge, he had evidence of ventriculomegaly and increased tone. At the first follow-up visit at 28 days CA, he was reported to have good focus, brief tracking, increased tone, jerky movements, and reflux. At 6 months 28 days CA, the Bayley MDI was 81 and the PDI was 65 (significant delay). Twin B's tone subsequently gradually improved, and by 9 months CA the neurologic findings were considered normal. By 19 months CA he had normal vision and hearing as well as normal neurologic findings, was walking and running, with good fine motor skills, and speech delay. The Bayley MDI, however, was 57 and the PDI was 74. He had received early intervention since hospital discharge and was referred at 19 months CA for speech therapy. His head growth is of interest. He was the smaller of the twins, with an initial head circumference at the 10th percentile. Head growth recovered and by 9 months 14 days CA, his head circumference was at the 50th percentile. Catch-up of head circumference in the first year of life has been shown to be associated with developmental recovery and higher IQ.[59,60] Recall that he had ventriculomegaly and an abnormal neurologic findings at discharge, which have been shown to be associated with abnormal neurologic outcome.[28] Although twin A does not have CP, he has significant cognitive and motor delay at 19 months CA. (For further details see summary in Table 17-1.)

The neonatal course for twin B was more severe with bilateral IVHs (grade 4 on the left and grade 2 on the right), seizures, and posthemorrhagic hydrocephalus requiring repeated ventricular taps by neurosurgery. Although the hydrocephalus resolved prior to discharge, he also had severe bronchopulmonary dysplasia requiring oxygen at discharge, and retinopathy of prematurity (ROP) with plus disease, which was treated with laser therapy. At discharge, twin B was reported to have seizures, tremors, increased tone, and questionable vision. At the first visit to follow-up at 1 month 27 days CA, he was noted to have motor asymmetry, torticollis, only brief tracking, increased tone, jerky movements, and seizures. This combination of multiple abnormal findings was very worrisome. At a visit at 4 month 26 days, the head circumference had dropped to the 15th percentile. By 6 months 28 days CA, tone in all four extremities was severely spastic, the Bayley MDI and PDI were both 49, and he had limited responses to visual or auditory stimuli. A diagnosis of spastic quadriplegia was made. Over the next few months he had limited head growth and by 11 months 18 days CA, his head circumference had fallen below the 3rd percentile. His weight gain was also dropping because of poor feeding and a gastric tube was recommended to facilitate feeds. His parents finally agreed and he underwent surgery prior to his 19 month 4 day CA visit. At that visit he was noted to have significantly increased tone in all four extremities with poor movement control. His diagnosis was severe spastic quadriplegia with dystonic movements, seizure disorder, and retardation.

17

Table 17-1 TWO-YEAR FOLLOW-UP OF EXTREMELY LOW-BIRTH-WEIGHT TWINS WITH
AND WITHOUT INTRAVENTRICULAR HEMORRHAGE

Mother: 31 years G1P2; IVF; married; 12th grade education		
	Medical and Neurologic Findings	
Age/Event	Twin A	Twin B
23$\frac{5}{7}$ wk gestation Discharge	520 g, no IVH, right ventriculomegaly, BPD $\uparrow$ extensor tone, O^2, hospitalized 111 days	630 g, IVH 4 Lt, IVH 2 Rt, $\uparrow$ posthemorrhagic hydrocephalus, tapped by neurosurgery, resolved, seizures, phenobarbital, retinopathy of prematurity with plus disease, Rx laser, tremors, $\uparrow$ tone, O$_2$, feeding problems, Zantac 117 days
Chronologic 4m 14d Corrected 28d	Suspect neurologic findings, good focus, brief tracking, $\uparrow$ tone, jerky movements, reflux, on O^2, EI, HC 10th %	Suspect neurologic findings, brief tracking, $\uparrow$ tone, jerky movements, seizures, phenobarbital, feeding problems, Zantac, on O$_2$, EI, HC 25th %
Chronologic 5m 18d Corrected 1m 27d	Suspect neurologic findings, tracks 180°, $\uparrow$ tone, jerky movements, on O^2, EI, HC 10th %	Suspect neurologic findings, torticollis Rt, eyes Rt, brief tracking, $\uparrow$ tone, jerky movements, seizures, phenobarbital, Zantac, on O$_2$, EI, HC 30th %
Chronologic 7m 7d Corrected 3m 16d	Suspect neurologic findings, tracks 180°, $\uparrow$ tone, on O^2, EI, HC 30th %	Suspect neurologic findings, poor tracking, $\uparrow$ tone uppers and lowers, jerky movements, feeding problems, seizures, phenobarbital, on O$_2$, EI, HC 40th %
Chronologic 8m 17d Corrected 4m 26d	Suspect neurologic findings, tracks 180°, mild $\uparrow$ tone, on O^2, EI, HC 30th %	Suspect neurologic findings, random eye movements, $\uparrow$ tone uppers and lowers, jerky movements, feeding problems, seizures, phenobarbital, on O^2, EI, HC 15th %
Chronologic 10m 19d Corrected 6m 28d	Suspect neurologic findings, tracks 180°, varying tone in legs, on O^2, EI, HC 30th % Bayley MDI 81, Bayley PDI 65	Abnormal neurologic findings, roving eye movements, $\uparrow$ tone uppers and lowers, jerky movements, seizures, phenobarbital, on O$_2$, EI Dx: spastic quadriplegia, MDI 49, PDI 49, HC 20th %
Chronologic 13m 5d Corrected 9m 14d	Normal neurologic findings, tracks 180°, O$_2$ at night only, EI, HC 50th %	Abnormal neurologic findings, poor tracking, $\uparrow$ tone, spastic quadriplegia, dyskinetic, movements, seizures, phenobarbital on O$_2$, EI, HC 10th %
Chronologic 15m 9d Corrected 11m 18d	Normal neurologic findings, tracks 180°, off oxygen, EI, HC 50th %, cruising	Abnormal neurologic findings, poor tracking, $\uparrow$ tone, spastic quadriplegia, jerky, dyskinetic movements, daily seizures/phenobarbital and Topomax, seizures, O$_2$ on standby, EI, PediaSure, wt and HC < 3rd %
Chronologic 16m 16d Corrected 13m 5d	Not seen	Abnormal neurologic findings, poor tracking, $\uparrow$ tone, spastic quadriplegia, dyskinetic movements, seizures, phenobarbital and Topomax, no O$_2$, EI, PediaSure, wt and HC < 3rd %
Chronologic 22m 25d Corrected 19m 4d	Normal neurologic findings, tracks 180°, walking, good pincer, good fine motor skills, not running, "Mama, Dada, baby," EI, HC 55th %, wt 3rd %, Bayley MDI 57, Bayley PDI 74, speech therapy recommended	Abnormal neurologic findings, poor tracking, smiles and laughs, nystagmus, esoptropia, seizures/ Phenobarbital and Zanagram, $\uparrow$ tone, spastic quadriplegia, dyskinetic movements, seizure disorder, EI, PT, OT, gastric tube feeds begun, PediaSure, wt and HC < 3rd %

EI, Early intervention; *HC*, head circumference; *Lt*, left; *MDI*, Mental Developmental Index; *OT*, occupational therapy; *PDI*, Psychomotor Developmental Index; *PT*, physical therapy; *Rt*, right; *wt*, weight; $\uparrow$, increased.

The twins were chosen for the 18- to 24-month presentation in this chapter for three reasons. The first was to illustrate some of the early neurologic findings seen in ELBW infants. Second, this is a twin set in which one has grade 4 IVH and the other has ventriculomegaly but no IVH, so their neurodevelopmental progress can be compared over time. Third, the twins had 9 to 10 assessments completed by 19 months CA so that the changes in neurologic and developmental status with increasing age were available.

Important Lessons for Diagnosis and Intervention

1. Monitoring head growth is an important component of the neurologic examination.
2. Persistence of multiple abnormal neurologic signs in the first 12 to 18 months is ominous.
3. Emergence of other findings (vision impairments, seizures, feeding issues) is associated with poor outcome.
4. Serial assessments are needed to ensure that appropriate interventions are in place.
5. Loss of abnormal neurologic findings in the first 12 months is associated with better neurologic outcome.

The 3- to 6-Year-Old Child

A conventional neurologic assessment[46] can be administered in conjunction with gross motor classification system at 3 to 6 years of age. By $3\frac{1}{2}$ years of age, intelligence and preacademic skills can be assessed, and CA is no longer used. By age 6 years (first grade), a variety of tests can be used to evaluate cognition, attention, and achievement.[22] Assessment may include the Beery Test of Vision Motor Integration,[61] an intelligence test such as the Wechsler Intelligence Scale for Children, 4th edition (WISC IV),[62] or Stanford-Binet Intelligence Scales,[63] and a receptive vocabulary test such as the Peabody Picture Vocabulary Test.[64] The assessment of behavior may include the Child Behavior Checklist[65] or the Connors Parent Rating Scales,[66] which are both parent interviews. A further assessment of functional domains can be obtained with the WeeFIM,[67] Vineland Adaptive Behavior Scales,[68] or Pediatric Evaluation of Disability Inventory (PEDI).[69] There are fewer outcome studies of ELBW infants evaluated at 3 of 6 years of age than at 18 to 24 months. Ment and associates[70] reported on a cohort of 337 preterm infants seen at $4\frac{1}{2}$ years of age as part of the follow-up of the Indomethacin Trial. Children who had received indomethacin had better outcomes than children who received saline; the rate of IQ less than 70 was 12% versus 17%, respectively.[70] Peterson and colleagues[60] reported on 128 VLBW children who underwent a comprehensive neuropsychological academic and behavioral assessment at 6.8 years of life. They reported that subnormal head circumference was significantly associated with lower IQ and poorer perceptual motor skills, academic achievement, and adaptive behavior. In addition, the VLBW cohort had significantly more cognitive and academic difficulties than term controls.

CASE HISTORY 2

This age of evaluation was chosen because it is the critical age of school entry, and success or failure in school for ex-ELBW infants may depend on the provision of appropriate support services as part of an Individualized Education Program (IEP). Baby B was born to a 37-year-old G4P4 married mother with a graduate degree and private health insurance. Delivery was at $24\frac{3}{7}$ weeks. Birth weight was 655 g, and complications included cardiomyopathy, bilateral pneumothoraces, seizures, bilateral grade 4 IVH, multiple ventricular taps to relieve pressure, and retinopathy of prematurity, which stabilized.

17

The discharge examination reported at 120 days was consistent with normal tone, good suck, and positive grasp, and the hydrocephalus was considered stable. After discharge, progressive hydrocephalus developed, however, and a shunt was placed on the right 2 months after discharge.

At 3 months CA, the baby presented with reflux, which was treated with ranitidine (Zantac). He was tracking to 180°, had slight head lag and increased tone, and when prone elevated to 90°. The shunt was functioning well and head circumference was at the 85th percentile. At 7 months CA, he still had increased tone in the lower extremities, slight head lag, some arching, but good grasp and release of the hands, and was cooing. Head circumference was at the 75th percentile. The Bayley MDI was 83 and PDI was 62. At 18 months CA the neurologic findings were consistent with mild spastic diplegia. He had increased tone, greater in the lower extremities, tight heel cords, and limited supination of the forearms. He had good sitting balance and could pull to stand but was not yet cruising. Head circumference was at the 95th percentile, and the shunt was functioning well. Bayley MDI was 95 and PDI less than 50 (significant delay). In this child's situation, we were confident with the diagnosis of classic spastic diplegia at 18 months CA. At 33 months, he presented with some additional findings. He had had two seizures since the last visit, and the neurologist's decision had been not to treat with anticonvulsants. He also had been diagnosed with farsightedness and was wearing glasses. He was now walking, wore bilateral ankle-foot orthoses (AFOs), had received two Botox injections, had an IEP, and was getting occupational therapy (OT) and physical therapy (PT). His head circumference was at the 98th percentile and the shunt was functioning fine. His test scores were as follows: Bayley MDI, 82; PDI, 70; Peabody Picture Vocabulary Test[64] 24th percentile; and Beery Vision Motor Index (VMI)[71] 4th percentile. The findings at 33 months demonstrate that additional neurosensory findings can manifest or be diagnosed at older ages than 18 months and that recovery of Bayley motor scores can occur between 18 and 33 months CA. This motor recovery is probably in part a response to the Botox injections, use of AFOs, and ongoing physical therapy and occupational therapy. His Peabody vocabulary score, however, is low. Language delays are frequent among ELBW infants and may still be evident at 33 to 36 months CA, despite early intervention. The low Beery VMI could reflect impaired fine motor function, but in a child with hydrocephalus this may represent a vision perception–motor integration problem. At 5 years 3 months CA he presented as a social and charming boy who walked independently with AFOs but had some minor problems with balance. His seizure disorder was now being treated with Tegretol, he was getting Botox injections every 8 months, he wore corrective lenses, and he continued to have findings consistent with a mild diplegia. He had an IEP and had been placed in an integrated kindergarten with children with and without disabilities. All of his test scores had improved since his last visit. His Wechsler Preschool and Primary Scale of Intelligence (WPPSI) IQ was 98, Peabody receptive vocabulary was at the 63rd percentile, Beery VMI was at the 16th percentile, and his mother's responses to the Child Behavior Checklist and the Connors Parent Rating Scales suggested no behavior problems. This is a wonderful example of excellent recovery of a child with bilateral grade 4 IVH. Why he is doing so well and twin A from the previous case history, with unilateral grade 4, is not doing well is not completely clear. Both boys reside in stable home environments and have received multiple support services. This difference points to the relatively poor predictive validity of neonatal cranial ultrasound. (This case is further summarized in Table 17-2.)

Table 17-2 FIVE-YEAR FOLLOW-UP OF EXTREMELY LOW-BIRTH-WEIGHT
INFANT: AN EXAMPLE OF RECOVERY OVER TIME

Mother: 36 years G4P4; married; graduate degrees; private insurance	
Age/Event	Medical and Neurologic Findings, Test Scores
24 3/7 wk gestation	655 g, BPD, cardiomyopathy, bilateral pneumothoraces, seizures, bilateral grade 4 IVH, multiple ventricular taps, ROP
Discharge	Normal tone, positive suck, positive grasp, hydrocephalus considered stable, hospitalized 120d
2m post discharge	Shunt placed for progressive hydrocephalus
CA 6m 18d CorA 3m 0d	Suspect neurologic findings, tracks 180°, EI, ↑ tone, slight head lag, prone 90°, HC 85th %, shunt functioning on right, reflux, on Zantac
CA 10m 21d CorA 7m 4d	Suspect neurologic findings, tracks 180°, shunt, ↑ tone lowers, slight head lag, likes to push back, some arching, prone 90°, good grasp and release, cooing, EI, PT, OT HC 75th %, Bayley MDI 83, Bayley PDI < 62
CA 21m 23d CorA 18m 5d	Abnormal neurologic findings, tracks 180°, ↑ tone lowers, mild uppers, limited supination of forearms, knee jerks 3+, ± Babinskis tight ankles, sits, pulls to stand; diagnosis: spastic diplegia, eating well, has asthma, eight episodes of otitis media, EI, PT, OT HC 95th %, Bayley MDI 95, Bayley PDI < 50
CA 36m 29d CorA 33m 11d	History of two seizures since last visit, not started on medication. Abnormal neurologic findings, consistent with mild spastic diplegia, has AFOs, getting Botox injections × 2, wears glasses for farsightedness, charming boy now walking, tracks 180°, has IEP and is getting OT and PT HC 98th %, Bayley MDI 82, Bayley PDI < 70, Peabody receptive vocabulary 24th %, Beery VMI 4th %
CA 5y 3m	Seizure disorder now treated with Tegretol, getting Botox q8m, tone in uppers appears normal, mild ↑ tone in lowers, ↓ balance but can walk independently, glasses, AFOs, IEP, and integrated kindergarten WPPSI IQ 98, Peabody receptive vocabulary 63rd %, Beery VMI 16th %, Child Behavior Checklist and Connors Parent Rating Scales within normal limits, HC 98th %

AFOs, Ankle-foot orthoses; *Beery VMI,* Beery Visual-Motor Integration (score); *CA,* chronologic age; *CorA,* correct age; *EI,* early intervention; *HC,* head circumference; *IEP,* Individualized Education Program; *MDI,* Mental Developmental Index; *OT,* occupational therapy; *PDI,* Psychomotor developmental index; *PT,* physical therapy; *WPPSI,* Wechsler Preschool and Primary Scale of Intelligence; ↑, increased.

Important Lessons for Diagnosis and Intervention

1. The outcome of infants with grade 4 IVH is not always ominous.
2. Persistent posthemorrhagic hydrocephalus may require shunting after discharge.
3. Recovery of Bayley cognitive and motor scores may continue during the first 5 years.
4. Follow-up outcomes at 5 to 6 years may provide a more stable quality indicator reflective of NICU care than 18- to 24-month outcomes.
5. Seizure disorders and sensory deficits may manifest late.
6. There can be a disconnect between motor impairments and cognitive impairments.

7. Diagnostic magnetic resonance imaging (MRI) prior to discharge may provide better neurologic prognostic information than cranial head ultrasound.
8. Provision of comprehensive support, therapeutic, and educational services is associated with recovery.

The School Age Child

By age 8 (third grade), intelligence, neuropsychological function, school performance, behavior problems, memory skills, sensorimotor function, language, functional skills, and learning disabilities can be identified.[22] A conventional neurologic assessment is administered.[46] Studies to school age have shown that preterm children have increased rates of clinically significant attention, thought, and social problems, anxiety, depression, withdrawn personality, and hyperactivity than term controls.[18,72-75] In addition, data suggest they are at increased risk of autism spectrum disorder (ASD). Limperopoulos and coworkers[76] reported that 25% of VLBW infants screen positive on the Modified Checklist for Autism in Toddlers (M-CHAT). The extremely low-gestational-age newborns (ELGAN) Study (<28 weeks) reported a 21% screen positive rate on the M-CHAT; the rate was 16% after exclusion of children with major neurosensory impairments; and 10% after exclusion of children with cognitive impairment.[77,78] One study of extremely preterm children with diagnostic confirmation reported that although 16% screened positive for ASD, 8% were diagnosed with ASD at 11 years.[79] Currently the American Academy of Pediatrics policy recommends screening of all children for ASD at 18 months and referral for ASD assessment for all those with positive screen results. Follow-up programs for high-risk infants should all be screening for ASD.

A number of studies have reported that approximately 50% of VLBW children require educational resources at school age. Vohr and associates[12] performed assessments at 8 years of age on ex-VLBW (600 to 1250 g) infants who participated in the longitudinal follow-up of the Indomethacin Trial. Within this cohort, rates of educational resource needs for children without IVH were 48%. However, rates for children with IVH ranged from 62% to 79%. The children with IVH also had significantly greater requirements for the number of individual resources needed, a self-contained classroom, and speech/language therapy. Within this cohort of VLBW children evaluated at 3, 4½, 6, and 8 years of age, significant improvement in cognitive and language test scores was observed between 3 and 8 years. Improvements in test scores were associated with higher maternal education, two-parent household, and early intervention services if the mother had less than a 12th grade education. Hack and colleagues[80] also reported that rates of impairment, defined as MDI or Kaufman Assessment Battery for Children (KABC) Mental Process Composite (MPC) score less than70 dropped from 39% at 20 months CA to 16% at 8 years for ELBW infants. A report by Luu and coworkers[81] demonstrated that preterm children continued to display catch-up gains on the Peabody Picture Vocabulary Test-Revised between 3 and 12 years of age. The average standardized score for preterms was 84.1 at 3 years and gained 1.2 points per year to 12 years.[81]

CASE HISTORY 3

Case report at school age. Table 17-3 shows the neurodevelopmental findings over 12 years for a boy born at 27 weeks of gestation who had normal cranial ultrasound findings during hospitalization. At 3 months CA he was noted to have increased tone, tremors, and jerky movements. Findings continued to be abnormal, and by 12 months CA a diagnosis of spastic diplegia was made. Note that between 6 and 12 months CA that developmental scores dropped and the Bayley MDI and PDI were both lower than 49 and remained lower than 49 at 18 months CA. Subsequently, steady improvement on cognitive skills can be observed, so that by 12 years his verbal IQ was 123, performance IQ was 106, and full-scale IQ was 116. He had exceptional vocabulary skills. His diagnosis remained spastic diplegia requiring multiple therapeutic and educational support services. He was, however, reported to have difficulty socializing with peers, and a provisional diagnosis of autism spectrum disorder was made.

17

Table 17-3 EIGHT-YEAR FOLLOW-UP OF INFANT WITH NORMAL CRANIAL ULTRASOUND FINDINGS

Mother: 30 years G2P3; married; partial college; private insurance		
Age/Event	**Medical and Neurologic Findings**	**Test Scores**
27 wk gestation	1040 g, RDS, PDA, bowel perforation, normal cranial ultrasound	
Discharge	Hospitalized 111 days, neurologic findings not reported	
3m CA	Suspect neurologic findings, tracks 180°, EI, ↑ tone, tremors, jerky movements	
6m CA	Suspect neurologic findings, tracks 180°, ↑ tone lowers, HC 60th %	Bayley MDI 63, Bayley PDI 73
12m CA	Abnormal neurologic findings, tracks 180°, ↑ tone lowers, mild uppers, limited supination of forearms, knee jerks 3+, ± Babinskis tight ankles, sits, pulls to stand; diagnosis: spastic diplegia, EI, PT, OT, HC 95th %	Bayley MDI 49, Bayley PDI < 49
18m	History of two seizures since last visit not placed on medication. Abnormal neurologic findings, consistent with mild spastic diplegia; has AFOs	Bayley MDI 49, Bayley PDI < 49
3y CA	q8m, tone in uppers appears normal, mild ↑ tone in lowers, ↓ balance but can walks with walker, ataxic, poor balance, poor fine motor skills, AFOs, IEP, Special Ed placement, HC 60th %, PT, OT	Peabody 2y 10m Beery VMI—unable to do Stanford Binet Intelligence Scale 83
4½y	Abnormal, CP, AFOs, walker, IEP, Special Ed placement, PT, OT	Peabody 4y 2m
6y 2m	Abnormal, CP, AFOs, walker IEP, Special Ed placement, PT, OT	Performance IQ 87 Beery VMI 5y 10m Verbal IQ 92 Full-scale IQ 89
8y	Abnormal, CP, AFOs, IEP, walker, Special Ed resources, PT, OT	Performance IQ 115 Verbal IQ 119 Full-scale IQ 119
12y	Abnormal, CP, AFOs, IEP, walker, Special Ed services Difficulties socializing, PT, OT	Verbal IQ 123 Performance IQ 106 Full-scale IQ 116 Peabody 33y 8m

AFOs, Ankle-foot orthoses; *Beery VMI,* Test of Vision Motor Integration (score); *CA,* chronologic age; *CP,* cerebral palsy; *EI,* early intervention; *HC,* head circumference; *IEP,* Individualized Education Program; *MDI,* Mental Developmental Index; *OT,* occupational therapy; *PDI,* Psychomotor Developmental Index; *Peabody,* Peabody Picture Vocabulary Test score; *PT,* physical therapy; ↑, increased; ↓, decreased.

Important Lessons for Diagnosis and Intervention

This child's history illustrates a number of important points:

1. Infants with normal neonatal cranial ultrasound findings can go on to have CP and have evidence of early and persistent motor delay.
2. Cognitive skills may improve with increasing age for children in a favorable home environment who receive comprehensive intervention and education support services. There was steady improvement in scores for this boy between 18 months and 12 years of age.
3. Despite a high IQ and excellent verbal skills at 12 years of age, he continued to need a number of resources within the school system, including occupational therapy and physical therapy.
4. At school age, ELBW children have a higher incidence of behavior problems requiring screening, diagnosis, intervention, and support.

The Adolescent and Young Adult

Adolescent outcome studies indicate that former ELBW infants are at increased risk for neurologic abnormalities, sensory impairments, lower IQs, motor impairments, and poor academic performance.[82-86]

As adolescents, ELBW children also have higher rates of health problems, especially asthma,[3,87,88] and they have also been shown to have a higher incidence of behavioral problems and psychopathology.[21] Saigal and coworkers[89] have investigated preferences of adolescents compared with professionals and parents relative to their health outcomes. They found that despite the higher rates of morbidities, both adolescents and their parents rated health-related quality of life higher than health care professionals. Although very preterm adolescents continue to display deficits in general cognition and higher level language skills in comparison with their term peers, significant catch-up in receptive vocabulary has been reported by 16 years of age.[26]

Outcome studies of VLBW infants as young adults are rare. These studies are extremely difficult to accomplish because of long-term tracking and the associated costs. Hack and colleagues[19] compared outcomes for VLBW infants at 20 years of age with those of term controls. VLBW adults were less likely to have graduated from high school or to be enrolled in a secondary school, and they had lower IQs, had more sensory impairments, and were shorter in stature. The findings of Saigal and coworkers[90] in a population of ELBW infants followed to young adulthood (22 to 25 years) in Canada were more favorable. These investigators found no significant differences between ELBW adults and controls in education or employment status. This better outcome may be related to the generally higher socioeconomic status of the Canadian population.

Important Lessons for Diagnosis and Intervention

The combination of optimal antenatal and neonatal care, a benign course in the NICU, an optimal home environment, and appropriate interventions can result in very good long-term outcomes for VLBW infants.

CASE HISTORY 4

Case report of young adult. The final case report presented in Table 17-4 is of a VLBW (1300 g) infant with a relatively benign course in the NICU, including normal cranial ultrasound findings. Her parents were married and college-educated, and had private insurance. She consistently did well during follow-up assessments on neurologic, developmental, and cognitive testing from 6 weeks to 6 years 11 months of age. At age 29 she did a medical school rotation in the NICU in which she was a VLBW patient, and later as a pediatric resident and fellow in pediatric neurology.

Table 17-4 ADULT OUTCOME OF VERY LOW-BIRTH-WEIGHT INFANT

Mother: 29 years G1P1; married; college; private insurance		
Age/Event	Medical and Neurologic Findings	Test Scores
31 wk gestation	1300 g, female, RDS, hyperbilirubinemia, apnea, feeding problems, normal cranial ultrasound	
Discharge	Hospitalized 45 days, neurologic findings normal	
6 wk CA	Normal neurologic findings, tracks 180°, minimal head lag, overall normal, HC <3rd %	
3m CA	Normal neurologic findings, tracks 180°, HC 25th %	
9m 21d CA	Normal neurologic findings, HC 45th %	Bayley MDI 11.7 m Bayley PDI 9.4 m
21.5m CA	Normal neurologic findings, HC 45th %	Bayley MDI 22.5 Bayley PDI 22.5
3y CA	Normal neurologic findings, HC 50th %	Stanford Binet IQ 132
6y 11m	Normal neurologic findings, HC 50th %	Stanford Binet IQ 111 Riley Motor Skills normal
29y	Presents in the WIH neonatal intensive care unit as a senior medical student. Calls to say she was in a follow-up study as an infant	
30y	Resident in pediatrics	Excellent outcome

CA, Chronologic age; *HC,* Head circumference; *MDI,* Mental Developmental Index; *PDI,* Psychomotor Developmental Index.

Gaps in Knowledge

1. Refinement of a systematic, easy-to-administer neurologic assessment in the first year of life to achieve better predictive validity
2. Identification of the specific environmental factors associated with recovery. We know that higher maternal education is an important predictor
3. Identification of genetic factors associated with recovery
4. Further investigation of postnatal interventions (massage, human milk, probiotics, thyroxine) associated with good outcomes and recovery
5. Further development and ease of obtaining magnetic resonance imaging prior to NICU discharge in an effort to identify focused interventions
6. Adolescent and adult outcome studies of infants at the limits of viability
7. Investigation of the relationships between neonatal morbidities and interventions and adult disease

Conclusions

ELBW infants without evidence of significant neonatal brain injury can recover from the stresses of preterm birth and prolonged NICU care when exposed to a nurturing home environment and comprehensive early intervention services. In contrast, ELBW infants in poor home environments with limited access to services do not do well. Meticulous longitudinal serial neurologic assessments, developmental assessments, and functional assessments are needed to evaluate ongoing neurodevelopmental status to ensure that appropriate intervention and educational services are in place, to evaluate changing neurodevelopmental status with increasing age, and

17

to better predict long-term outcome. Assessment at school age provides more reliable outcome data than preschool assessment.

References

1. National Institutes of Health (NIH). Consensus Development Conference: effects of corticosteroids for fetal maturation on perinatal outcomes. *Am J Obstet.* 1995;173:246-248.
2. El-Metwally D, Vohr B, Tucker R. Survival and neonatal morbidity at the limits of viability in the mid 1990s: 22 to 25 weeks. *J Pediatr.* 2000;137:616-622.
3. Fanaroff AA, Hack M, Walsh MC. The NICHD neonatal research network: changes in practice and outcomes during the first 15 years. *Semin Perinatol.* 2003;27:281-287.
4. Hintz SR, Poole WK, Wright LL, et al. Changes in mortality and morbidities among infants born at less than 25 weeks during the post-surfactant era. *Arch Dis Child Fetal Neonatal Ed.* 2005;90: F128-F133.
5. Hintz SR, Kendrick DE, Vohr BR, et al. Changes in neurodevelopmental outcomes at 18 to 22 months' corrected age among infants of less than 25 weeks' gestational age born in 1993-1999. *Pediatrics.* 2005;115:1645-1651.
6. Blakely ML, Lally KP, McDonald S, et al. Postoperative outcomes of extremely low birth-weight infants with necrotizing enterocolitis or isolated intestinal perforation: a prospective cohort study by the NICHD Neonatal Research Network. *Ann Surg.* 2005;241:984-989.
7. Laptook AR, O' Shea TM, Shankaran S, et al. Adverse neurodevelopmental outcomes among extremely low birth weight infants with a normal head ultrasound: prevalence and antecedents. *Pediatrics.* 2005;115:673-680.
8. Shankaran S, Johnson Y, Langer JC, et al. Outcome of extremely-low-birth-weight infants at highest risk: gestational age < or = 24 weeks, birth weight < or = 750 g, and 1-minute Apgar < or = 3. *Am J Obstet Gynecol.* 2004;191:1084-1091.
9. Vohr BR, Wright LL, Dusick AM, et al. Center differences and outcomes of extremely low birth weight infants. *Pediatrics.* 2004;113:781-789.
10. Walsh MC, Morris BH, Wrage LA, et al. Extremely low birthweight neonates with protracted ventilation: mortality and 18-month neurodevelopmental outcomes. *J Pediatr.* 2005;146:798-804.
11. Schmidt B, Asztalos EV, Roberts RS, et al. Impact of bronchopulmonary dysplasia, brain injury, and severe retinopathy on the outcome of extremely low-birth-weight infants at 18 months: results from the trial of indomethacin prophylaxis in preterms. *JAMA.* 2003;289:1124-1129.
12. Vohr BR, Allan WC, Westerveld M, et al. School-age outcomes of very low birth weight infants in the indomethacin intraventricular hemorrhage prevention trial. *Pediatrics.* 2003;111:e340-e346.
13. Vohr BR, Msall ME, Wilson D, et al. Spectrum of gross motor function in extremely low birth weight children with cerebral palsy at 18 months of age. *Pediatrics.* 2005;116:123-129.
14. Doyle LW, Anderson PJ. Improved neurosensory outcome at 8 years of age of extremely low birthweight children born in Victoria over three distinct eras. *Arch Dis Child Fetal Neonatal Ed.* 2005;90:F484-F488.
15. Litt J, Taylor HG, Klein N, et al. Learning disabilities in children with very low birthweight: prevalence, neuropsychological correlates, and educational interventions. *J Learn Disabil.* 2005;38: 130-141.
16. Marlow N, Wolke D, Bracewell MA, et al. Neurologic and developmental disability at six years of age after extremely preterm birth. *N Engl J Med.* 2005;352:9-19.
17. Sherlock RL, Anderson PJ, Doyle LW. Neurodevelopmental sequelae of intraventricular haemorrhage at 8 years of age in a regional cohort of ELBW/very preterm infants. *Early Hum Dev.* 2005;81: 909-916.
18. Taylor HG, Klein N, Minich NM, et al. Middle-school-age outcomes in children with very low birthweight. *Child Dev.* 2000;71:1495-1511.
19. Hack M, Flannery DJ, Schluchter M, et al. Outcomes in young adulthood for very-low-birth-weight infants. *N Engl J Med.* 2002;346:149-157.
20. Hack M, Klein N. Young adult attainments of preterm infants. *JAMA.* 2006;295:695-696.
21. Hack M, Youngstrom EA, Cartar L, et al. Behavioral outcomes and evidence of psychopathology among very low birth weight infants at age 20 years. *Pediatrics.* 2004;114:932-940.
22. Vohr BR, Wright LL, Hack M, et al. Follow-up care of high-risk infants. *Pediatrics.* 2004;114(Suppl 5):1377-1397.
23. Chamnanvanakij S, Margraf LR, Burns D, et al. Apoptosis and white matter injury in preterm infants. *Pediatr Dev Pathol.* 2002;5:184-189.
24. Perlman JM. Summary proceedings from the neurology group on hypoxic-ischemic encephalopathy. *Pediatrics.* 2006;117:S28-S33.
25. Shalak L, Perlman JM. Hemorrhagic-ischemic cerebral injury in the preterm infant: current concepts. *Clin Perinatol.* 2002;29:745-763.
26. Luu TM, Ment LR, Schneider KC, et al. Lasting effects of preterm birth and neonatal brain hemorrhage at 12 years of age. *Pediatrics.* 2009;123:1037-1044.
27. Papile LA, Burstein J, Burstein R, et al. Incidence and evolution of subependymal and intraventricular hemorrhage: a study of infants with birth weights less than 1,500 gm. *J Pediatr.* 1978;92: 529-534.
28. Ment LR, Vohr B, Allan W, et al. The etiology and outcome of cerebral ventriculomegaly at term in very low birth weight preterm infants. *Pediatrics.* 1999;104:243-248.

29. Ancel PY, Livinec F, Larroque B, et al. Cerebral palsy among very preterm children in relation to gestational age and neonatal ultrasound abnormalities: the EPIPAGE cohort study. *Pediatrics.* 2006;117:828-835.
30. Ment LR, Oh W, Ehrenkranz RA, et al. Low-dose indomethacin and prevention of intraventricular hemorrhage: a multicenter randomized trial. *Pediatrics.* 1994;93:543-550.
31. Schmidt B, Davis P, Moddemann D, et al. Long-term effects of indomethacin prophylaxis in extremely-low-birth-weight infants. *N Engl J Med.* 2001;344:1966-1972.
32. Yeh TF, Lin YJ, Lin HC, et al. Outcomes at school age after postnatal dexamethasone therapy for lung disease of prematurity. *N Engl J Med.* 2004;350:1304-1313.
33. Jobe AH. Postnatal corticosteroids for preterm infants: do what we say, not what we do. *N Engl J Med.* 2004;350:1349-1351.
34. Piecuch RE, Leonard CH, Cooper BA, et al. Outcome of infants born at 24-26 weeks' gestation: II. Neurodevelopmental outcome. *Obstet Gynecol.* 1997;90:809-814.
35. Pinto-Martin JA, Riolo S, Cnaan A, et al. Cranial ultrasound prediction of disabling and nondisabling cerebral palsy at age two in a low birth weight population. *Pediatrics.* 1995;95:249-254.
36. Prevalence and characteristics of children with cerebral palsy in Europe. *Dev Med Child Neurol.* 2002;44:633-640.
37. Vohr BR, Wright LL, Dusick AM, et al. Neurodevelopmental and functional outcomes of extremely low birth weight infants in the National Institute of Child Health and Human Developmental Neonatal Research Network, 1993-1994. *Pediatrics.* 2000;105:1216-1226.
38. Bax MC. Terminology and classification of cerebral palsy. *Dev Med Child Neurol.* 1964;11: 295-297.
39. Wood E, Rosenbaum P. The gross motor function classification system for cerebral palsy: a study of reliability and stability over time. *Dev Med Child Neurol.* 2000;42:292-296.
40. Russell DJ, Avery LM, Rosenbaum P, et al. Improved scaling of the Gross Motor Function Measure for children with cerebral palsy: evidence of reliability and validity. *Phys Ther.* 2000;80:873-885.
41. Drillien CM. Abnormal neurologic signs in the first year of life in low-birthweight infants: possible prognostic significance. *Dev Med Child Neurol.* 1972;14:575-584.
42. Vohr BR, Garcia-Coll C, Mayfield S, et al. Neurologic and developmental status related to the evolution of visual-motor abnormalities from birth to 2 years of age in preterm infants with intraventricular hemorrhage. *J Pediatr.* 1989;115:296-302.
43. Paneth N, Qiu H, Rosenbaum P, et al. Reliability of classification of cerebral palsy in low-birthweight children in four countries. *Dev Med Child Neurol.* 2003;45:628-633.
44. Palisano R, Rosenbaum P, Walter S, et al. Development and reliability of a system to classify gross motor function in children with cerebral palsy. *Dev Med Child Neurol.* 1997;39:214-223.
45. Bayley N. *Bayley Scales of Infant Development-II.* San Antonio, TX: Psychological Corporation; 1993.
46. Amiel-Tison C. Neuromotor status. In: Taeusch HW, Yogman MW, eds. *Follow-up management of the high-risk infant.* Boston: Little: Brown & Company; 1987.
47. Berlin CI, Hood L, Morlet T, et al. Auditory neuropathy/dys-synchrony: diagnosis and management. *Ment Retard Dev Disabil Res Rev.* 2003;9:225-231.
48. Joint Committee on Infant Hearing; American Academy of Audiology; American Academy of Pediatrics; American Speech-Language-Hearing Association; and Directors of Speech and Hearing Programs in State Health and Welfare Agencies. Year 2000 position statement: principles and guidelines for early hearing detection and intervention programs. *Pediatrics.* 2000;106:798-817.
49. Madden C, Wiley S, Schleiss M, et al. Audiometric, clinical and educational outcomes in a pediatric symptomatic congenital cytomegalovirus (CMV) population with sensorineural hearing loss. *Int J Pediatr Otorhinolaryngol.* 2005;69:1191-1198.
50. Morton CC, Nance WE. Newborn hearing screening—a silent revolution. *N Engl J Med.* 2006; 354:2151-2164.
51. Nance WE, Lim BG, Dodson KM. Importance of congenital cytomegalovirus infections as a cause for pre-lingual hearing loss. *J Clin Virol.* 2006;35:221-225.
52. Pass RF, Fowler KB, Boppana SB, et al. Congenital cytomegalovirus infection following first trimester maternal infection: symptoms at birth and outcome. *J Clin Virol.* 2006;35:216-220.
53. Moeller MP. Early intervention and language development in children who are deaf and hard of hearing. *Pediatrics.* 2000;106:E43.
54. Yoshinaga-Itano C. From screening to early identification and intervention: Discovering predictors to successful outcomes for children with significant hearing loss. *J Deaf Stud Deaf Educ.* 2003;8: 11-30.
55. Ment LR, Vohr B, Allan W, et al. Change in cognitive function over time in very-low-birth-weight infants. *JAMA.* 2003;289:705-711.
56. Blasco PA. Preterm birth: to correct or not to correct. *Dev Med Child Neurol.* 1989;31:816-821.
57. Lems W, Hopkins B, Samson JF. Mental and motor development in preterm infants: the issue of corrected age. *Early Hum Dev.* 1993;34:113-123.
58. Bayley N. *Bayley Scales of Infant Development-III.* San Antonio, TX; Psychological Corporation; 2006.
59. Hack M, Breslau N. Very low birth weight infants: effects of brain growth during infancy on intelligence quotient at 3 years of age. *Pediatrics.* 1986;77:196-202.
60. Peterson J, Taylor HG, Minich N, et al. Subnormal head circumference in very low birth weight children: neonatal correlates and school-age consequences. *Early Hum Dev.* 2006;82:325-334.
61. Beery K. *Developmental Test of Visual Motor Integration,* 4th ed. Parsippany, NJ: Modern Curriculum Press; 1997.

17

62. Wechsler D. *The Wechsler Intelligence Scale for Children.* 4th ed. San Antonio, TX: The Psychological Corporation; 2003.
63. Roid G. *The Stanford-Binet Intelligence Scales.* 5th ed. Ithasca, Ill: Riverside Publishing; 2003.
64. Dunn L. *Peabody Picture Vocabulary Test.* 3rd ed. Circle Pines, MN: American Guidance Service; 1997.
65. Achenbach TM. *Child Behavior Checklist 2-3.* Burlington, VT: University of Vermont, Department of Psychiatry; 1992.
66. Conners CK. *Connors Parent Rating Scales Revised.* San Antonio, TX: Psychological Corporation; 1996.
67. Ottenbacher KJ, Msall ME, Lyon N, et al. The WeeFIM instrument: its utility in detecting change in children with developmental disabilities. *Arch Phys Med Rehabil.* 2000;81:1317-1326.
68. Sparrow S, Balla D, Cicchetti D. *Vineland Adaptive Behavior Scales: Interview Edition, Survey Form Manual.* Circle Pines, MN: American Guidance Service; 1984.
69. *Pediatric Evaluation of Disability Inventory (PEDI).* Nashville, TN: Ellsworth and Vandermeer Press, Lt; 1997.
70. Ment LR, Vohr B, Allan W, et al. Outcome of children in the indomethacin intraventricular hemorrhage prevention trial. *Pediatrics.* 2000;105:485-491.
71. Beery K. *Developmental Test of Visual-Motor Integration.* 3rd ed. Los Angeles: Western Psychological Services; 1989.
72. Botting N, Powls A, Cooke RW, et al. Attention deficit hyperactivity disorders and other psychiatric outcomes in very low birthweight children at 12 years. *J Child Psychol Psychiatry.* 1997;38: 931-941.
73. Gardner F, Johnson A, Yudkin P, et al. Behavioral and emotional adjustment of teenagers in mainstream school who were born before 29 weeks' gestation. *Pediatrics.* 2004;114:676-682.
74. Grunau RE, Whitfield MF, Fay TB. Psychosocial and academic characteristics of extremely low birth weight (< or =800 g) adolescents who are free of major impairment compared with term-born control subjects. *Pediatrics.* 2004;114:e725-e732.
75. Dahl LB, Kaaresen PI, Tunby J, et al. Emotional, behavioral, social, and academic outcomes in adolescents born with very low birth weight. *Pediatrics.* 2006;118:e449-459.
76. Limperopoulos C, Bassan H, Sullivan NR, et al. Positive screening for autism in ex-preterm infants: prevalence and risk factors. *Pediatrics.* 2008;121:758-765.
77. Kuban KC, O'Shea TM, Allred EN, et al. Positive screening on the Modified Checklist for Autism in Toddlers (M-CHAT) in extremely low gestational age newborns. *J Pediatr.* 2009;154:535-540 e531.
78. O'Shea TM, Allred EN, Dammann O, et al. The ELGAN study of the brain and related disorders in extremely low gestational age newborns. *Early Hum Dev.* 2009;85:719-725.
79. Johnson S, Hollis C, Kochhar P, et al. Autism spectrum disorders in extremely preterm children. *J Pediatr.* 2010;156:525-531 e522.
80. Hack M, Taylor HG, Drotar D, et al. Poor predictive validity of the Bayley Scales of Infant Development for cognitive function of extremely low birth weight children at school age. *Pediatrics.* 2005;116:333-341.
81. Luu TM, Vohr BR, Schneider KC, et al. Trajectories of receptive language development from 3 to 12 years of age for very preterm children. *Pediatrics.* 2009;124:333-341.
82. Doyle LW, Ford GW, Rickards AL, et al. Antenatal corticosteroids and outcome at 14 years of age in children with birth weight less than 1501 grams. *Pediatrics.* 2000;106:E2.
83. Hack M, Taylor HG, Klein N, et al. School-age outcomes in children with birth weights under 750 g. *N Engl J Med.* 1994;331:753-759.
84. Rushe TM, Rifkin L, Stewart AL, et al. Neuropsychological outcome at adolescence of very preterm birth and its relation to brain structure. *Dev Med Child Neurol.* 2001;43:226-233.
85. Saigal S, den Ouden L, Wolke D, et al. School-age outcomes in children who were extremely low birth weight from four international population-based cohorts. *Pediatrics.* 2003;112:943-950.
86. Saigal S, Hoult LA, Streiner DL, et al. School difficulties at adolescence in a regional cohort of children who were extremely low birth weight. *Pediatrics.* 2000;105:325-331.
87. Anand D, Stevenson CJ, West CR, et al. Lung function and respiratory health in adolescents of very low birth weight. *Arch Dis Child.* 2003;88:135-138.
88. Korhonen P, Laitinen J, Hyodynmaa E, et al. Respiratory outcome in school-aged, very-low-birth-weight children in the surfactant era. *Acta Paediatr.* 2004;93:316-321.
89. Saigal S, Stoskopf BL, Feeny D, et al. Differences in preferences for neonatal outcomes among health care professionals, parents, and adolescents. *JAMA.* 1999;281:1991-1997.
90. Saigal S, Stoskopf B, Streiner D, et al. Transition of extremely low-birth-weight infants from adolescence to young adulthood: comparison with normal birth-weight controls. *JAMA.* 2006;295:667-675.

Index